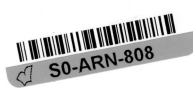

American Cancer Society
Atlas of
Clinical Oncology

Series Volumes

Blumgart, Fong, Jarnagin	*Hepatobiliary Cancer*
Cameron	*Pancreatic Cancer*
Carroll, Grossfeld, Reese	*Prostate Cancer*
Char	*Tumors of the Eye and Ocular Adnexa*
Clark, Duh, Jahan, Perrier	*Endocrine Tumors*
Eifel, Levenback	*Cervical, Vulvar and Vaginal Cancer*
Fuller	*Uterine and Endometrial Cancer*
Ginsberg	*Lung Cancer*
Grossbard	*Malignant Lymphomas*
Ozols	*Ovarian Cancer*
Pollock	*Soft Tissue Sarcomas*
Posner, Vokes, Weichselbaum	*Cancer of the Upper Gastrointestinal Tract*
Prados	*Brain Cancer*
Raghavan	*Germ Cell Tumors*
Shah	*Head and Neck Cancer*
Silverman	*Oral Cancer*
Sober, Haluska	*Skin Cancer*
Steele, Richie	*Kidney Tumors*
Volberding	*Cancer in the Immunocompromised Host*
Wiernik	*Adult Leukemias*
Willett	*Cancer of the Lower Gastrointestinal Tract*
Winchester, Winchester	*Breast Cancer*
Yasko	*Bone Tumors*

American Cancer Society

Atlas of
Clinical Oncology

Editors

GLENN D. STEELE JR, MD
University of Chicago

THEODORE L. PHILLIPS, MD
University of California

BRUCE A. CHABNER, MD
Harvard Medical School

Managing Editor

TED S. GANSLER, MD, MBA
Director of Health Content, American Cancer Society

American Cancer Society
Atlas of
Clinical Oncology

Skin Cancer

Arthur J. Sober, MD
Frank G. Haluska, MD, PhD

both of
Massachusetts General Hospital
Harvard Medical School
Boston, Massachusetts

2001
BC Decker Inc
Hamilton • London

BC Decker Inc
20 Hughson Street South
P.O. Box 620, L.C.D. 1
Hamilton, Ontario L8N 3K7
Tel: 905-522-7017; 1-800-568-7281
Fax: 905-522-7839
E-mail: info@bcdecker.com
Website: www.bcdecker.com

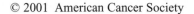

ISBN 1–55009–108-5
Printed in Canada

Sales and Distribution

United States
BC Decker Inc
P.O. Box 785
Lewiston, NY 14092-0785
Tel: 905-522-7017; 1-800-568-7281
Fax: 905-522-7839
E-mail: info@bcdecker.com
Website: www.bcdecker.com

Canada
BC Decker Inc
20 Hughson Street South
P.O. Box 620, L.C.D. 1
Hamilton, Ontario L8N 3K7
Tel: 905-522-7017; 1-800-568-7281
Fax: 905-522-7839
E-mail: info@bcdecker.com
Website: www.bcdecker.com

Foreign Rights
John Scott & Company
International Publishers' Agency
P.O. Box 878
Kimberton, PA 19442
Tel: 610-827-1640
Fax: 610-827-1671

**U.K., Europe, Scandinavia,
Middle East**
Harcourt Publishers Limited
Customer Service Department
Foots Cray High Street
Sidcup, Kent
DA14 5HP, UK
Tel: 44 (0) 208 308 5760
Fax: 44 (0) 181 308 5702
E-mail: cservice@harcourt_brace.com

Australia, New Zealand
Harcourt Australia Pry. Limited
Customer Service Department
STM Division
Locked Bag 16
St. Peters, New South Wales, 2044
Australia
Tel: (02) 9517-8999
Fax: (02) 9517-2249
E-mail: stmp@harcourt.com.au
Website: www.harcourt.com.au

Japan
Igaku-Shoin Ltd.
Foreign Publications Department
3-24-17 Hongo
Bunkyo-ku,Tokyo, Japan 113-8719
Tel: 3 3817 5680
Fax: 3 3815 6776
E-mail: fd@igaku.shoin.co.jp

**Singapore, Malaysia, Thailand,
Philippines, Indonesia, Vietnam,
Pacific Rim**
Harcourt Asia Pte Limited
583 Orchard Road
#09/01, Forum
Singapore 238884
Tel: 65-737-3593
Fax: 65-753-2145

Notice: The authors and publisher have made every effort to ensure that the patient care recommended herein, including choice of drugs and drug dosages, is in accord with the accepted standard and practice at the time of publication. However, since research and regulation constantly change clinical standards, the reader is urged to check the product information sheet included in the package of each drug, which includes recommended doses, warnings, and contraindications. This is particularly important with new or infrequently used drugs.

Contributors

MICHAEL B. ATKINS, MD
Associate Professor of Medicine
Harvard Medical School
Division of Hematology/Oncology
Beth Israel Deaconess Medical
  Center
Boston, Massachusetts
*Melanoma: Chemotherapy,
  Cytokine Therapies, and
  Biochemotherapy*

C. KOMEN BROWN, MD, PhD
University of Pittsburgh
School of Medicine
University of Pittsburgh Cancer
  Institute
Pittsburgh, Pennsylvania
Adjuvant Therapy for Melanoma

SOLA X. CHENG
Investigator
Brigham and Women's Hospital
Harvard Medical School
Boston, Massachusetts
*Treatment of Primary Cutaneous
  Lymphomas*

DIANE S. CHIU, MD
Department of Dermatology
Harvard Medical School
Boston, Massachusetts
Basal Cell Carcinoma

A. BENEDICT COSIMI, MD
Professor of Surgery
Department of Surgery
Massachusetts General Hospital
Harvard Medical School
Boston, Massachusetts
*Surgical Management of
  Cutaneous Melanoma*

KATALIN FERENCZI, MD
Harvard Medical School
Brigham and Women's Hospital
Boston, Massachusetts
Cutaneous Lymphoma

MICHELE A. GADD, MD
Assistant Professor of Surgery
Harvard Medical School
Division of Surgical Oncology
Massachusetts General Hospital
Boston, Massachusetts
*Lymphatic Mapping and Sentinel
  Lymph Node Biopsy*

JARED A. GOLLOB, MD
Assistant Professor of Medicine
Harvard Medical School
Associate Director of Biologic
  Therapy Program
Beth Israel Deaconess Medical
  Center
Boston, Massachusetts
*Melanoma: Chemotherapy,
  Cytokine Therapies, and
  Biochemotherapy*

ALLAN C. HALPERN, MD
Memorial Sloan-Kettering
  Cancer Center
New York, New York
Risk Assessment

FRANK G. HALUSKA, MD, PhD
Director, Melanoma Assessment
  Unit
Hematology/Oncology Division
Massachusetts General Hospital
Assistant Professor of Medicine
Harvard Medical School
Boston, Massachusetts
*Genetics of Skin Cancer,
  Immunotherapy for Melanoma*

HARLEY A. HAYNES, MD
Professor of Dermatology
Harvard Medical School
Vice-Chairman
Department of Dermatology
Brigham and Women's Hospital
Co-Director, Cutaneous
  Oncology Unit
Dana Farber Cancer Institute
Boston, Massachusetts
*Merkel Cell (Cutaneous
  Neuroendocrine) Carcinoma*

DAVID HILL, PhD
Centre for Behavioural Research
  in Cancer
Professional Fellow
University of Melbourne
Victoria, Australia
Prevention of Skin Cancer

VINCENT C. HO, MD
Professor of Dermatology
Division of Dermatology
University of British Columbia
Vancouver, British Columbia
Melanoma: Biopsy Techniques

JOHN M. KIRKWOOD, MD
Professor and Vice-Chairman for
    Clinical Research
Department of Medicine
University of Pittsburgh School of
    Medicine
Director, Melanoma Center
University of Pittsburgh Cancer
    Institute
Pittsburgh, Pennsylvania
Adjuvant Therapy for Melanoma

SUSAN E. KROWN, MD
Professor of Medicine
Weill Medical College of Cornell
    University
Attending Physician and Member
Memorial Sloan-Kettering Cancer
    Center
New York, New York
Kaposi's Sarcoma

THOMAS S. KUPPER, MD
Fitzpatrick Professor of
    Dermatology
Harvard Medical School
Chair, Department of Dermatology
Brigham and Women's Hospital
Boston, Massachusetts
*Cutaneous Lymphoma, Treatment
    of Primary Cutaneous
    Lymphomas*

RICHARD G.B. LANGLEY, MD
Assistant Professor
Division of Dermatology
Department of Medicine
Dalhousie University
QEII Health Sciences Center
Halifax, Nova Scotia
Clinical Presentation: Melanoma

ASHFAQ A. MARGHOOB, MD
Memorial Sloan-Kettering Cancer
    Center
New York, New York
Risk Assessment

ROBIN MARKS, MBBS, MPH,
    FRACP, FACD
Professor of Dermatology
University of Melbourne
Director of Dermatology
St. Vincent's Hospital
Director of Research and Training
Skin and Cancer Foundation
Victoria, Australia
Prevention of Skin Cancer

PHILLIP H. MCKEE, MD, FRCPATH
Associate Professor
Harvard Medical School
Director, Dermatopathology
Brigham and Women's Hospital
Consultant Dermatopathologist
Children's Hospital
Boston, Massachusetts
*Cutaneous Lymphoma, Merkel Cell
    (Cutaneous Neuroendocrine)
    Carcinoma*

GREGG M. MENAKER, MD
Instructor in Dermatology
Harvard Medical School
Director, Dermatologic Surgery Unit
Massachusetts General Hospital
Boston, Massachusetts
Basal Cell Carcinoma

RADHA MIKKILINENI, MD, MSc
Post-Doctoral Fellow
Brown University
Providence, Rhode Island
Epidemiology

MARTIN C. MIHM JR., MD
Professor of Pathology
Harvard Medical School
Boston, Massachusetts
Clinical Presentation: Melanoma

PATRICIA L. MYSKOWSKI, MD
Associate Professor of
    Dermatology
Weill Medical College of Cornell
    University
Memorial Sloan-Kettering Cancer
    Center
New York, New York
Kaposi's Sarcoma

HOSSAMELDIN NAEEM, MD
Research Fellow in Dermatology
Harvard Medical School
Clinical and Research Fellow
Brigham and Women's Hospital
Dana Farber Cancer Institute
Boston, Massachusetts
*Treatment of Primary Cutaneous
    Lymphomas*

PAUL NGHIEM, MD, PhD
Instructor in Dermatology
Harvard Medical School
Cutaneous Oncology Unit
Dana Farber Cancer Institute
Department of Dermatology
Brigham and Women's Hospital
Boston, Massachusetts
*Merkel Cell (Cutaneous
    Neuroendocrine) Carcinoma*

JOSE R. PEÑA, MD
University of Louisiana at
    Shreeveport Medical School
Director
Mohs/Dermatologic Surgery
University of Louisiana
Shreeveport, Louisiana
*Treatment of Nonmelanoma Skin
    Cancer*

JUNE K. ROBINSON, MD
Professor of Medicine
(Dermatology) and Pathology
Loyola University Chicago
Program Leader of Skin Cancer
Program
Cardinal Bernardin Cancer Center
Maywood, Illinois
Squamous Cell Carcinoma

DANA SACHS, MD
Memorial Sloan-Kettering Cancer
Center
New York, New York
Risk Assessment

ARTURO SAAVEDRA, MD
Harvard Medical School
Brigham and Women's Hospital
Boston, Massachusetts
*Treatment of Nonmelanoma Skin
Cancer*

ARTHUR J. SOBER, MD
Professor of Dermatology
Harvard Medical School
Associate Chief of Dermatology
Massachusetts General Hospital
Boston, Massachusetts
*Clinical Presentation: Melanoma,
Uncommon Cutaneous
Malignancies*

KENNETH K. TANABE, MD
Associate Professor of Surgery
Harvard Medical School
Chief, Division of Surgical
Oncology
Massachusetts General Hospital
Boston, Massachusetts
*Lymphatic Mapping and Sentinel
Lymph Node Biopsy*

ABEL TORRES, MD, JD
Vice-Chairman for Education
Department of Dermatology
Harvard Medical School
Director, Mohs/Dermatologic
Surgery Center
Dana-Farber Cancer Institute
Brigham and Women's Hospital
Boston, Massachusetts
*Treatment of Nonmelanoma Skin
Cancer*

HENSIN TSAO, MD, PHD
Instructor, Harvard Medical School
Department of Dermatology
Massachusetts General Hospital
Boston, Massachusetts
Genetics of Skin Cancer

JENNIFER F. TSENG, MD
Research Fellow
Harvard Medical School
Department of Surgery
Massachusetts General Hospital
Boston, Massachusetts
*Lymphatic Mapping and Sentinel
Lymph Node Biopsy*

C.C. WANG, MD, FACR
Harvard Medical School
Massachusetts General Hospital
Boston, Massachusetts
Radiation Therapy

MARTIN A. WEINSTOCK, MD, PHD
Professor of Dermatology
Brown University
Chief of Dermatology
VA Medical Center
Providence, Rhode Island
Epidemiology

MARNI C. WISEMAN, MD
Division of Dermatology
University of British Columbia
Vancouver, British Columbia
Melanoma: Biopsy Techniques

DAVID A. WRONE, MD
Clinical Fellow
Department of Dermatology
Harvard Medical School
Boston, Massachusetts
*Uncommon Cutaneous
Malignancies*

SIXUN YANG, MD, PHD
Hematology/Oncology Division
Massachusetts General Hospital
Harvard Medical School
Boston, Massachusetts
Immunotherapy for Melanoma

Contents

Preface

As we enter the Twenty-first Century, malignancies of the skin are by far the most common form of cancer encountered in the United States and Canada. Well over one million cases are detected each year. Unlike occult internal malignancies, cancers of the skin are located on the external surface, readily accessible for diagnosis. All that is required for recognition is awareness of the clinical features specific for each type of skin cancer, an index of suspicion, and examination of the patient's skin surface.

This volume was written to provide all medical professionals with a knowledge base that will assist in the recognition and management of both very common and less common forms of skin cancer. But it also acknowledges that some forms of skin cancer present challenges of diagnosis and therapy because of their propensity to metastasize, and ultimately to threaten the patient's life. Recently, advances have been made in developing new modalities of diagnosis and treatment for these conditions, and this volume reviews the progress in these areas. We have chosen to emphasize the visual aspects of skin cancer, since dermatology is a visual discipline. Consequently, this volume is richly illustrated in color; text is used primarily where illustrations would be of less value. In addition to diagnostic features, the epidemiologic, therapeutic, and preventative aspects of skin cancer are discussed. To accomplish our objectives, we recruited an outstanding group of clinician-scientists who contributed their expertise to the undertaking. This volume should complement more general textbooks of dermatology and more specific skin cancer monographs.

We would like to acknowledge the following sources of support in the preparation of this volume: The Marion Gardner Jackson Trust, Bank of Boston, Trustee, and the Cancer Research Institute for their financial support: Jennifer Mallory and Paula Presutti of BC Decker Inc for their technical support; and Brian Decker for his constant encouragement and guidance.

AJS
FGH
December 2000

Epidemiology

RADHA MIKKILINENI, MD, MSc
MARTIN A. WEINSTOCK, MD, PhD

Cutaneous malignancies are extremely common and have represented an increasingly larger burden to society over the past several decades. Malignant melanoma (MM), the keratinocyte carcinomas (KCs) (basal cell carcinoma [BCC] and squamous cell carcinoma [SCC]), and mycosis fungoides (MF), a variant of cutaneous lymphoma (CL), have all increased significantly in incidence over the past decades. Malignant melanoma and the KCs are etiologically linked to ultraviolet (UV) radiation exposure whereas risk factors for MF have yet to be elucidated. Identifying risk factors for disease, modifying risk factors to reduce disease incidence, and monitoring trends in disease are the critical roles epidemiology plays in relation to these skin cancers.

CUTANEOUS MALIGNANT MELANOMA

Sources of Data

Melanoma is notable for its rapid rise in incidence worldwide over the past several decades, its frequent occurrence in young adults, its high mortality rates in advanced disease, and the large contribution of sun exposure—a preventable risk factor—to its etiology. These characteristics make melanoma both relevant and amenable to study by population health methods.

The cancer registries of countries worldwide routinely include melanoma, and estimates of incidence generally arise from these registries. Most countries, including the United States, have regional registries, which provide information considered representative of the general population of their nation. The Surveillance, Epidemiology, and End Results (SEER) program of the National Cancer Institute (NCI) compiles information on cancer incidence from 12 different regional registry sites across the United States and covers about 14 percent of the population.[1] Under-registration of melanoma is of concern in population-based registry estimates of incidences.[2] Much of melanoma diagnosis and treatment occurs in the outpatient setting, and pathology specimens may be sent to laboratories outside the registries' coverage areas. Since much of the registries' information on melanoma is derived from hospitals and laboratories within their geographic area, the incidence estimates of melanoma could under-represent the actual rates. A number of studies have evaluated the magnitude of this problem in the United States. The degree of under-reporting has been estimated as between 10 and 21 percent[3,4] and depends on the balance between improvements in the ascertainment methods used and changes in health care delivery that increase the difficulty of ascertainment.

Other sources of incidence data include record linkage systems, in which the majority of individuals in a community receive most (if not all) of their medical care from a single provider. This is the case for certain communities (such as Rochester, Minnesota) as well as for special populations (such as clients of health maintenance organizations [HMOs]).[5] Incidence rates derived from this latter population, though, may not be generalizable to the US population since the "pre-paid" health plan participants may not be similar enough to the general population. Scandinavian countries have unique nationwide registries. This makes melanoma registration in these countries more uniform and less susceptible but not immune to problems of under-reporting. The completeness of registry information on melanoma in many developing countries is limited by funding, by limited health services, and by the low relative priority of this disease.[6]

Another factor that complicates the interpretation of melanoma incidence is the choice of the standard population used to calculate rates. Since skin cancer is more common in elderly people, if the World Standard Population is used to calculate rates, age-adjusted rates for melanoma in the United States are lower than if the 1970 US Standard Population is used. The World Standard Population represents younger age groups to a greater extent than the standard populations of developed countries, which disproportionately represent older age groups. Consequently, when comparing incidence rates between countries or studies it is important to take into account the standard population used in the derivation of rates.

Mortality data for melanoma is generally accurate, and studies attempting to assess the accuracy of death certification confirm this.[7]

Incidence

Melanoma incidence has increased rapidly in white populations over the past 60 years. The oldest cancer registry in the United States, the Connecticut Tumor Registry, has been tracking melanoma since 1935, and this registry revealed an increase in melanoma incidence from 1.0 per 100,000 from 1935 to 1939 to 16 per 100,000 in 1996. In 1973, the NCI's SEER program began tracking most cancers, including melanoma. There was an increase in incidence from 6.4 per 100,000 in 1973 to 16 per 100,000 in 1996 (SEER Cancer Statistics Review, 1973 to 1996) (Figure 1–1). From 1973 to 1994, there was an overall percent increase of 120 percent, with an increase of 154 percent and 90 percent in men and women, respectively.[8] The annual rate of increase of melanoma incidence over this time period was 4.3 percent, and the continued rise in melanoma incidence has been longer than that for any of the other leading sites of cancer (Figure 1–2).

International incidence data reflect similar trends in the white populations of New Zealand, Australia, and Europe, but no great increases in the nonwhite populations of East and South Asia and South America.[9] The highest world rates are recorded in Australia, New Zealand, and Israel, but the incidence has also been steadily rising in the northern European nations, including the United Kingdom, Ireland, and the Nordic countries.[10] Table 1–1 summarizes selected recent incidence data. There are limited data on the incidence of melanoma in nonwhite populations because the burden of this disease in Africans, South Asians, East Asians, and Hispanics is substantially less than in individuals of European origin. Nonetheless, some data exist and provide a stark contrast to the disease incidence data for Caucasians. Increased pigmentation is protective, and a large US study analyzing the incidence of melanoma in darker-skinned individuals showed African Americans as having the lowest incidence, followed by Hispanics and Asians.[11] A SEER data analysis of rates and trends from 1973 to 1994 shows the incidence of melanoma to have increased in African American men from 0.6 per 100,000 to 1.0 per 100,000, representing an annual increase of 0.7 percent.[1] In contrast, African American women actually had an annual percent decrease of 1.3 percent, with rates remaining relatively stable at 0.7 per 100,000 in 1994.[1] Incidence rates were 1.5 per 100,000 and 0.9 per 100,000 in females and males, respectively, in the French West Indies.[12] This information must be interpreted in light of the characteristics of the study population compared to those of the general population of Martinique. The study population was 77 percent black and 23 percent white as opposed to the general population, which was 96 percent black and 4 percent white. Therefore, the incidence rates of melanoma in the West Indian black population are likely even lower. Melanoma incidence derived from cancer registries in India are quite low, with rates of 0.5 per 100,000 and 0.2 per 100,000 in males and females, respectively, in Bombay in 1988.[6]

In the last decade of the twentieth century, the increase in incidence was still apparent, but recent studies suggest a decline in the rate of increase in certain subgroups.[13,14] Researchers in Scotland, the United States, and Australia note rate stabilization, and in recent years, a decline in incidence, particularly in women.[8,15,16] These changes in trends could reflect the success of skin cancer prevention strate-

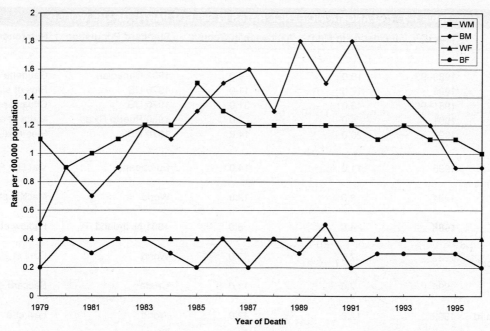

Figure 1–1. Trends in cancer incidence from 1979 to 1995. All rates are age-adjusted to the 1970 US Standard Population. Incidence data are derived from the Surveillance, Epidemiology and End Results (SEER) Cancer Incidence Public-Use Database, 1973 to 1996. WM = white male; BM = black male; WF = white female; BF = black female. (Adapted from Wingo PA, Ries LA, Rosenberg HM, et al. Cancer incidence and mortality, 1973–1995: a report card for the U.S. Cancer. 1998;82:1197–207.

gies. Educational programs may have increased public awareness of the dangers of sunlight exposure and may have resulted in behavioral changes that are reducing the risk of melanoma. Reports on future trends in melanoma incidence, particularly in highly afflicted populations, are eagerly anticipated.

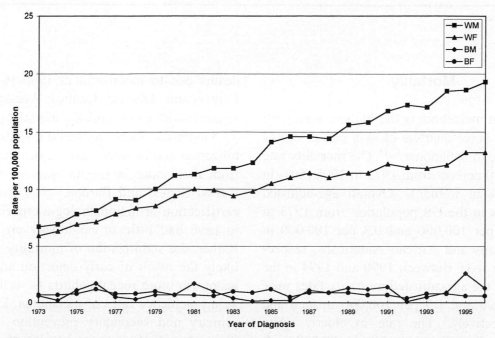

Figure 1–2. Melanoma incidence in the United States, 1973 to 1996. All rates are age-adjusted to the 1970 US Standard Population. Incidence data are derived from the Surveillance, Epidemiology, and End Results (SEER) Cancer Incidence Public-Use Database, 1973 to 1996. (BF = black female; BM = black male; WF = white female; WM = white male.)

Table 1–1. MELANOMA INCIDENCE RATES IN SELECT PARTS OF THE WORLD					
Location	Year	Incidence in Men*	Incidence in Women*	Standard Population	Reference
North America					
Canada	1989–93	10.0	9.0	1991 Canadian	Gaudette et al, 1998
United States	1996	17.0	11.0	1970 US	Ries et al, 1997
Kauai (HA)	1981–90	43.0	31.0	1970 US	Chuang et al, 1999
Puerto Rico	1991	4.0	2.0	1950 Puerto Rican	Matta et al, 1998
Connecticut	1996	20.0	14.0	1970 US	Ries et al, 1997
Europe					
Netherlands	1995	11.0	14.0	European	Van Der Rhee et al, 1999
United Kingdom					
Scotland	1994	8.0	12.0	World	MacKie et al, 1997
Ireland					
N. Ireland	1988	4.0	8.0	1981 N. Ireland	Pedlow et al, 1997
Italy					
Central Italy	1987	7.0	7.0	World	Carli et al, 1994
France					
Paris	1994	7.0	11.0	Crude	Baccard et al, 1997
Switzerland					
Canton of Vaud	1992	12.0	12.0	World	Levi et al, 1995
Australia	1989	30.0	24.0	World	Jelfs et al, 1994
N. Queensland	1996–7	49.0	42.0	World	Buettner et al, 1998
South Australia	1990	25.0	26.0	World	Jones et al, 1992
Tasmania	1990	23.0	32.0	World	Jones et al, 1992
Middle East					
Israel	1989	8.0	8.0	World	Iscovich et al, 1995
Africa					
South Africa					
Cape Town	1995	28.0	22.0	World	Saxe et al, 1998
India					
Bombay	1988	0.5	0.2	World	Nair et al, 1998

* Per 100,000 population.

Mortality

Mortality from melanoma is the highest among all skin diseases. Three-quarters of skin cancer deaths are attributable to melanoma.[17,18] The mortality rate increased by 40 percent from 1973 to 1995 (50% in men and 20% in women).[8] Overall age-adjusted mortality rates in the US population from 1973 to 1996 are 2.5 per 100,000 and 0.3 per 100,000 in white Americans and African Americans, respectively[1] (Figure 1–3). Between 1990 and 1994 in the United States, the age-adjusted mortality rates were 3.1 per 100,000 and 1.5 per 100,000 in men and women, respectively.[1] The rate in elderly white males over 65 years of age was 11 per 100,000, with the steepest rise in rate over this time period occurring in advanced age groups. There were 7,276 deaths due to melanoma in 1996 (CDC Wonder; Centers for Disease Control Wonder, an online resource with cause-specific mortality data).

Numerous studies around the world suggest stabilization and in some cases, a decline in mortality from melanoma in recent years in Australia, the United States, and Europe.[19–21] Changes in death certification or histopathologic criteria are thought to have had little or no impact on these trends. Rather, the stabilization of mortality rates is more likely the result of early detection and removal of lesions in more recent cohorts as well as the stabilizing incidence rates of melanoma. Efforts at both primary and secondary prevention of melanoma have intensified in recent decades, and it is encouraging to observe the subsequent decline in melanoma mortality.[15]

Gender

Consistent gender differences in melanoma incidence, mortality, and anatomic site distribution have been reported. The incidence rates of melanoma in North America are higher in men than in women; moreover, the rates of rise in incidence have also been higher in men.[22] In contrast, incidence rates in women in the United Kingdom and Norway have been noted to be higher than those in men.[23–25]

Mortality is also greater in men than in women, in a fairly consistent pattern worldwide. Lesions in women tend to be thinner at diagnosis than those in men, which may contribute to longer survival times for women. Women continue to have better prognoses even after adjusting for tumor thickness and anatomic site. Diagnosis of earlier lesions in women has been related to a number of behavioral factors that vary between the sexes. For instance, female attire may expose more skin overall than male attire and make skin lesions more obvious. In addition, women may be more aware of and receptive to preventive health behaviors and education.[23]

The anatomic distribution of melanoma also varies by gender. Men have a greater frequency of melanoma on the trunk and back whereas women have the disease more frequently on a lower limb.

This contributes to the gender difference in mortality as trunk melanoma has a worse prognosis than leg or thigh melanoma.[26] Elder found that melanoma of the ear occurred six times more often in men than in women and occurred twice as often on the scalp, neck, and face in men than in women.[26] Rates of occurrence on the trunk were 5.3 per 100,000 and 2.3 per 100,000 in males and females, respectively, whereas lower-limb melanoma occurred at rates of 1.1 per 100,000 and 3.3 per 100,000 in men and women, respectively.

Socioeconomic Differences

A positive association between melanoma risk and socioeconomic status (SES) has been reported.[27,28] Kirkpatrick and colleagues analyzed melanoma cases in Washington state from 1974 to 1985 and found an increasing risk of melanoma with rising income in individuals aged 30 to 69 years.[29] In people over 70 years of age, an inverse association was detected, primarily due to a high incidence of lentigo maligna melanoma in these individuals.[29] This histologic subtype of melanoma is unique in that it occurs most often on chronically sun-exposed sites. Some individuals of a lower SES may work outdoors and have greater long-term sun exposure. Others may

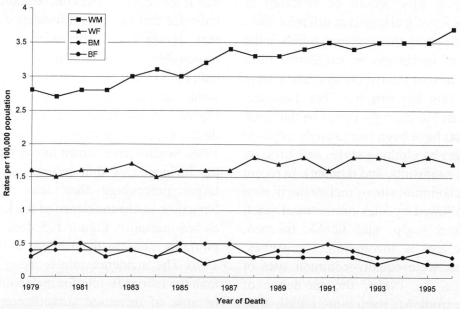

Figure 1–3. Melanoma mortality in the United States, 1979 to 1996. Rates are age-adjusted to the 1970 US Standard Population. Mortality data are derived from CDC Wonder. WM = white male; WF = white female; BM = black male; BF = black female.

have less opportunity for intense sun exposure, due to economic barriers to sunny vacations. Higher-income groups are thought to have more intense intermittent sun exposure because they normally work indoors and tend to have recreational sun exposure and high UV sun exposure on holidays. This type of sun exposure is thought to primarily result in the other histologic subtypes of melanoma, such as superficial spreading and nodular melanoma.

Another study analyzed the relationship between socioeconomic status and melanoma incidence, using SEER registry data from 1973 to 1993.[30] The authors concluded that education, as opposed to income, is the primary determinant of melanoma risk. Education is thought to influence behavior and to thus alter melanoma risk. Disease prognosis and survival are also thought to be influenced by socioeconomic factors. Affluent individuals have better 5-year survival rates; this survival advantage persists after controlling for other major prognostic factors.[31]

Anatomic Sites

It is thought that intense intermittent sunlight exposure is a primary risk factor for melanoma in temperate climates and that the most common anatomic sites of disease are those that receive this type of exposure. If this is so, then changes in behavior and clothing styles over time would be reflected in changing frequencies of melanoma at different sites. The findings of one study that analyzed trends in the site distribution of melanoma in successive birth cohorts since the turn of the twentieth century were consistent with this hypothesis.[13] For instance, melanoma has been increasingly found on the trunk and back, sites that have been increasingly exposed because of changes in clothing styles and lifestyle (sunny vacations, swimsuits, and tanning). In recent cohorts, the most common site of melanoma in men was the trunk, followed by sites on the head (ears, lips, eyelids, face, scalp, and neck). In men, melanoma of the legs is uncommon. For women, the legs and trunk were equally common sites of occurrence. Since the 1960s, the incidence of melanoma on the trunk has risen more rapidly than has melonoma incidence at other sites.[32] Elwood and Gallagher looked at incidence by site in indi-

viduals younger than 50 years of age and found that the highest incidence rate (per unit area of skin) was that of intermittently exposed skin and that the highest density of melanoma in both sexes was on the back. In individuals over 50 years of age, the highest numbers of melanoma were found on chronically sun-exposed sites such as the face.[33]

Latitude Gradients

Melanoma generally has higher incidence rates in white populations that live closer to the equator.[34] This is true in North America and Australia, where individuals who reside closer to the equator have progressively higher rates of melanoma than those who live farther away.[2] In Europe, however, higher rates are found in northern countries such as Scandinavia, Norway, and the United Kingdom, and lower rates are found in the countries of the Mediterranean, presumably due to the protective role of greater pigmentation in the more southerly populations.[9]

Surveillance Bias

There has been much debate about the validity of the reported melanoma incidence increases.[35] It is possible that some of the rise is due to surveillance artifact, but much of the literature suggests that the trends are real.[13,36] The concomitant rise in mortality indicates that the rise in incidence is at least partly real. If increased surveillance alone had been responsible for the increased incidence rates, then, with the greater detection of early lesions, mortality would have decreased or stayed the same over time. Figure 1–4 and Table 1–2 depict trends in Breslow thickness of melanoma in men and women since 1988. Studies have shown that in terms of thickness, the incidence of thin lesions has increased by a larger percentage than that of thick lesions. Nonetheless, the incidence of thick tumors has risen, as has mortality. Figure 1–5 depicts incidence and mortality rates in the United States from 1973 to 1996. The incidence rate is rising at a greater rate than the mortality rate for melanoma, which may be because of increased surveillance and removal of early lesions that might never have progressed. Nonetheless, mortality also continued to rise over

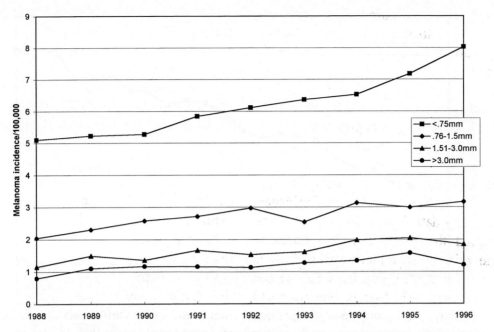

Figure 1–4. Melanoma incidence in the United States in men, by Breslow thickness, 1988 to 1996. All rates are age-adjusted to the 1970 US Standard Population. Incidence data are derived from the Surveillance, Epidemiology and End Results (SEER) Cancer Incidence Public-Use Database, 1973 to 1996.

the past few decades. Recently, however, both incidence and mortality rates appear to be stabilizing.

KERATINOCYTE CANCERS

Keratinocyte carcinomas (KCs) include basal cell carcinoma and squamous cell carcinoma, the two most common forms of skin cancer. The descriptive epidemiology of KCs must be interpreted in light of the limitations of the data sources. Keratinocyte carcinomas are not routinely included in cancer registries, hampering our ability to calculate their incidence and prevalence accurately and monitor trends.[2] There are potentially significant problems with under-registration of KCs in these registries that may be greater than the corresponding problems with melanoma. The effects of under-registration of KCs, the resultant underestimation of KCs, and the impact of surveillance bias on rates have yet to be quantified. Other methods used to evaluate the occurrence of KCs include self-reporting, studies within pre-paid health plans (HMOs), and skin cancer surveys that are either nationwide or within specific regions. This latter method has provided the majority of incidence data on KCs, but survey meth-

ods used in these studies are known to vary widely between nations, complicating the direct comparison of worldwide data. Some of these complications arise from variation in the method by which KC cases are ascertained by different surveys. Keratinocyte carcinomas can be enumerated by either counting individuals with cancer or counting all incident cancers. This latter method would count all cancers, even multiple cancers in a single individual, as separate incident cancers. Two Australian studies

Table 1–2. MELANOMA INCIDENCE IN US WOMEN, BY BRESLOW THICKNESS*				
	Breslow Thickness (mm)			
Year	**< 0.75**	**0.75–1.5**	**1.51–3.0**	**> 3.0**
1988	4.5	1.68	0.78	0.52
1989	4.5	1.91	0.84	0.59
1990	4.28	1.86	0.97	0.55
1991	4.76	2.14	1.05	0.6
1992	4.51	1.97	0.97	0.54
1993	4.92	1.93	1.00	058
1994	5.38	1.84	0.77	0.66
1995	5.76	2.13	1.01	0.65
1996	5.94	2.17	1.02	0.62

*All rates are age-adjusted to the 1970 US Standard Population. Incidence data are derived from the Surveillance, Epidemiology and End Results (SEER) Cancer Incidence Public-Use Database, 1973 to 1996.

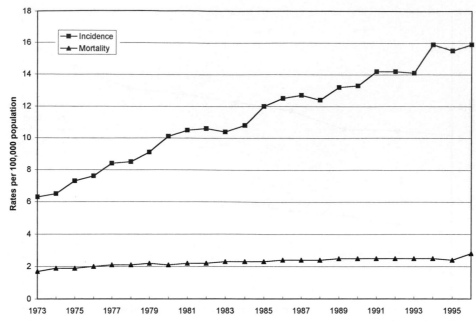

Figure 1–5. Melanoma incidence and mortality in the United States, 1973 to 1996. All rates are age-adjusted to the 1970 US Standard Population. Incidence data are derived from the Surveillance, Epidemiology and End Results (SEER) Cancer Incidence Public-Use Database, 1973 to 1996.

are notable because their study methods were particularly stringent.[37,38] These studies were population-based longitudinal studies in which subjects were surveyed and examined for skin cancer at two different time periods. Subjects first completed a questionnaire about any skin cancers they had been treated for in the past and then underwent systematic skin examination by dermatologists. Patients were examined once during each survey period. Biopsies were performed for all suspicious lesions, and the specimens were examined by one dermatopathologist. The incidence of KC was then calculated by counting all KCs diagnosed between surveys and all KCs diagnosed at the second survey (Table 1–3).

Squamous cell carcinoma (SCC) and basal cell carcinoma (BCC) are often grouped together in studies, further limiting the conclusions that can be drawn about the epidemiology of each. From 1977 to 1978, the National Cancer Institute (NCI) conducted surveys covering eight geographic regions in the United States to assess the incidence of KCs. The age-adjusted KC incidence rate was 233 per 100,000 in white Americans and 3.4 per 100,000 in African Americans.[39] Scotto and colleagues estimated the annual incidence of KCs at approximately 500,000 cases in the early 1980s.[39] A more recent

projection by Miller and Weinstock was between 900,000 and 1.2 million cases in 1994.[40]

Squamous Cell Carcinoma

Incidence

Despite the limitations outlined above, some conclusions may be drawn from the available data. Similar to melanoma, SCC has been steadily rising in incidence over the past several decades. Two NCI surveys of KCs took place; one was conducted in 1971 and 1972, and the other was conducted in 1977 and 1978, to allow for comparisons in rates over time.[41] A comparison of SCC rates between these two time periods suggested increases of 5 percent in males and 15 percent in females, but these increases were not statistically significant. A few American studies aim specifically to analyze the incidence of SCC in well-defined populations (see Table 1–3). The highest rates of SCC incidence in the world occur in Australia, as do the highest rates of melanoma.

The incidence of SCC has been rising worldwide over the past decades.[42–44] It has been increasing at rates between 3 and 10 percent per year.[42–45] As in the case of rising melanoma incidence, the etiology of the rise of KCs in Caucasians is thought to be a consequence of increased UV light exposure. These increases have been 2- to 3-fold in most studies that compare rates from the 1980s to the early 1990s.[32,44,46-49] Evidence now exists regarding the efficacy of daily sunscreen use in reducing the incidence of SCC. The Nambour Skin Cancer Prevention Trial aimed to investigate the effectiveness of daily sunscreen application in reducing the incidence of SCC in members of a Queensland community over a period of 4.5 years. The study revealed that the use of daily sunscreen had no harmful effect on individuals over this time period and that the incidence of SCC was significantly reduced in the daily sunscreen group compared to the no-daily-sunscreen group.[38] The study results provide strong additional evidence to support the long-suspected etiologic link between UV exposure and subsequent SCC.

Gender and racial differences in SCC incidence exist. Gender differences are fairly consistent worldwide, with a greater SCC occurrence in men than in women. Rate ratios of SCC incidence in men compared to women range between 2.0 and 3.4 in the United States.[2] A study of SCC incidence in Hispanics in New Mexico in 1977 to 1978 revealed a rate that was less than 10 percent and about 20 percent of the rates in Anglo-American males and females, respectively.[50]

Anatomic Sites

The majority of SCCs occur on the head, neck, and upper extremities.[32,39,45,51] The Rochester Epidemi-ology Project study found 66 percent of SCCs on the head and neck in women versus 73 percent on the head and neck in men. Men were also more likely to have multiple tumors than women and more frequent occurrence on the ears.[52] This latter site of SCC occurrence also results in greater mortality than SCC at other anatomic sites.[52,53] Squamous cell carcinoma arose on the lower extremities at a rate of 10 percent in men and 17 percent in women in the Swiss canton of Vaud study.[54]

The anatomic site differences in the occurrence of SCC in darker-pigmented individuals are striking and point toward differing etiologies of SCC. In Africans, East Asians, and South Asians, SCC frequently occurs in areas of chronic injury or irritation. These sites include chronic leg ulcers, burn scars, skin infections, or sites of irritation from tight clothing.[55-59] There is a propensity for SCC to occur on the lower extremities in these populations, a site that also tends to be the most common location of repeated cutaneous injury.

Basal Cell Carcinoma

Basal cell carcinoma is the most common skin cancer in white populations around the world.[42] Estimates of BCC incidence and prevalence vary widely among different populations. Similar constraints to those imposed on the interpretation of SCC rates apply to the accuracy of BCC rates. Since sun exposure is important in the etiology of BCC, much of the variation in incidence rates may reflect variations in geog-

Table 1–3. KERATINOCYTE CANCER INCIDENCE RATES							
Location	Year	SCC in Men*	SCC in Women*	BCC in Men*	BCC in Women*	Standard Population	Reference
Rochester (MN)	1990–1992	191	71	—	—	1990 US	Gray et al, 1997
Kauai (HI)	1983–1987	153	92	576	298	1980 US	Chuang et al, 1995
New Hampshire	1993–1994	78	31	117	53	1970 US	Karagas et al, 1999
North Humberside, UK	1978–1991	29	21	116	104	1991 England and Wales	Ko et al, 1994
Canton of Vaud, Switzerland	1991–1992	287	254	613	690	World	Levi et al, 1995
Geraldton, Western Australia	1987–1992	775	501	7,067	3,379	World	English et al, 1997
Nambour, Australia	1986	436	347	1,962	1,561	World	Green et al, 1996

BCC = basal cell carcinoma; SCC = squamous cell carcinoma.
* Per 10^5 population.

raphy, sun exposure, pigmentation, and behavior. Nonetheless, studies regarding the incidence and prevalence of BCC in the majority of white populations tend to concur in terms of the general magnitude and demographics of this cancer. Table 1–3 contains data on recent estimates of BCC incidence rates.

The incidence of BCC has also risen over the past decades. The magnitude of the increase has been fairly large across multiple populations in different countries. Most studies report a 20 to 80 percent increase.[41,60,61] These incidence increases may be due in part to greater public awareness and to vigilance on the part of both patients and physicians. Trends in BCC incidence were analyzed in Australia over a 10-year period from 1985 to 1995 by means of a nationwide household survey.[62] Researchers reported an increase in BCC of 19 percent, compared to a rise in SCC of 93 percent and a decline in the BCC-SCC ratio from 4:1 to 2.5:1. When analyzed in greater detail, it is clear that most of the increase was due to a rise in rates in elderly people; rates of BCC in the young had actually decreased.[62] A large rise in BCC incidence was also evident in elderly people in a New Hampshire study, but detailed analysis of trends in younger age groups was precluded by small numbers.[61]

Skin cancer prevention has been a major health concern over the past 20 years in Australia. The attitudes of the young toward sunlight have undergone substantial changes, and so has their behavior, as indicated by a decreased incidence of sunburn over time.[63] It is hoped that the trends noted above are the results of the enormous public health efforts that have been mounted to stem the rising tide of skin cancer. Many other highly affected countries have lagged behind Australia in terms of widespread skin cancer prevention efforts. Whether or not trends in these countries will eventually correlate with the Australian experience remains to be seen.

Prevalence

In 1997, 8,730 BCCs were diagnosed in a US population consisting of 99,554 individuals who presented to the skin cancer screening program sponsored by the American Academy of Dermatology. This figure overestimates prevalence as participation in screening is voluntary and as individuals who have noted suspicious lesions are more apt to present at screenings. Staples and colleagues estimated that in 1995, more than 190,000 Australians were treated for BCC, not including treatment of multiple tumors in an individual.[62] They also estimated that between 0.5 and 2.0 percent of the population are annually treated for BCC in Australia, with variations dependent on the distance to the equator.

Gender and Anatomic Site

Men generally have higher rates of BCC; sex ratios of incidence are between 1.3 and 1.9 in North America.[2] This sex distribution has varied over time and is different for younger individuals. One study in tropical Australia reports a sex ratio of 1.3:1 for cohorts born before 1945 but reports a ratio of 0.8:1 in younger cohorts.[64] These differences may be the result of different sunlight exposure patterns or different thresholds for seeking medical attention.[62] Seventy to 90 percent of BCCs are located on the face, head, and neck—the sites of chronic sun exposure.[2] These anatomic predilections are consistent between the sexes, except that women tend to have a greater frequency of BCC on the lower extremities and men tend to have more on the ear. This latter aspect of site distribution could be the result of the typical differences in clothing and hair styles between the sexes. Changes in anatomic site distribution over time have also been noted. In cohorts born after 1945 in Australia, BCC occurs more commonly on the back and proportionately less commonly on the head and neck. In a comparison between BCC sites of Kauai (Hawaii) residents and Minnesota residents, the former had significantly more lesions on the trunk and back than the latter.[65] These changes in site distributions are attributed to the warm weather in Kauai and Australia, resulting in greater outdoor activity combined with less clothing coverage.

Mortality of Keratinocyte Carcinomas

Malignant melanoma is responsible for almost 75 percent of deaths attributable to skin cancer.[18] The contribution of KCs to skin cancer mortality is less significant than that of melanoma, except in elderly people and among nonwhite racial groups. When mortality does result from KCs, it is generally due to SCC.[52,53,66] A useful approach to mortality from SCC is an analysis of the manner in which this tumor kills, namely, by metastasis. It has been estimated that almost 75 percent of the mortality from SCC in the United States occurs in individuals with metastatic disease.[67] The mortality of BCC is low, and if death results, it is usually due to direct extension to and invasion of vital organs.[68] Only about 0.03 percent of BCCs are thought to metastasize, but this potential does increase with tumor size.[53,69] Most of the morbidity and mortality of BCC occurs in individuals over 75 years of age and is thought to be primarily due to failure of the patient to bring the lesion to clinical attention.[70]

There is limited information on trends in the mortality of KCs and even less on trends in the mortalities of SCC and BCC taken individually. In Australia, a decline in mortality from KCs has occurred since 1930, an annual average decrease of 10 percent in men and 17 percent in women.[42] When corrections were made for misclassification errors, a decline in mortality from KC was noted in the United States from 1969 to 1988.[67] Deaths result from melanoma more often than from KCs, even though KCs are at least 10 to 25 times more common than melanoma.[40] Thus, despite the low mortality of KCs, the absolute numbers of deaths may represent a substantial burden to society. The importance of KCs and their impact on public health may increase if KC incidence rates continue to rise.

Impact of Skin Cancer in Older and Younger Subpopulations

The epidemiology of melanoma and KCs has been studied in elderly people. Individuals aged over 65 years and diagnosed with melanoma tend to have lower 5-year survival rates: 64 percent overall, compared to 78 percent in younger age groups.[71] This difference has been attributed to delays in identification and subsequent referral of skin lesions in elderly people.[72] Factors accounting for delays include the presence of less obvious lesions (such as nodular and amelanotic melanomas) or lesions located in sites that are difficult to observe. Other factors that prevent patients from seeking care include psychiatric, visual, or verbal impairments. Moreover, it is contended that skin cancer preventive efforts are less effective in reaching the elderly populations.[71] Finally, elderly people present with a different proportion of histogenetic melanoma subtypes than the young.[71] Superficial spreading melanoma is the most common subtype in both groups but is proportionately less common in elderly people. Elderly individuals tend to have a greater predominance of the other subtypes, some of which carry worse prognoses.

The impact of KCs is greater in elderly people than in young people, in terms of contribution to skin cancer mortality. In fact, 90 percent of skin cancer deaths in young white individuals are due to melanoma whereas only a minority of skin cancer deaths in people over 85 years of age is attributable to melanoma.[18] The worldwide median age at the presentation of melanoma is 48 years (Balch et al, 1985). Therefore, it is appropriate to measure the impact of melanoma by assessing the years of potential life lost (YPLL) due to melanoma. Strikingly, in adults, melanoma ranks second only to leukemia in the number of years of life lost per death. The YPLL of melanoma is estimated at 17. The excess premature mortality caused by melanoma emphasizes the need for early detection of melanoma and for continued preventive efforts.[73]

CUTANEOUS LYMPHOMAS

Cutaneous lymphomas (CLs) include T- and B-cell lymphomas and their clinical variants. In general, T-cell lymphomas are more common than the B-cell lymphomas of the skin. The most common variant of cutaneous T-cell lymphoma (CTCL) is mycosis fungoides (MF). Thus, studies have focused on the epidemiology of this variant. Data on incidence and mortality are sparse, and the etiology of cutaneous lymphoma is unknown.

Studies show that under-registration of cutaneous lymphoma occurs, limiting the accuracy of incidence estimates. One Israeli study compared cutaneous lymphoma incidence rates derived from cancer registries with those obtained from these registries plus various other sources that included hospitals, outpatient offices, and pathology labs. The study's authors found substantial under-reporting of CL when registry data alone was used, versus a combination of additional data sources. The rates derived from multiple sources were 24 percent higher for non-MF cutaneous lymphoma and 49 percent higher for MF than the respective Israeli Cancer Registry rates.[74] The accuracy of the registration of CL by the US SEER program registry was also evaluated by estimating the under-reporting that occurred at one of the SEER program registry sites, and it was found that 84 percent of all CLs were reported to the registries.[75] Under-registration may occur because early CL rarely results in hospitalization and is therefore less likely to be registered unless outpatient laboratories and centers are routinely surveyed for cases. Moreover, MF has an indolent course; hence, it is possible for afflicted individuals to die from other causes before their MF has progressed.[75]

Comparisons of incidence rates among different populations or countries is complicated by the differing methods of acquiring this data. There are variations between countries in the reporting practices of disease, as well as the use of different denominators and time periods over which rates are calculated.[74]

The accuracy of cause-of-death certification for MF has also been called into question. In one report, only 60 percent of the deaths attributable to MF were actually certified as caused by MF.[76] Substantial misclassification in the cause-of-death coding of MF exists; hence, MF mortality statistics are also difficult to interpret.[76] Misclassification of the cause of death can occur if advanced stages of MF are confused with other forms of lymphoma. Deaths may also be falsely attributed to other malignancies or disease processes that result in death but that occur as a consequence of MF or the treatment of MF. Mycosis fungoides may also increase case fatality from other disorders (for example, by limiting a patient's ability to tolerate aggressive treatments).

Incidence

In the United States, the incidence of MF in men is more than twice that in women. It occurs more frequently in African Americans than in white Americans and more commonly in elderly people than in the young.[75,77] Table 1–4 summarizes reported incidence rates of CL and MF in several studies.

The incidence rates of MF increased from 1973 through 1984 but have since stabilized.[75,77] In the United States, the age-adjusted rate in 1973 of MF was 0.2 per 100,000, compared to 0.5 per 100,000 in 1984 and 1992. Improvements in disease detection through more precise disease definitions and more sensitive molecular tests may have accounted for the rising incidence rates through the 1980s. Changes in exposure to an as yet unidentified risk factor for MF could also have contributed to these trends.

Mortality

Mortality is greater among men than among women, and it increases with age. It is also higher among blacks than among whites worldwide.[78,79] There is considerable variation in mortality rates among different countries. Some of these differences can be attributed to variations in case ascertainment, but

Table 1–4. CUTANEOUS LYMPHOMA INCIDENCE RATES					
Location	Year	Variant	Incidence*	Standard Population	Reference
United States (SEER)	1973–1992	MF	0.36	1970 US	Weinstock et al, 1999
Rochester (MN)	1970–1984	CTCL	0.9	1980 US	Chuang et al, 1990
Los Angeles (CA)	1973-1984	MF	0.16	1970 US	Bernstein et al, 1989
Norway	1960–1980	CTCL	0.13	Crude	McFadden et al, 1983
England and Wales	1981	MF	0.13	Crude	Slevin et al, 1987
Netherlands	1974–1980	CTCL	0.14	Crude	Hamminga et al, 1982
Israel	1985–1993	CL	0.9	World	Iscovich et al, 1997
Western Australia	1960–1969	CL	0.15	World	Dougan et al, 1981

CL = cutaneous lymphoma; CTCL = cutaneous T-cell lymphoma; MF = mycosis fungoides; SEER = Surveillance, Epidemiology and End Results; US = United States.

again, differing exposures to etiologic agents could also have an effect. In the United States, mortality from MF has declined by 22 percent from 1979 to 1991.[75] This decline was evident in African Americans and in whites, but the rate declined to a greater extent in women compared to men.[75] The decline in mortality may be the result of earlier disease diagnosis and treatment, resulting in an improved prognosis, or it could reflect the changing biology of MF.[75]

CONCLUSION

Monitoring trends in incidence, mortality, and changing frequencies of disease allows clinicians to evaluate the relative success or failure of measures implemented to control disease. The continued study of skin cancer from a public-health perspective is compelling, given the large burden to society these illnesses impose in terms of morbidity, mortality, and cost.

REFERENCES

1. Ries LAG, Kosary CL, Hankey BF, et al, editors. SEER cancer statistics review, 1973–1994. Bethesda, (MD): National Cancer Institute; 1997. NIH Publication No. 97-2789). p. 305–18.
2. Weinstock MA. Ultraviolet radiation and skin cancer: epidemiologic data from the United States and Canada. In: Young AR, Björn LO, Moan J, Nultsch W, editors. Environmental UV photobiology. New York: Plenum Press; 1993. p. 295–344.
3. Karagas MR, Thomas DB, Roth GJ, et al. The effects of changes in health care delivery on the reported incidence of cutaneous melanoma in western Washington State. Am J Epidemiol 1991;133:58–62.
4. West DW, Zippin C, Lum D, et al. An epidemiologic study of unreported cutaneous malignant melanoma among residents of Alameda and Contra Costa counties. 1991. (Unpublished study.)
5. Popescu NA, Beard CM, Treacy PJ, et al. Cutaneous malignant melanoma in Rochester, Minnesota: trends in incidence and survivorship, 1950 through 1985. Mayo Clin Proc 1990;65:1293–302.
6. Nair MK, Varghese C, Mahadevan S, et al. Cutaneous malignant melanoma—clinical epidemiology and survival. J Indian Med Assoc 1998;96:19–20.
7. Weinstock MA, Reynes JF. Validation of cause of death certification for outpatient cancers: the contrasting cases of melanoma and mycosis fungoides. Am J Epidemiol 1998;148:1184–6.
8. Hall IH, Miller DR, Rogers JD, Bewerse B. Update on the incidence and mortality from melanoma in the United States. J Am Acad Dermatol 1999;40:35–42.
9. Parkin DM, Muir CS, Whelan SL, et al, editors. Cancer incidence in five continents. Vol. VI. Lyon (France): International Agency for Research on Cancer; 1992.
10. Franceschi S, La Vecchia C, Negri E, Levi F. Increases in mortality from cutaneous melanoma in southern Europe. Int J Cancer 1992;51:160–2.
11. Cress RD, Holly EA. Incidence of cutaneous melanoma among non-Hispanic whites, Hispanics, Asians, and blacks: an analysis of California cancer registry data. Cancer Causes Control 1997;8:246–52.
12. Garsaud P, Boisseau-Garsaud AM, Ossondo M, et al. Epidemiology of cutaneous melanoma in the French West Indies (Martinique). Am J Epidemiol 1998;147:66–8.
13. Dennis LK, White E, Lee JAH. Recent cohort trends in malignant melanoma by anatomic site in the United States. Cancer Causes Control 1993;4:93–100.
14. Van Der Rhee HJ, Van Der Spek-Keijser LMT, Van Westering R, Coebergh JWW. Increase in and stabilization of incidence and mortality of primary cutaneous malignant melanoma in western Netherlands, 1980–95. Br J Dermatol 1999;140:463–7.
15. Marks R. Two decades of the public health approach to skin cancer control in Australia: why, how and where are we now? Australas J Dermatol 1999;40(1):1–5.
16. MacKie RM. Incidence, risk factors and prevention of melanoma. Eur J Cancer 1998;34, Suppl 3:S3–6.
17. Centers for Disease Control. Deaths from melanoma—United States, 1973–1992. MMWR 1995;44:337, 343–47.
18. Weinstock MA. Death from skin cancer among the elderly: epidemiologic patterns. Arch Dermatol 1997;133:1207–9.
19. Roush GC, McKay L, Holford TR. A reversal in the long-term increase in deaths attributable to malignant melanoma. Cancer 1992;69:1714–20.
20. Scotto J, Pitcher H, Lee JAH. Indications of future decreasing trends in skin-melanoma mortality among whites in the United States. Int J Cancer 1991;49:490–7.
21. Thörn M, Sparén P, Bergström R, Adami H-O. Trends in mortality rates from malignant melanoma in Sweden 1953-1987 and forecasts up to 2007. Br J Cancer 1992;66:563–7.
22. Ries LAG, Hankey BF, Miller BA, et al, editors. Cancer statistics review 1973–88. Bethesda (MD): National Cancer Institute; 1991. NIH Publication No. 91-2789.
23. Streetly A, Markowe H. Changing trends in the epidemiology of malignant melanoma: gender differences and their implications for public health. Int J Epidemiol 1995;24:897–907.

24. Bentham G, Aase A. Incidence of malignant melanoma of the skin in Norway, 1955–1989: associations with solar ultraviolet radiation, income and holidays abroad. Int J Epidemiol 1996;25:1132–8.

25. Elwood JM, Swerdlow AJ, Cox B. Trends in incidence and mortality from cutaneous melanoma in England and Wales. Trans Menzies Found 1989;15:131–5.

26. Elder DE. Skin Cancer: melanoma and other specific nonmelanoma skin cancers. Cancer 1995; 75; Suppl 1:245–56.

27. Lee JAH, Strickland D. Malignant melanoma: social status and outdoor work. Br J Cancer 1980;41:757–63.

28. Gallagher RP, Elwood JM, Threlfall WJ, et al. Occupation and risk of cutaneous melanoma. Am J Ind Med 1986;9:289–94.

29. Kirkpatrick CS, Lee JAH, White E. Melanoma risk by age and socio-economic status. Int J Cancer 1990;46:1–4.

30. Harrison RA, Haque AU, Roseman JM, Soong S. Socioeconomic characteristics and melanoma incidence. Ann Epidemiol 1998;8:327–33.

31. MacKie RM, Hole DJ. Incidence and thickness of primary tumours and survival of patients with cutaneous malignant melanoma in relation to socioeconomic status. BMJ 1996;312:1125–8.

32. Glass AG, Hoover RN. The emerging epidemic of melanoma and squamous cell skin cancer. JAMA 1989;262:2097–100.

33. Elwood JM, Gallagher RP. Site distribution of malignant melanoma. Can Med Assoc J 1983;128:1400–4.

34. Swerdlow AJ. International trends in cutaneous melanoma. Ann N Y Acad Sci 1990;609:235–51.

35. Dennis LK. Analysis of the melanoma epidemic, both apparent and real. Arch Dermatol 1999;135:275–80.

36. Armstrong BK. The epidemiology of melanoma: where do we go from here? In: Gallagher RP, Elwood JM, editors. Epidemiological aspects of cutaneous malignant melanoma. Boston: Kluwer Academic Publishers, 1994. p. 307–23.

37. English DR, Kricker A, Heenan PJ, et al. Incidence of non-melanocytic skin cancer in Geraldton, Western Australia. Int J Cancer 1997;73:629–33.

38. Green A, Beardmore G, Hart V, et al. Skin cancer in a Queensland population. J Am Acad Dermatol 1988; 10:1045–52.

39. Scotto J, Fears TR, Fraumeni JF. Incidence of non-melanoma skin cancer in the United States. Washington (DC): Public Health Service, 1983. NIH Publication No. 83-2433.

40. Miller DL, Weinstock MA. Nonmelanoma skin cancer in the United States: incidence. J Am Acad Dermatol 1994;30:774–8.

41. Fears TR, Scotto J. Changes in skin cancer morbidity between 1971–72 and 1977–78. J Natl Cancer Inst 1982;69:365–70.

42. Marks R, Staples M, Giles GG. Trends in non-melanocytic skin cancer treated in Australia: the second national survey. Int J Cancer 1993;53:585–90.

43. Gray DT, Suman VJ, Su DWP, et al. Trends in the population-based incidence of squamous cell carcinoma of the skin first diagnosed between 1984 and 1992. Arch Dermatol 1997;133:735–40.

44. Levi F, Franceschi S, Te V-C, et al. Trends of skin cancer in the Canton of Vaud, 1976–1992. Br J Cancer 1995;72:1047–53.

45. Gallagher RP, Ma B, McLean DI, et al. Trends in basal cell carcinoma, squamous cell carcinoma, and melanoma of the skin from 1973 through 1987. J Am Acad Dermatol 1990;23:413–21.

46. Ko CB, Walton S, Keczkes K, et al. The emerging epidemic of skin cancer. Br J Dermatol 1994;130:69–72.

47. Osterlind A, Hou-Jensen K, Jensen OM. Incidence of cutaneous malignant melanoma in Denmark 1978–1982. Anatomic site distribution, histologic types, and comparison with non-melanoma skin cancer. Br J Cancer 1988;58:385–91.

48. Nelemans PJ, Kiemeney LALM, Rampen FHJ, et al. Trends in mortality from malignant cutaneous melanoma in the Netherlands, 1950–1988. Eur J Cancer 1993;29A:107–11.

49. MacKie RM, et al. Cutaneous malignant melanoma, Scotland, 1979–89. Lancet 1992;339:971–5.

50. Macdonald EJ, Heinze EB. Epidemiology of cancer in Texas: incidence analyzed by type, ethnic group, and geographic location. New York: Raven Press, 1978.

51. Chuang T-Y, Reizner GT, Elpern DJ, et al. Squamous cell carcinoma in Kauai, Hawaii. Int J Dermatol 1995;34:393–7.

52. Osterlind A, Hjalgrim H, Kulinsky B, Frentz G. Skin cancer as a cause of death in Denmark. Br J Dermatol 1991;125:580–2.

53. Weinstock MA, Bogaars HA, Ashley M, et al. Non-melanoma skin cancer mortality: a population-based study. Arch Dermatol 1991;127:1194–7.

54. Levi F, LaVecchia C, Te V-C, Mezzanotte G. Descriptive epidemiology of skin cancer in the Swiss canton of Vaud. Int J Cancer 1988;42:811–6.

55. Chakravorty RC, Dutta-Choudhuri R. Malignant neoplasms of the skin in eastern India: an analysis of cases seen at its Chittaranjan Cancer Hospital, Calcutta, during the years 1963–65 inclusive. Indian J Cancer 1968;5:133–44.

56. Yeh S. Relative incidence of skin cancer in Chinese in Taiwan with special reference to arsenical cancer. Natl Cancer Inst Monogr 1963;10:81–107.

57. Tada M, Miki Y. Malignant skin tumors among dermatology patients in university hospitals of Japan. J Dermatol 1984;11:313–21.

58. Camain R, Tuyns AJ, Sarrat H, et al. Cutaneous cancer in Dakar. J Natl Cancer Inst 1972;48:33–49.

59. Yakubu A, Mabogunje OA. Squamous cell carcinoma of the skin in Africans. Trop Geogr Med 1995;47:91–3.

60. Dahl E, Åberg M, Rausing A, Rausing E-L. Basal cell carcinoma: an epidemiologic study in a defined population. Cancer 1992;70:104–8.

61. Karagas MR, Greenberg RE, Spencer SK, et al. Increase in incidence rates of basal cell and sqaumous cell skin cancer in New Hampshire, USA. Int J Cancer 1999;81:555–9.

62. Staples M, Marks R, Giles G. Trends in the incidence of non-melanocytic skin cancer treated in Australia 1985–1995: Are primary prevention programs starting to have an effect? Int J Cancer 1998;78:144–8.

63. Hill D, White V, Marks R, Borland R. Changes in sun-related attitudes and behaviors, and reduced sunburn prevalence in a population at high risk of melanoma. Eur J Cancer Prev 1993;2:447–56.

64. Czarnecki D, Collins N, Nash C. Basal cell carcinoma in tropical Australia. Int J Dermatol 1992;31:398–9.

65. Reizner GT, Chuang T-Y, Elpern DJ, et al. Basal cell carcinoma in Kauai, Hawaii: the highest documented incidence in the United States. J Am Acad Dermatol 1993;29:184–9.

66. Dunnje Jr, Levin EA, Linden G, Harzfeld L. Skin cancer as a cause of death. Calif Med 1965;102:361–3.

67. Weinstock MA. Nonmelanoma skin cancer mortality in the United States, 1969 through 1988. Arch Dermatol 1993;129:1286–90.

68. Lever WF, Lever GS. Histopathology of the skin. 6th ed. Philadelphia: J.B.Lippincott; 1983.

69. Sahl WJ, Snow SN, Levine NS. Giant basal cell carcinoma: report of two cases and review of the literature. J Am Acad Dermatol 1994;30:856–9.

70. Sahl WJ. Basal cell carcinoma: influence of tumor size on mortality and morbidity. Int J Dermatol 1995;34.

71. McHenry PM, Hole DJ, MacKie RM. Melanoma in people aged 65 and over in Scotland, 1979–1989. BMJ 1992;304:746–9.

72. Harland CC, Marsden RA. Melanoma in people aged 65 and over [letter]. BMJ 1992;304:1055.

73. Albert VA, Koh HK, Geller AC, et al. Years of potential life lost: another indicator of the impact of cutaneous malignant melanoma on society. J Am Acad Dermatol 1990;23:308–10.

74. Iscovich J, Paltiel O, Azizi E, et al. Cutaneous lymphoma in Israel, 1985–1993: a population-based incidence study. Br J Cancer 1998;77:170–3.

75. Weinstock MA, Gardstein BA. Twenty-year trends in the reported incidence of mycosis fungoides and associated mortality. Am J Public Health 1999;89:1240–4.

76. Weinstock MA, Reynes JF. Validation of cause-of-death certification for outpatient cancers: the contrasting cases of melanoma and mycosis fungoides. Am J Epidemiol 1998;148:1184–6.

77. Weinstock MA, Horm JW. Mycosis fungoides in the United States: increasing incidence and descriptive epidemiology. JAMA 1988;260:42–6.

78. Greene MH, Dalager NA, Lamberg SI, et al. Mycosis fungoides: epidemiologic observations. Cancer Treat Rep 1979;63:597–606.

79. Weinstock MA. Epidemiology of mycosis fungoides. Semin Dermatol 1994;13:154–9.

2

Genetics of Skin Cancer

HENSIN TSAO, MD, PhD
FRANK G. HALUSKA, MD, PhD

Cancer is essentially a genetic disease. A series of mutations, either inherited or acquired, accumulate and affect the cell's ability to proliferate, invade, and survive. Figure 2–1 illustrates this process. A single cell (yellow cell) may acquire a mutation that confers a growth advantage over its normal counterparts (green cells). With time, the proportion of cells that carry this mutation increases; thus, there is clonal expansion of the yellow cell. A second mutation (red cell) may further drive proliferation and lead to continued expansion of another subclone. Conversely, mutations in other genes can result in the early demise of the cell (blue cell). Tumor formation results from a series of selection pressures that favor growth and survival. Even though a given cancer may be derived from a single cell, numerous subclones probably exist within the tumor, representing different levels of selection. Tumors are thus clonally derived but genetically heterogeneous.

There are three large categories of genes that affect cellular proliferation and survival. Growth-promoting genes, or oncogenes, were originally identified as viral genes that "transform" a normal cell to a malignant cell. Subsequent molecular studies have shown that almost all virally encoded oncogenes have counterparts in the human genome

(proto-oncogenes). A partial list of known oncogenes is provided in Table 2–1. Many proto-oncogenes are tightly regulated growth-signaling molecules that become mutated or amplified and overcome the normal restraints imposed by cellular homeostasis; these proto-oncogenes are thus "activated" and become oncogenes. In general, oncogenes are genetically dominant, in that mutation of one allele is sufficient to produce the phenotype. (A diploid cell has two copies, or alleles, of every autosomal gene.) One of the first oncogenes to be isolated was the *RAS* oncogene; activating mutations in *RAS* have been reported in up to 30 percent of cutaneous melanomas.

A second class of genes negatively regulate cell growth or promote cell death and are termed tumor suppressor genes (TSGs). A partial list of the known TSGs is provided in Table 2–2. Unlike oncogenes, both alleles of the TSG must be inactivated for complete loss of function. Tumor suppressors often inhibit cell division, down-regulate growth signals, or promote cell death. Inactivated TSGs have been shown to be prominently involved in skin cancer—for example, the *PTC* gene in basal cell carcinomas, the *CDKN2A* gene in cutaneous melanoma, and the *p53* gene in squamous cell carcinomas.

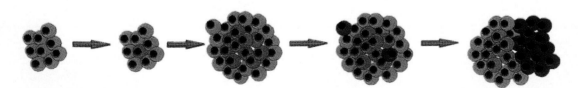

Figure 2–1. Selection of mutant clones in the formation of tumors.

Table 2–1. PARTIAL LISTING OF COMMONLY MUTATED ONCOGENES		
Oncogene	**Affected Malignancies**	**Protein Function**
Growth factor		
v-sis	Glioma, fibrosarcoma	PDGF
Receptor tyrosine kinases		
EGFP	Squamous cell carcinomas	EGF receptor
TRK	Colon cancer	NGF receptor
NEU	Neuroblastoma, breast cancer	Related to EGF receptor
RET	MEN 2A, MEN 2B	GDNF receptor
Nonreceptor tyrosine kinases		
SRC	Colon cancer	Tyrosine protein kinase
BCR/ABL	CML	Tyrosine protein kinase
Membrane G proteins		
HRAS	Colon, lung, pancreatic cancer	G protein
KRAS	AML, thyroid cancer, melanoma	G protein
NRAS	Melanoma	G protein
Serine/threonine protein kinase		
v-raf	Sarcoma	Serine/threonine protein kinase
Nuclear proteins		
MYC	Neuroblastoma, lung cancer	Transcription factor
LMYC	Lung cancer	Transcription factor
v-fos	Osteosarcoma	Transcription factor

AML = acute myelogenous leukemia; CML = chronic myelogenous leukemia; EGF = epidermal growth factor; GDNF = glial-derived neurotrophic factor; MEN = multiple endocrine neoplasia; NGF = nerve growth factor; PDGF = platelet-derived growth factor.

A third class of cancer-related genes, the mutator genes or caretaker genes, do not directly affect cell division or cell death; rather, these genes maintain the integrity of the human genome. When the genetic caretaker function is lost, mutations accumulate much more rapidly. An exemplary skin-associated caretaker defect is xeroderma pigmentosum (XP). In XP, cutaneous malignancies arise within the first decade of life, due to a failure to repair ultraviolet (UV)–induced genetic lesions. Oncogenes are thus more likely to be activated and tumor suppressor genes are more prone to be abrogated with a caretaker-deficient phenotype.

Mechanism of Genetic Damage in Skin Cancer

In the genetic analysis of cancer, the types of mutations also give us clues to the mechanism of genetic injury. For instance, transitions from CC pairs to TT pairs in the DNA (CC-to-TT mutations) are signatures of UV damage. Various mechanisms of mutations exist to damage the genome. Most cancers are aneuploid, reflecting a fundamental genomic instability. On karyotypic analysis, the somatic loss or gain of chromosomes is commonly seen in solid cancers. Although chromosomal translocations are

Table 2–2. PARTIAL LIST OF TUMOR SUPPRESSOR GENES		
Gene	**Cancer Syndrome**	**Function**
RB1	Familial retinoblastoma	Transcriptional regulator
APC	Familial adenomatous polyposis	Down-regulator of β-catenin
NF-1	Neurofibromatosis 1	GTPase
NF-2	Neurofibromatosis 2	Cytoskeletal protein
PTEN/MMAC1	Cowden disease	Phosphatase, cytoskeletal protein
TP53	Li-Fraumeni syndrome	Transcription factor
CDKN2A	Familial melanoma	CDK inhibitor
BRCA1,2	Familial breast cancer	(Not fully understood)
VHL	Von Hippel Lindau syndrome	Transcriptional regulator

CDK = cyclin-dependent kinase; GTPase = guanosine triphosphatase.

also seen in solid tumors, recurrent translocations frequently cause leukemias and lymphomas. The site of these translocations can be reproducibly identified, and many genes affected by these large chromosomal shifts have been isolated. Certain tumors also contain amplifications of genes that favor growth. Larger amplifications can be observed on cytogenetic analysis; observing more limited gene amplification requires molecular analysis. The insertion of viral sequences into the genome can lead to cancer although this is uncommon. Human papillomavirus, for instance, can cause both benign proliferations of keratinocytes and malignant degeneration of the cervical epithelium. Viral proteins can induce neoplasms by binding normal host proteins and interrupting growth inhibition.

Most cancers also involve mutations that exist at a much finer level of resolution. Whole genes or parts of genes can be deleted. Within the gene, small stretches of sequences or a single base pair can be lost. Alternatively, segments of deoxyribonucleic acid (DNA) or single base pairs can also be inserted into a gene, thereby inactivating its function. Insertions and deletions frequently change the reading frame of the encoded gene, resulting in premature termination of the translated product or in a completely unrelated amino acid sequence. Finally, single base pair substitutions usually change the amino acid sequence of a protein product (missense mutation) or bring about a premature stop codon (nonsense mutation). Missense mutations do not necessarily imply a loss of function since conservative amino acid changes can represent a polymorphism or an alternative sequence that retains normal function. For instance, a common polymorphism in the melanoma predisposition gene, *CDKN2A*, changes an alanine to a threonine at position 148, seemingly without altering the p16 protein function.

Identification of Cancer-Causing Genes

So how are cancer-related genes isolated? Two general approaches (Figure 2–2) have been used to answer this question. When a mutation in a cell leads to increased growth (oncogenic transformation), positive selection will lead to a preferential enrichment of the cell population with the mutation. This

enrichment provides a natural functional strategy to identify oncogenes. Furthermore, when expressing oncogenic proteins, cells often undergo alterations in their growth and morphologic phenotype. For example, the oncogene *RAS* was originally isolated on the basis of its ability to "transform" primary and immortalized fibroblasts into tumorigenic fibroblastic cell lines with an altered spindle-shape morphology and an ability to create tumors in mice. Deoxyribonucleic acid sequences that confer this phenotypic change can thus be identified, and the mutations can be detected. Since this approach relies on the presence rather than the absence of a gene that produces a phenotype, researchers have been able to discover many human oncogenes through functional approaches. Functional strategies for identifying tumor suppressor genes are much less effective. Sequences of DNA that suppress growth are difficult to assess since growth inhibition and/or cell death precludes further expansion of the cell population for molecular analysis.

A more generally applicable approach involves positional cloning of cancer-related genes. Genes affected by chromosomal translocations in hematologic malignancies (eg, the *C-MYC* oncogene involved in the chromosome 8/14 translocation of Burkitt's lymphoma) represent the earliest successful positional efforts. Unlike cytogenetic analyses of the leukemias and lymphomas, cytogenetic analyses of solid tumors have been complicated by the large

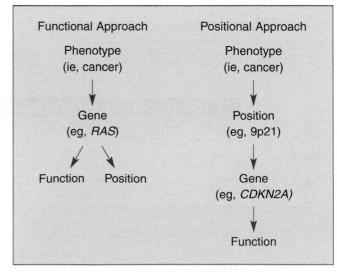

Figure 2–2. Approaches to the identification of cancer-related genes.

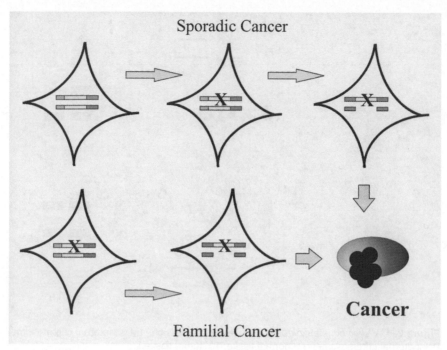

Figure 2–3. The two-hit hypothesis. In sporadic cancers, both copies of a tumor suppressor gene need to be inactivated for tumor formation. In familial cancers, one mutated gene is inherited, and every cell is thus genetically handicapped. A second mutational event in any cell can lead to the early formation of tumors at many foci.

numbers of chromosomal aberrations and the lack of a clear pattern of recurrence. Thus, other positional approaches have been used to identify TSGs in solid tumors. A major advance in our understanding of tumor suppressor mechanisms was made in studies of familial retinoblastoma and the molecular basis for this cancer syndrome. A heritable cancer syndrome, such as nevoid basal cell carcinoma syndrome, usually presents at an earlier age compared with the general population and leads to multiple tumors in one or more organ sites. A paradigm to explain these features was first hypothesized by Alfred Knudson in the early 1970s.[1] Studying the epidemiology of familial and sporadic retinoblastoma, Knudson constructed a model in which he proposed that two mutational events were required for retinoblastoma formation (the "two-hit hypothesis") (Figure 2–3). He suggested that in familial retinoblastoma, the first mutation is inherited in the germline (ie, in every cell of the body) while the second event occurs in the tumor-forming cells. Since every cell is genetically altered, more tumors develop at an earlier age. He speculated that in sporadic retinoblastoma, both mutations have to occur

in the same cell for a tumor to develop; thus, the frequency is reduced and the onset is delayed.

The molecular correlate of the two-hit hypothesis is a loss of heterozygosity (LOH) within the tumor (Figure 2–4). In LOH analysis, the loss of genetic material within the tumor is compared to the intact genetic material from somatic tissue. As shown in Figure 2–4, DNA is extracted from the tumor specimen, and peripheral blood leukocyte DNA is obtained from a blood specimen. The TSG of interest is represented by the box along with two flanking markers: markers *A* and *B* from the mother and markers *a* and *b* from the father. In this example, *A* and *a* are polymorphic (ie, they differ by DNA sequence and can thus be distinguished by size or sensitivity to restriction enzymes and visualized on a gel). Marker *A* is in close proximity to the gene while marker *B* is much farther away. Since normal cells (such as peripheral blood leukocytes) contain two copies of every non-X gene, markers *A*, *a*, *B*, and *b* can be separated; the individual in Figure 2–4 is thus heterozygous for markers *Aa* and *Bb*. If the TSG is deleted along with marker *A* in the tumor, only marker *a* will be apparent—thus, a loss of heterozygosity, diagnosed as two

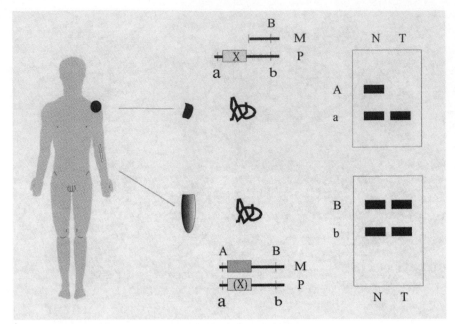

Figure 2–4. Loss of heterozygosity. (See text for discussion.) (M = maternal chromosome; P = paternal chromosome; N = normal tissue; T = tumor tissue.)

bands becoming one on the upper gel. Genetic events more complex than deletion have been described to explain the mechanics of LOH. The remaining copy of the gene can be either normal and mutated in the tumor (sporadic cancer) or previously inactivated by an inherited mutation (familial cancer). A marker farther away (marker Bb) will retain heterozygosity (lower gel). Using this approach with numerous polymorphic markers, investigators can map regions of LOH and obtain positional information to identify tumor suppressor loci.

Another positional approach uses pedigrees with hereditary cancer. If familial cancer is suspected and well-defined kindreds are available, the cancer phenotype can be treated as any mendelian disorder, and linkage analysis can be used to better define the position of the tumor suppressor gene. Linkage analysis is based on the observation that a patient can inherit known markers with their disease gene if the markers are in proximity to the gene. The probability of inheriting this marker with the disease gene is a function of the genetic distance between the two loci. Markers farther away from the disease gene will undergo recombination events and will independently segregate from the disease gene. The likelihood that this marker is close to the disease gene can be expressed as the *lod score*, or the logarithm

of the odds that the marker and the disease gene locus are linked. A lod score of greater than 3 (or 1000:1 in favor of linkage) is usually accepted as the threshold of significance. For example, the locus for a familial melanoma gene was linked to chromosome 9p21, with a maximal lod score of over 12.[2] In other words, the likelihood that one of the markers was close to a melanoma-predisposing gene was greater than 10^{12}:1. Negative lod scores exclude linkage for the region where the lod score is less than –2.0. Although negative lod scores are not as useful as positive lod scores, the information can redirect efforts to more likely candidate TSG loci.

Once a disease gene is located, a map of the region is generated. This map, like all other maps, is a representation of the area of interest. Various types of maps exist (eg, genetic, physical, radiation hybrid), and a discussion of how information is extracted from these maps is beyond the scope of this chapter. In its simplest form, however, a map is a linear arrangement of markers or clones from which various genes can be identified. The DNA sequence of candidate genes is then compared with the sequence of genes derived from the tumor specimen or the genes carried by individuals with hereditary cancers. The identification of a mutation, which cosegregates with the disease phenotype and which is not found in a comparable population of normal individuals, is evidence suggestive of a disease gene.

This introduction is not meant to be an exhaustive treatment on cancer genetics or disease gene identification. Those requiring more detailed explication should refer to the third and fourth items listed in the References section.[3,4] The following sections will examine some recent developments in the genetics of the major cutaneous malignancies— basal cell carcinoma, squamous cell carcinoma, and cutaneous melanoma. Clinical, pathologic, and treatment discussions can be found in the chapters that focus on individual cancers.

SURVEY OF GENES INVOLVED IN THE MAJOR CUTANEOUS MALIGNANCIES

Genetics of Basal Cell Carcinoma

Basal cell carcinoma (BCC) is the most common cancer, with over 750,000 estimated cases per year. Although most BCCs are sporadic, inherited forms have been described in nevoid basal cell carcinoma syndrome (NBCCS) (Mendelian Inheritance of Man [MIM] number 109400), Bazex-Dupre-Christol syndrome (MIM 301845), and Rombo syndrome (MIM 180730). Except for NBCCS, the genetics of these syndromes are largely unexplored given the rarity of the disorders.

Nevoid basal cell carcinoma syndrome is an autosomal dominant disease characterized by the rapid development of numerous BCCs early in the affected individual's life. About 80 to 90 percent of Caucasian individuals with NBCCS will develop BCCs by a median age of 20 years.[5,6] Patients can develop from 1 to > 1,000 BCCs (median, 8 BCCs).[6]

Clinically, the BCCs appear as small brown papules that resemble skin tags, moles, or hemangiomas. These tumors are predominantly distributed on the face (especially periorbital areas, eyelids, nose, malar region, and upper lip), neck, and back, followed by the chest and upper limbs.[5,7] The BCCs can become more aggressive after adolescence, and exceptional cases have been reported to metastasize.[7] Basal cell carcinomas have been described in African American NBCCS kindreds although these cancers occur at a lower frequency than in Cau-

casian families.[6] The histology of BCCs associated with NBCCS is indistinguishable from that of typical BCCs. Milia and epidermal cysts have been described in about half of the cases,[5,7] and palmar and plantar pits occur in 65 to 80 percent of individuals; rare BCCs have been reported to develop within these pits.[5,7]

PTC

Through extensive linkage analysis, several groups mapped the gene for NBCCS to chromosome 9q22-31.[8–12] Concurrent with the linkage studies, deletional analyses of tumor specimens found that about 70 percent of sporadic BCCs also exhibited LOH on chromosome 9q.[13,14] Thus, both linkage and LOH data converged to provide strong evidence for a BCC-related TSG on 9q.

In 1996, two groups demonstrated germline mutations of the *PATCHED* (*PTC*) gene from NBCCS patients and in somatic DNA from sporadic BCCs.[15,16] In recent studies, 15 to 39 percent of affected individuals from NBCCS families were found to harbor mutations in the *PTC* gene.[17,18] Furthermore, *PTC* mutations have also been found in sporadic medulloblastomas, breast carcinomas, meningiomas, and one colon cancer cell line.[19,20]

The *PTC* gene is involved in development of organisms from fruit flies (*Drosophila*) to mammals. In *Drosophila*, mutations in the *PTC* gene cause segmental patterning defects;[21] hence, the derivation of the name *PATCHED*. The PTC protein binds and inhibits a transmembrane protein, SMOOTHENED (SMO) (Figure 2–5).[22] However, this inhibition can be relieved when the soluble protein SONIC HEDGEHOG (SHH) binds PTC. Inhibition of SMO signaling is apparently critical for tumor suppression (ie, SMO signaling is growth promoting) (see Figure 2–5). Consequently, changes that increase SMO signaling, such as loss of PTC[15–17,19,20] or activating mutations of SMO,[23,24] have been shown to be associated with human cancer.

TP53

The *TP53* gene encodes for a protein designated p53, which has been termed "guardian of the genome" since it responds to genotoxic insults by (1) arresting

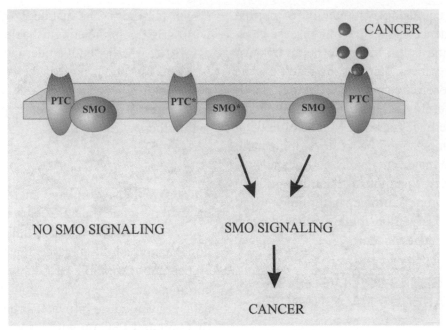

Figure 2–5. The PATCHED (PTC) and SMOOTHENED (SMO) pathways. Smoothened signaling is normally inhibited by PTC in the cell membrane. Mutations in either PTC or SMO (PTC*, SMO*) that prevent this interaction lead to increased SMO signaling and growth promotion. Alternatively, excessive SONIC HEDGEHOG (SHH) relieves the inhibition of SMO by PTC and can also induce skin cancer.

cell division to effect DNA repair or (2) inducing apoptosis when genetic damage becomes irreparable (Figure 2–6). Mutations in *TP53* have been described in BCCs although reported rates have ranged from 0 to 60 percent.[25–29] Many of the mutations are CC-to-TT or C-to-T changes at dipyrimidine sites consistent with UV damage. Differences in the reported rates may reflect technical limitations. Since BCC cell lines are not readily available, most studies rely on BCC specimens derived from clinical biopsies. Since *TP53* mutations have been frequently detected in UV-damaged premalignant keratinocytes, contaminating keratinocytes in BCC specimens may yield false-positive mutations.

RAS

Activating *RAS* mutations are among the most common genetic lesions in human cancer. Mutations in the *RAS* gene have been reported in BCCs although these events occur in less than 10 percent of BCCs.[30–33] The *RAS* proteins regulate intracellular signal transduction and are active when guanosine triphosphate (GTP) is bound. The *RAS* signal is attenuated by the hydrolysis of this GTP to guano-sine diphosphate (GDP). Mutations in *RAS* frequently alter the rate of hydrolysis, thus leading to an "activated" protein that inappropriately promotes cell growth and survival. (Discussion of the complex *RAS* signaling pathways is beyond the scope of this chapter.)[34] One class of proteins (GTPase-activating proteins, or GAP proteins) down-regulates *RAS* by increasing the hydrolysis of GTP to GDP. There is an isolated report of rare nonsense mutations of the *GAP* gene in BCCs.[35]

Genetics of Squamous Cell Carcinoma

Squamous cell carcinoma (SCC) is the second most common skin cancer after BCC. Unlike BCCs, SCCs can arise from precursor lesions called actinic keratoses (AKs). Most AKs and SCCs occur on sun-exposed sites, thus implicating UV damage as the primary source of genetic injury. There are no known well-described syndromes that specifically involve hereditary SCCs. Related epithelial tumors, such as keratoacanthomas, can occur in a familial setting (eg, Ferguson-Smith syndrome [OMIM 132800]). Xeroderma pigmentosum (XP) patients develop SCCs and will be discussed later.

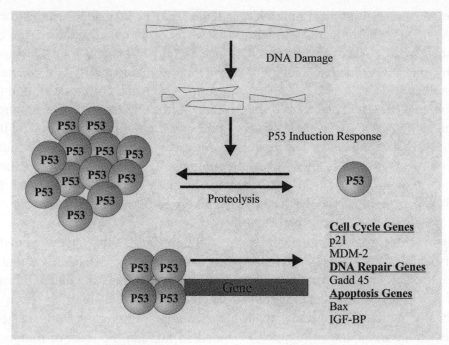

Figure 2–6. The p53 response. The normal amounts of p53 in a cell are maintained at a low level through transcriptional regulation and ongoing proteolysis. When DNA damage occurs (such as with ultraviolet or x-ray irradiation), the levels of p53 increase. The p53 tetramerizes and leads to the increased transcription of cell cycle genes, DNA repair genes, and apoptosis genes.

Genetic studies of AKs and sporadic SCCs have revealed allelic loss at chromosomes 9p, 13q, 17p, 17q, and 3p.[14,36] Except for *TP53*, which lies on chromosome 17p, the targets for mutations at the other chromosome sites are unknown.

TP53

Inactivation of the tumor suppressor gene *TP53* appears to play a pivotal role in the pathogenesis of AKs and SCCs. Brash and colleagues found that 14 of 24 (58%) invasive SCCs of the skin contain mutations in *TP53*. Many of the alterations were CC-to-TT mutations that are diagnostic of UV injury.[37,38] Other studies have also found similar mutations of *TP53*, albeit at lower rates in different series.[27,39]

How does loss of p53 lead to SCC? Two observations have helped elucidate a potential mechanism. First, p53 mutations can occur in early precancerous AKs and SCC in situ lesions.[40–42] Therefore, early inactivation of p53 contributes to later malignant degeneration, and mutations in p53 alone are not sufficient to induce neoplastic transformation. Second, in p53-deficient murine skin, UV irradiation leads to a diminished apoptotic response when compared to normal wild-type p53 murine skin. Ziegler and colleagues have thus proposed that the skin possesses a p53-dependent response to DNA damage, a response that aborts precancerous cells. If this response is abrogated in a cell by an earlier p53 mutation, UV irradiation can select for clonal expansion of the p53-mutated cell and act as both tumor initiator and promoter.[40]

Genetics of Cutaneous Melanoma

Although cutaneous melanoma (CM) is the least common of the major cutaneous malignancies, it is responsible for most deaths attributable to skin cancer. In 2000, an estimated 47,700 new cases of invasive melanoma will develop in the United States, with an estimated 7,700 deaths.[43] A familial variant of CM has long been recognized. Greene and Fraumeni estimated that 8 to 12 percent of melanomas arise in patients with a family history of the disease.[44] The recognition of atypical moles and multiple melanomas in a familial setting led to the first descriptions of a genetic cancer syndrome involving melanocytic tumors. Clark and colleagues[45] and Lynch and colleagues[46] independently described the

BK mole syndrome and familial atypical multiple-mole melanoma (FAMMM) syndrome, respectively. The knowledge of the genetic basis of CM has been greatly advanced by our recent understanding of these familial melanomas.

Familial melanoma (FM) is characterized by multiple CMs in the setting of atypical moles (see Figures 3–16, 3–17, 3–18, 4–6, and 4–7). The mode of inheritance is controversial and is most likely polygenic.

Distinguishing between atypical (or dysplastic) moles and CMs is often difficult. Clinical characteristics of atypical nevi include a larger mole (> 5 to 10 mm) with both macular and palpable components. The border and color may both be irregular although shades of blue and gray suggest possible melanoma. Occasionally, patients can present with more than 100 moles on the trunk and extremities.

In individuals with a history of FM, the cumulative risk of developing a CM has been estimated to be around 50 percent by the age of 50 years.[47,48] Familial melanoma patients tend to develop cancer at an earlier age compared to the general population[49] and have an increased relative risk of developing a second primary melanoma.[48,50]

CDKN2A

The first tumor suppressor gene isolated and shown to be significantly involved in melanoma was *CDKN2A*. In the early 1990s, two lines of investigation—deletional analyses of somatic tumors lines[51] and linkage analysis of melanoma-prone kindreds[2,52,53]—led to the localization of a melanoma tumor suppressor on 9p21. With this positional information, Kamb and colleagues[54] and Nobori and colleagues[55] refined the area of involvement on chromosome 9p21 and isolated a previously identified cell cycle regulatory gene, *CDKN2A* (previously designated *p16*). Hussussian and colleagues demonstrated germline mutations of *CDKN2A* in 92 percent of CM patients from chromosome 9p21–linked FM kindreds,[56] thus formally establishing the molecular basis of a subset of FM cases. Subsequent studies reported an overall *CDKN2A* germline mutation rate approaching 40 percent among kindreds, demonstrating linkage to chromo-

some 9p21 or stringent criteria for familial cases. However, in unlinked families, the overall germline rate is only 7 percent.[57] In Queensland, Australia, where the incidence of CM is the highest in the world, Aitken and colleagues found that only 10 percent of the highest-risk FM kindreds (those with four or more family members) and 0.2 percent of all CM cases harbored *CDKN2A* mutations.[58] These findings suggest that *CDKN2A* is involved in only a small subset of melanoma-prone kindreds and is unlikely to play a significant role on a population-wide basis.

Studies have subsequently shown that *CDKN2A* is homozygously deleted in about 50 percent of melanoma cell lines and mutated in about 15 percent of melanoma cell lines.[54,55,59–64] Fewer primary melanoma specimens have been genetically examined so far, and the rates of mutations reported for these specimens range from 2 to 33 percent.[65–69]

The *CDKN2A* locus is complex. It contains four exons that encode for two alternative transcripts (Figure 2–7); p16 is a splice product of exons 1α, 2, and 3, while p14ARF (p19ARF in mice) is the product of exons 1β, 2, and 3. The p14ARF transcript is translated in an alternative reading frame, thereby producing a second protein, p14ARF, which has no amino acid sequence homology to p16.[70] S-phase entry is dependent on the phosphorylation of the retinoblastoma (RB) protein by a cyclin-dependent protein kinase, CDK4. The p16 binds and inhibits CDK4, thus blocking cell cycle progression at G_1/S. In the absence of p16, CDK4 functions unchecked to phosphorylate RB, thus triggering increased S-phase entry; p16 is a G_1/S "brake" on the cell cycle engine. The other product of *CDKN2A*, p14/p19ARF, has been shown more recently to bind and inhibit MDM2, a protein that accelerates degradation of p53.[71,72] Without p14/p19ARF, the amount of p53 in the cell is diminished. Thus, by affecting the pRb and p53 pathways, loss of *CDKN2A* can impact both cell cycling and apoptosis.

CDK4

A second gene on the retinoblastoma pathway that has been linked to CM is *CDK4*. As described earlier, the protein kinase activity of CDK4 is responsi-

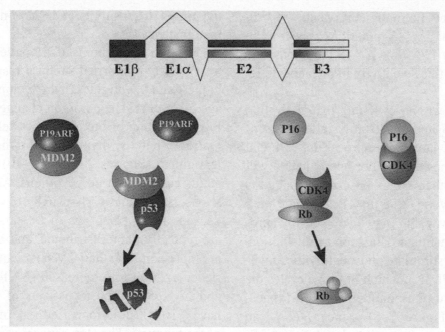

Figure 2–7. The *CDKN2A* gene and pathways (E-exon). (See text for discussion.)

ble for the ability of RB to promote cell cycle progression. Since p16 negatively regulates CDK4, any mutation that renders CDK4 resistant to p16 will produce the same functional consequence as loss of p16. Mutations in the p16-binding region of CDK4 have been found in CM. Substitutions at codons 22[73] and 24[73,74] of CDK4 have been described in sporadic and familial forms[75] of CM.

In our current understanding, the two genes known to contribute to hereditary melanoma—*CDKN2A* and *CDK4*—interact with one another both genetically and biochemically. The importance of this checkpoint in melanoma tumorigenesis (in contrast with other tumors) is still unknown.

PTEN/MMAC1

Deletions in the chromosome 10q region have been described for various tumors, including gliomas and melanomas. In 1997, several groups identified a novel tumor suppressor gene located on chromosome 10q23 variously designated as *PTEN* or *MMAC1*.[76,77] Deletions and mutations in *PTEN/MMAC1* have been described in about 30 percent of CMs.[78,79] Moreover, mutations in this gene have also been implicated in Cowden disease, a cutaneous, breast, and thyroid cancer syndrome;[80] Bannayan-Zonana syndrome, a condition defined by extensive and disparate hamar-

tomas;[81] and juvenile polyposis coli, a disorder characterized by diffuse hamartomatous polyps of the gastrointestinal tract.[82] Thus, *PTEN/MMAC1* appears to be a critical tumor suppressor involved in the development of various cancers.

The full function of the PTEN protein is still unknown. The protein shares homologies with the cytoskeletal protein, tensin, and a class of enzymes known as protein phosphatases. Protein phosphatases reverse the action of protein kinases and regulate the function of proteins by removing covalently attached phosphate groups from serine/threonine/tyrosine residues (ie, by dephosphorylation). Unlike other protein phosphatases, however, PTEN can also remove phosphate groups attached to lipid substrates. Recent studies suggest that PTEN may be involved in the cellular apoptotic response; thus, loss of *PTEN/MMAC1* may result in the failure of apoptosis in the cancerous cell.

RAS

Alterations in *RAS* have been described in primary melanomas, melanoma metastases, and cultured melanoma cell lines.[83] The frequency of mutations has reportedly ranged from approximately 5 to 30 percent. As benign moles have been shown to harbor *RAS* mutations, *RAS* mutations alone are probably insufficient to induce the malignant phenotype.[84] In cutaneous melanoma, *NRAS* mutations appear to be more common than *HRAS* or *KRAS* mutations; the molecular basis for this selectivity in melanocytes is currently unknown.

More recently, we have found that activating mutations in *NRAS* and inactivating alterations of *PTEN/MMAC1* are largely reciprocal in CM cell lines; that is, cell lines that harbor one mutation will rarely contain the other.[85] This observation suggests that *RAS* and *PTEN/MMAC1* may be epistatic on a single genetic pathway that may be universally abrogated in CM. Biochemical data support this notion, as RAS is known to stimulate phosphatidylinositol 3-phosphate kinase (PI-3K), which in turn elevates the intracellular levels of phosphatidylinositol 3-triphosphate (PIP_3)[86–88] (Figure 2–8). Since *PTEN* can dephosphorylate PIP_3 to form phosphatidylinositol 2-biphosphate (PIP_2),[89] loss of *PTEN* activity will simulate increased *RAS* activity. Elevated PIP_3 levels affect various effector molecules, including the protein kinase AKT,[90] which can phosphorylate BAD and which releases BcL-2.[91] BcL-2 can generate antiapoptotic signals that ultimately favor cell survival.

Genetics of Xeroderma Pigmentosum

Xeroderma pigmentosum (XP) is an autosomal recessive complex of disorders, characterized by intense photosensitivity and early onset of cutaneous malignancies.

The initial symptoms of XP patients include photosensitivity (abnormal sunburn response) and photodistributed lentigines, which appear around the age of 2 years. The common changes of dermatoheliosis (thinning of the epidermis, telangiectasia formation, patchy hyper/hypopigmentation, solar lentigines) (Figures 2–9 and 2–10) seen in normal adults can be seen in XP infants. Actinic keratoses, BCCs, SCCs, and CMs usually develop in the first decade, at a median age of 8 years. These cancers are typically photodistributed, and BCCs and SCCs are more common than CMs. Patients with XP experience a 2,000-fold increased risk for BCCs, SCCs, and CMs compared to patients of similar age and have a 10,000-fold increased risk of SCC on the tip of the tongue.[92] The skin cancers can be massive and disfiguring. Most patients with XP die at an earlier age because of their malignancies.

Seven genes responsible for the XP phenotype have been identified (*XPA* to *XPG*). Mutations in

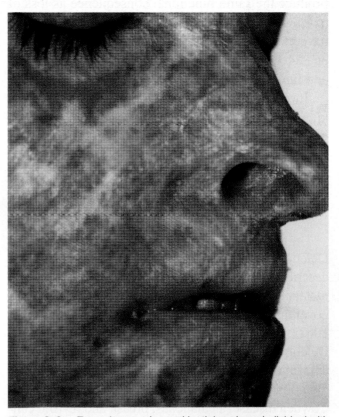

Figure 2–9.   Extensive scarring and lentigines in an individual with xeroderma pigmentosum. (Courtesy of Dr. Kenneth Kraemer, National Cancer Institute.)

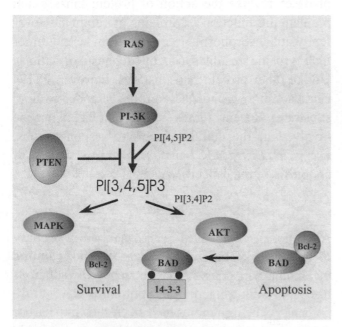

Figure 2–8.   The RAS/PTEN pathway. (See text for discussion.)

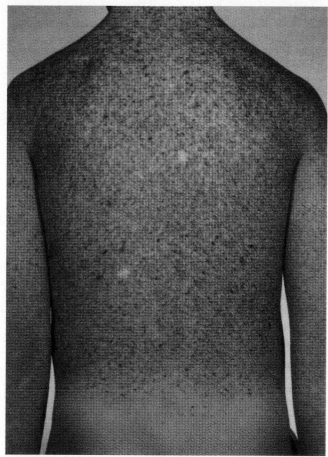

Figure 2–10. Confluent photodistributed lentigines in a xeroderma pigmentosum patient. (Courtesy of Dr. Kenneth Kraemer, National Cancer Institute.)

each gene leads to slightly different phenotypes. For instance, *XPA* mutations lead to the most severe variant, with skin cancers and frequent neurologic decay. On the other hand, *XPC* mutations are the most common and are associated with skin cancers but with rare neurologic findings.

The *XP* genes are all components of a UV-responsive DNA repair engine known as nucleotide excision repair (NER). The conservation of NER genes from yeast to humans suggests that the system is critical for the survival of all eukaryotes. Briefly, UV irradiation induces certain types of DNA damage (cyclobutane pyrimidine dimers and [6-4]pyrimidine-pyrimidone product), which, if uncorrected, can propagate and lead to carcinogenic mutations. The various *XP* genes encode for proteins that recognize injured DNA (XPA and XPE), unwind the coiled DNA structure to expose the lesion (XPB and XPD), and repair the damaged DNA strand (XPF and XPG).

Since these NER proteins function as genomic caretakers, the formation of tumors in XP results from the mutagenic inactivation of tumor suppressors and the activation of oncogenes. The actual genes targeted for mutations are largely unknown although some studies have shown that two of these targets include *TP53*[93,94] and *RAS.*[95]

CONCLUSION

The skin is a unique organ for studying the interaction between environmental carcinogenesis and hereditary cancer susceptibility. Ultraviolet signature mutations have been detected in *CDKN2A, CDK4,* and *TP53*, suggesting that excessive sun exposure is mechanistically involved in the formation of certain skin cancers such as cutaneous melanoma, basal cell carcinomas, and squamous cell carcinomas. Furthermore, when the machinery for mutation repair is itself genetically abrogated, such as in xeroderma pigmentosum, these skin cancers form at a greatly exaggerated rate. An understanding of the molecular events underlying early neoplastic transformation in the skin may lead to more effective chemoprevention.

REFERENCES

1. Knudson A. Mutation and cancer: a statistical study. Proc Natl Acad Sci U S A 1971;68:820–3.
2. Cannon-Albright LA, Goldgar DE, Meyer LJ, et al. Assignment of a locus for familial melanoma, MLM, to chromosome 9p13-p22. Science 1992; 258:1148–52.
3. Vogelstein B, Kinzler KW. The genetic basis of human cancer. New York: McGraw Hill; 1998.
4. Strachan T, Read AP. Human molecular genetics. Oxford (UK): BIOS Scientific Publishers; 1996.
5. Shanley S, Ratcliffe J, Hockey A, et al. Nevoid basal cell carcinoma syndrome: review of 118 affected individuals. Am J Hum Genet 1994;50:282–90.
6. Kimonis VE, Goldstein AM, Pastakia B, et al. Clinical manifestations in 105 persons with nevoid basal cell carcinoma syndrome. Am J Hum Genet 1997;69: 299–308.
7. Gorlin RJ. Nevoid basal cell carcinoma syndrome. Medicine 1987;66:98–110.
8. Wicking C, Berkman J, Wainwright B, et al. Fine genetic mapping of the gene for nevoid basal cell carcinoma syndrome. Genomics 1994;22:505–11.

9. Gailani MR, Bale SJ, Leffell DJ, et al. Developmental defects in Gorlin syndrome related to a putative tumor suppressor gene on chromosome 9. Cell 1992;69:111–7.

10. Farndon PA, Del Mastro RG, Evans DG, et al. Location of gene for Gorlin syndrome. Lancet 1992;339: 581–2.

11. Reis A, Kuster W, Linss G, et al. Localisation of gene for the naevoid basal-cell carcinoma syndrome. Lancet 1992;339:617.

12. Goldstein AM, Stewart C, Bale AE, et al. Localization of the gene for the nevoid basal cell carcinoma syndrome. Am J Hum Genet 1994;54:765–73.

13. Quinn AG, Sikkink S, Rees JL. Delineation of two distinct deleted regions on chromosome 9 in human non-melanoma skin cancers. Genes Chromosomes Cancer 1994;11:222–5.

14. Quinn AG, Sikkink S, Rees JL. Basal cell carcinomas and squamous cell carcinomas of human skin show distinct patterns of chromosome loss. Cancer Res 1994;54:4756–9.

15. Johnson RL, Rothman AL, Xie J, et al. Human homolog of patched, a candidate gene for the basal cell nevus syndrome. Science 1996;272:1668–71.

16. Hahn H, Wicking C, Zaphiropoulous PG, et al. Mutations of the human homolog of *Drosophila* patched in the nevoid basal cell carcinoma syndrome. Cell 1996;85:841–51.

17. Aszterbaum M, Rothman A, Johnson RL, et al. Identification of mutations in the human PATCHED gene in sporadic basal cell carcinomas and in patients with the basal cell nevus syndrome. J Invest Dermatol 1998;110:885–8.

18. Wicking C, Shanley S, Smyth I, et al. Most germ-line mutations in the nevoid basal cell carcinoma syndrome lead to a premature termination of the PATCHED protein, and no genotype-phenotype correlations are evident. Am J Hum Genet 1997;60: 21–6.

19. Xie J, Johnson RL, Zhang X, et al. Mutations of the PATCHED gene in several types of sporadic extracutaneous tumors. Cancer Res 1997;57:2369–72.

20. Raffel C, Jenkins RB, Frederick L, et al. Sporadic medulloblastomas contain PTCH mutations. Cancer Res 1997;57:842–5.

21. Hooper JE, Scott MP. The *Drosophila* patched gene encodes a putative membrane protein required for segmental patterning. Cell 1989;59:751–65.

22. Stone DM, Hynes M, Armanini M, et al. The tumor-suppressor gene patched encodes a candidate receptor for sonic hedgehog. Nature 1996 Nov 14;384: 129–34.

23. Xie J, Murone M, Luoh SM, et al. Activating smoothened mutations in sporadic basal-cell carcinoma. Nature 1998;391:90–2.

24. Reifenberger J, Wolter M, Weber RG, et al. Missense mutations in SMOH in sporadic basal cell carcinomas of the skin and primitive neuroectodermal tumors of the central nervous system. Cancer Res 1998;58:1798–803.

25. Rady P, Scinicariello F, Wagner RF Jr, et al. p53 mutations in basal cell carcinomas. Cancer Res 1992;52: 3804–6.

26. Shea CR, McNutt NS, Volkenandt M, et al. Overexpression of p53 protein in basal cell carcinomas of human skin. Am J Pathol 1992;141:25–9.

27. Moles JP, Moyret C, Guillot B, et al. p53 gene mutations in human epithelial skin cancers. Oncogene 1993;8:583–8.

28. Konishi K, Yamanishi K, Ishizaki K, et al. Analysis of p53 gene mutations and loss of heterozygosity for loci on chromosome 9q in basal cell carcinoma. Cancer Lett 1994;79:67–72.

29. Ziegler A, Leffell DJ, Kunala S, et al. Mutation hotspots due to sunlight in the p53 gene of non-melanoma skin cancers. Proc Natl Acad Sci U S A 1993;90:4216–20.

30. van der Schroeff JG, Evers LM, Boot AJ, et al. Ras oncogene mutations in basal cell carcinomas and squamous cell carcinomas of human skin. J Invest Dermatol 1990;94:423–5.

31. Lieu FM, Yamanishi K, Konishi K, et al. Low incidence of Ha-ras oncogene mutations in human epidermal tumors. Cancer Lett 1991;59:231–5.

32. Campbell C, Quinn AG, Rees JL. Codon 12 Harvey-ras mutations are rare events in nonmelanoma human skin cancer. Br J Dermatol 1993;128:111–4.

33. Wilke WW, Robinson RA, Kennard CD. H-ras-1 gene mutations in basal cell carcinoma: automated direct sequencing of clinical specimens. Mod Pathol 1993; 6:15–9.

34. Campbell SL, Khosravi-Far R, Rossman KL, et al. Increasing complexity of ras signaling. Oncogene 1998;17:1395–413.

35. Friedman E, Gejman PV, Martin GA, et al. Nonsense mutations in the C-terminal SH2 region of the GTPase activating protein (GAP) gene in human tumours. Nat Genet 1993;5:242–7.

36. Rehman I, Takata M, Wu YY, et al. Genetic change in actinic keratoses. Oncogene 1996;12:2483–90.

37. Brash DE, Rudolph JA, Simon JA, et al. A role for sunlight in skin cancer: UV-induced p53 mutations in squamous cell carcinoma. Proc Natl Acad Sci U S A 1991;88:10124–8.

38. Dumaz N, Stary A, Soussi T, et al. Can we predict solar ultraviolet radiation as the causal event in human tumours by analysing the mutation spectra of the p53 gene? Mutat Res 1994;307:375–86.

39. Kubo Y, Urano Y, Yoshimoto K, et al. p53 gene mutations in human skin cancers and precancerous

lesions: comparison with immunohistochemical analysis. J Invest Dermatol 1994;102:440–4.

40. Ziegler A, Jonason AS, Leffell DJ, et al. Sunburn and p53 in the onset of skin cancer. Nature 1994;372: 773–6.

41. Taguchi M, Watanabe S, Yashima K, et al. Aberrations of the tumor suppressor p53 gene and p53 protein in solar keratosis in human skin. J Invest Dermatol 1994;103:500–3.

42. Campbell C, Quinn AG, Ro YS, et al. p53 mutations are common and early events that precede tumor invasion in squamous cell neoplasia of the skin. J Invest Dermatol 1993;100:746–8.

43. Greenlee RT, Murray T, Bolden S, et al. Cancer statistics, 2000. CA Cancer J Clin 2000;50:7–33.

44. Greene MH, Fraumeni JF Jr. The hereditary variant of malignant melanoma. In: Clark WH Jr, Goldman LI, Mastrangelo MJ, editors. Human malignant melanoma. New York: Grune Stratton; 1979: p. 139–66.

45. Clark WH Jr, Reimer RR, Green M, et al. Origin of familial malignant melanoma from heritable melanocytic lesions: the B-K mole syndrome. Arch Dermatol 1978;114:723–8.

46. Lynch HT, Frichot BC III, Lynch JF. Familial atypical multiple mole-melanoma syndrome. J Med Genet 1978;15:352–6.

47. Tucker MA, Fraser MC, Goldstein AM, et al. Risk of melanoma and other cancers in melanoma-prone families. J Invest Dermatol 1993;100:350S–5S.

48. Greene MH, Clark WHJ, Tucker MA, et al. High risk of malignant melanoma in melanoma-prone families with dysplastic nevi. Ann Intern Med 1985;102: 458–65.

49. Goldstein AM, Fraser MC, Clark WHJ, et al. Age at diagnosis and transmission of invasive melanoma in 23 families with cutaneous malignant melanoma/ dysplastic nevi. J Natl Cancer Inst 1994;86:1385–90.

50. Carey WPJ, Thompson CJ, Synnestvedt M, et al. Dysplastic nevi as a melanoma risk factor in patients with familial melanoma. Cancer 1994;74:3118–25.

51. Fountain JW, Karayiorgou M, Ernstoff MS, et al. Homozygous deletions within human chromosome band 9p21 in melanoma. Proc Natl Acad Sci U S A 1992;89:10557–61.

52. Nancarrow DJ, Mann GJ, Holland EA, et al. Confirmation of chromosome 9p linkage in familial melanoma. Am J Hum Genet 1993;53:936–42.

53. Gruis NA, Sandkuijl LA, Weber JL. Linkage analysis in Dutch familial atypical multiple mole-melanoma (FAMMM) syndrome families. Effect of nevus count. Melanoma Res 1993;3:271–7.

54. Kamb A, Gruis N, Weaver-Feldhaus J, et al. A cell cycle regulator potentially involved in genesis of many tumor types. Science 1994;264:436–40.

55. Nobori T, Miura K, Wu DJ, et al. Deletions of the cyclin-dependent kinase-4 inhibitor gene in multiple human cancers. Nature 1994;368:753–6.

56. Hussussian CJ, Struewing JP, Goldstein AM, et al. Germline p16 mutations in familial melanoma. Nat Genet 1994;8:15–21.

57. Haluska FG, Hodi FS. Molecular genetics of familial cutaneous melanoma. J Clin Oncol 1998;16:670–82.

58. Aitken J, Welch J, Duffy D, et al. CDKN2A variants in a population-based sample of Queensland families with melanoma. J Natl Cancer Inst 1999;91:446–52.

59. Pollock PM, Yu F, Qiu L, et al. Evidence for u.v. induction of CDKN2 mutations in melanoma cell lines. Oncogene 1995;11:663–8.

60. Bartkova J, Lukas J, Guldberg P, et al. The p16-cyclin D/Cdk4-pRb pathway as a functional unit frequently altered in melanoma pathogenesis. Cancer Res 1996;56:5475–83.

61. Flores JF, Walker GJ, Glendening JM, et al. Loss of the $p16^{INK4a}$ and $p15^{INK4b}$ genes, as well as neighboring 9p21 markers, in sporadic melanoma. Cancer Res 1996;56:5023–32.

62. Luca M, Xie S, Gutman M, et al. Abnormalities in the CDKN2 ($p16^{INK4}$/MTS-1) gene in human melanoma cells: relevance to tumor growth and metastasis. Oncogene 1995;11:1399–1402.

63. Maelandsmo GM, Florenes VA, Hovig E, et al. Involvement of the pRb/p16/cdk4/cyclinD1 pathway in the tumorigenesis of sporadic malignant melanomas. Br J Cancer 1996;73:909–16.

64. Castellano M, Pollock PM, Walters MK, et al. CDKN2A/p16 is inactivated in most melanoma cell lines. Cancer Res 1997;57:4868–75.

65. Gruis NA, Weaver-Feldhaus J, Liu Q, et al. Genetic evidence in melanoma and bladder cancers that p16 and p53 function in separate pathways of tumor suppression. Am J Pathol 1995;146:1199–1207.

66. Healy E, Sikkink S, Rees JL. Infrequent mutation of $p16^{INK4}$ in sporadic melanoma. J Invest Dermatol 1996;107:318–21.

67. Piccinin S, Doglioni C, Maestro R, et al. p16/CDKN2 and CDK4 gene mutations in sporadic melanoma development and progression. Int J Cancer 1997;74:26–30.

68. Kumar R, Rozell BL, Louhelainen J, et al. Mutations in the CDKN2A (p16ink4a) gene in microdissected sporadic primary melanoma. Int J Cancer 1998;75: 193–8.

69. Ruiz A, Puig S, Lynch M, et al. Retention of the CDKN2A locus and low frequency of point mutations in primary and metastatic cutaneous malignant melanoma. Int J Cancer 1998;76:312–6.

70. Liggett WHJ, Sidransky D. Role of the p16 tumor suppressor gene in cancer. J Clin Oncol 1998;16: 1197–1206.

71. Zhang Y, Xiong Y, Yarbrough WG. ARF promotes MDM2 degradation and stabilizes p53: ARF-INK4a locus deletion impairs both the Rb and p53 tumor suppression pathways. Cell 1998;92:725–34.

72. Pomerantz J, Schreiber-Agus N, Liegeois NJ, et al. The Ink4a tumor suppressor gene product, p19Arf, interacts with MDM2 and neutralizes MDM2's inhibition of p53. Cell 1998;92:713–23.

73. Tsao H, Benoit E, Sober AJ, et al. Novel mutations in the p16/CDKN2A binding region of the cyclin-dependent kinase-4 (CDK4) gene. Cancer Res 1997;58:109–13.

74. Wolfel T, Hauer M, Schneider J, et al. A p16^{INK4a}-insensitive CDK4 mutant targeted by cytolytic T lymphocytes in a human melanoma. Science 1995;269: 1281–4.

75. Zuo L, Weger J, Yang Q, et al. Germline mutations in the p16^{INK4a} binding domain of CDK4 in familial melanoma. Nat Genet 1996;12:97–9.

76. Li J, Yen C, Liaw D, et al. PTEN, a putative tyrosine phosphatase gene mutated in human brain, breast and prostate cancer. Science 1997;275:1943–7.

77. Steck PA, Pershouse MA, Jasser SA, et al. Identification of a candidate tumour suppressor gene, MMAC1, at chromosome 10q23.3 that is mutated in multiple advanced cancers. Nat Genet 1997;15:356–62.

78. Guldberg P, Thor Straten P, Birck A, et al. Disruption of the MMAC1/PTEN gene by deletion or mutation is a frequent even in malignant melanoma. Cancer Res 1997;57:3660–3.

79. Tsao H, Zhang X, Benoit E, et al. Identification of PTEN/MMAC1 alterations in uncultured melanomas and melanoma cell lines. Oncogene 1998;16: 3397–402.

80. Liaw D, Marsh DJ, Li J, et al. Germline mutations of the PTEN gene in Cowden disease, an inherited breast and thyroid cancer syndrome. Nat Genet 1997;16:64–7.

81. Marsh DJ, Dahia LM, Zheng Z, et al. Germline mutations in PTEN are present in Bannayan-Zonana syndrome. Nat Genet 1997;16:333–4.

82. Olschwang S, Serova-Sinilnikova OM, Lenoir GM, et al. PTEN germ-line mutations in juvenile polyposis coli. Nat Genet 1998;18:12–4.

83. Herlyn M, Satyamoorthy K. Activated ras: yet another player in melanoma? Am J Pathol 1996;149:739–44.

84. Carr J, Mackie RM. Point mutations in the N-ras oncogene in malignant melanoma and congenital naevi. Br J Dermatol 1994;131:72–7.

85. Tsao H, Zhang X, Fowlkes K, et al. Relative reciprocity of NRAS and PTEN/MMAC1 alterations in cutaneous melanoma cell lines. Cancer Res 2000; 60:1800–4.

86. Kodaki T, Woscholski R, Hallberg B, et al. The activation of phosphatidylinositol 3-kinase by Ras. Curr Biol 1994;4:798–806.

87. Downward J, de Gunzburg J, Riehl R, et al. p21 ras-induced responsiveness of phosphatidylinositol turnover to bradykinin is a receptor number effect. Proc Natl Acad Sci U S A 1988;85:5774–8.

88. Downward J. Role of phosphoinositide-3-OH kinase in ras signaling. Adv Second Messenger Phosphoprotein Res 1997;31:1–10.

89. Maehama T, Dixon JE. The tumor suppressor, PTEN/MMAC1, dephosphorylates the lipid second messenger, phosphatidylinositol 3,4,5-triphosphate. J Biol Chem 1998;273:13375–8.

90. Franke TF, Kaplan DR, Cantley LC, et al. Direct regulation of the akt proto-oncogene product by phosphatidylinositol-3,4-bisphosphate. Science 1997; 275:665–8.

91. del Peso L, Gonzalez-Garcia M, Page C, et al. Interleukin-3-induced phosphorylation of BAD through the protein kinase akt. Science 1997;278:687–9.

92. Bootsma D, Kraemer KH, Cleaver JE, et al. Nucleotide excision repair syndromes: xeroderma pigmentosum, Cockayne syndrome, and trichothiodystrophy. In: Vogelstein BV, Kinzler K, editors. The genetic basis of human cancer. New York: McGraw-Hill; 1998. p. 245–74.

93. Williams C, Ponten F, Ahmadian A, et al. Clones of normal keratinocytes and a variety of simultaneously present epidermal neoplastic lesions contain a multitude of p53 gene mutations in a xeroderma pigmentosum patient. Cancer Res 1998;58:2449–55.

94. Giglia G, Dumaz N, Drougard C, et al. p53 mutations in skin and internal tumors of xeroderma pigmentosum patients belonging to the complementation group C. Cancer Res 1998;58:4402–9.

95. Daya-Grosjean L, Robert C, Drougard C, et al. High mutation frequency in ras genes of skin tumors isolated from DNA repair deficient xeroderma pigmentosum patients. Cancer Res 1993;53:1625–9.

3

Risk Assessment

DANA SACHS, MD
ASHFAQ A. MARGHOOB, MD
ALLAN C. HALPERN, MD

The early detection of cancers of the skin can significantly decrease morbidity, mortality, and cost associated with treating advanced disease.[1] Identifying individuals at high risk for developing skin cancer can help clinicians focus screening and educational efforts to prevent skin cancer and to detect cancers at a curable stage. This chapter reviews the risk factors for the development of skin cancer. Emphasis is placed on the risk factors that can be elucidated from a routine history and physical examination.

There are a few rare genetic syndromes that increase an individual's risk for developing skin cancer (Table 3–1). Given the rarity of these syndromes, they will not be discussed in this chapter. However, the identification of these syndromes has helped researchers locate genes that (when mutated or disregulated) can result in skin cancer. The recognition of the roles of the patched gene in basal cell nevus syndrome, *p53* mutations in squamous cell carcinoma, and *p16* or *CDKN2A* (cyclin-dependent kinase) mutations in melanoma raises the possibility of genetic testing as a risk assessment tool for the future. In particular, more recent understanding of the deletions or mutations of the p16 gene in melanoma cell lines suggests that opportunities exist for future genetic screening in families prone to melanoma.[2]

This chapter is designed to assist the practitioner in recognizing the known major skin cancer risk factors. This knowledge can help identify individuals that would benefit most from skin cancer screening and prevention efforts (Table 3–2).

PATIENT HISTORY: HELPING TO IDENTIFY RISK FACTORS

Age

The incidence of skin cancer increases with age.[3–7] The passage of time may provide more opportunities for the initiation and promotion of cutaneous tumors. In addition, immune surveillance is decreased in older individuals. Aging is associated with a decreased ability to repair deoxyribonucleic acid (DNA).[8,9] This decreased ability to repair DNA may lead to the incorporation of mutations into the cellular DNA, ultimately rendering a skin cell malignant.[8]

Despite the high incidence and prevalence of skin cancer in elderly people, an increasing number of younger people are developing cancers of the skin.[10,11] In fact, melanoma is the leading cause of years of potential life lost due to cancer.[12]

Sun Exposure and Skin Type

Ultraviolet radiation from the sun is the most important environmental exposure known to cause skin cancer.[13,14] The evidence linking skin cancer and sun

Table 3–1. GENETIC SYNDROMES WITH INCREASED RISK OF SKIN CANCERS

Xeroderma pigmentosum
Nevoid basal cell carcinoma syndrome
Epidermolysis bullosa
Epidermodysplasia verruciformis
Dyskeratosis congenita
Familial melanoma (familial multiple mole and melanoma [FAMMM])

Table 3–2. RELATIVE RISK ASSESSMENT			
Assessment	MM	BCC	SCC
Patient History			
Age	inc	inc	inc
Sun exposure			
Intermittent (recreational)	2–3	1.7–5.0	inc
Constant (occupational)	0.25–5.00	1.4	inc
Childhood	3.3	2.8–3.9	inc
Adulthood	2.5	inc	inc
Sunburn	1.4–4.6	1.7–2.4	1.5
Skin type I	1–5	2–3	2
PUVA therapy	1–5	4–5	8.6–100.0
Tanning lamp exposure	1.0–7.7	NA	NA
Geography	inc	1.5	1.8–2.4
History of prior skin cancer	3–17	2.8	inc
Family history of skin cancer	8	6.7	inc
Socioeconomic status	1.3–1.6	NA	NA
Immunosuppression	2–8	1.4–10.0	5–250
Chemical carcinogen exposure	NA	4.6	2.8–3.9
X-ray therapy	NA	3–4	3–4
Physical examination			
Pigmentary characteristics			
Light hair	2–10	2–9	1.6–12.5
Light eyes	2–3	1.6–1.9	1.8
Fair complexion	2–18	inc	inc
Freckles	3–20	1.7–2.9	1.7–2.9
Melanocytic nevi			
Congenital melanocytic nevi	5–15	NA	NA
Number of nevi (common)	2–64	1.6–1.7	NA
Atypical (dysplastic) nevi	2–1269	NA	NA
Nevus sebaceous	NA	5–20	NA
Ulcers and scars	NA	NA	inc

BCC = basal cell carcinoma; increased risk but absolute relative risk not known; MM = malignant melanoma; NA= no answer or not applicable; PUVA = psoralen plus ultraviolet A; SCC = squamous cell carcinoma.

exposure is derived from clinical, epidemiologic, and basic science studies.[7,14,15] Skin cancer may develop if a cell is rendered unable to repair sun-induced DNA damage, as is seen in the rare genetic disorder xeroderma pigmentosum. Patients with this disorder develop multiple basal cell carcinomas, squamous cell carcinomas, and all melanomas at a young age.

Even though sun exposure has been determined to be a significant environmental factor contributing to skin cancer, it is often difficult to obtain histories that accurately measure the amount of ultraviolet exposure an individual has had in the course of his or her life. Furthermore, specifics such as intensity, duration, action spectrum, and frequency of ultraviolet exposure leading to the development of skin cancer have not been fully elucidated. The type of sun exposure, whether it is intermittent or chronic, and the age when sun exposure occurs appear to influence the development of skin cancer.

Most melanomas are believed to be related to ultraviolet exposure.[14,16,17] Intermittent sun exposure (ie, bursts of high-intensity ultraviolet exposure as received during recreational and vacation activities) has consistently been linked to melanoma, with a relative risk of approximately 3.[13,18–21] In contrast, occupational or chronic exposure to the sun has been determined to have a more varied pattern with regard to melanoma risk.[17,21] Some studies have shown an increased risk of melanoma[22] whereas others have shown occupational exposure to confer a protective effect against melanoma, especially in those who tan well.[20,23–25]

Sun exposure during childhood is another important risk factor for developing melanoma. Migrant studies demonstrate that individuals who spent their childhood in sunny locations have an increased risk for melanoma.[26–29] One large migration study compared melanoma rates between those born in Australia and those who immigrated to Australia and found that migration before the age of 15 years was associated with an increased risk for melanoma. In contrast, emigration after age 15 was associated with a decreased risk of melanoma.[27] Furthermore, epidemiologic studies addressing the association between childhood sunburn and melanoma support childhood sun exposure as a risk factor with a relative risk of 2.[25]

Fitzpatrick skin types describe an individual's propensity to burn and tan in response to ultraviolet sun exposure (Table 3–3). Patients with a propensity to sunburn and an inability to tan (type I) have the greatest risk for developing melanoma. Blistering or peeling sunburns, painful sunburns, and sunburns in childhood are all risk factors for melanoma, carrying a relative risk of 1.40 to 4.60.[21,30,31]

In addition to the link between ultraviolet exposure and melanoma, sun exposure is also an important environmental risk factor for the development of nonmelanoma skin cancer[18,19] (Figure 3–1). Both basal cell carcinoma (BCC) and squamous cell carcinoma (SCC) have a propensity to arise on sun-exposed skin and occur most commonly in light-skinned individuals (types I and II).

Evidence suggests that cumulative and chronic sun exposure is more important in the pathogenesis of SCC than in that of BCC.[32,33] Actinic keratoses, also known as solar keratoses, have been linked to chronic ultraviolet (UV) exposure. They are the most common precursor lesions for nonmelanoma skin cancer.[34] Clinically, they are rough red scaly papules on sun-exposed skin. Their prevalence is known to increase with age, and they are seen more commonly in men than in women (Figure 3–2).

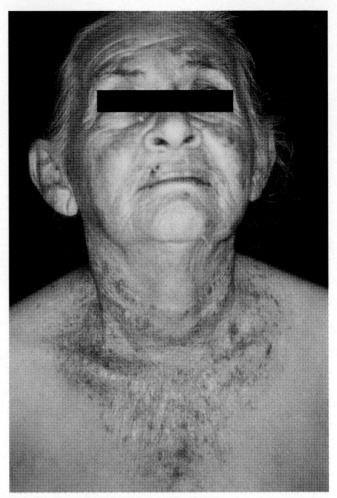

Figure 3–1.   Multiple actinic keratoses and squamous cell carcinomas in a patient with chronic sun exposure.

Table 3–3. CLASSIFICATION OF SKIN TYPE		
Type	Description	Population Affected
I	Always burn; never tan	White (Celtic)
II	Always burn; usually tan	White
III	Burn sometimes; always tan	White
IV	Rarely burn; always tan	White
V	Sunburn and tan after extreme UV exposure	Dark-skinned (Latino, etc.)
VI	Sunburn and tan after extreme UV exposure	Black

UV = ultraviolet.
Adapted from Coopman et al. Photodamage and photoaging in: Arndt, LeBoit, Robinson, Wintroub, editors. Cutaneous medicine and surgery: an integrated program in dermatology. Philadelphia: WB Saunders Co.; 1996. p. 739.

In contrast, basal cell carcinoma appears to be linked to intermittent sun exposure[14] (Figure 3–3). The associations of SCC with chronic UV exposure and BCC with intermittent UV exposure are further suggested by the temporal, geographic, and anatomic patterns of these tumors.[35] Furthermore, evidence suggests that BCC, but not SCC, may be related to sunburn incurred in childhood.[33] Therefore, intermittent UV exposure is a risk factor shared by both BCC and melanoma.[30]

The action spectrum of UV light resulting in the development of BCC, SCC, and melanoma has not been clarified. It had long been believed that ultraviolet B (UVB) radiation was the main trigger for all three skin cancers. However, recent evidence indicates that ultraviolet A (UVA) radiation may play an important role in the development of some of these malignancies.[36,37]

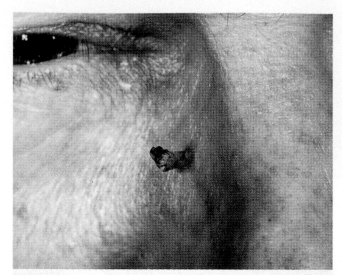

Figure 3–2. Five variants of actinic keratosis have been described: erythematous, keratotic papular, verrucous, pigmented, and cutaneous horn. The patient shown has a cutaneous horn.

Psoralen plus Ultraviolet A Radiation Therapy

Psoralen followed by exposure to UVA radiation, a combination known as PUVA, is a therapeutic modality used to treat a variety of dermatoses such as psoriasis, atopic dermatitis, and mycosis fungoides. Many studies have documented a link between the therapeutic use of PUVA and the subsequent development of cutaneous malignancies. It is well documented that PUVA increases the risk for

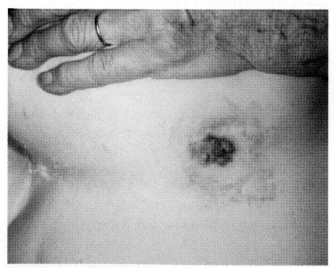

Figure 3–3. Superficial basal cell carcinoma arising in a site that is more likely to receive intermittent sun exposure than chronic sun exposure.

developing squamous cell carcinoma.[38,39] An increase in the number of SCC was noted at 2 years in PUVA-treated patients as compared to the general population, and at 10 years of follow-up, there was a 10-fold increase in the incidence of squamous cell carcinoma. They showed a PUVA-related dose-dependent increase in squamous cell carcinomas.[40] In addition to this study, meta-analysis of nine studies found the incidence of SCC in patients exposed to high-dose PUVA to be 14-fold higher than in patients exposed to low-dose PUVA. High-dose PUVA was defined as more than 200 treatments or as doses greater than 1,000 J/cm^2, depending on the study.[39]

The evidence linking PUVA to BCC and to melanoma is less clear. Psoralen plus UVA has been shown to increase the number of BCCs in patients who receive more than 250 PUVA treatments,[41] but conclusive evidence linking PUVA to BCC is lacking.[42]

More significant, one recent study showed that patients treated with PUVA had more than a fivefold increased risk for developing melanoma. (It should be noted that one patient had three of the reported melanomas.[43]) However, Swedish follow-up studies with PUVA failed to corroborate this increased risk for developing melanoma.[44,45]

Tanning Lamp Exposure

As stated above, UV exposure is a known risk factor for the development of cutaneous malignancies. The use of tanning lamps that emit UVA, UVB, or both UVA and UVB radiation are becoming increasingly popular, especially among young persons. In fact, approximately 25 million Americans use sunbeds each year.[46] Hence, it is reasonable to question whether tanning lamps contribute to skin cancer. Some data exist suggesting that exposure to tanning lamps is a risk factor for developing skin cancer. However, people who use tanning lamps often have other confounding variables, such as high-risk behavior with regard to sun exposure, lighter skin, and higher socioeconomic status.[46,47] A recent Swedish case-control study found an elevated odds ratio of 1.8 for developing melanoma after regular sunbed use of up to 250 exposures. After 250 exposures, however, the odds ratio of developing melanoma was not significant.[48]

Geographic Factors

Researchers and epidemiologists have observed that Caucasian individuals living closer to the equator have a greater risk for skin cancer compared to Caucasians living at higher latitudes. However, this is not always consistent, as evidenced by higher rates of melanoma in Scandinavia compared to the Mediterranean countries. The explanation for this difference is most likely the confounding issue of skin phototype and the fact that northern Europeans frequently vacation in southern climates. [25]

In addition to latitude, the thinning stratospheric ozone layer may play a role in risk assessment. This thinning is believed to be caused by increased chlorofluorocarbons in the environment. Ozone, formed in the stratosphere, prevents 100 percent of ultraviolet C (UVC) and 85 percent of UVB radiation from reaching Earth's surface. On the other hand, UVA is not blocked by the ozone layer; this accounts for the fact that 90 to 95 percent of solar radiation reaching the surface of Earth is UVA.

It is estimated that a 5 percent decrease in the ozone layer will increase the incidence of melanoma by 5 to 8 percent, that of basal cell carcinoma by 10 percent, and that of squamous cell carcinoma by 20 percent.[49] The Environmental Protection Agency (EPA) estimated that a 1 percent decrease in ozone will lead to a 4 to 6 percent increase in the lifetime incidence of BCC and SCC.[50] However, because ozone depletion is a relatively recent event, it is unlikely to explain the epidemic in skin cancer that we are currently witnessing. Since many skin cancers have a latency period of 5 to over 15 years, it will be another 10 to 15 years before the effects of ozone depletion are seen.

History of Prior Skin Cancer

Patients with a history of melanoma are at risk for developing multiple additional primary melanomas.[51] The incidence of multiple primary melanoma has been reported to be between 2 and 17 percent, and because of heightened screening in these individuals, their subsequent melanomas are significantly thinner in Breslow depth than their first melanomas.[51,52] In addition, a prior history of BCC and/or SCC is also associated with a higher risk of developing

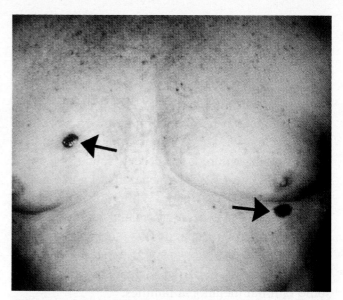

Figure 3–4. This patient has a melanoma in situ (left chest) and a basal cell carcinoma (right chest). Patients with skin cancer are often at risk for developing multiple skin cancer.

melanoma, with a relative risk ranging from 2.8 to 17[53–55] (Figure 3–4).

Patients with a history of BCC or SCC are also at increased risk for developing additional primary nonmelanoma skin cancers.[56] In fact, approximately 50 percent of patients with BCC or SCC will develop another new skin cancer within 5 years[56–58] (Figure 3–5).

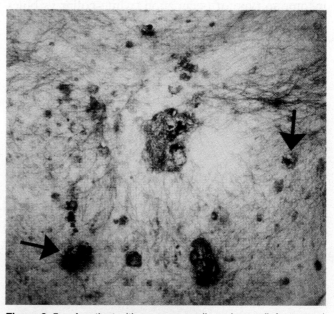

Figure 3–5. A patient with squamous cell carcinoma (left sternum) and basal cell carcinoma (right chest).

Family History of Skin Cancer

A family history of melanoma in a first-degree relative (parent, grandparent, sibling, child, aunt, or uncle) is a significant risk factor for melanoma, with a relative risk of 2.50 to 5.00.[54,59,60] A family history of melanoma can be elicited in approximately 1 of 10 melanoma patients.[61] Approximately 20 percent of melanoma kindreds have been found to have a mutation of the *CDKN2A* gene, also known as the *p16* tumor suppressor gene. While no specific phenotypic traits have been associated with *CDKN2A* mutations, there are shared traits (such as dysplastic nevi, fair skin, and sun sensitivity) that may account for some of the increased melanoma risk seen in some familial melanoma families.[62–64]

Family history is also a risk factor for BCC and SCC.[65,66] A family history of nonmelanoma skin cancer was associated with a significantly increased risk of BCC in an Italian case-control study (an odds ratio of 6.7)[67] and in a Swedish study (a relative risk of 11).[65] One study that reviewed risk factors for multiple BCCs found that the two most significant risk factors were a family history of BCC and sunburn after 60 years of age[65] (Figure 3–6).

Occupation and Socioeconomic Status

Socioeconomic status has been studied under different definitions that range from educational to income to type of occupation (white-collar vs blue-collar). The incidence of melanoma appears to be higher among the upper socioeconomic classes.[68–70]

Interestingly, the Surveillance, Epidemiology, and End Results (SEER) database revealed that a high school degree was associated with a higher incidence of melanoma but that the income of an individual was not.[71] Furthermore, a case-control study that examined American Cancer Society data demonstrated that melanoma risk was higher for those in higher-paying versus lower-paying occupations and for those in white-collar versus blue-collar occupations. The relative risks for these groups were 1.58 and 1.33, respectively.[72]

There are several hypotheses that attempt to explain why individuals in higher socioeconomic classes are at greatest risk for melanoma. White-collar workers and individuals with higher-paying jobs may travel more frequently to sunny climates, thereby increasing their exposure to intermittent bursts of intense UV light and increasing the incidence of sunburn, both known risk factors for melanoma.[14] Furthermore, individuals with higher education levels may have a greater awareness of health-related issues, which may facilitate improved skin cancer detection.

Socioeconomic status data is less clear-cut for nonmelanoma skin cancer. In general, occupational exposure to sunlight is thought to be an important cause of SCC and some BCCs.[73] A prospective study by Robinson and colleagues stated that both BCC and SCC were more common in the lower socioeconomic strata.[74]

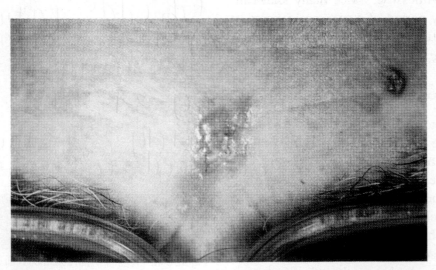

Figure 3–6.   Two basal cell carcinomas on the forehead of an elderly patient.

Immunosuppression

Basal cell carcinoma and squamous cell carcinoma frequently occur in patients who have received solid organ transplants. In contrast to the general population, organ transplant recipients develop more SCCs than BCCs. Furthermore, the immunosuppressed patients tend to develop multiple primary skin cancers, many of which behave in a more aggressive manner than they do in the nonimmunosuppressed population.[75,76] The high rates of skin cancer in immunosuppressed patients underscores the importance of immune surveillance for preventing the development of skin cancers in response to sun exposure and human papillomavirus infections.[77]

The nature of immunosuppressive therapy may affect skin cancer rates in transplant recipients. Kidney transplant recipients receiving cyclosporine, azathioprine, and prednisolone had a 2.8 times higher risk of SCC, compared to patients receiving azathioprine and prednisolone.[78]

Both kidney transplant and heart transplant recipients are at increased risk for developing skin cancer.[79] However, heart transplant recipients have a 2.9 times higher risk of cutaneous malignancy, compared to kidney transplant recipients.[78] A retrospective review of nearly 300 heart transplantation patients showed a cumulative risk for the development of either SCC or BCC to be 3 percent at 1 year, 21 percent at 5 years, and 35 percent at 10 years.[80]

Melanoma has also been found to be increased in the immunosuppressed population (although to a lesser extent than SCC), with a relative risk of 4.[81–83]

Chemical Carcinogen Exposure

Exposure to chemical carcinogens is another risk factor for skin cancer. Arsenic in Fowler's solution, Donovan's solution, and Asiatic pills was once used as a medicinal agent for a host of nondermatologic and dermatologic conditions, including psoriasis, asthma, syphilis, eczema, and dermatitis herpetiformis (Figure 3–7). Today, arsenic is found in certain industrial workplaces, such as those in the mining, agricultural, forestry, and manufacturing sectors. It has also been found in contaminated well water on the southwest coast of Taiwan. The affected Taiwanese have been noted to have an endemic peripheral vascular disease known as "blackfoot disease," but they also have other malignant neoplasms of the skin, lung, liver, and bladder.[84]

Arsenic can be absorbed transcutaneously or through the respiratory and gastrointestinal tract. The precise molecular events induced by arsenic that lead to skin cancer are not known. Arsenic is, however, a known powerful chromosome-altering agent. In vitro studies have shown an increased rate of sister chromatid exchanges. The pertinent history would include a history of exposure to contaminated well water, an occupational history of arsenic exposure, or other symptoms of arsenism.

Bowen's disease (squamous cell carcinoma in situ) and basal cell carcinoma are the most common skin cancers seen in the setting of arsenic exposure (Figure 3–8). Multiple skin cancers can be present on both sun-exposed and sun-protected cutaneous sites. Furthermore, there appears to be a direct correlation between the amount of arsenic exposure and the development of skin cancer.[76]

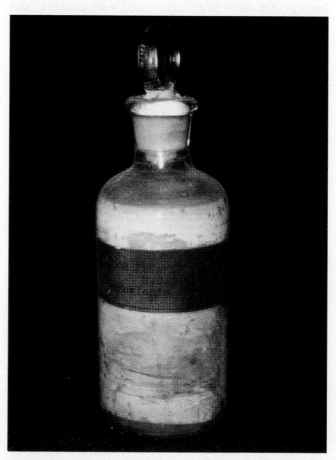

Figure 3–7. An old medicinal bottle of Fowler's solution.

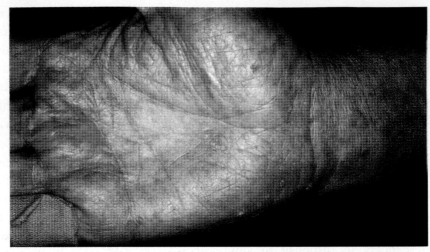

Figure 3–8. Arsenical keratoses on the hand of a patient with chronic arsenism.

There have been reports of SCC arising from exposure to polycyclic aromatic hydrocarbons, products of the combustion and distillation of carbonaceous materials. These carcinogens are contained in coal tar, pitch, paraffin oil, petroleum-based lubricating oil, and soot.[85] Pesticides and insecticides have been associated with cancers, and it has been suggested that a connection may exist between melanoma and pesticides.[86]

Ionizing Radiation Therapy

Ionizing radiation has been known to be a skin carcinogen for many years. Most of the evidence derives from populations of patients treated with radiation for benign skin conditions such as tinea capitis and acne. The latency period for skin malignancies in these populations is approximately 25 to 30 years.[87] The most common tumors seen are BCC and SCC. Radiation was used to treat tinea capitis until the 1960s. The relative risk for skin cancer (BCC and SCC) in two major populations with tinea capitis treated with radiation was determined to be approximately 3.[88,89]

PHYSICAL EXAMINATION: LOOKING FOR SIGNS

Pigmentary Characteristics

Pigmentary characteristics, or constitutive skin color, has been studied as a risk factor for melanoma and for nonmelanoma skin cancers. Individuals with a fair complexion, light eyes, and light hair are at increased risk for developing skin cancers.

Light hair (blond or red) carries a relative risk of 2 to 3 for melanoma, a relative risk of 2 for BCC, and a relative risk of 12.5 for SCC.[21,31,90–93]

Blue eye color has been associated with a relative risk for melanoma of 1.55 to 3.07.[21,61,90,93] Blue and green eye colors have been associated with a relative risk for BCC of 1.8 and 1.9, respectively.[67]

A fair or pale complexion has been associated with a relative risk for melanoma of 1.7 to 18.4.[21] A fair or pale complexion and a medium complexion were both associated with a relative risk for BCC of 1.1.[67]

Photodamage

"Photodamage" is a general term used to describe the physical changes induced by chronic sun exposure. Photodamage can manifest as a number of different cutaneous lesions and may be difficult to quantitate beyond mild, moderate, and severe. Chronic actinic damage is easier to assess in individuals of skin phototypes I and II. Freckles (discussed below) and actinic keratoses have been studied as risk factors for skin cancer. The chance of an untreated actinic keratosis transforming into SCC is unknown. However, it has been estimated that there is a 10 percent chance that an actinic keratosis in a patient with multiple actinic keratoses will transform into an SCC over a 10-year period.[94] Actinic keratoses are not obligate precursors of SCC, but they may be seen as risk markers for skin cancer.

Other lesions suggestive of photodamage that have been less extensively studied include poikilodermatous changes (uneven skin pigmentation), Favre-Racouchot disease (cysts and comedones), and rhytides (wrinkles). Any or all of these findings should alert the clinician to extensive photodamage even if the history is negative for extensive exposure.

Freckling

Freckles are associated with an increased risk for melanoma (a reported relative risk of 20)[93,95–97] (Figure 3–9). In an epidemiologic study of childhood melanoma in Australia, heavy facial freckling was found to be one of the strongest determinants of melanoma risk, along with the presence of large nevi,

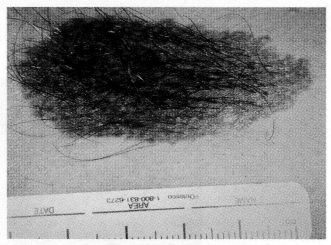

Figure 3–10. Medium congenital nevus with hypertrichosis. Note the fairly symmetrical and homogenous appearance.

a family history of melanoma, and an inability to tan.[98,99] Furthermore, freckling has been associated with an increased risk for both BCC and SCC, with odds ratios ranging from 1.7 to 2.9.[7,32,33,66,100–102]

Congenital Melanocytic Nevi

Congenital melanocytic nevi, which generally grow in proportion to the growth of the child, are often classified according to the size they are predicted to reach in adulthood. A small congenital melanocytic nevus will be less than 1.5 cm in greatest diameter in adulthood, a medium nevus will measure between 1.5 and 19.9 cm, and a large congenital melanocytic nevus will measure 20 cm or more[103,104] (Figures 3–10 to 3–12).

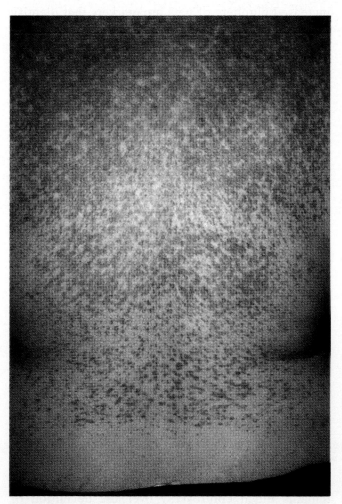

Figure 3–9. Extensive freckling across the back of a patient with skin phototype I.

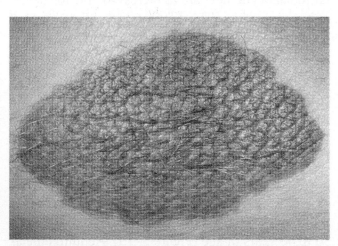

Figure 3–11. Medium congenital nevus with a mammillated surface. Note the fairly symmetrical and homogenous appearance.

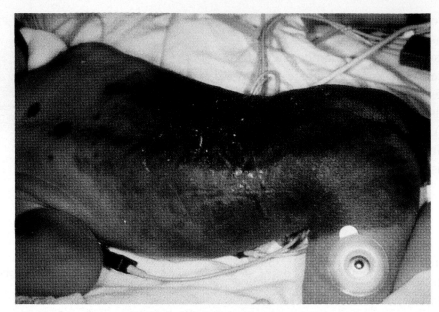

Figure 3–12. Large congenital nevus. This patient is at elevated risk for melanoma or neurocutaneous melanoma because the nevus involves the posterior midline.

Any congenital melanocytic nevus can give rise to melanoma (albeit rarely).[105] The risk of melanoma appears to be roughly proportional to the size of the nevus. The lifetime risk of melanoma developing in congenital nevi less than 20 cm in diameter is estimated to be between 0 and 6.3 percent.[104,106] However, much controversy still surrounds the issue of whether congenital nevi less than 20 cm in diameter are truly lesions at high risk for developing melanoma. Two recent studies evaluating medium-sized congenital nevi did not reveal an increased risk for melanoma in nevi of this size.[103,107] In contrast, it is well established that patients with large congenital melanocytic nevi are at increased risk for developing melanoma. The lifetime risk of developing cutaneous melanoma in patients with large nevi is estimated to be between 4.5 and 10 percent, with a relative risk in the range of 101 to 1,046.[108–113]

Acquired "Common" Melanocytic Nevi

The total number of melanocytic nevi in an individual is one of the strongest measurable predictors of melanoma development. Common melanocytic nevi begin to appear at 6 months of age, increase in number during puberty, and are maximally expressed by 30 to 40 years of age (Figure 3–13). Acquired melanocytic nevi may be contiguous with melanoma, and increased numbers of nevi are markers that identify persons at increased risk for developing melanoma. The relative risk of melanoma increases linearly as the number of nevi increases[53,54,59,114,115] (Figure 3–14). The relative risk for melanoma in patients with 11 to 25 nevi was 1.6; for those with 26 to 50 nevi, it was 4.4; for those with 51 to 100 nevi, it was 5.4; and for patients with more than 100 nevi, the relative risk was 9.8.[114]

In addition to increasing melanoma risk, higher numbers of nevi appear to indicate a greater risk for the development of basal cell carcinoma. A case-control study with BCC patients and controls revealed that females with BCC had significantly higher nevus counts.[116] High nevus counts have not been reported to be a risk factor for SCC.

Atypical (Dysplastic) Nevi

An atypical nevus is a type of acquired melanocytic nevus. Unlike common acquired nevi, atypical nevi are frequently asymmetric and have irregular borders, multiple colors, and diameters greater than 5 mm[117,118] (Figure 3–15). The term "dysplastic nevus" is often used to denote an atypical nevus. From the clinical and histologic perspectives, there remains much controversy over the definition of dysplastic nevi.[119]

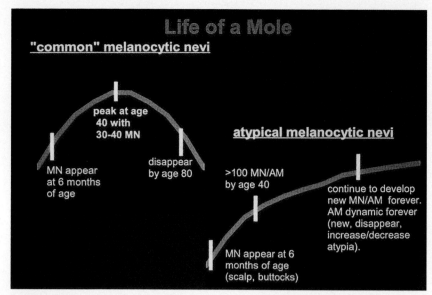

Figure 3–13.   Graph depicting the natural history of "common" and dysplastic nevi.

Dysplastic nevi, independently of the total number of nevi, are a powerful risk factor for the development of melanoma.[117] One study that examined the number and type of nevi in individuals revealed that patients with one clinically dysplastic nevus had a twofold increase in melanoma risk while those with more than 10 dysplastic nevi had a 12-fold increased risk[115] (Figures 3–14, and 3–16 to 3–18).

Not all patients with dysplastic nevi are at equal risk for developing melanoma; the risk varies, depending on the personal and family histories of melanoma. Kraemer and colleagues classified patients with dysplastic nevi into five groups, according to the presence of melanoma: type A, sporadic dysplastic nevi; type B, familial dysplastic nevi; type C, sporadic dysplastic nevi with melanoma; type D1, familial dysplastic nevi and one family member with melanoma; and type D2, familial dysplastic nevi and two or more family members who have had melanoma.[120] The risk for

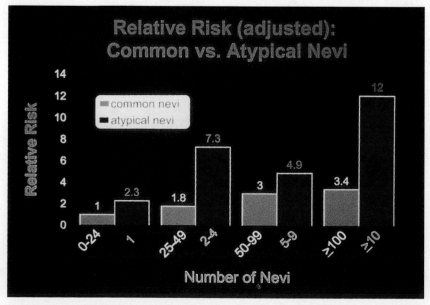

Figure 3–14.   Graph showing that the relative risk for developing melanoma depends on the number and the type of nevi present.

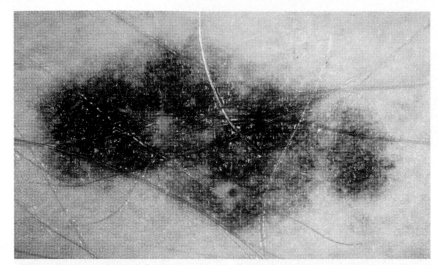

Figure 3–15. This biopsy-proven atypical nevus has clinical features that are often seen in melanoma: irregular borders, variegated pigmentation, and asymmetry.

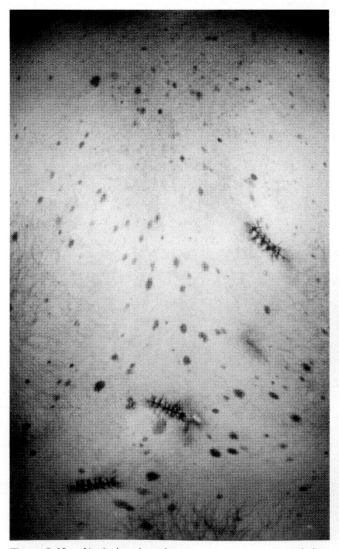

Figure 3-16. Atypical nevi can be seen on non-sun-exposed sites such as the buttocks.

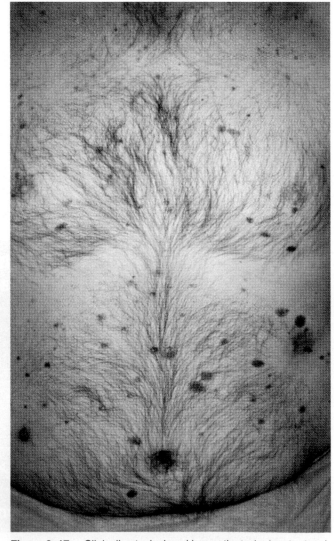

Figure 3–17. Clinically atypical nevi in a patient who has had multiple excisions of nevi.

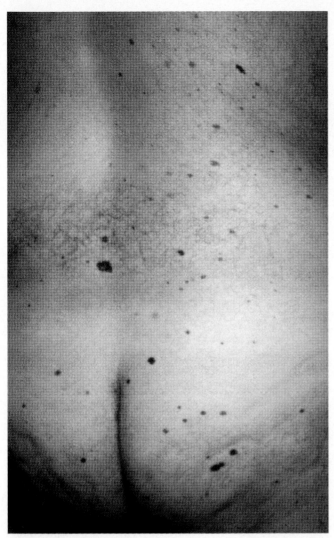

Figure 3–18. Atypical nevi can be seen on non-sun-exposed sites such as the buttocks.

melanoma increased from type A to type D2. Patients in the D2 category had a lifetime melanoma risk of over 80 percent.

Rigel and colleagues characterized patients with atypical nevi into four risk groups based on the presence or absence of a personal and/or family history of melanoma.[121] Patients in group 0 (atypical nevi and no personal or family history of melanoma) were estimated to have a relative risk (RR) for melanoma of 2 to 92. Patients in group I (atypical nevi and only a personal history of melanoma) were estimated to have a RR for melanoma of 8 to 127. Patients in group II (atypical nevi and no personal history of melanoma but one family member with melanoma) were estimated to have a RR of 33 to 444. Patients in group III (atypical nevi and two or

more family members with a history of melanoma) were found to have the highest risk of melanoma, with RR ranging from 85 to 1269.[122]

Nevus Sebaceous

Nevus sebaceous (nevus sebaceous of Jadassohn) is a benign lesion present at birth and usually located on the scalp. It ranges from a smooth and hairless plaque to a verrucous and nodular plaque and typically has a yellow to orange color (Figure 3–19). Because of the high incidence of benign and malignant tumors developing within them, nevi sebaceous are often excised in late childhood or early adulthood. On rare occasions, extensive lesions may be associated with epilepsy, mental retardation, and other neurologic defects.[123]

Basal cell carcinoma (BCC) has been reported to be clinically evident in 5 to 7 percent of cases of nevus sebaceous. However, a recent retrospective analysis of 596 cases of nevus sebaceous found that BCCs were present in only 0.8 percent of cases, lower than previously reported. This discrepancy may be due to a number of trichoblastomas that were initially categorized as BCCs.[124] It is rare for squamous cell carcinoma (SCC) to be found in these tumors.[123] Other tumors that have been reported to arise within nevi sebaceous include syringocystadenoma papilliferum, trichoblastoma, nodular hidrade-

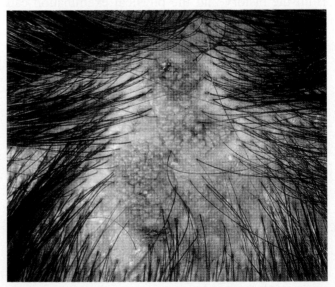

Figure 3-19. Nevus sebaceous, with basal cell carcinoma arising at the inferior margin.

noma, syringoma, sebaceous epithelioma, chondroid syringoma, and trichilemmoma.

Burn Scars, Heat Injury, and Chronic Ulcers

Malignant transformation is known to occur in scars and chronic ulcers. While SCC is the most common malignancy arising at these sites, BCC, melanoma, malignant fibrous histiocytoma, liposarcoma, and osteogenic sarcoma have also been reported. It is estimated that 2 percent of SCCs arise within chronic scars. Squamous cell carcinomas arising in ulcers (Marjolin's ulcer) are more common in men and have a latency period of approximately 35 years (from the time of injury until the time of malignant transformation). The mortality rate rises as the period of latency increases, and lesions on the extremities have a worse prognosis, with rates of metastasis approaching 30 percent.[125]

Melanoma arising in a burn scar is a rare event. Recently, three cases of melanoma arising in burn scars were reported from Tunisia. The latency period of the melanoma ranged from 47 to 70 years. The authors proposed several hypotheses for the development of this melanoma and suggested that the natural history of this "secondary melanoma" is different from that of classic melanoma in that the fibrotic barrier of the scar prevents tumor spread.[126]

CONCLUSION

Both the history and the physical examination can help identify individuals at risk for developing skin cancer. The history can help determine the individual's phototype (skin type), demographics, occupational and recreational history of UV light exposure, personal and family history of skin cancer, and exposure to chemical carcinogens. The physical examination gives clues to an individual's risk for skin cancer by revealing hair and eye color, complexion type, presence of freckles and melanocytic nevi, and actinic damage as shown by the presence of actinic or solar keratoses.

REFERENCES

1. Freedberg K, Koh H. Screening for malignant melanoma and nonmelanoma skin cancer: a cost-effectiveness analysis. Clin Res 1990;38:712A.
2. Piepkorn M. Melanoma genetics: an update with focus on the CDKN2A (p16)/ARF tumor suppressors. J Am Acad Dermatol 2000;42:705–22.
3. Weinstock MA. Epidemiology of melanoma. Cancer Treat Res 1993;65:29–56.
4. Kopf A. Computer analysis of 3531 basal-cell carcinomas of the skin. J Dermatol 1979;6:267–81.
5. Kaldor J, Shugg D, Young B, et al. Non-melanoma skin cancer: ten years of cancer-registry-based surveillance. Int J Dermatol 1993;53:886–91.
6. Aubry F, MacGibbon B. Risk factors of squamous cell carcinoma of the skin. Cancer 1985;55:907–11.
7. Kricker A, Armstrong B, English D. Sun exposure and non-melanocytic skin cancer. Cancer Causes Control 1994;5:367–92.
8. Gilchrest B, Eller M, Geller A, Yaar M. The pathogenesis of melanoma induced by ultraviolet radiation. N Engl J Med 1999;340:1341–8.
9. Wei Q. Effect of aging on DNA repair and skin carcinogenesis: a minireview of population-based studies. Symposium Proceedings. J Invest Dermatol 1998;3:19–22.
10. Roudier-Pujol C, Auperin A, Nguyen T, et al. Basal cell carcinoma in young adults: not more aggressive than in older patients. Dermatology 1999;199:119–23.
11. LeSueur B, Silvis N, Hansen R. Basal cell carcinoma in children: report of 3 cases. Arch Dermatol 2000; 136:370–2.
12. Albert V, Koh H, Geller A, et al. Years of potential life lost: another indicator of the impact of cutaneous malignant melanoma on society. J Am Acad Dermatol 1990;23:308–10.
13. Grob J, Stern R, Mackie R, Weinstock M. Epidemiology, causes, and prevention of skin diseases. Cambridge: Blackwell Sciences; 1997.
14. Armstrong B, Kricker A. Epidemiology of sun exposure and skin cancer. Cancer Surv 1996;26:133–53.
15. Camplejohn R. DNA damage and repair in melanoma and non-melanoma skin cancer. Cancer Surv 1996; 26:193–206.
16. Scotto J, Fears T. The association of solar ultraviolet and skin melanoma incidence among Caucasians in the United States. Cancer Invest 1987;5:275–83.
17. Elwood J. Melanoma and sun exposure. In: Grob J, Stern R, Mackie R, Weinstock W, editors. Epidemiology, causes, and prevention of skin diseases. Cambridge (UK): Blackwell Sciences; 1997. p. 48–95.
18. Elwood J. Melanoma and sun exposure: contrasts between intermittent and chronic exposure. World J Surg 1992;16:157–65.
19. Nelemans P, Rampen F, Ruiter D, Verbeek A. An addition to the controversy on sunlight exposure and melanoma risk: a meta-analytical approach. J Clin Epidemiol 1995;48:1331–42.
20. Walter S, King W, Marrett L. Association of cutaneous

malignant melanoma with intermittent exposure to ultraviolet radiation: results of a case-control study in Ontario, Canada. Int J Epidemiol 1999;28:418–27.

21. Evans R, Kopf A, Lew R, et al. Risk factors for the development of malignant melanoma—I: Review of case-control studies. J Dermatol Surg Oncol 1988; 14:393–408.

22. Dubin N, Pasternack BS, Moseson M. Simultaneous assessment of risk factors for malignant melanoma and non-melanoma skin lesions, with emphasis on sun exposure and related variables. Int J Epidemiol 1990;19:811–9.

23. Osterlind A, Tucker M, Stone B, Jensen O. The Danish case-control study of cutaneous malignant melanoma. II. Importance of UV-light exposure. Int J Cancer 1988;42:319–24.

24. Westerdahl J, Olsson H, Ingvar C. At what age do sunburn episodes play a crucial role for the development of malignant melanoma? Eur J Cancer 1994;30A:1647–54.

25. Balch C, Houghton A, Sober A, Soong S. Cutaneous melanoma. 3rd ed. St. Louis: Quality Medical Publishing; 1998.

26. Autier P, Dore J, Gefeller O, et al. EORTC Melanoma Co-operative Group. Melanoma risk and residence in sunny areas. Br J Cancer 1997;76:1521–4.

27. Khlat M, Vail A, Parkin M, Green A. Mortality from melanoma in migrants to Australia: variation by age at arrival and duration of stay. Am J Epidemiol 1992; 135:1103–13.

28. Mack T, Floderus B. Malignant melanoma risk by nativity, place of residence at diagnosis, and age at migration. Cancer Causes Control 1991;2:401–11.

29. Green A, Bain C, McLennan R, Siskind V. Risk factors for cutaneous melanoma in Queensland. Recent Results Cancer Res 1986;102:76–97.

30. Rosso S, Zanetti R, Pippione M, Sancho-Garnier H. Parallel risk assessment of melanoma and basal cell carcinoma: skin characteristics and sun exposure. Melanoma Res 1998;8:573–83.

31. Lock-Andersen J, Drzewiecki K, Wulf H. Eye and hair colour, skin type and constitutive pigmentation as risk factors for basal cell carcinoma and cutaneous malignant melanoma: a Danish case-control study. Acta Derm Venereol 1999;79:74–80.

32. Vitasa B, Taylor H, Strickland P, et al. Association of nonmelanoma skin cancer and actinic keratosis with cumulative solar ultraviolet exposure in Maryland watermen. Cancer 1990;65:2811–7.

33. Gallagher R, Hill G, Bajdik C, et al. Sunlight exposure pigmentation factors, and risk of nonmelanocytic skin cancers. II. Squamous cell carcinoma. Arch Dermatol 1995;131:164–9.

34. Schwartz R. Premalignant keratinocytic neoplasms. J Am Acad Dermatol 1996; 35:223–42.

35. Gallagher R, Ma B, McLean D, et al. Trends in basal cell carcinoma, squamous cell carcinoma, and melanoma of the skin from 1973 through 1987. J Am Acad Dermatol 1990;23:413–21.

36. Setlow R. Spectral regions contributing to melanoma: a personal view. J Invest Dermatol 1999;4:46–9.

37. Stern RS, Laird N. Skin Cancer after PUVA treatment for psoriasis. Cancer 1994;73:2759–64.

38. Cockayne S, August P. PUVA photocarcinogenesis in Cheshire. Clin Exp Dermatol 1997;22:300–4.

39. Stern R, Lunder E. Risk of squamous cell carcinoma in methoxsalen (psoralen) and UV-A radiation (PUVA). A meta-analysis. Arch Dermatol 1998;134:1582–5.

40. Stern R, Liebman E, Vakeva L. Oral psoralen and ultraviolet-A light PUVA treatment of psoriasis and persistent risk of nonmelanoma skin cancer. PUVA follow-up study. J Natl Cancer Inst 1998;90:1278–84.

41. McKenna KE, Patterson CC, Handley JH. Cutaneous neoplasms following PUVA therapy for psoriasis. Br J Dermatol 1996;134:639–42.

42. Studniberg H, Weller P. PUVA, UVB, psoriasis, and nonmelanoma skin cancer. J Am Acad Dermatol 1993;29:1013–22.

43. Stern R, Nichols K, Vakeva L. Malignant melanoma in patients treated for psoriasis with methoxsalen (psoralen) and ultraviolet A radiation (PUVA). N Engl J Med 1997;336:1041–5.

44. Lindelof B, Sigurgeirsson B, Tegner E, et al. PUVA and cancer risk: the Swedish follow-up study. Br J Dermatol 1999;141:108–12.

45. Hannuksela-Svahn A, Pukkala E, Koulu L, et al. Cancer incidence among Finnish psoriasis patients treated with 8-methoxypsoralen bath PUVA. J Am Acad Dermatol 1999;40:694–6.

46. Swerdlow A, Weinstock M. Do tanning lamps cause melanoma? An epidemiologic assessment. J Am Acad Dermatol 1998;38:89–98.

47. Autier P, Dore J, Lejeune F, et al. Cutaneous malignant melanoma and exposure to sunlamps or sunbeds: an EORTC multicenter case-control study in Belgium, France and Germany. EORTC Melanoma Cooperative Group. Int J Cancer 1994;58:809–13.

48. Westerdahl J, Ingvar C, Masback A, et al. Risk of cutaneous malignant melanoma in relation to use of sunbeds: further evidence for UV-A carcinogenicity. Br J Cancer 2000;82:1593–9.

49. Coldiron B. Update on ozone depletion. Skin Cancer Found J 1993;11:10–1.

50. Environmental Protection Agency. Regulatory impact analysis; protection of stratospheric ozone. Washington (DC): U.S. Environmental Protection Agency; 1988.

51. Marghoob A, Slade J, Kopf A, et al. Risk of developing multiple primary cutaneous melanomas in patients with the classic atypical-mole syndrome: a case-control study. Br J Dermatol 1996;135:704–11.

52. Johnson TM, Hamilton T, Lowe L. Multiple primary melanomas. J Am Acad Dermatol 1998;39:422–7.

53. Reynolds P, Austin D. Epidemiologic-based screening strategies for malignant melanoma of the skin. In: Engstrom P, Anderson P, Mortenson L, editors. Advances in cancer control: epidemiology and research. New York: Alan R Liss; 1984. p. 245–54.

54. Holman C, Armstrong B. Pigmentary traits, ethnic origin, benign nevi, and family history as risk factors for cutaneous malignant melanoma. J Natl Cancer Inst 1984;72:257–66.

55. Marghoob A, Slade J, Salopek T, et al. Basal cell and squamous cell carcinomas are important risk factors for cutaneous malignant melanoma. Cancer 1995; 75:707–14.

56. Karagas M, Stukel T, Greenberg R, et al. Risk of subsequent basal cell carcinoma and squamous cell carcinoma of the skin among patients with prior skin cancer. JAMA 1992 267:3305–10.

57. Marghoob A, Kopf A, Bart R, et al. Risk of another basal cell carcinoma developing after treatment of a basal cell carcinoma. J Am Acad Dermatol 1993; 28:22–8.

58. Frankel D, Hanusa B, Zitelli J. New primary non-melanoma skin cancer in patients with a history of squamous cell carcinoma of the skin. J Am Acad Dermatol 1992;26:720–6.

59. Green A, MacLennan R, Siskind V. Common acquired naevi and the risk of malignant melanoma. Int J Cancer 1985;35:297–300.

60. Cutler C, Foulkes W, Brunet J, et al. Cutaneous malignant melanoma in women is uncommonly associated with a family history of melanoma in first-degree relatives: a case-control study. Melanoma Res 1996;6:435–40.

61. Sober A, Kang S, Barnhill R. Discerning individuals at elevated risk for cutaneous melanoma. Clin Dermatol 1992;10:15–20.

62. Greene M. The genetics of hereditary melanoma. Cancer 1999;86:1644–57.

63. Rhodes A, Weinstock M, Fitzpatrick T, et al. Risk factors for cutaneous melanoma: a practical method of recognizing predisposed individuals. JAMA 1987; 258:3146–54.

64. Weinstock MA, Brodsky GL. Bias in the assessment of family history of melanoma and its association with dysplastic nevi in a case-control study. J Clin Epidemiol 1998;51:1299–303.

65. Wallberg P, Kaaman T, Lindberg M. Multiple basal cell carcinoma. A clinical evaluation of risk factors. Acta Derm Venereol 1998 78:127–9.

66. Hogan D, Lane P, Wong D. Risk factors for squamous cell carcinoma of the skin in Saskatchewan, Canada. J Dermatol Sci 1990;1:97–101.

67. Naldi L, DiLandro A, D'Avanzo B, Parazzini F. Host-related and environmental risk factors for cutaneous basal cell carcinoma: evidence from an Italian case-control study. J Am Acad Dermatol 2000;42:446–52.

68. Lee J, Strickland D. Malignant melanoma: social status and outdoor work. Br J Cancer 1980;41:757–63.

69. Gallagher R, Elwood J, Threlfall W, et al. Occupation and risk of cutaneous melanoma. Am J Ind Med 1986;9:289–94.

70. MacKie R, Hole D. Incidence and thickness of primary tumours and survival of patients with cutaneous malignant melanoma in relation to socioeconomic status. BMJ 1996;312:1125–8.

71. Harrison R, Haque A, Roseman J, Soong S. Socioeconomic characteristics and melanoma incidence. Ann Epidemiol 1998;8:327–33.

72. Pion I, Rigel D, Garfinkel L, et al. Occupation and the risk of malignant melanoma. Cancer 1995;75:637–44.

73. Beral V, Robinson N. The relationship of malignant melanoma, basal and squamous skin cancers to indoor and outdoor work. Br J Cancer 1981;44:886–91.

74. Robinson J, Altman J, Rademaker A. Socioeconomic status and attitudes of 51 patients with giant basal and sqaumous cell carcinoma and paired controls. Arch Dermatol 1995;131:428–31.

75. Veness M. Aggressive skin cancers in a cardiac transplant recipient. Australas Radiol 1997;41:363–6.

76. Johnson TM, Rowe DE, Nelson BR, Swanson NA. Squamous cell carcinoma of the skin (excluding lip and oral mucosa). J Am Acad Dermatol 1992;25:467–84.

77. McGregor J, Proby C. The role of papillomaviruses in human non-melanoma skin cancer. Cancer Surv 1996;26:219–36.

78. Jensen P, Hansen S, Moller B, et al. Skin cancer in kidney and heart transplant recipients and different long-term immunosuppressive therapy regimens. J Am Acad Dermatol 1999;40:177–86.

79. Euvrard S, Kanitakis J, Pouteil-Nobel C, et al. Comparative epidemiologic study of premalignant and malignant epithelial cutaneous lesions developing after kidney and heart tranplantation. J Am Acad Dermatol 1995;33:222–9.

80. Lampros T, Cobanoglu A, Parker F, et al Squamous and basal cell carcinoma in heart transplant recipients. J Heart Lung Transplant 1998;17:586–91.

81. Hintner H, Fritsch P. Skin neoplasia in the immuno-deficient host. The clinical spectrum: Kaposi's sarcoma, lymphoma, skin cancer and melanoma. Curr Probl Dermatol 1989;18:210–7.

82. Greene M, Young T, Clark WJ. Malignant melanoma in renal-transplant recipients. Lancet 1981;1:1196–9.

83. Rockley P, Trieff N, Wagner RJ, Tyring S. Nonsunlight risk factors for malignant melanoma. Part II: Immunity, genetics, and workplace prevention. Int J Dermatol 1994;33:462–7.

84. Lin T, Huang Y. Arsenic species in drinking water, hair, fingernails, and urine of patients with blackfoot disease. J Toxicol Environ Health 1998;53:85–93.

85. Everall J, Dowd P. Influence of environmental factors excluding ultraviolet radiation on the incidence of skin cancer. Bull Cancer 1978;65:241–8.

86. Burkhart CG, Burkhart CN. Melanoma and insecticides: is there a connection? J Am Acad Dermatol 2000;42:302–3.

87. Hood I, Young J. Late sequelae of superficial irradiation. Head Neck Surg 1984;7:65–72.

88. Modan B, Alfondary E, Shapiro D, et al. Factors affecting the development of skin cancer after scalp irradiation. Radiat Res 1993;134:125–8.

89. Shore R, Albert R, Reed M, et al. Skin cancer incidence among children irradiated for ringworm of the scalp. Radiat Res 1984;100:192–204.

90. Zanetti R, Rosso S, Martinez C, et al. The multicentre south European study 'Helios.' I: Skin characteristics and sunburns in basal cell and squamous cell carcinomas of the skin. Br J Cancer 1996;73:1440–6.

91. Grulich A, Bataille V, Swerdlow A, et al. Naevi and pigmentary characteristics as risk factors for melanoma in a high-risk population: a case-control study in New South Wales, Australia. Int J Cancer 1996;67:485–91.

92. Marrett L, King W, Walter S, From L. Use of host factors to identify people at high risk for cutaneous malignant melanoma. Can Med Assoc J 1992;147:445–53.

93. Bliss JM, Ford D, Swerdlow AJ, et al. Risk of cutaneous melanoma associated with pigmentation characteristics and freckling: systematic overview of 10 case-control studies. The International Melanoma Analysis Group (IMAGE). Int J Cancer 1995;62:367–76.

94. Freedberg I, Eisen A, Wolff K, et al. Dermatology in general medicine. 5th ed. Vol. I. New York: McGraw-Hill; 1999. p. 826.

95. Rodenas JM, Delgado-Rodriguez M, Herranz MT, et al. Sun exposure, pigmentary traits, and risk of cutaneous malignant melanoma: a case-control study in a Mediterranean population. Cancer Causes Control 1996;7:275–83.

96. Dubin N, Moseson M, Pasternak B. Epidemiology of malignant melanoma: pigmentary traits, ultraviolet radiation, and the identification of high-risk populations. Recent Results Cancer Res 1986;102:56–75.

97. Gallagher RP, McLean DI, Yang CP, et al. Suntan, sunburn, and pigmentation factors and the frequency of acquired melanocytic nevi in children. Similarities to melanoma: the Vancouver Mole Study. Arch Dermatol 1990;126:770–6.

98. Whiteman DC, Valery P, McWhirter W, Green AC. Risk factors for childhood melanoma in Queensland, Australia. Int J Cancer 1997;70:26–31.

99. McLean DI, Gallagher RP. "Sunburn" freckles, cafe-au-lait macules, and other pigmented lesions of schoolchildren: the Vancouver Mole Study. J Am Acad Dermatol 1995;32:565–70.

100. Gallagher R, Hill G, Bajdik C, et al. Sunlight exposure, pigmentary factors, and risk of nonmelanocytic skin cancer. I. Basal cell carcinoma. Arch Dermatol 1995;131:157–63.

101. Hogan D, To T, Gran L, et al. Risk factors for basal cell carcinoma. Int J Dermatol 1989;28:591–4.

102. English D, Armstrong B, Kircker A, et al. Demographic characteristics, pigmentary and cutaneous risk factors for squamous cell carcinoma of the skin: a case-control study. Int J Cancer 1998;76:628–34.

103. Sahin S, Levin L, Kopf A, et al. Risk of melanoma in medium-sized congenital melanocytic nevi: a follow-up study. J Am Acad Dermatol 1998 39:428–33.

104. Marghoob A, Kopf A, Bittencourt F. Moles present at birth: their significance. Skin Cancer Found J 1999;17:36–98.

105. Ceballos P, Ruiz-Maldonado R, Mihm M. Melanoma in children. New Engl J Med 1995;332:656–62.

106. Rhodes A, Melski J. Small congenital nevocellular nevi and the risk of cutaneous melanoma. J Pediatr 1982;100:219–24.

107. Swerdlow A, English J, Qiao Z. The risk of melanoma in patients with congenital nevi: a cohort study. J Am Acad Dermatol 1995;32:595–9.

108. Ruiz-Maldonado R, Orozco-Covarrubias M. Malignant melanoma in children: a review. Arch Dermatol 1997;133:363–71.

109. Sober A, Burstein J. Precursors to skin cancer. Cancer 1995;75:645–50.

110. Rhodes A. Pigmented birthmarks and precursor melanocytic lesions of cutaneous melanoma identifiable in childhood. Pediatr Clin North Am 1983;30:435–63.

111. Egan C, Oliveria S, Elenitsas R, et al. Cutaneous melanoma risk and phenotypic changes in large congenital nevi: a follow-up study of 46 patients. J Am Acad Dermatol 1998;39:923–32.

112. DeDavid M, Orlow S, Provost N, et al. A study of large congenital melanocytic nevi and associated malignant melanomas: review of cases in the New York University Registry and the world literature. J Am Acad Dermatol 1997;36:409–16.

113. Marghoob A, Bittencourt J, Kopf A, Bart R. Large congenital melanocytic nevi. Curr Probl Dermatol 2000;12(3):146–52.

114. Holly E, Kelly J, Shpall S, Chiu S. Number of melanocytic nevi as a major risk factor for malignant melanoma. J Am Acad Dermatol 1987;17:459–68.

115. Tucker MA, Halpern A, Holly EA, et al. Clinically recognized dysplastic nevi. A central risk factor for cutaneous melanoma. JAMA 1997;277:1439–44.

116. Lock-Andersen J, Drzewiecki K, Wulf H. Naevi as a risk factor for basal cell carcinoma in Caucasians: a Danish case-control study. Acta Derm Venereol 1999;79:314–9.

117. Halpern A, DuPont G, Elder D, et al. Dysplastic nevi as risk markers of sporadic (nonfamilial) melanoma. Arch Dermatol 1991;127:995–9.

118. Marghoob A. The dangers of atypical mole (dysplastic nevus) syndrome. Postgrad Med 1999;105:147–64.

119. Resnik K, Ackerman A. Melanoma risk in individuals with clinically atypical nevi? Dermatopathol Pract Concept 1995;1:269–76.

120. Kraemer K, Greene M. Dysplastic nevus syndrome. Familial and sporadic precursors of cutaneous melanoma. Dermatol Clin 1985;3:225–37.

121. Rigel D, Rivers J, Friedman R, Kopf A. Risk gradient for malignant melanoma in individuals with dysplastic nevi. Lancet 1988;1:352–3.

122. Slade J, Marghoob A, Salopek T, et al. Atypical mole syndrome: risk factor for cutaneous malignant melanoma and implications for management. J Am Acad Dermatol 1995;32:479–94.

123. Elder D, Elenitsas R, Jaworsky C, Johnson B. Lever's histopathology of the skin. 8th ed. Philadelphia: Lippincott-Raven; 1997. p. 763–4.

124. Cribier B, Scrivener Y, Grosshans E. Tumors arising in nevus sebaceus: a study of 596 cases. J Am Acad Dermatol 2000;42:263–8.

125. Phillips T, Salman S, Bhawan J, Rogers G. Burn scar carcinoma: diagnosis and management. Dermatol Surg 1998;22:561–5.

126. Ghazi J, Hamouda B. Melanoma arising in burn scars: report of 3 observations and a literature review. Arch Dermatol 1999;135:1551–2.

Clinical Presentation: Melanoma

RICHARD G. B. LANGLEY, MD
MARTIN C. MIHM JR, MD
ARTHUR J. SOBER, MD

The ability to directly inspect the skin and mucous membranes provides a unique opportunity to diagnose and excise melanoma at an early and curable stage. The increasing incidence of melanoma and the prognostic importance of establishing an early diagnosis underscore the importance of recognizing the clinical features of melanoma. Since there is an inverse relationship between the depth of invasion of melanoma and survival, it is important to recognize the early clinical features of melanoma to facilitate early diagnosis and timely excision of melanoma when there is a higher chance for cure. The majority of melanomas can be diagnosed by clinical examination, and it is essential that all physicians understand the basic clinical features of melanoma. The major focus of this chapter is to outline the clinical presentation of primary cutaneous melanoma.

HISTORY

The clinical assessment of a patient with a suspected melanoma begins with an evaluation of risk factors and a history of the lesion in question. Central risk factors include phenotypic[1] and genetic factors[2] and environmental exposure to solar radiation.[3,4] The major risk factors for the development of melanoma are summarized in Table 4–1. Patients at increased risk for melanoma can be identified and educated for primary prevention, and certain high-risk patients can be observed for early detection.

SIGNS AND SYMPTOMS

A change in an existing nevus or the development of a new pigmented lesion is a cardinal symptom of melanoma and should be viewed with particular suspicion. A history of persistent and sustained change is characteristic of melanoma. Benign lesions may also undergo change; however, such change is often transient and has an underlying cause, such as trauma to an existing nevus (Figure 4–1). The rate of change is also important. Change in melanoma is typically observed over a period of months or years. In contrast, benign lesions may develop or change over a period of days. For example, suspicion of melanoma may arise when folliculitis develops within a pre-

Table 4–1. RISK FACTORS FOR CUTANEOUS MELANOMA
Pigmentary characteristics
Blue eyes
Blond, fair, or red hair
Light complexion
Response to sun exposure
Freckling tendency
Inability to tan
Tendency to sunburn
Upper socioeconomic status
Family history of melanoma
Family history of dysplastic nevi
P16 mutation
Nevi
Melanocytic nevi (increased number of nevi)
Dysplastic nevi (risk directly related to number)
Changing mole
Itching or painful mole
Congenital nevus
History of prior melanoma
Immunosuppression

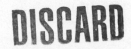

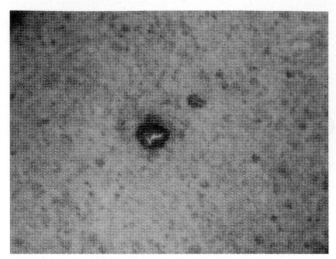

Figure 4–1. Irritated nevus. This patient presented with an acute change in a pre-existing nevus located on her arm. The changes included pain and erythema of 1 day's duration, and there was an antecedent history of trauma to the nevus. The symptoms and clinical changes spontaneously resolved within a week.

existing nevus; or inflammatory skin lesions such as pyogenic granulomas may arise de novo (Figure 4–2). The common presenting symptoms and signs of cutaneous melanoma are summarized below.

Pruritus

The presence of itching has been noted in approximately 25 percent of patients with early melanoma.[5]

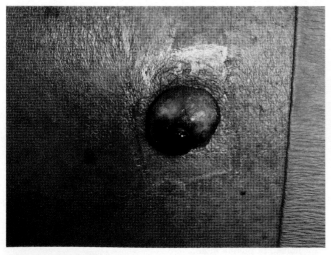

Figure 4–2. Pyogenic granuloma. This friable pink nodule developed abruptly on the thigh of a pregnant patient. Pyogenic granulomas may be misdiagnosed as nodular melanomas. (Reproduced with permission from Langley RG, Sober AJ. Clinical recognition of melanoma and its precursors. Hematol/Oncol Clin North Am 1998;12:699–715.)

The presence of pruritus, while nonspecific, can be important, particularly if the pruritus occurs in a changing nevus. Although some patients may present with pain or bleeding, early cutaneous melanoma is usually asymptomatic. In fact, such symptoms are usually associated with more advanced disease with a poorer prognosis[5] (Table 4–2).

Change in Size

A change in size is a useful early sign of cutaneous melanoma and occurs in approximately 70 percent of cases.[5] Change in size is noted as either a centrifugal spreading of the lesion (so-called radial growth) or an increase in height (vertical growth). The clinical appearance of radial or centrifugal growth often correlates with the microscopic radial-growth phase of melanoma, in which malignant cells remain in situ, confine themselves to the epidermis, or invade the superficial dermis. At the point of dermal invasion, the lesion appears clinically as a macule or minimally raised plaque. The recognition of melanoma at this point is critical to improving patient survival because melanoma diagnosed and excised at this point is highly curable. Neoplastic cells eventually penetrate deeper into the dermis, with both horizontal and vertical growth in the lesion. Vertical growth presents clinically as a papule or nodule within a pre-existing lesion seen as a pigmented flare or as a discrete solitary nodule. In contrast, nodular melanomas evolve de novo in vertical growth and appear clinically as a papule or nodule in previously normal skin.

Table 4–2. PERCENTAGE OF PATIENTS PRESENTING WITH SIGNS AND SYMPTOMS OF MELANOMA, BY CLARK LEVEL				
	Clark Level of Invasion*			
Sign or Symptom	II	III	IV	V
Size	71	58	64	83
Color	55	55	54	64
Elevation	36	60	67	80
Bleeding	10	26	42	54
Ulcer	4	13	27	43
Tenderness	9	11	15	18
Itching	25	24	36	43

*Values represent fraction responding affirmatively to the presence or absence of a symptom.
Reproduced with permission from Wick MM, Sober AJ, Fitzpatrick TB, et al. Clinical characteristics of early cutaneous melanoma. Cancer 1980;45:2684.

Change in Color and Change in Shape

Color change is another useful finding in early melanoma and is usually noted as an area of progressive darkening. Variegation in pigment pattern may be prominent, with hues of tan, brown, black, pink, red, or white. The distribution of colors in a melanoma is often haphazard. Focal areas of darkening, particularly when noted in an eccentric location, are viewed with particular suspicion (Figure 4–3). Pink or red discoloration in a nevus or in surrounding skin suggests potential malignancy.

Another characteristic of early melanoma is a change in shape, often with asymmetry. The borders can be irregular with prominent indentations or notches.

CLINICAL EXAMINATION

The clinical examination of a patient with a suspected melanoma includes a complete skin examination (including scalp, palms, soles, buttocks, and genitalia) and regional lymph node palpation. A complete skin examination is the standard of care in patients with suspected melanoma as cutaneous melanomas can occur in the mucosa or on any cutaneous surface. The most common areas for melanoma to develop vary by sex and race (Figure 4–4). In white males, melanoma most commonly develops on the trunk (particularly the upper back) whereas the lower legs and upper back are the favored locations in females.

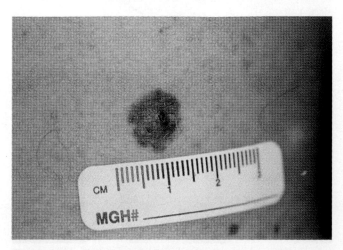

Figure 4–3. Early superficial spreading melanoma. This patient presented with a focal, eccentric, dark black macule within a pre-existing nevus.

In blacks and Asians, melanoma develops most commonly in an acral location, especially on palms and soles but also on mucosal sites.

Patients should be examined in a properly lit setting (direct light and at a tangential angle to the skin). Magnification is often helpful in examining suspicious lesions for distinctive coloration and surface changes. The dermatoscope, a handheld illuminated magnifier (10×) that is used after applying oil to the lesion, appears to improve diagnostic accuracy for the physician with sufficient training in its use.[6,7]

Examining a pigmented lesion to determine if it is benign or malignant requires a careful clinical assessment of its features, including size, color, border, and surface characteristics. Asymmetry is a hallmark of early melanoma. Asymmetry is identified by the lack of similarity in shape and (often) color when an axis is visualized through a lesion and opposite segments are compared (Figure 4–5, *A*). In contrast, benign pigmented lesions are usually round and symmetric.

Border irregularity is another key clinical feature of melanoma. The border of a melanoma has indentations that are discrete, sharp, and variable (see Figure 4–5, *B*). Benign pigmented lesions have borders that are regular and smooth (Figure 4–6, lesion on right). The borders of atypical nevi can be irregular; however, they lack the discrete, sharp cut-off seen in melanoma borders, and instead fade almost imperceptibly into normal skin (Figure 4–7; see also Figure 4–6, lesion on left).

Color change in melanoma exhibits variability and irregularity (see Figure 4–5, *C*). Variegation can be marked in later lesions whereas early lesions may have only focal darkening in an eccentric location. Benign pigmented lesions typically have uniform color. When variable, they tend to have order and to lack both the complexity and the haphazard dispersion of color that are identified with melanoma.

Size can be a helpful guide in distinguishing benign and malignant pigmented lesions as most melanomas are often larger lesions, measuring greater than 6 mm in size (see Figure 4–5, *D*).

The "ABCD" mnemonic has been widely used to help patients and health professionals remember the characteristic clinical features of melanoma[8] (A, asymmetry; B, border; C, color; D, diameter)

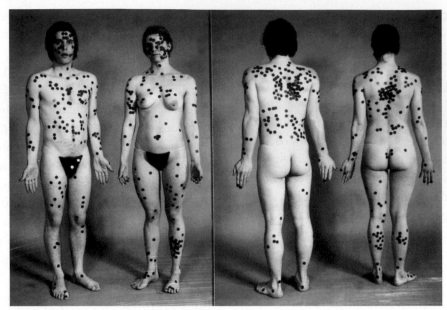

Figure 4–4.   Anatomic site distribution of primary cutaneous melanoma, by sex. (Courtesy of the Melanoma Clinical Cooperative Group)

(see Figure 4–5). It is important to recognize that although ABCD is a helpful mnemonic, its components are not definitive clinical diagnostic criteria. While the majority of melanomas may be diagnosed with such criteria, cutaneous melanomas may have all, some, or none of these clinical fea-

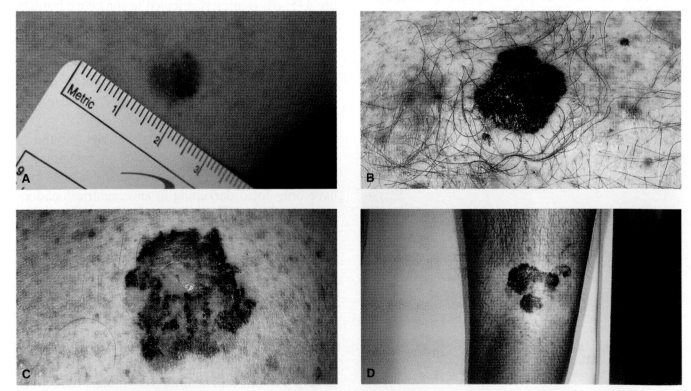

Figure 4–5.   "ABCDs" of melanoma. *A,* Asymmetry: the shape of one half of the lesion does not match that of the other half. *B,* Border: the border is irregular, uneven, or notched. *C,* Color: the color is variegated, with different shades of tan, brown, black, red, or pink. *D,* Diameter: the diameter is usually > 6 mm in melanomas; a change in size is an important early sign.

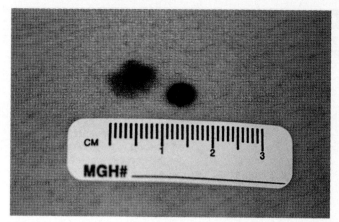

Figure 4–6. Dysplastic nevus (left) and compound nevus (right). Compare the compound nevus (right), which is a small, well-circumscribed, uniformly pigmented papule, with the dysplastic nevus (left), which has minimal color variegation (from tan to brown) and a border fading into the surrounding skin.

tures. For example, nodular melanomas are characteristically symmetric, with regular borders, and can be uniform in color or amelanotic. Size greater than 6 mm lacks validation and is not an absolute criterion as melanomas smaller than 6 mm are well recognized. In addition, there is a subset of melanomas that may be exceedingly difficult or impossible to diagnose on clinical examination alone as they lack the conventional clinical features of melanoma. Two subsets of lesions were defined in a study of clinically unsuspected melanomas: one group of melanomas clinically mimicked basal cell carcinomas; the other presented as lesions with hyperkeratotic or verrucous features such as seborrheic keratoses or verruca vulgaris.[9] The majority of these lesions (9 of 13) were amelanotic. We have identified several cases of clinically unsuspected melanomas that have mimicked basal cell carcinomas, benign nevi, and even eczematous dermatitis.[10] In the absence of the conventional clinical features of melanoma, the history of a persistently changing lesion or new lesion in a high-risk patient should be viewed with suspicion, and reassessment or biopsy should be performed. Several other clues are helpful. First, any verrucous scalp nevus with a clinical diagnosis of verruca vulgaris or seborrheic keratosis but on biopsy is histologically a dermal nevus is suspect. If the biopsy specimen shows atypia, the entire lesion should be removed. Second, any eczema resistant to usual therapeutic mea-

sures should be suspected as Bowen's disease, amelanotic melanoma, or possibly a T-cell dyscrasia, and a biopsy should be performed.

CLASSIFICATION

Four classic melanoma growth patterns with distinct clinical and pathologic features have been described (Table 4–3): superficial spreading, nodular, acral lentiginous, and lentigo maligna melanomas.

Superficial Spreading Melanoma

Superficial spreading melanoma (SSM) is the most common type of cutaneous melanoma (~70%), and can occur in any location on the skin. It frequently arises in a precursor nevus or dysplastic nevus and has a prolonged period of superficial or radial growth of 1 to 7 years.

Superficial spreading melanoma may arise in a nevus as a focal area of darkening or may develop as an irregular extension into the surrounding skin (Figures 4–8 and 4–9). It may also develop de novo as a darkly pigmented macule or barely raised plaque. Variegation in color is a key feature of melanoma, and SSM may become striking, with various hues of tan, brown, black, red, gray, and white (see Figure 4–5, *B* and *C*). The pigment can also be distributed irregularly or haphazardly. While the skin markings in the lesion remain intact initially, they can be lost with progression of SSM, and the surface may appear glossy. If regression is present, it may be recognized clinically as a gray or white area and can be enhanced with a Wood's lamp (long-wave

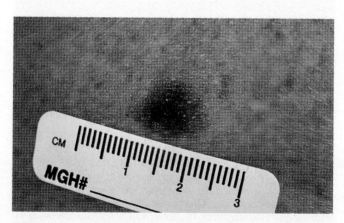

Figure 4–7. Dysplastic nevus. Note the central darker brown pigmentation and the tan-brown border fading into the surrounding skin.

Table 4–3. COMPARISONS OF CLINICAL FEATURES OF CUTANEOUS MELANOMA

Type of Melanoma	Frequency (%)	Duration before Diagnosis (yr)	Mean Age at Diagnosis	Site	Clinical Features
Radial-growth phase					
Superficial spreading melanoma	70	1–7	Mid-40s	Any site; lower legs in females, back in both sexes	Raised border on palpation or inspection; pink white, grays, and blues in brown lesion
Acral lentiginous melanoma (including subungual melanoma)	10	1–10	60s	Sole, palms, mucous membranes, subungual sites	Flat; irregular border; predominately dark brown to black with highly irregular border with areas of regression; brown-tan macular lesions with variation in pigment pattern; raised nodules within flat areas; brown, or black, may be amelanotic
Lentigo maligna melanoma	5	5–50	70s	Nose, cheeks, temples	Flat, pigmentary flare, showing shades of tan, brown, to dark brown, often with black flecks; gray areas associated with regression
No radial-growth phase					
Nodular melanoma	15	< 1	Mid- to late 40s	Any site	Nodule arises in apparently normal skin or in nevus; brown black; may have bluish hues; sometimes reddish plaques may be amelanotic

Adapted from Sober AJ. In: Soter NA, Baden HP, editors. Pathophysiology of dermatologic diseases. New York: McGraw-Hill; 1984.

ultraviolet). Irregularity of the borders of an SSM is an important finding, and sharp notching is often evident (see Figures 4–8 and 4–5, *B* and *C*). As the lesion enlarges radially, notching and irregularity of the border may become pronounced. The development of a raised papule or nodule may indicate the vertical-growth phase (ie, the lesion has begun deeper invasion and has acquired metastatic potential) (Figure 4–10; see also Figure 4–9; histologic features are illustrated in Figure 4–11).

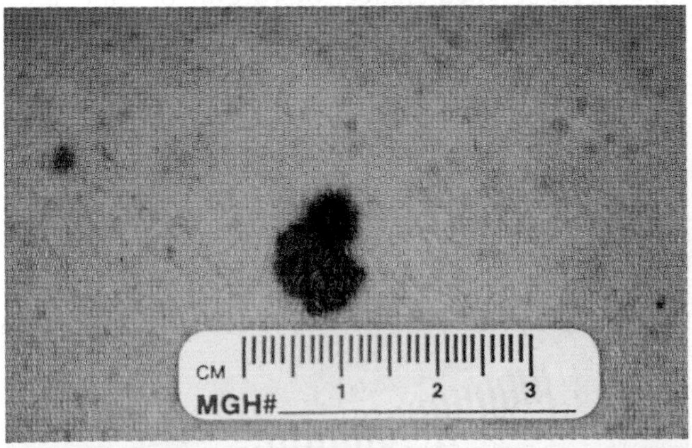

Nodular Melanoma

Nodular melanoma appears clinically as a papule or a nodule in the vertical-growth phase. In the majority of cases, nodular melanoma arises from clinically normal skin. Less frequently, it arises from a nevus,

Figure 4–8. Superficial spreading melanoma. A highly characteristic lesion with asymmetry, color variegation with shades of light brown and black, and irregularity of the border. (Reproduced with permission from Langley RG, Fitzpatrick TB, Sober AJ. Clinical characteristics. In: Balch CM, Houghton AN, Sober AJ, Soong SJ, editors. Cutaneous melanoma. 3rd ed. St. Louis: Quality Medical Publishing; 1998.)

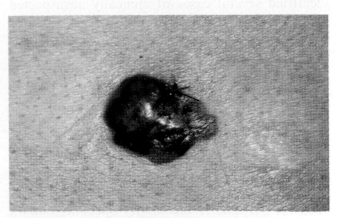

Figure 4–9. An invasive cutaneous melanoma arising in a nevus. Remnants of the nevus can be seen as the tan-brown areas on the left and inferior portion of the lesion.

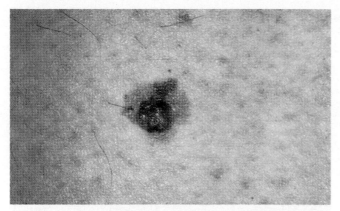

Figure 4–10. Superficial spreading melanoma, 1.0 mm in thickness, Clark level IV. A nodule is arising within the lesion, indicating a vertical-growth phase.

but by definition, no pre-existing radial-growth phase or spreading pigmented flare is detectable. It represents approximately 15 percent of melanomas and occurs most commonly on the trunk (in males) and legs (in females), with a peak incidence in the fifth decade. Nodular melanomas have a rapid onset and usually develop over several months.

In contrast to the other major forms of melanoma, nodular melanomas lack the conventional criteria (ABCD) that are helpful in the clinical diagnosis of the other subtypes of melanoma. Nodu-lar melanoma often presents as a symmetric papule or nodule with regular borders (Figure 4–12). The color is often uniform and is usually blue black or bluish red. Approximately 5 percent of cases are amelanotic (Figure 4–13). Nodular melanomas can also present as polypoid lesions with a stalk. Nodular melanoma (particularly when amelanotic) can be very difficult to diagnose clinically and may be confused with thrombosed hemangioma, pyogenic granuloma, blue nevus, eccrine poroma, and pigmented basal cell carcinoma, for example. (The histology of nodular melanoma is illustrated in Figure 4–14.)

Acral Lentiginous Melanoma

Acral lentiginous melanomas (ALMs) account for 5 to 10 percent of all melanomas and arise on acral locations, including palms, soles, and beneath the nail plate.

Location alone does not define ALMs; they are also characterized by the histology of the radial-growth phase (see below). Nodular melanomas and SSMs can also occur in acral locations. The majority of melanomas seen in Asians and blacks are ALMs; however, the site-specific incidence is similar in all races. The peak incidence is in the sixth

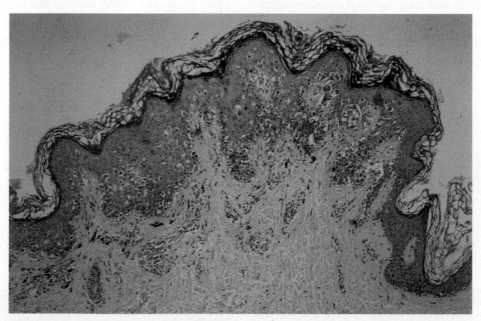

Figure 4–11. Superficial spreading melanoma: extensive proliferation of epithelioid cells that are focally contiguous along the dermoepidermal junction and that extend in a pagetoid array broadly up to the granular cell layer. These cells, whether singly disposed or in nests, all have uniform malignant change. There is no evidence of invasion in this in situ example.

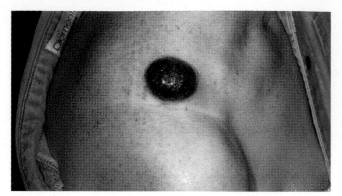

Figure 4–12. Nodular melanoma, invasive to Clark anatomic level V, with a measured depth of 42 mm. This striking advanced lesion arose de novo on the shoulder of a 51-year-old patient who unfortunately had regional node metastasis at the time of presentation.

decade, and ALM presents most frequently on the plantar surface of the foot. Acral lentiginous melanomas evolve slowly, with a prolonged radial-growth phase. Patients with ALMs may neglect these lesions, possibly because of the difficulty of examining them in locations such as the plantar foot, and may present with lesions measuring several centimeters in diameter.

The clinical characteristics of ALM are similar to the other types of melanoma when in radial-growth phase. It may initially present as a tan, brown, blue-black, or black macule. If neglected, an ALM may become quite large and may have striking asymmetry and irregular borders (Figures 4–15 and 4–16). The vertical-growth phase may be recognized in a papule or nodule that can be blue, black, or amelan-

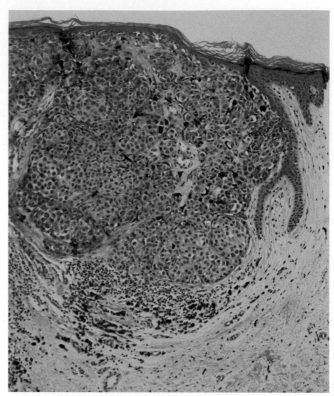

Figure 4–14. Nodular melanoma: an expansile nodule of epithelioid melanoma cells is defined by the hyperplastic epidermis, which envelops it on one side. Note the multifocal intraepidermal involvement over the nodule. There is no evidence of a radial-growth phase beyond the nodular component of the lesion. The lesion is invasive to Clark level III and has a measured depth of 0.7 mm.

otic. There are often significant delays in the diagnosis, and ulceration may be present, portending a poorer prognosis. When ALM is amelanotic, it may be misdiagnosed as a benign lesion because it may

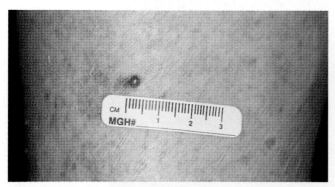

Figure 4–13. This 69-year-old patient presented with an asymptomatic pink papule on the right pretibial area. The biopsy specimen revealed an amelanotic melanoma invasive to Clark anatomic level IV, with a measured depth of 2.9 mm. (Reproduced with permission from Langley RG, Fitzpatrick TB, Sober AJ. Clinical characteristics. In: Balch CM, Houghton AN, Sober AJ, Soong SJ, editors. Cutaneous melanoma. 3rd ed. St. Louis: Quality Medical Publishing; 1998.)

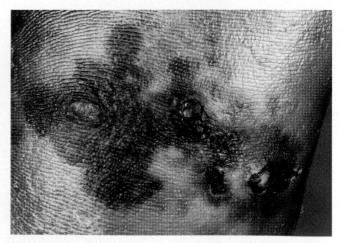

Figure 4–15. Acral lentiginous melanoma, vertical-growth phase. This highly asymmetric and darkly pigmented lesion on this black woman's plantar foot had marked border irregularity.

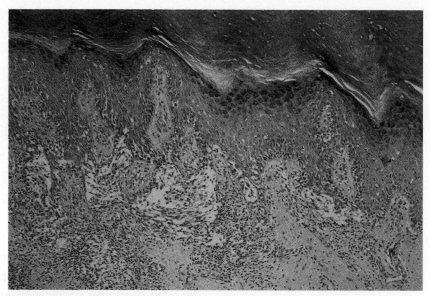

Figure 4–16. Acral lentiginous melanoma. Note the very hyperplastic rete ridges with almost fingerlike projections and the presence of strikingly malignant melanocytes with cytoplasm filled with melanin granules contiguously disposed along the basilar region. Focal pagetoid spread is associated with melanoma in situ in this region of the cutaneous surface of the body.

have a flesh-colored appearance resembling a clavus, wart, or pyogenic granuloma.

Subungual melanoma is a type of ALM that occurs most frequently on the thumb or great toe. The initial appearance may be nondescript, simply a brown to black discoloration in the nail bed, in a periungual location, or in the nail matrix. The pigmentation may extend as a longitudinal pigmented band and may resemble a benign lesion such as a nevus, which can be difficult to differentiate from a subungual

melanoma by clinical examination alone (Figure 4–17). Extension of pigmentation beyond the cuticle onto the skin of the proximal nail fold is an important diagnostic sign (known as Hutchinson's sign) associated with melanoma, and should prompt an excisional biopsy. With progression, ulceration can occur, with loss of the nail plate (Figure 4–18). Subungual melanoma may resemble (and be misdiagnosed as) a subungual hematoma, onychomycosis, paronychia, ingrown toenail, nevus, wart, or pyogenic granuloma.

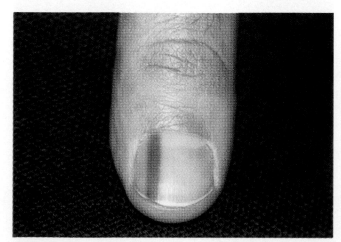

Figure 4–17. Melanonychia striata. This 35-year-old male presented with a recent-onset, linear, narrow, light brown pigmentation on the thumbnail. Biopsy of this lesion revealed a nevus.

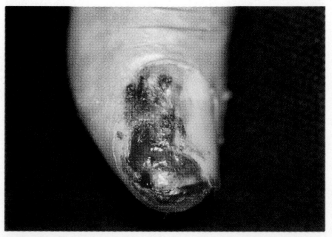

Figure 4–18. Advanced-stage subungual melanoma. There is partial loss of the nail plate due to the tumor, which occupies a portion of the nail bed.

Subungual hematomas are common and are important to differentiate. These lesions are often acutely painful, and there is usually a history of trauma at the site. They may appear as discrete black, maroon, or multicolored lesions located within the nail bed or matrix. A diagnostic and therapeutic procedure involves piercing the nail with a large-bore needle or the tip of a heated paper clip to release the blood in symptomatic cases of recent onset. The nail should be re-examined because a subungual hematoma will gradually resolve, with clearing of the discoloration of the proximal portion as the nail plate grows out.

Lentigo Maligna Melanoma

Lentigo maligna melanoma (LMM) typically occurs on chronically sun-exposed and photodamaged skin, particularly on the head and neck, with the nose and cheek being favored locations. It comprises approximately 4 to 15 percent of all melanomas and occurs predominately in elderly patients, with a peak incidence in the seventh decade.

The tumor can be present for long periods (5 to 15 years) in its precursor form (lentigo maligna) before invasion occurs. In the precursor form, it gradually enlarges and extends peripherally with markedly irregular borders with prominent notching; it can become large, measuring several centimeters or more (Figure 4–19). The coloration of lentigo maligna is

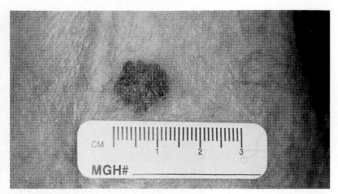

Figure 4–20. Lentigo maligna. This was a flat (macular) lesion with prominent color variation.

typically tan brown, with differing shades throughout (Figure 4–20). It appears as a stain in the skin, usually with the same reflectance as the adjacent non-pigmented skin. Early lentigo maligna may sometimes be difficult to distinguish clinically from solar

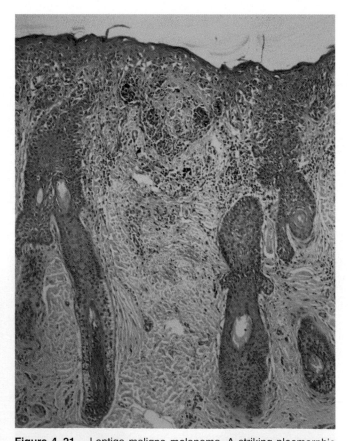

Figure 4–21. Lentigo maligna melanoma. A striking pleomorphic population of hyperchromatic melanocytes is present along the basilar region of the epidermis and the external root sheath of the hair follicle. Focal pagetoid spread is observed. Note the presence of invasive nests of hyperchromatic melanocytes in the papillary dermis, associated with chronic inflammatory cells. The lesion is invasive to Clark level II and has a measured depth of 0.3 mm.

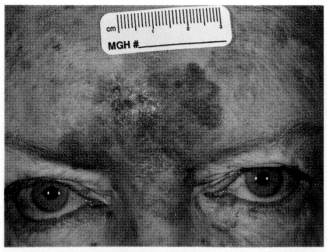

Figure 4–19. Lentigo maligna melanoma. This 80-year-old patient presented with a slowly enlarging lesion with asymmetry and tan, brown, and dark brown colors.

lentigines or pigmented actinic keratosis. These lesions have a dull reflectance when compared to lentigo maligna. As the lesion enlarges, the pigmentation may appear mottled with flecks of dark brown or black pigmentation. Gray or white areas appear as sites of partial regression. Lentigo maligna may eventuate into LMM, but the exact percentage of this transformation is not known. The risk of developing LMM from lentigo maligna is believed to vary by age: the lifetime risk has been calculated as 4.7 percent at 45 years of age and a 2.2 percent for a 65-year-old.[11] A striking characteristic of early LMM is its flatness. A discrete papular or nodular area usually signals that invasion has occurred and may indicate the presence of the vertical-growth phase. Lentigo maligna melanoma tends to be considerably variable in color (with hues of tan, brown, black, or blue gray) and can be amelanotic. These tumors can have extremely convoluted borders with prominent notching and indentation (histology is depicted in Figure 4–21). Amelanotic variants of lentigo maligna and LMM rarely occur. These lesions are usually mistaken for Bowen's disease or eczema.

REFERENCES

1. Rhodes AR, Weinstock MA, Fitzpatrick TB, et al. Risk factors for cutaneous melanoma. A practical method of recognizing predisposed individuals. JAMA 1987;258:3146–54.

2. Piepkorn M. Melanoma genetics: an update with focus on the CDKN2A p1 tumor suppressors. J Am Acad Dermatol 2000;42:705–22.

3. Langley RG, Sober AJ. A clinical review of the evidence for the role of ultraviolet radiation in the etiology of cutaneous melanoma. Cancer Invest 1997;15:561–7.

4. Elwood JM. Melanoma and sun exposure. Semin Oncol 1996;23:650–66.

5. Wick MM, Sober AJ, Fitzpatrick TB, et al. Clinical characteristics of early cutaneous melanoma. Cancer 1980;45:2684–6.

6. Steiner A, Pehamberger H, Wolff K. In vivo epiluminescence microscopy of pigmented skin lesions. II. Diagnosis of small pigmented skin lesions and early detection of malignant melanoma. J Am Acad Dermatol 1987;17:584–91.

7. Binder M, Schwarz M, Winkler A, et al. Epiluminescence microscopy. A useful tool for the diagnosis of pigmented skin lesions for formally trained dermatologists. Arch Dermatol 1995;131:286–91.

8. Friedman RJ, Rigel DS, Kopf AW. Early detection of malignant melanoma: the role of physician examination and self-examination of the skin. CA Cancer J Clin 1985;35:130–51.

9. Andersen WK, Silvers DN. "Melanoma? It can't be melanoma!" A subset of melanomas that defy clinical recognition. JAMA 1991;266:3463–5.

10. Langley RG, Fitzpatrick TB, Sober AJ. Clinical characteristics. In: Balch CM, Houghton AN, Sober AJ, Soong SJ, editors. Cutaneous melanoma. St. Louis: Quality Medical Publishing, Inc.; 1998.

11. Weinstock MA, Sober AJ. The risk of progression of lentigo maligna to lentigo maligna melanoma. Br J Dermatol 1987;116:303–10.

5

Basal Cell Carcinoma

GREGG M. MENAKER, MD

DIANE S. CHIU, MD

Basal cell carcinoma (BCC) is the most common cutaneous malignancy. Although this tumor very rarely metastasizes, it is capable of extensive tissue destruction and local invasion. Its cells are thought to be derived from the basal cell layer of the epidermis and the outer root sheath of the hair follicle. Synonyms for BCC include *basal cell epithelioma*, *basalioma*, and *rodent ulcer*.

EPIDEMIOLOGY AND RISK FACTORS

In white races, BCC is the most common malignant tumor. Each year, an estimated 900,000 new cases are diagnosed in the United States, with incidence rates as high as 300 per 100,000 population.[1] There is evidence of a striking increase in the incidence of non-melanoma skin cancer in North America during the past two decades.[1,2] The lifetime risk of developing BCC in the United States is 30 percent.[1,2] This disease is more common with increasing age, its incidence typically beginning after the age of 30 years and peaking at the age 70 years.[3] In recent years, however, BCC has become more common in young adults. Men make up just over half of all patients with BCC.[4,5]

Exposure to ultraviolet (UV) light is thought to be a major risk factor in the development of BCC. About 85 percent of tumors occur on sun-exposed areas, particularly the head and neck, while approximately 15 percent of tumors occur on skin protected from sun exposure.[6,7] Recent studies have suggested that intermittent high-dose sun exposure in childhood and adolescence may be more important than cumulative lifetime radiation exposure.[6,8,9] Therefore, the pattern of UV exposure significant to the development of BCC may be more similar to that of malignant melanoma than to that of squamous cell carcinoma (SCC).

While the nose is the most commonly involved site for BCC, the eyelids, the inner canthi, and postauricular areas are also frequently involved. Basal cell carcinoma is uncommon on the dorsa of the hands and the forearms. The palms, the soles, and the vermilion border of the lips are rarely involved. There is a strong correlation between BCC and anatomic areas associated with an increased density of pilosebaceous follicles, with tumors occurring almost exclusively on hair-bearing skin. In contrast, the distribution and prevalence of SCC is clearly linked to areas exposed to UV light.

Individuals with light skin color, blond or red hair, blue or green eyes, an inability to tan, a tendency to freckle easily, and a family history of skin cancer are at increased risk for BCC.[3,10] The incidence is increased in individuals of Celtic ancestry whereas those of southern European descent have a decreased risk.[8,9] Significant outdoor exposure, particularly in outdoor occupations such as farming, has also been regarded as a risk factor.[3,10] Basal cell carcinoma is extremely uncommon in darker-skinned races (African Americans, Asians, Native Americans, etc.).

Skin damaged by ionizing radiation, thermal injury, vaccination scars, and chronic inflammation is more susceptible to the development of BCC.[3,11–14] Various benign and malignant cutaneous tumors have also been associated with BCC, including melanoma, SCC, keratoacanthoma, neurofibroma, seborrheic keratosis, nevus sebaceous, linear epidermal nevus, nevomelanocytic nevus, infundibular cyst, pilomatricoma, hemangioma, and condyloma acuminatum.[13–18] Arsenic present in drinking water or in preparations such as Fowler's solution is another proven risk factor for BCC.[19]

Immunocompromised patients have an increased BCC risk that is postulated to be the result of impaired cell-mediated immunity as well as of increased susceptibility to oncogenic viruses.[20] Patients with acquired immunodeficiency syndrome (AIDS) or those receiving immunosuppressive drugs following solid organ transplantation are at increased risk for both BCC and SCC.[21,22] After renal transplantation, the overall incidence of SCC is 250 times higher compared to that of the general population, while that of BCC is 10 times higher.[22] In these patients, the tumors may also be more aggressive, with an increased likelihood of recurrence or metastasis.

PATHOGENESIS

The tumor cells of BCC are basophilic, with compact nuclei and a relatively small amount of cytoplasm. Their morphology is similar to the cells of the basal layer of the epidermis and its appendages. Recent studies with antikeratin antibodies demonstrated that BCC possesses a keratin pattern that resembles that of the outer root sheath of the hair follicle below the isthmus and/or the bulge region of the vellus hair follicle, rather than that of the basal cell epithelium.[23,24] This supports the theory that these tumors are follicularly derived and may help to explain their almost exclusive occurrence in hair-bearing skin. Basal cell carcinoma is capable of differentiating into various adnexal and epithelial structures, a feature most likely derived from pleuripotential immature epithelial cells. Tumor maturation is stroma dependent, being governed by the connective tissue in its proximity.[25] It is widely believed that the failure of BCC to grow in tissue culture may be related to its stromal dependence. The characteristic peripheral palisade of tumor cells is produced by the interaction with the dermis.

On histopathologic sections, stromal retraction is often observed around the tumor. This finding was once regarded as a fixation artifact. However, immunostaining of the peritumoral lacunae with laminin, type IV collagen, and bullous pemphigoid antibodies revealed the presence of laminin and type IV collagen on the stroma side of the lacunae, but an absence of bullous pemphigoid antigen. Therefore, loss of bullous pemphigoid antigen may contribute to the characteristic stromal retraction seen in association with some types of BCC.[26]

Basal cell carcinoma also is associated with increased collagenase production by fibroblasts, which decreases the number of anchoring fibrils and the collagen content in the basement membrane zone.[14] In addition, the number of hemidesmosomes is diminished, and the expression of bullous pemphigoid antigens, epiligrin, and the $\alpha_6\beta_4$ integrins is altered, resulting in a further weakening of the basement membrane zone and thus facilitating tumor invasion.[14,27,28]

Several of the genodermatoses are associated with an increased incidence and an earlier age of onset of BCC. The most studied of these include basal cell nevus syndrome (or Gorlin's syndrome), albinism, and xeroderma pigmentosum. Examination of these inherited syndromes has helped elucidate the pathophysiology and molecular genetics of BCC.

Nevoid basal cell carcinoma syndrome (NBCCS), also known as basal cell nevus syndrome or Gorlin's syndrome, is an autosomal dominant disorder of developmental anomalies, characterized by numerous BCCs (possibly hundreds), beginning as early as 2 years of age.[29–31] Other features include palmar and plantar pits, odontogenic keratocysts of the jaw, calcification of soft tissues such as the falx cerebri, calcified ovarian fibromas, spina bifida occulta, rib abnormalities, scoliosis or kyphosis, macrocephaly with characteristic facies (including frontal bossing, broad nasal root, and hypertelorism), and mental deficiency. Medulloblastoma and cardiac fibroma are other tumors associated with this syndrome. Genetic analysis has localized the responsible gene to chromosome 9q22.[31–33] This site is the location for the human homologue of the *"patched"* gene, originally identified in *Drosophila* to encode a protein involved in tissue organization.[34] The exact mechanism for neoplasia is unclear, but the gene is thought to play a prenatal role in embryonal structural development as well as a postnatal role as a tumor suppressor gene. Studies of sporadic BCC as well as NBCCS-associated tumors have demonstrated a high frequency of allelic loss at chromosome 9q22, suggesting the probability of a tumor suppressor gene at this site.[31–33]

The patched (PTCH) gene product functions as a transmembrane receptor for the sonic hedgehog (SHH) protein. Overexpression of SHH has been found to induce the development of BCC in mice as well as to induce the development of BCC-like features in transgenic human skin.[35, 36] Thus, SHH is thought to inhibit PTCH function. Additionally, the binding of SHH to PTCH is also thought to prevent normal inhibition by PTCH of a 7-span transmembrane protein known as *smoothened* (SMO). Mutations in the SMO gene, localized to chromosome 7q32, have been found in sporadic BCCs.[37,38] Furthermore, skin abnormalities similar to BCCs have developed in transgenic murine skin overexpressing mutant SMO.[38]

Ultraviolet radiation–induced mutation of the *p53* tumor suppressor gene has also been implicated in the development of cutaneous malignancies.[39,40] The majority of nonmelanoma skin cancers, including over 50 percent of BCCs and 90 percent of SCCs, have been shown to contain specific *p53* mutations associated with ultraviolet B (UVB) exposure.[41]

Xeroderma pigmentosum is an autosomal recessive disorder characterized by an inability to repair deoxyribonucleic acid (DNA) damage induced by UV radiation. This failure of DNA repair leads to the persistence of mutagenic pyrimidine (thymine) dimers. Patients show extreme photosensitivity and develop widespread cutaneous tumors, including BCCs, SCCs, and malignant melanomas. These patients have a 1,000-fold higher incidence of cutaneous malignancy, compared to the normal population.[42,43]

People with various forms of albinism exhibit defective or absent tyrosinase, which impairs the ability to produce melanin. This confers decreased photoprotection against UV radiation, and patients are subsequently at increased risk for developing multiple skin tumors upon exposure to UV light.

CLINICAL SUBTYPES AND PATHOLOGIC FEATURES

Characteristic cells of BCC resemble those of the basal cell layer of the epidermis but generally have a larger nucleus-cytoplasm ratio and do not exhibit intercellular bridges. The nuclei are usually oval or elongated and are nonanaplastic in appearance.

Basal cell carcinomas are associated with many histologic patterns that behave differently and have variable outcomes and prognoses. Tumors may be classified as nodular, superficial, micronodular, morpheaform, infiltrating, pigmented, metatypical, and fibroepitheliomas of Pinkus, with a significant proportion showing mixed patterns.

Nodular Basal Cell Carcinoma

The most common form of BCC, accounting for over 50 percent of tumors, is the nodular type. These are the typical dome-shaped pearly papules and nodules with rolled translucent borders and telangiectasias (Figure 5–1, *A*). They frequently become crusted or ulcerated and are often seen in conjunction with actinically damaged skin. The lesions generally enlarge slowly and are also known as rodent ulcers (see Figure 5–1, *B*). Histopathologically, these tumors are composed of large well-defined nodular aggregates of basophilic neoplastic cells. There is peripheral palisading of nuclei and retraction of the tumor from surrounding stroma (see Figure 5–1, *C* to *E*). A cystic appearance may also be appreciated when mucin is present in large aggregates.

Superficial Basal Cell Carcinoma

Superficial BCC presents clinically as erythematous scaly papules or plaques, most commonly on the trunk or extremities. It also occasionally presents on other sun-exposed areas such as the head and neck. These lesions are usually well defined, often with a slightly elevated border, and they exhibit slow centrifugal growth (Figure 5–2, *A* to *C*). There may be areas of erosion or crusting. These tumors can become invasive over time. Histologically, atypical basaloid cells show a broad attachment to the overlying epidermis and hair follicle epithelium. Tumor islands are relatively small. Peripheral palisading is present and stromal retraction is seen (see Figure 5–2, *D*).

Micronodular Basal Cell Carcinoma

Micronodular tumors are poorly defined indurated firm plaques that are associated with an increased incidence of recurrence. Histologically, these lesions

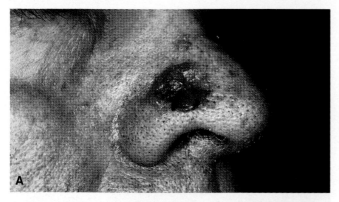

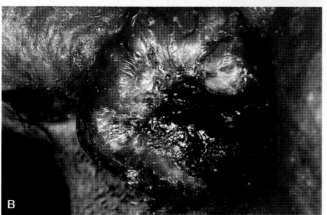

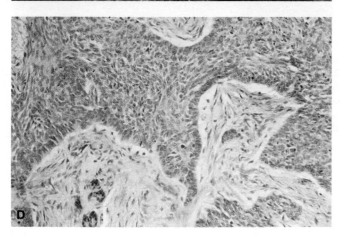

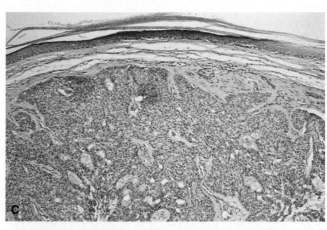

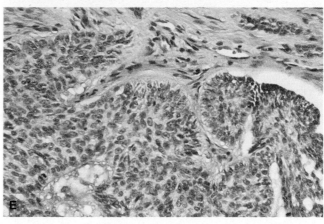

Figure 5–1. *A*, Nodular basal cell carcinoma (BCC) of the nose, presenting as a pearly plaque with a rolled translucent border, telangiectases, and central crusting. *B*, Classic rodent ulcer form of BCC. *C*, Histopathologic micrograph of nodular BCC (hematoxylin and eosin; ×100 original magnification), demonstrating a large well-defined aggregate of basophilic cells. *D*, Histopathologic micrograph of nodular BCC (hematoxylin and eosin; ×200 original magnification), demonstrating the peripheral palisading of tumor cell nuclei. *E*, Histopathologic micrograph of nodular BCC (hematoxylin and eosin; ×320 original magnification). There is peripheral palisading of nuclei as well as stromal retraction. Tumor cells are oval-shaped and have a large nucleus-cytoplasm ratio.

appear similar to nodular BCC, but with smaller rounded nests (approximately the size of hair bulbs) that exhibit minimal palisading. Stromal retraction is also uncommon, and the tumor nodules are asymmetric and widely dispersed (Figure 5–3).

Morpheaform (Sclerosing) Basal Cell Carcinoma

Morpheaform BCC (also known as sclerosing, fibrosing, or desmoplastic BCC) is generally the

most diagnostically and therapeutically challenging subtype. It accounts for up to 5 percent of all BCCs and tends to be more aggressive, sometimes invading deeply into muscle and fat. Clinically, it resembles a scar or a small patch of scleroderma and appears as a whitish to yellowish fibrotic plaque with poorly defined margins (Figure 5–4). No particular anatomic site is preferred, and the lesions rarely ulcerate or bleed. Aggregates of tumor cells are small, thin, and elongated, with sharp angulated ends. The surrounding stroma is densely fibrotic.

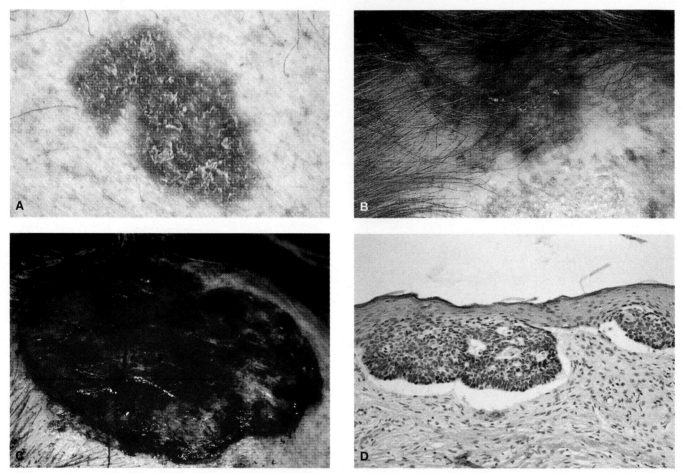

Figure 5–2. *A,* Superficial basal cell carcinoma (BCC) of the trunk, presenting as a well-defined erythematous scaly plaque. Clinically, it may be confused with eczema, psoriasis, or Bowen's disease. *B,* Superficial BCC of the forehead, presenting as a well-defined erythematous scaly plaque with a slightly elevated border and some areas of surface crusting. *C,* Post–Mohs' micrographic surgery defect of the superficial BCC depicted in Figure 5–2, *B*. Though slow growing, these lesions can become quite extensive and occasionally may become invasive. *D,* Histopathologic micrograph of superficial BCC (hematoxylin and eosin; x200 original magnification), demonstrating the broad attachment of the small basaloid tumor cell nests to the overlying epidermis. Peripheral palisading and stromal retraction are also evident.

Peripheral palisading is generally absent, and stromal retraction is rare.

Infiltrating Basal Cell Carcinoma

Histologically, infiltrating BCC lies somewhere between the nodular and morpheaform subtypes although it is clinically often classified together with morpheaform BCC. On examination, these tumors are whitish yellow, poorly defined, and often difficult to differentiate from the surrounding skin (Figure 5–5, *A*). Histologically, the tumor lobules are irregular, angulated, and jagged, with elongated strands that invade into the deep dermis and occasionally into the subcutaneous fat and muscle. The surrounding stroma is fibrotic, although not as sclerotic as in mor-

pheaform BCC. Peripheral palisading and stromal retraction is rarely seen (see Figure 5–5, *B*).

Pigmented Basal Cell Carcinoma

Pigmented basal cell carcinoma is a fairly common BCC variant, especially in dark-skinned people. Clinically, the lesions are fairly well-defined papules or plaques with a translucent or pearly appearance and range in color from pink to dark brown or black. They may be confused with other lesions such as malignant melanomas, seborrheic keratoses, or benign melanocytic nevi (Figure 5–6, *A*). Histologically, their features are similar to those of nodular BCCs with variable amounts of melanin present within the basaloid cells and macrophages. The melanin is produced by benign melanocytes found interspersed within the tumor (see Figure 5–6, *B*).

Metatypical Basal Cell Carcinoma

The metatypical BCC has clinical and histologic features of both BCC and SCC. It tends to be more aggressive than other forms of BCC and can grow with the speed of SCC, with a higher incidence of metastasis (Figure 5–7, *A*).[44,45] Metatypical BCC cells are larger and possess a paler nucleus and more eosinophilic cytoplasm than the cells of other forms of BCC. Peripheral palisading and stromal retraction are absent. These lesions may exhibit prominent mitotic activity, with dyskeratosis. Keratin pearls may occasionally be seen (see Figure 5–7, *B*).

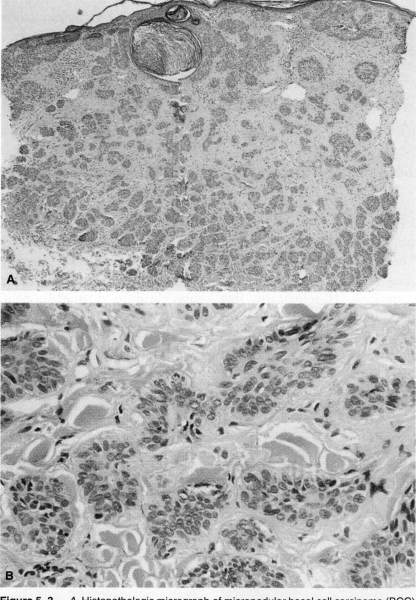

Figure 5–3. *A,* Histopathologic micrograph of micronodular basal cell carcinoma (BCC) (hematoxylin and eosin; x50 original magnification). Microscopically, these lesions appear similar to nodular BCC but display smaller rounded nests approximately the size of hair bulbs. The tumor nodules are widely dispersed and asymmetric. *B,* Histopathologic micrograph of micronodular BCC, (hematoxylin and eosin; x320 original magnification). In contrast to nodular BCC these small rounded tumor nests exhibit minimal palisading of nuclei. Stromal retraction is also uncommon.

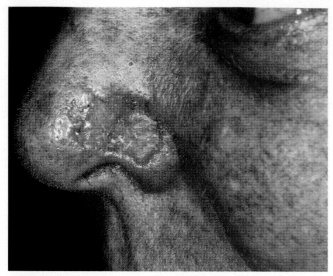

Figure 5–4. Morpheaform basal cell carcinoma (BCC) of the nose, presenting as a fibrotic whitish yellow plaque with poorly defined margins. Often diagnostically challenging, it may resemble a scar or a small patch of scleroderma.

Fibroepithelioma of Pinkus

An unusual variant of BCC, fibroepithelioma of Pinkus was first described in 1953 and is most commonly seen in the lumbosacral area.[46] The lesions appear as pink to flesh-colored, sessile, dome-shaped nodules that may resemble a fibroepithelial polyp or seborrheic keratosis. Histologically, this tumor exhibits features of both superficial BCC and reticulated seborrheic keratosis. Branching strands of basaloid cells proliferate symmetrically and can extend deep into the dermis. This thin honeycomb

pattern of cells surrounds a fibromucinous stroma. Stromal retraction is uncommon, but peripheral palisading is seen. Horn cysts are sometimes present. Although originally considered premalignant, fibroepithelioma of Pinkus may evolve into an ulcerative and invasive BCC (Figure 5–8).

DIAGNOSIS

The differential diagnosis of BCC depends on the subtype. Nodular BCC (the most common nodular form) must be distinguished from intradermal nevus, sebaceous hyperplasia, and molluscum contagiosum. Surface scaling or crusting can cause the lesion to be confused with keratoacanthoma, SCC, or verruca vulgaris. Pigmented BCC must be differentiated from malignant melanoma. Superficial BCC may look like nummular eczema, psoriasis, actinic keratosis, Bowen's disease, or seborrheic keratosis. Morpheaform and infiltrating BCCs usually present the greatest diagnostic challenge. They are often difficult to detect clinically as they resemble a scar or a small patch of scleroderma.

Histologically, BCC can exhibit cutaneous appendageal differentiation resembling hair follicles or apocrine, eccrine, and sebaceous glands, which may lead to diagnostic confusion. We recently observed a large (5 cm) ulcerated plaque with hemorrhagic scale crust, telangiectasias, and a thick pearly nodular border on the temple of an elderly patient seen at Massachusetts General Hospital (Fig-

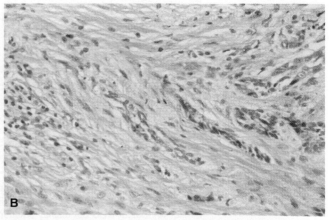

Figure 5–5. *A,* Infiltrating basal cell carcinoma (BCC) of the chest, presenting as a sclerotic plaque that may be difficult to differentiate from surrounding normal skin. Clinically, this lesion is indistinguishable from the morpheaform subtype, and they are often classified together. *B,* Histopathologic micrograph of infiltrating BCC (hematoxylin and eosin; x320 original magnification), depicting irregular tumor lobules with elongated strands that invade into the deep dermis and occasionally into the subcutaneous fat and muscle. The surrounding stroma is fibrotic.

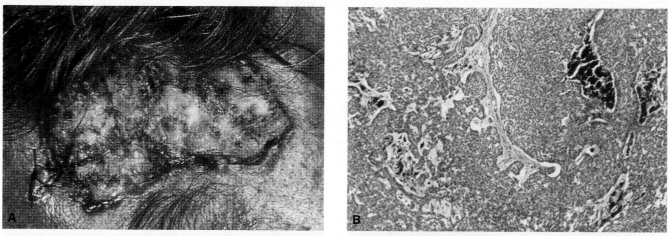

Figure 5–6. *A,* Pigmented basal cell carcinoma (BCC) presenting as a well-defined plaque with a pearly rolled border that is brown black. The central portion of the lesion ranges in color from pink to black and displays some superficial ulceration. *B,* Histopathologic micrograph of pigmented BCC (hematoxylin and eosin; x200 original magnification). Melanin is present within the tumor cells and in macrophages.

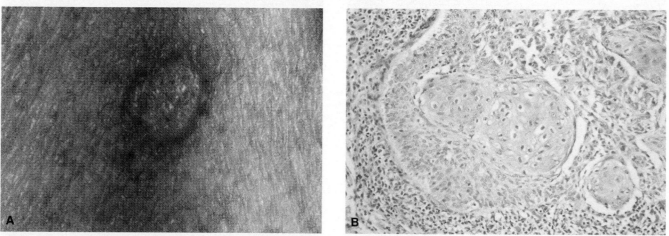

Figure 5–7. *A,* Metatypical basal cell carcinoma (BCC) of the neck. This lesion has clinical and histopathologic features of both BCC and squamous cell carcinoma. *B,* Histopathologic micrograph of metatypical BCC depicts larger tumor cells with paler nuclei and more eosinophilic cytoplasm (hematoxylin and eosin; x320 original magnification).

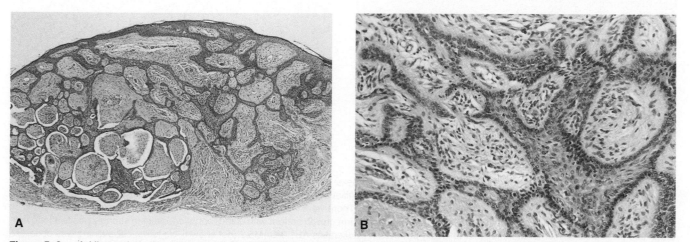

Figure 5–8. *A,* Histopathologic micrograph of fibroepithelioma of Pinkus (x50 original magnification). This tumor resembles both superficial BCC and reticulated seborrheic keratosis. The branching strands of basaloid cells can extend deep into the dermis. *B,* Histopathologic micrograph of fibroepithelioma of Pinkus (hematoxylin and eosin; x200 original magnification) depicts peripheral palisading and fibromucinous stroma.

ure 5–9, *A*). The initial biopsy of the lesion showed findings most consistent with invasive adenocarcinoma thought to be secondary to metastasis, although a primary adnexal tumor could not be ruled out (see Figure 5–9, *B* and *C*). However, since the clinical examination of the lesion was most suggestive of a BCC, another biopsy was performed. This biopsy showed tumor consistent with the nodular

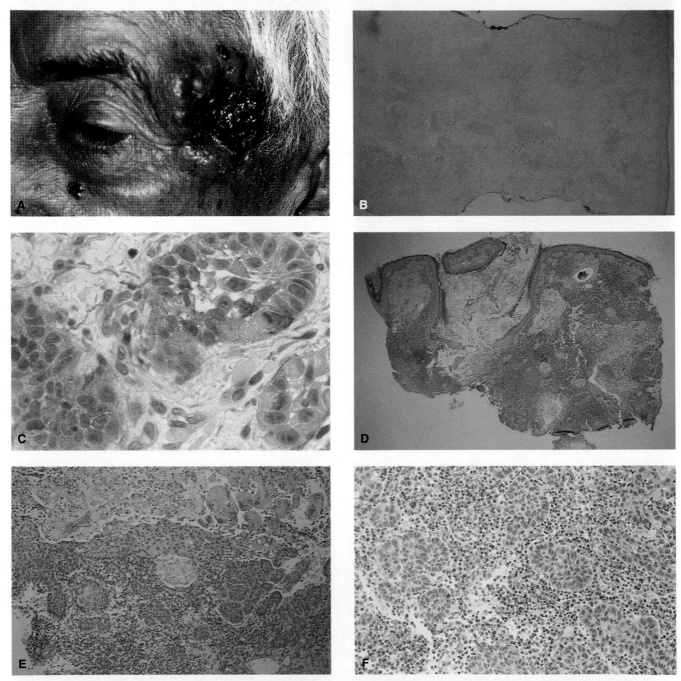

Figure 5–9.   Case study of a basal cell carcinoma with marked adnexal differentiation. *A*, An elderly patient presenting with a 5-cm ulcerated nodule on the right temple. *B*, *C*, Histopathologic micrographs of the initial skin biopsy specimen revealed findings most consistent with invasive adenocarcinoma (hematoxylin and eosin; x50 original magnification). There were no changes of the overlying epidermis or superficial dermis. In the deeper dermis, cytologically atypical tumor cells displayed a cribriform growth pattern with gland formation, staining strongly positive for cytokeratin 903 and epithelial membrane antigen and focally positive for cytokeratins AE1.3/CAM5.2 (not shown). No tumor cell staining was observed for carcinoembryonic antigen (CEA) or prostate-specific antigen. These results most supported a metastatic process although a primary adnexal tumor could not be ruled out. *D*, *E*, *F*, Histopathologic micrographs of the specimen from the second skin biopsy show tumor consistent with BCC (nodular and metatypical), with marked adnexal differentiation (hematoxylin and eosin; original magnification: *D*, x50; *E*, x200; *F*, x320).

and metatypical types of BCC, with marked adnexal differentiation (Figure 5–9, *D* to *F*). It was noted that the tumor morphology was distinctly different from that of the initial biopsy specimen. Thus, when pathologic findings do not corroborate with the clinical examination, clinicopathologic correlation is vital, and repeat sampling may be necessary.

The "gold standard" for diagnosis of any BCC is skin biopsy. A recent study found no significant difference between a punch biopsy and a shave biopsy in determining the histologic subtype of BCC.[47] The texture of a BCC upon manipulation is generally soft and friable. With small tumors (< 1 cm), primary BCCs may appear to be completely removed after a biopsy. However, the incidence of residual BCC in patients with no clinical evidence of residual tumor after biopsy is 66 percent.[48] Thus, it is important to adequately treat all patients who appear to be "cured" after biopsy.

COURSE AND PROGNOSIS

The untreated BCC typically runs a slowly progressive course of peripheral extension, invasion, and destruction of adjacent tissue (Figure 5–10). In those lesions that involve the face, severe mutilation (particularly of the nose and eyes) may occur. Invasive tumors may extend into the skull, sinuses, dura, and brain and may cause death if neglected. Dissemination of BCC is exceptionally rare and is often associated with recurrent lesions that are unresponsive to repeated surgical treatment or radiotherapy.[49] Also, metastasis may depend on the size of the original lesion and the depth of tumor invasion.[4,50] Tumors greater than 3 cm in diameter have a 2 percent incidence of metastasis and/or death. This increases to 25 percent in those lesions more than 5 cm in diameter, and to 50 percent in lesions more than 10 cm in diameter.[51] Histologic subtype is poorly correlated with the development of metastasis. The reported incidence of metastasis ranges from 0.0028 to 0.1 percent; the most common sites involve lymph nodes, lung, and bone via lymphatic or hematogenous spread.[52–54] Once the diagnosis of metastasis has occurred, the median survival is 8 months.[52]

A patient with one BCC should be observed for both local recurrence and emergence of new tumors.

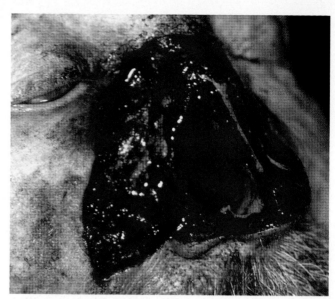

Figure 5–10. Post–Mohs' micrographic surgery defect showing extensive involvement of the nose by basal cell carcinoma.

After 5 years, recurrent lesions appear in about 9 percent of conventionally treated primary lesions and in 1 percent of primary lesions treated with Mohs' micrographic surgery.[55] The prognosis and recurrence rates for recurrent BCC are much worse; the 5-year recurrence rate was 20 percent for recurrent lesions treated with all non-Mohs' modalities and approximately 6 percent for those treated with Mohs' micrographic surgery.[56] Lesions of the nose and ears are most likely to recur, and the time course of recurrence is usually within 3 years of treatment.[55] Unlike SCC, there is no premalignant stage of BCC equivalent to actinic keratoses. Following treatment of one BCC, the risk of developing a subsequent tumor within 5 years is 45 percent.[57]

ACKNOWLEDGMENTS

Thomas J. Flotte, MD, for preparation of histopathologic slides; Lyn M. Duncan, MD, for preparation of histopathologic slides (Figure 5–9, *B* to *F*); and Erin M. Bowler, BS, for preparation of clinical photographs.

REFERENCES

1. Miller DL, Weinstock MA. Nonmelanoma skin cancer in the United States: incidence. J Am Acad Dermatol 1994;30:774–8.

2. Lear JT, Smith AG. Basal cell carcinoma. Postgrad Med J 1997;73:538–42.

3. Goldberg LH. Basal cell carcinoma. Lancet 1996;347: 663–7.

4. Randle HW. Basal cell carcinoma: identification and treatment of the high-risk patient. Dermatol Surg 1996;22:255-61.

5. Chuang TY, Popescu A, Su WPD, Chute CG. Basal cell carcinoma. A population based incidence study in Rochester, Minnesota. J Am Acad Dermatol 1990; 22:413–7.

6. Gallagher RP, Hill GB, Bajdik CD, et al. Sunlight exposure, pigmentary factors, and risk of nonmelanocytic skin cancer. 1. Basal cell carcinoma. Arch Dermatol 1995;131:157–63.

7. Franceschi S, Levi F, Randimbison L, La Vecchia C. Site distribution of different types of skin cancer: new aetiological clues. Int J Cancer 1996;67:24–8.

8. Kricker A, Armstrong BK, English DR, Heenan PJ. A dose response curve for sun exposure and basal cell carcinoma. Int J Cancer 1995;60:482–8.

9. Kricker A, Armstrong BK, English DR, Heenan PJ. Does intermittent sun exposure cause basal cell carcinoma? A case control study in Western Australia. Int J Cancer 1995;60:489–94.

10. Hogan DJ, To T, Gran L, et al. Risk factors for basal cell carcinoma. Int J Dermatol 1989; 28:591–4.

11. Escudero Nafs FJ, Guarch Troyas R, Perez Montejano-Sierra M, Colas San Juan C. Basal cell carcinoma in a vaccination scar. Plast Reconstr Surg 1995;95: 199–200

12. Stromberg BV, Klingman R, Schluter WW. Basal cell burn carcinoma. Ann Plast Surg 1990;24:186–8.

13. Johnson TM, Tschen J, Ho C, et al. Unusual basal cell carcinomas. Cutis 1994;54:85–92.

14. Miller SJ. Biology of basal cell carcinoma (Part I). J Am Acad Dermatol 1991;24:1–13.

15. Rao BK, Freeman RG, Poulos EG, et al. The relationship between basal cell epithelioma and seborrheic keratosis. A study of 60 cases. J Dermatol Surg Oncol 1994;20:761–4.

16. Coskey RJ, Mehregan AH. The association of basal cell carcinomas with other tumors. J Dermatol Surg Oncol 1987;13:553–5.

17. Ikeda I, Ono T. Basal cell carcinoma origination from an epidermoid cyst. J Dermatol 1990;17:643–6.

18. Boyd AS, Rapini RP. Cutaneous collision tumors. Am J Dermatopathol 1994;16:253–7.

19. Yeh S, How SW, Lin CS. Arsenical cancer of skin. Cancer 1968;21:312–39.

20. Oram Y, Orengo I, Griego RD, et al. Histologic patterns of basal cell carcinoma based upon patient immunostatus. Dermatol Surg 1995;21:611–4.

21. Wang CY, Brodland DG, Su WP. Skin cancers associated with acquired immunodeficiency syndrome. Mayo Clin Proc 1995;70:766–72.

22. Hartevelt MM, Barinck JN, Koote AM, et al. Incidence of skin cancer after renal transplantation in the Netherlands. Transplantation 1990;49:506–9.

23. Asada M, Schaart FM, de Almeida HL Jr, et al. Solid basal cell epithelioma (BCE) possibly originates from the outer root sheath of the hair follicle. Acta Derm Venereol 1993;73:286–92.

24. Kruger K, Blume-Peytavi U, Ortanos CE. Basal cell carcinoma possibly originates from the outer root sheath and/or the bulge region of the vellus hair follicle. Arch Dermatol Res 1999;291:253–9.

25. Van Scott EJ, Reinertson RP. The modulating influence of the stromal environment on epithelial cells studied in human autotransplants. J Invest Dermatol 1961;36:109–17.

26. Merot Y, Faucher F, Didierjean L, Saurat JH. Loss of bullous pemphigoid antigen in peritumoral lacunae of basal cell epitheliomas. Acta Derm Venereol 1984;64:209–13.

27. Korman NJ, Hrabovsky SL. Basal cell carcinomas display extensive abnormalities in the hemidesmosome anchoring fibril complex. Exp Dermatol 1993;2: 139–44.

28. Sollberg S, Peltonen J, Uitto J. Differential expression of laminin isoforms and β4 integrin epitopes in the basement zone of normal human skin and basal cell carcinomas. J Invest Dermatol 1992;98:864–70.

29. Gorlin RJ. Nevoid basal cell carcinoma syndrome. Dermatol Clin 1995;13:113–25.

30. Gutierrez MM, Mora RG. Nevoid basal cell carcinoma syndrome. J Am Acad Dermatol 1986;15:1023–30.

31. Shanley S, Ratcliffe J, Hockey A, et al. Nevoid basal cell carcinoma syndrome: review of 118 affected individuals. Am J Med Genet 1994;50:282–90.

32. Gailani MR, Bale SJ, Leffell DJ, et al. Developmental defects in Gorlin syndrome related to a putative tumor suppressor gene on chromosome 9. Cell 1992;69:111–7.

33. Shanley SM, Dawkins H, Wainwright BJ, et al. Fine deletion mapping on the long arm of chromosome 9 in sporadic and familial basal cell carcinomas. Hum Mol Genet 1995;4:129–33.

34. Gailani MR, Stahle-Backdahl M, Leffell DJ, et al. The role of the human homologue of *Drosophila* patched in sporadic basal cell carcinomas. Nat Genet 1996;13:78–81.

35. Oro AE, Higgins KM, Hu Z, et al. Basal cell carcinomas in mice overexpressing sonic hedgehog. Science 1997;276:817–21.

36. Fan H, Oro AE, Scott MP, Khavari PA. Induction of basal cell carcinoma features in transgenic human skin expressing sonic hedgehog. Nat Med 1997;3: 788–92.

37. Reifenberger J, Wolter M, Weber RG, et al. Missense mutations in SMOH in sporadic basal cell carcino-

mas of the skin and primitive neuroectodermal tumors of the central nervous system. Cancer Res 1998;58:1798–803.

38. Xie J, Murone M, Luoh SM, et al. Activating smoothened mutations in sporadic basal-cell carcinoma. Nature 1998;391:90–2.

39. Maltzman W, Czyzyk L. Ultraviolet irradiation stimulates levels of p53 cellular tumor antigen in nontransformed mouse cells. Mol Cell Biol 1984;4:1689–94.

40. Urano Y, Asano T, Yoshimoto K, et al. Frequent p53 accumulation in the chronically sun-exposed epidermis and clonal expansion of p53 mutant cells in the epidermis adjacent to basal cell carcinoma. J Invest Dermatol 1995;104:928–32.

41. Ziegler A, Jonason AS, Leffell DJ, et al. Sunburn and p53 in the onset of skin cancer. Nature 1994;372: 773–6.

42. Kraemer KH, Lee MM, Scotto J. Xeroderma pigmentosum: cutaneous, ocular, and neurologic abnormalities in 830 published cases. Arch Dermatol 1987;123:241–50.

43. Kraemer KH, Lee MM, Andrews AD, Lambert WC. The role of sunlight and DNA repair in melanoma and nonmelanoma skin cancer: the xeroderma pigmentosum paradigm. Arch Dermatol 1994;130:1018–21.

44. Borel DM. Cutaneous basosquamous carcinoma: review of the literature and report of 35 cases. Arch Pathol 1973;95:293–7.

45. Farmer ER, Helwig EB. Metastatic basal cell carcinoma: a clinicopathologic study of 17 cases. Cancer 1980;46:748–57.

46. Pinkus H. Premalignant fibroepithelial tumors of the skin. Arch Dermatol Syph 1953;67:598–615.

47. Russell EB, Carrington PR, Smoller BR. Basal cell carcinoma: a comparison of shave biopsy versus punch biopsy techniques in subtype diagnosis. J Am Acad Dermatol 1999;41:69–71.

48. Holmkvist KA, Rogers GS, Dahl PR. Incidence of residual basal cell carcinoma in patients who appear tumor free after biopsy. J Am Acad Dermatol 1999; 41:600–5.

49. Amonette RA, Salasche SJ, Chesney TM, et al. Metastatic basal cell carcinoma. J Dermatol Surg Oncol 1981;7:397–400.

50. Lo JS, Snow SN, Reizner GT, et al. Metastatic basal cell carcinoma: report of twelve cases and a review of the literature. J Am Acad Dermatol 1991;24:715–9.

51. Snow SN, Sahl W, Lo JS, et al. Metastatic basal cell carcinoma: report of five cases. Cancer 1994;73: 328–35.

52. von Domarus H, Stevens PJ. Metastatic basal cell carcinoma. J Am Acad Dermatol 1984;10:1043–60.

53. Cotran RS. Metastasizing basal cell carcinomas. Cancer 1961;14:1036–40.

54. Paver K, Poyzer K, Burry N, Deakin M. Letter: The incidence of basal cell carcinoma and their metastases in Australia and New Zealand. Australas J Dermatol 1973;14:53.

55. Rowe DE, Carroll RJ, Day CL. Long-term recurrence rates in previously untreated (primary) basal cell carcinoma: implications for patient follow-up. J Dermatol Surg Oncol 1989;15:315–28.

56. Rowe DE, Carroll RJ, Day CL. Mohs surgery is the treatment of choice for recurrent (previously treated) basal cell carcinoma. J Dermatol Surg Oncol 1989;15:424–31.

57. Marghoob A, Kopf AW, Bart RS, et al. Risk of another basal cell carcinoma developing after treatment of a basal cell carcinoma. J Am Acad Dermatol 1993;28: 22–8.

Pott's observation...

6

Squamous Cell Carcinoma

JUNE K. ROBINSON, MD

In the United States, there are approximately 200,000 new cases of cutaneous squamous cell carcinoma (SCC) each year. While most SCCs can be cured, many become locally invasive and destructive. Some are capable of metastases and cause death in 2,300 people per year. About 25 percent of the yearly skin cancer deaths are attributed to SCC. It has been estimated that a Caucasian male born in 1994 has a 9 to 14 percent chance of developing an SCC within his lifetime. The estimate for a white woman ranges from 4 to 9 percent.[1] Those at increased risk have the fair-skinned phenotype, excessive cumulative ultraviolet (UV) radiation overexposure, advancing age, an outdoor vocation or avocation, and residence in sunbelt latitudes.

ETIOLOGY

Chemical Carcinogenesis

The first recognition that chemical exposure in the workplace could cause human cancer was the report by Percival Pott in 1775 of an excess incidence of SCC of the scrotum among young chimney sweeps in London[2] (Figure 6–1). Pott attributed those tumors to soot. Latter studies confirmed Pott's observation and demonstrated that the chemical agents in soot responsible for scrotal cancer in the "climbing boys" were polycyclic aromatic hydrocarbons, particularly benzo[a]pyrene.[3] In this century, polycyclic aromatic hydrocarbons are used in cutting oils, and workers develop cutaneous SCC from such exposure.[4] Other occupational SCCs may be identified in the future and will probably be first recognized by clinicians, who obtain a detailed history of occupational exposure having a latent period of 20 to 25 years. The polycyclic hydrocarbon carcinogens are potent photosensitizers, with action spectra primarily in the long UV range (eg, promotion of tumor formation by croton oil after a single UV exposure in mice).[5]

More recently, etiologic associations in pesticide workers and patients who have received arsenical medications have been established between arsenic

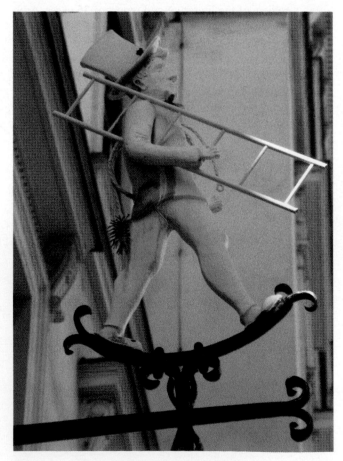

Figure 6–1. Eighteenth-century sign depicting a chimney sweep.

and cancers (SCCs) of the skin, lung, and liver.[6] Arsenical keratosis occurs years after a person ingests sufficient quantities of arsenic. Usually, patients either have intentionally taken arsenic as medication (eg, Fowler's solution, Asiatic pill) to treat diseases such as asthma or have unintentionally consumed arsenic in pesticide-contaminated well water. Typically, arsenical keratoses are flesh-colored papules with heavy spicules of scale, 2 to 3 mm in size, that develop on the palms and soles (Figure 6–2). They are usually painless but feel rough to the touch. Since arsenic exposure increases the risk of developing internal carcinomas (eg, gastrointestinal or genitourinary), arsenical keratoses provide a cutaneous marker for susceptibility to internal malignancy. These keratoses first occur after about 2 years of arsenic exposure (minimum total exposure of 0.5 to 1.0 g) and can transform into SCC after a latency of at least 10 years. Lesions of Bowen's disease (SCC in situ) occur on unexposed areas of the body.

Photocarcinogenesis

Currently, the single environmental carcinogen with the greatest impact on cancer incidence is exposure to UV light, which is often a combination of occupational and recreational exposure. Control of excessive exposure to UV light means attempting to alter the lifestyles and behaviors of millions of individuals. In experimental animals, the carcinogenic-action spectrum ranges primarily between 280 and 320 nm (ultraviolet B [UVB]), the acute erythrogenic or sunburn spectrum. Squamous cell carcinoma affects primarily sun-exposed sites such as the face, head, and neck. Pigmentary traits, such as hair and eye color and the tendency to sunburn, are strong independent indicators of the risk for SCC. In SCC, the adjusted odds ratio (OR) ranges from 1.6 for people with fair hair to 13.0 for those with red hair. Pale eye color is associated with a risk of 1.8 for SCC, and a skin type that always burns and never tans has an OR of 2.0 for SCC.[7]

The risk of SCC (Figure 6–3, red line) increases with increasing sun exposure beyond a threshold of 70,000 cumulated hours of exposure in a lifetime. Odds ratios for SCC were up to eight or nine times those of the control group for the highest exposure

(200,000 hours). Basal cell carcinoma (BCC) (see Figure 6–3, blue line) exhibited a twofold increased risk for lower exposures (8,000 to 10,000 cumulated hours in a lifetime), with a plateau and a slightly decreased risk for the highest exposures. People involved in outdoor work showed a significantly increased risk of SCC (an OR of 1.6 for more than 54,000 cumulated hours of exposure in a lifetime). Squamous cell carcinoma develops if people expose themselves to higher doses of UV for prolonged periods of time. Skin type modulates the response: people who tan poorly have an increased risk even if moderately exposed.[8] Patients with psoriasis who receive long-term psoralen and ultraviolet A (PUVA) therapy to treat the skin disease are especially prone to develop SCC and have an incidence

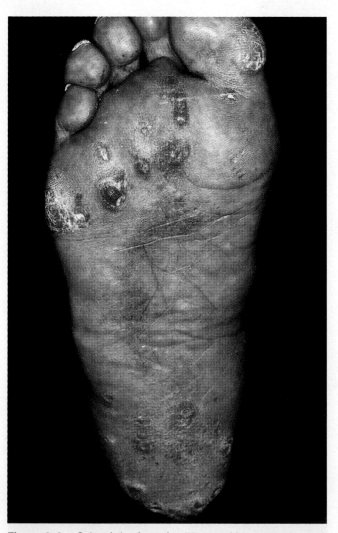

Figure 6–2. Sole of the foot of a 70-year-old woman who took Fowler's solution for asthma as a child. Numerous arsenical keratoses are on the heel, ball, and arch of the foot.

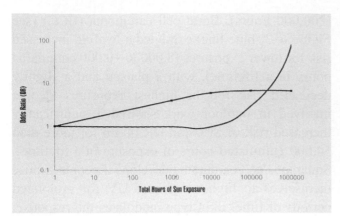

Figure 6–3. Dose-response curves for risk of basal cell carcinoma (blue) and squamous cell carcinoma (red) in relation to the number of hours of sun exposure in a lifetime. Points fitted and displayed are tenths of the log-transformed scale in the observed range. (Reproduced with permission from Zanetti R, Rosso S, Martinez C, et al. The multicentre south European study "Helios." I: Skin characteristics and sunburns in basal cell and squamous cell carcinomas of the skin. Br J Cancer 1996; 73:1440–6.)

of 2.36 times the expected incidence.[9] The carcinogenic risk of PUVA is dose related, with its risk of SCC being 12.8 times greater for patients receiving higher doses than for those receiving low doses. A surprising number of tumors develop on skin that is not usually exposed to the sun but that was exposed to UV light during the course of PUVA therapy (Figure 6–4). Squamous cell carcinomas due to PUVA therapy tend to be of the well-differentiated type.

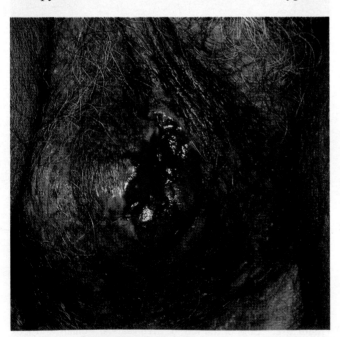

Figure 6–4. Scrotal well-differentiated squamous cell carcinoma in a patient undergoing psoralen plus ultraviolet A (PUVA) therapy.

Thermal Burn Scars and Other Environmental Risk Factors

While most cutaneous SCCs develop in areas exposed to solar radiation, they may also form in areas subjected to chronic inflammation or trauma. Marjolin first reported the occurrence of SCC in scars, hence the term "Marjolin's ulcer." Chronic radiodermatitis (Figure 6–5), discoid lupus erythematosus, or other chronic ulcers may predispose to development of SCC. Tobacco use has been associated with SCC of the lip.

THE BIOLOGIC CONTINUUM OF SQUAMOUS CELL CARCINOMA

Actinic Keratosis

Epidemiologic, clinical, histopathologic, and molecular evidence indicates that actinic (solar) keratosis represents an early stage in the biologic continuum ranging from carcinoma "in situ" to invasive SCC (Figure 6–6). Actinic keratosis (AK) most often results from chronic overexposure to the sun's UV rays in susceptible people and is very common. The estimated rate of progression of an individual AK lesion to SCC is from 0.1 to 10.0 percent.[10,11] People

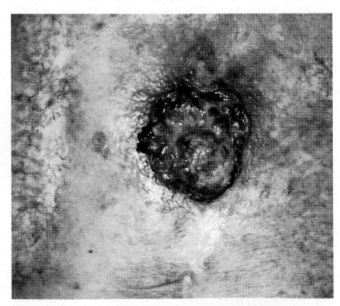

Figure 6–5. Well-differentiated squamous cell carcinoma arising from the chest wall of a woman treated 15 years ago with a radical mastectomy and radiation therapy. The tumor arose in the chronic radiodermatitis and is bound to the underlying ribs.

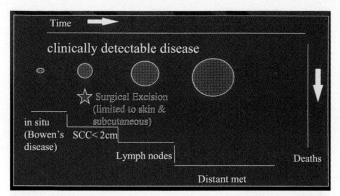

Figure 6–6. The biologic continuum of squamous cell carcinoma.

with more than 10 AK lesions have a cumulative probability of 14 percent of developing an SCC within 5 years.[12]

Actinic keratoses are usually seen as multiple lesions in sun-exposed areas of the skin in persons in or past middle life who have fair complexions. The lesions are seen most commonly on the face, the dorsa of the hands, and the bald portions of the scalp in men (Figure 6–7). Usually, the lesions measure less than 1 cm in diameter. They are erythematous, are often covered by adherent scales, and except for the hypertrophic form, show little or no elevation above the surrounding skin surface. Some actinic keratosis lesions are pigmented and show peripheral spreading, making clinical differentiation from lentigo maligna (melanoma in situ) difficult (Figure 6–8). Some AK lesions have marked hyperkeratosis and clinically form cutaneous horns. The proliferative form of AK lesion, an erythematous macule with poorly defined borders, enlarges over time and can spread along the surface of the skin, reaching up to 3 to 4 cm in size (Figure 6–9). It grows around hair follicles to the level of sebaceous glands and may be very difficult to differentiate from SCC in situ.[13]

On the lower lip, the lesion that is analogous to actinic keratosis is actinic cheilitis or solar cheilitis. Clinically, actinic cheilitis appears as dry, fissured, and crusted lips, often with a gray-white discoloration and an atrophic appearance. The vermilion area of the lower lip may become indistinct, with a loss of the normal mucocutaneous junction. The patient may complain of irritation and burning discomfort (Figure 6–10). Actinic cheilitis is a premalignant condition in which carcinomatous changes occur. Many years may elapse before invasive SCC develops within actinic cheilitis. Treatment of the condition may prevent the progression to invasive SCC. The removal or destruction of the damaged epithelium can be accomplished by several methods, including topical 5-fluorouracil, cryosurgery, and carbon dioxide (CO_2) laser vaporization.[14]

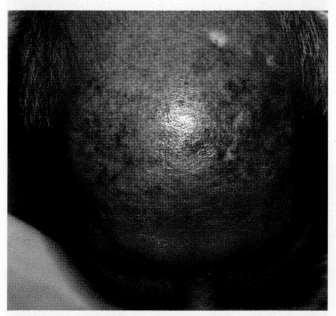

Figure 6–7. A band of actinic keratosis covers the upper forehead and extends to the line that once represented the frontal hairline. The erythematous macules are rough to the touch.

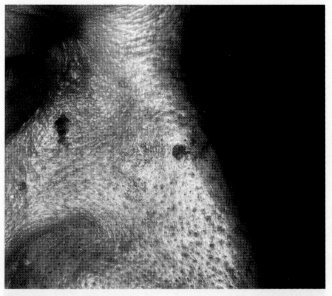

Figure 6–8. A 2-mm pigmented macular lesion on the nasal dorsum of this man fades into a lighter brown area toward the midline of the nose. The variation in pigmentation resembles lentigo maligna. The biopsy specimen showed a pigmented actinic keratosis.

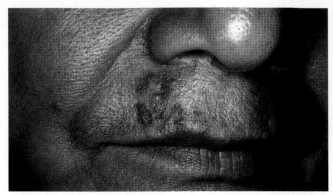

Figure 6–9. Proliferative actinic keratosis on the upper lip of a woman.

Bowen's Disease

Bowen's disease (SCC in situ) has a slow course over a period of years, but it may progress to invasive SCC. It may result from exposure to ionizing radiation, solar radiation, PUVA, or arsenic ingestion. The clinical patterns most commonly seen are (a) chronic crusted (Figure 6–11) or ulcerated plaques with a nodular component and well-defined borders and (b) a minimally elevated flesh-colored plaque with only slight scale (Figure 6–12). This indolent process typically presents as a well-demarcated scaly plaque.

In the early phase, the slow growing erythematous scaly patch of Bowen's disease may resemble psoriasis, eczema, or actinic keratosis; but since the diameter exceeds 0.5 cm, it is too large to be an AK lesion. If someone has a new onset of what looks like psoriasis in only one digit, it is reasonable to assume that it is not psoriasis (Figure 6–13). When the clinically suspected disease does not respond to

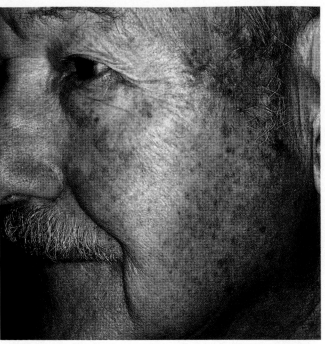

Figure 6–11. The chronic scaling plaque on the left preauricular cheek of this 67-year-old man is Bowen's disease, and the lesion of the nasal tip is an actinic keratosis.

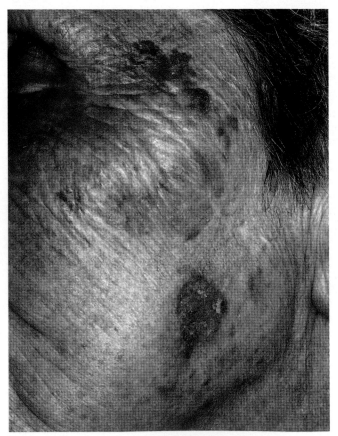

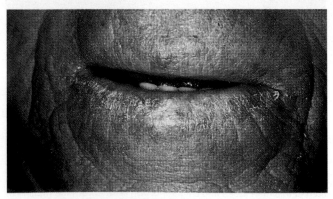

Figure 6–10. Actinic cheilitis on the lower lip of a 78-year-old man who worked outdoors. The central white area is leukoplakia.

Figure 6–12. Bowen's disease on the left cheek of an 82-year-old woman is a minimally elevated flesh-colored plaque with only slight scale.

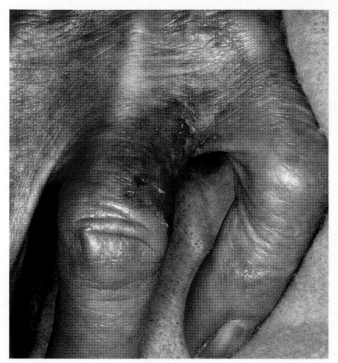

Figure 6–13. A solitary scaling plaque of Bowen's disease in the finger web of the fourth and fifth digits in a 78-year-old female.

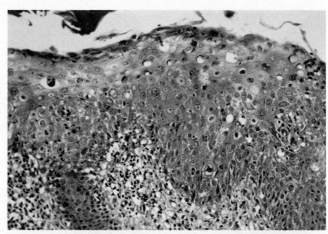

Figure 6–14. Pathologic presentation of Bowen's disease, an intraepidermal squamous cell carcinoma (SCC) or SCC in situ. Cells show individual keratinization. These dyskeratotic cells are large and round and have homogeneous, strongly eosinophilic cytoplasm and a hyperchromatic nucleus. While the border between the epidermis and the dermis appears sharp, the atypical cells in Bowen's disease frequently extend into the follicular infundibula and cause replacement of the follicular epithelium by atypical cells down to the entrance of the sebaceous duct. (Courtesy of Brian J. Nickoloff, MD, PhD, Professor of Pathology, Loyola University, Chicago.)

usual treatment, performing a biopsy may help to make the diagnosis of Bowen's disease (Figure 6–14). The average reported delay from onset of disease to diagnosis is 5 to 8 years.[15] Patients with Bowen's disease do not appear to be at any unusually high general cancer risk; however, there is an increased risk of invasive SCC of the skin and lip,[16] likely due to the common risk factor of UV light.

Erythroplasia of Queyrat

When SCC in situ occurs on the penis, it is known as erythroplasia of Queyrat and occurs almost exclusively in uncircumcised men. It is not associated with internal malignancies but is associated with a higher incidence of locally invasive SCC than Bowen's disease. Classically, the primary lesion consists of solitary or multiple erythematous velvet-textured plaques on the glans penis (Figure 6–15). Since the skin of the glans does not keratinize, there is no scale production. The asymptomatic lesion has a velvety red appearance with sharply demarcated edges and may be a slightly infiltrated plaque. Occasional cases may extend to the distal urethra (see Figure 6–15). Less commonly, lesions are located on

the shaft or on the coronal sulcus (Figure 6–16). Progression to invasive SCC of the penis has been observed in up to 30 percent of patients, with metastases in about 20 percent of patients. Squamous cell carcinoma of the penis represents less than 1 percent of all cancers in men in the United States. In China

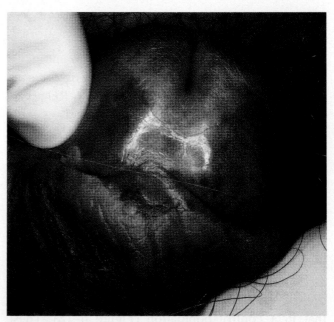

Figure 6–15. Erythroplasia of Queyrat with multiple erythematous velvet-textured plaques on the glans penis extends to the distal urethra.

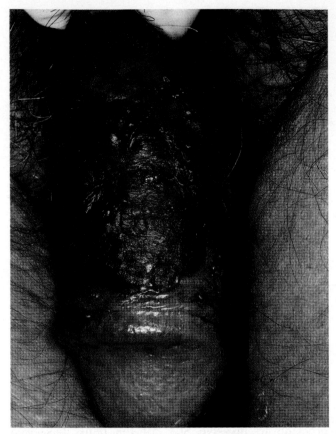

Figure 6–16. Less commonly, lesions of erythroplasia of Queyrat are located on the shaft of the penis.

and Vietnam, however, SCC of the penis represents 12 to 15 percent of cancers.

Squamous Cell Carcinoma

The majority of SCCs occur on the head and neck, with a disproportionate number arising on the ears, scalp, and neck of men[17] (Figure 6–17). Relatively few occur on the trunk, and fewer occur in people under 30 years of age, which indicates that prolonged cumulative UV radiation exposure is important to the process of developing SCC. The highest risk factors for the development of SCC are the presence of AK for prior nonmelanoma skin cancer.[18]

Immunosuppressed patients (eg, organ transplant recipients and patients with chronic lymphomas) and patients undergoing long-term PUVA therapy are especially prone to develop SCC. The risk of SCC in transplantation patients ranges from 20 to 253 times that in a control population (Figure 6–18). These patients are at greater risk if they are mismatched for

donor human leukocyte antigen (HLA), compared with HLA-matched patients. As the duration of immunosuppression approaches 3 to 5 years after transplantation, the risk of skin cancer increases. In contrast to the BCC-SCC ratio of 4:1 in the normal population, the ratio in transplantation patients ranges from 1:1.2 to 1:3. Squamous cell carcinomas in immunocompromised patients tend to occur on sun-exposed skin, tend to be more aggressive clinically, and have a greater chance of metastasis.

Squamous cell carcinomas at high risk for metastases are those that grow rapidly, are aneuploid, reach a size greater than 2 cm, invade deeply and reach a thickness of 6 mm, are recurrent after previous treatment, or are located in high-risk areas such as the ear, the vermilion of the lip, and the columella of the nose[19–22] (Figure 6–19). Immunocompromised patients are also likely to develop metastases.[23–25]

Early invasive SCC arising from AK may be subtle and difficult to distinguish clinically from SCC in situ (Figure 6–20). Keratoses that undergo rapid

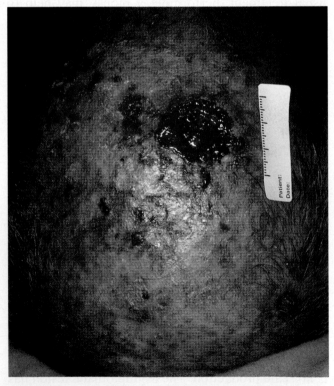

Figure 6–17. The bald scalp of this 54-year-old man with lymphoma gave rise to a poorly differentiated squamous cell carcinoma (SCC) and multiple actinic keratoses. Since his platelet count was 24,000 and since he was not responding to chemotherapy for the lymphoma, he was referred to radiation therapy to treat this potentially lethal SCC.

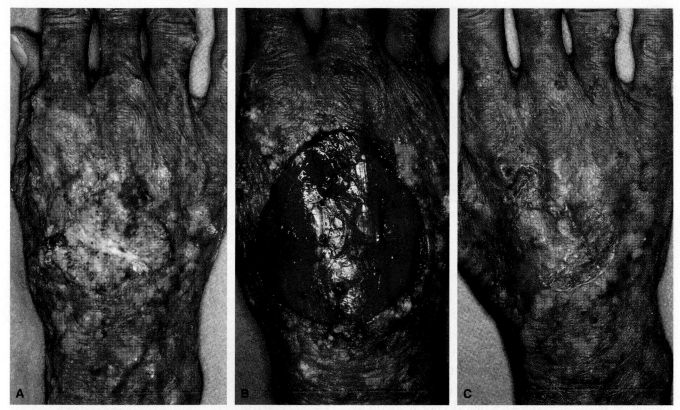

Figure 6–18. *A,* A well-differentiated squamous cell carcinoma of the dorsum of the right hand of a renal transplantation patient. *B,* The tumor was resected with Mohs' surgery, and the defect was reconstructed with a split-thickness skin graft. *C,* The patient had full functional use of the hand 1 year after the surgery.

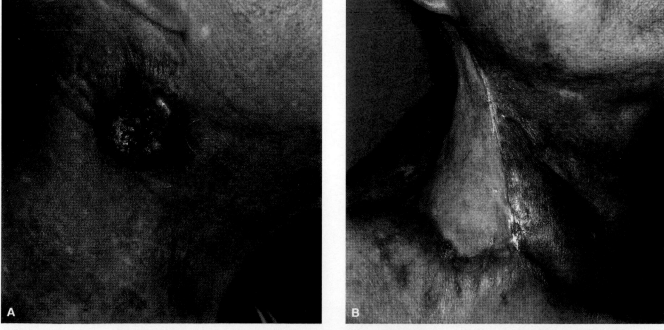

Figure 6–19. *A,* This 79-year-old man had a history of rapid progression over the preceding 2 weeks in this moderately differentiated squamous cell carcinoma (SCC). At presentation, the tumor (4.0 x 2.9 x 2.7 cm in volume) on the right side of the neck was bound to muscle. There was no palpable lymphadenopathy. *B,* The patient was treated with wide local excision and modified radical ipsilateral neck dissection, then was primarily reconstructed with a flap from the right pectoralis major muscle. The surgical specimen showed infiltration of the skeletal muscle and lymphovascular invasion by the SCC, but 14 lymph nodes were free of tumor.

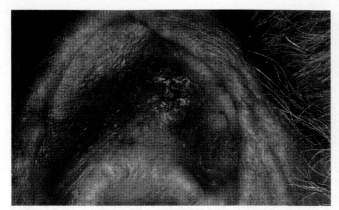

Figure 6–20. Early invasive squamous cell carcinoma arising in an actinic keratosis of the ear.

growth or spontaneous ulceration or that start to hurt may be SCCs. Classically, SCC is a papular lesion that is erythematous, hyperkeratotic with ill-defined margins, and often ulcerated even when small. If the hyperkeratotic scale is removed, the tumor often bleeds. A biopsy is needed to distinguish early lesions of SCC from BCC and AK lesions. A biopsy should be performed on AKs that do not respond to usual therapeutic efforts (eg, lesions that persist after a course of topical 5-fluorouracil or after cryosurgery with the application of liquid nitrogen to the lesion).

Occasionally, an SCC may assume a mushroom-like configuration with a crusted keratotic crater, mimicking a keratoacanthoma (Figure 6–21). Pathologically, this morphologic variant is usually a well-differentiated SCC.

Verrucous carcinoma, a low-grade SCC, occurs in the following four common locations: the aerodigestive area, including the lip; the plantar area of the

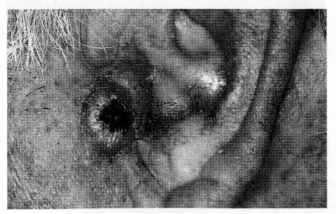

Figure 6–21. The mushroomlike configuration of squamous cell carcinoma, mimicking a keratoacanthoma.

feet (epithelioma cuniculatum); the anourogenital area (Buschke-Löwenstein tumor), and other cutaneous sites. This tumor has a wartlike appearance and tends to be slow growing and not deeply invasive (Figure 6–22). Verrucous carcinoma of anogenital mucosa occurs most commonly on the glans penis (Figure 6–23). It occurs more commonly in uncircumcised men and presents as a large cauliflower-like lesion. Human papillomavirus 6 (HPV-6) seems to play a role in the development of this tumor. Verrucous carcinoma of the feet (epithelioma cuniculatum) is an ulcerated exophytic tumor with sinuses draining a foul-smelling discharge. The tumor causes bleeding, pain, and difficulty in walking (Figure 6–24). The

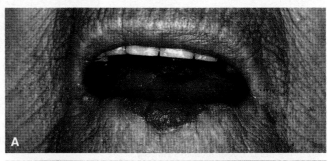

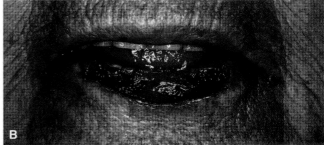

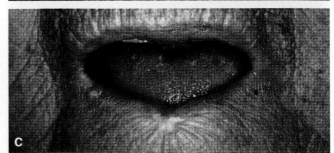

Figure 6–22. *A,* Recurrent verrucous squamous cell carcinoma on the lower lip of a 72-year-old woman. *B,* The tumor was resected with Mohs' surgery, resulting in a defect (4.0 x 2.1 cm) that spared the underlying muscle. The defect was allowed to heal by second intention. *C,* The lip was healed and fully functional 2 months after surgery. Six months after surgery, the scar is firm, and wound contraction is at its peak, which causes the slight central depression. During the 2 years following surgery, tissue remodeling will contribute to improvement in the lip's function and appearance, and the depression may improve over the next year.

sinuses are characterized as being like a rabbit burrow, or cuniculate. The tumor usually involves the skin overlying the first metatarsal head but may also occur elsewhere on the foot.

Carcinoma of the lip, which is the second most common head and neck tumor, is most often SCC. It usually begins as a rough scaling of fissured area of the lower lip that may progress to a white patch (leukoplakia). Neglect of these tumors can allow them to evolve into large, fungating, and deeply ulcerated lesions.

THE BIOLOGIC BEHAVIOR OF CUTANEOUS SQUAMOUS CELL CARCINOMA

The four patterns of invasion of SCC consist of two locally invasive patterns and two pathways of metastasis. A squamous cell carcinoma may invade locally by infiltrating deeply through the subcutaneous adipose tissues, but on reaching the fasciae or capsular planes, muscle, perichondrium, or periosteum, the tumor fans out laterally and ceases to penetrate deeper tissues (Figure 6–25). Squamous cell carcinoma may also spread along blood vessels or nerves, like a train running along a track (Figure 6–26). Perineural invasion is particularly difficult to determine pathologically as the spindle cells of the SCC wrap around the nerve bundle. Lastly, SCCs may metastasize locally or to regional lymph nodes. Less often, they metastasize by hematogenous spread.

Pathology

Squamous cell carcinoma of the skin consists of masses of proliferating atypical keratinocytes

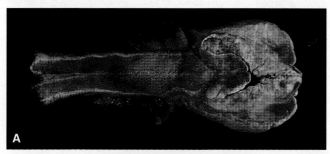
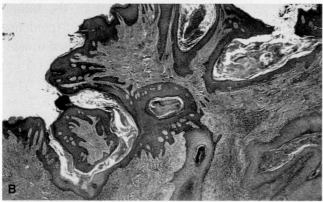
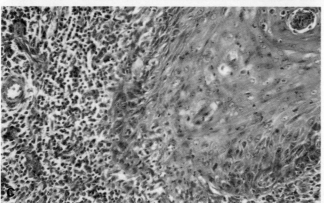

Figure 6–23. *A*, A 49-year-old man underwent amputation of the penis for a verrucous carcinoma that arose from the glans penis and invaded the distal two-thirds of the penis. *B*, A low-power view of the tumor demonstrates the papillomatous proliferation supported on a stalk; however, the tumor extends below the stalk into the urethra. *C*, A high-power view of the invading border of the squamous cell carcinoma shows the well-differentiated keratinocytes. The tumor invades with broad bulbous downward proliferations that may contain keratin-filled cysts. The tumor invades by "bulldozing" rather than "stabbing." (Courtesy of Brian J. Nickoloff, MD, PhD, Professor of Pathology, Loyola University, Chicago.)

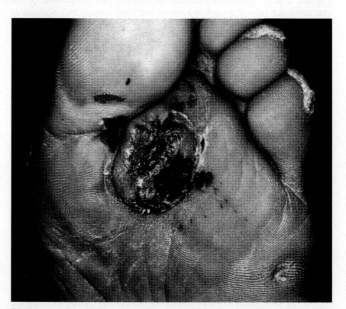

Figure 6–24. Verrucous carcinoma of the foot (epithelioma cuniculatum) is an ulcerated exophytic tumor with sinuses draining a foul-smelling discharge.

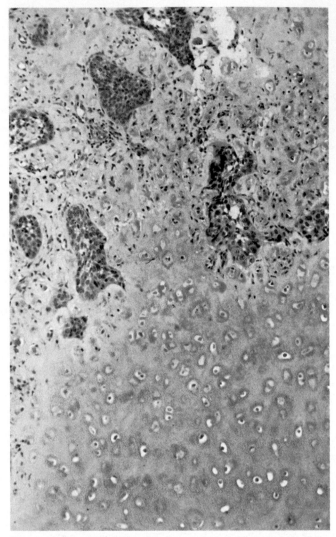

Figure 6–25. Well-differentiated squamous cell carcinoma of the ear fans out over the perichondrium but may invade the surface of the cartilage.

extending into the dermis from the overlying epidermis. The atypia is manifested by cells with large nuclear-cytoplasmic ratios, varying degrees of nuclear pleomorphism, prominent nucleoli, multinucleated cells, and mitotic figures that may appear atypical. There may be individual cell keratinization and small foci of incomplete keratinization termed "keratin pearls" (Figure 6–27). The surrounding inflammatory infiltrate in SCC is variable in extent and composition, depending on the type of lesion. Invasive lesions are accompanied by a relatively heavy infiltrate of small lymphocytes.

The number of atypical squamous cells is higher in the more poorly differentiated tumors that have a greater risk of metastasis (Figure 6–28). No keratin

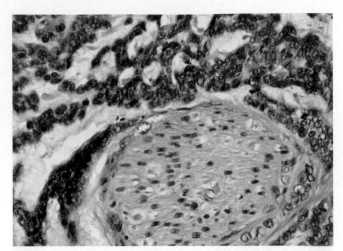

Figure 6–26. Perineural spread of squamous cell carcinoma.

pearls are present in poorly differentiated SCC. Keratinization occurs in small cell groups. Spindle cell SCC is an undifferentiated variant of the tumor. Other variants of SCC that have a higher incidence of metastases are acantholytic (adenoid) and mucin-producing SCC. A tumor size in excess of 1.5 cm correlates with the risk of metastasis for these types of tumor.

Verrucous carcinoma, a low-grade SCC, displays papillomatosis and a deep dermal extension of well-differentiated squamous epithelium. There is only occasional evidence of individual cell keratinization, and mitotic activity is low.

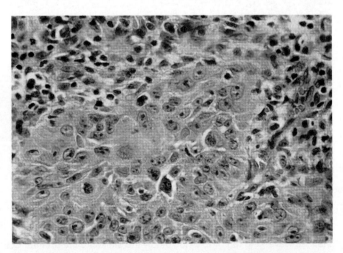

Figure 6–27. Pathologic presentation of a well-differentiated squamous cell carcinoma shows dermal invasion by epidermal masses, whose cells are predominately mature squamous cells showing relatively slight atypicality. Nuclear pleomorphism and an occasional mitotic figure are present. (Courtesy of Brian J. Nickoloff, MD, PhD, Professor of Pathology, Loyola University, Chicago.)

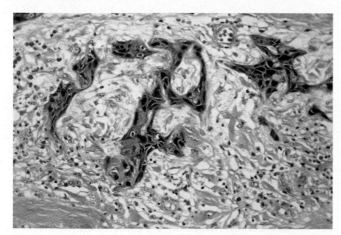

Figure 6–28. A poorly differentiated squamous cell carcinoma shows an absence of keratinization. (Courtesy of Brian J. Nickoloff, MD, PhD, Professor of Pathology, Loyola University, Chicago.)

Biologic Course

There is natural variation in SCC; however, if left untreated, SCC continues to grow and invades at a variable rate, depending on the degree of differentiation, the pre-existing condition from which the tumor arose, and the immunologic status of the patient. Squamous cell carcinomas that are not associated with UV exposure and that are secondary to inflammatory or degenerative processes are high-risk tumors. Thus, the rate of metastasis in SCC arising in osteomyelitic sites was 31 percent (20% in radiation-induced skin cancer, and 18% in carcinomas in burn scars). Furthermore, SCC arising from glabrous skin (such as that on the glans penis and from the oral mucosa) and the lips have a high rate of metastasis unless recognized and adequately treated at an early stage. Carcinoma of the lower lip has a metastatic rate of about 16 percent, and death occurs in about half of these patients as the result of metastases.

Other variables associated with the risk of local recurrence and metastasis after treatment are location, size, depth, histologic differentiation, perineural involvement, immunosuppression status, and prior treatment. Squamous cell carcinoma of the ear and lip are a higher risk. Those tumors with a diameter greater than 2 cm have nearly three times the rate of metastasis of those less than 2 cm in diameter. Tumors up to 4 mm in depth are low-risk tumors, and those of greater depth than 4 mm are of higher

risk. Histologic differentiation is a significant prognostic factor: well-differentiated SCCs have a better prognosis than poorly differentiated ones. Poorly differentiated SCCs have double the local recurrence after treatment and three times the metastatic rate. Poorly differentiated SCCs make up only about 13.7 percent of the SCCs reported. Perineural invasion is a histologic indicator of a biologically aggressive tumor; perineural invasion in SCC of the lip may have a metastatic rate of 80 percent.

Last, immunosuppressed patients have a 2 to 3 percent risk of metastasis; however, the greatly increased number of SCCs developed by these patients confers an overall metastatic rate of almost 13 percent.[26] As these prognostic variables coexist in a patient, the therapeutic considerations become more radical (eg, immunosuppressed patient with a recurrent poorly differentiated SCC greater than 2 cm in diameter invading bone, as shown in Figure 6–29). A previously treated tumor that recurs locally has a metastatic rate of 25 percent. After metastasis of SCC, the 5-year survival is 26.8 percent.[19] This

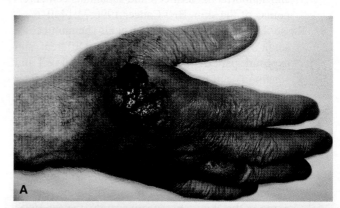

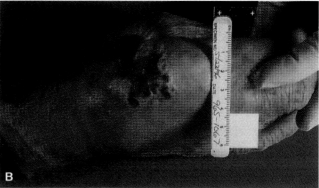

Figure 6–29. *A,* This right-handed immunosuppressed patient had a recurrent poorly differentiated squamous cell carcinoma > 2 cm in diameter that invaded the underlying bone. There was no palpable lymphadenopathy. *B,* The hand was amputated.

ominous survival rate lends increasing importance to early detection and adequate initial therapy of SCC.

REFERENCES

1. Miller DL, Weinstock MA. Non-melanoma skin cancer in the United States: incidence. J Am Acad Dermatol 1994;50:774–8.

2. Pott P. Chiururgical observation relative to the cataract, the polyps of the nose, the cancer of the scrotum, the different kinds of ruptures, the mortification of the toes and feet. London: Hawes, Clarke and Collins; 1775.

3. Kennaway EL. On the cancer-producing factor in tar. BMJ 1924;1:564–7.

4. Tsuji T, Otake N, Kobayashi T, Milua N. Multiple keratoses and squamous cell carcinoma from cutting oils. J Am Acad Dermatol 1992;27:767–8.

5. Epstein JH. Photocarcinogenesis: a review. Natl Cancer Inst Monogr 1978;50:13–25.

6. Mabuchi K, Lilienfeld AM, Snell LM. Lung cancer among pesticide workers exposed to inorganic arsenicals. Arch Environ Health 1979;34:312–20.

7. Zanetti R, Rosso S, Martinez C, et al. The multicentre south European study 'Helios.' I: Skin characteristics and sunburns in basal cell and squamous cell carcinomas of the skin. Br J Cancer 1996;73:1440–6.

8. Rosso S, Martinez C, Tormo MJ, et al. The multicentre south European study 'Helios.' II: Different sun exposure patterns in the aetiology of basal cell and squamous cell carcinomas of the skin. Br J Cancer 1996;73:1447–54.

9. Stern RS, Lunder EJ. Risk of squamous cell carcinoma and methoxsalen (psoralen) and UV-A radiation (PUVA). A meta-analysis. Arch Dermatol 1998; 134:1582–5.

10. Marks R, Rennie G, Selwood TS. Malignant transformation of solar keratosis to squamous cell carcinoma in the skin: a prospective study. Lancet 1988; 1:795–7.

11. Dobson JM, De Spain J, Hewett JE, Clark DP. Malignant potential of actinic keratosis and the controversy over treatment: a patient oriented perspective. Arch Dermatol 1991;127:1029–31.

12. Moon TE, Levine N, Cartmel B, et al. Effect of retinol to prevent squamous cell skin cancer in moderate-risk subjects. Cancer Epidemiol Biomarkers Prev 1997;6:949–56.

13. Schwarze HP, Loche F, Gorguet MC, et al. Invasive cutaneous squamous cell carcinoma associated with actinic keratosis. Dermatol Surg 1999;25:587–9.

14. Robinson JK. Actinic cheilitis: a prospective study comparing four treatment methods. Arch Otolaryngol Head Neck Surg 1989;115:848–52.

15. Lee MM, Wick MM. Bowen's disease. Clin Dermatol 1993;11:43–6.

16. Jarger AB, Gramkow A, Hjalgrim H, et al. Bowen disease and risk of subsequent malignant neoplasms. Arch Dermatol 1999;135:790–3.

17. Franceschi S, Levi F, Randimbison L, La Vecchia C. Site distribution of different types of skin cancer; new etiologic clues. Int J Cancer 1996;67:24–8.

18. English DR, Armstrong BK, Kricker A, et al. Demographic characteristics, pigmentary and cutaneous risk factors for squamous cell carcinoma of the skin: a case control study. Int J Cancer 1998;76: 628–34.

19. Rowe DE, Carroll RJ, Day CI. Prognostic factors for local recurrence, metastasis and survival rates in squamous cell carcinoma of the skin, ear, and lip. J Am Acad Dermatol 1992;26:1–26.

20. Kwa RE, Campana K, Moy RL. Biology of cutaneous squamous cell carcinoma. J Am Acad Dermatol 1992;26:1–26.

21. Johnson TM, Rowe DE, Nelson BR. Squamous cell carcinoma of the skin (excluding the lip and oral mucosa). J Am Acad Dermatol 1992;26:467–84.

22. Robinson JK, Rademaker AW, Goolsby C, et al. Prognostic significance of DNA ploidy in non-melanoma skin cancer. Cancer 1996;77:284–91.

23. Euvardi D, Kanitakis J, Pouteil-Nobel C, el al. Comparative epidemiologic study of premalignant and malignant epithelial cutaneous lesion developing after kidney and heart transplantation. J Am Acad Dermatol 1995;33:222–9.

24. Jensen P, Hansen S, Moller B, et al. Skin cancer in kidney and heart transplant recipients and different long term immunosuppressive therapy regimens. J Am Acad Dermatol 1999;40:177–86.

25. Weimar VM, Ceilley RI, Goeken JA. Aggressive biologic behavior of basal and squamous cell cancers in patients with chronic lymphocytic leukemia or chronic lymphocytic lymphoma. J Dermatol Surg Oncol 1979;5:609–14.

26. Mullen D, Silverberg SG, Penn I. Squamous cell carcinoma of the skin and lip in renal homograft recipients. Cancer 1976;37:729–34.

7

Cutaneous Lymphoma

KATALIN FERENCZI, MD

PHILLIP H. McKEE, MD, FRCPATH

THOMAS S. KUPPER, MD

Primary cutaneous lymphomas are a heterogeneous group of diseases in terms of clinical, histologic, and immunophenotypic manifestations. In addition, they vary in biologic potential, ranging from an indolent process without metastatic potential (such as pagetoid reticulosis) to high-grade tumors with substantial mortality (such as Sézary syndrome).

Because of their heterogeneity, classifying cutaneous lymphomas has been difficult, and there is still no universally accepted scheme. In the past, histologic criteria were used to classify lymphomas. Only the updated Kiel[1] and the revised European-American lymphoid neoplasms (REAL)[2] classifications acknowledge that cutaneous lymphomas may be considered separately; however, neither provides extensive information about the biologic behavior of cutaneous lymphomas.

For many years, dermatologists have observed that lymphomas limited to the skin behave differently from those involving both skin and internal organs at first presentation. The European Organization for Research and Treatment of Cancer (EORTC) classification,[3] the first scheme that deals separately with primary cutaneous lymphomas, is based on a combination of clinical, histologic, and immunophenotypic criteria (Table 7–1). A major advantage of the EORTC classification scheme is that it recognizes that distinguishing between primary and secondary cutaneous lymphomas is essential for proper clinical management. Primary and secondary cutaneous lymphomas are different entities in terms of molecular characteristics, clinical aspects, biologic behavior, and prognosis and thus require markedly different therapeutic approaches.

PRIMARY CUTANEOUS LYMPHOMA

The term "primary cutaneous lymphoma" is used to describe lymphoma presenting in the skin and showing no evidence of extracutaneous manifestations at diagnosis and within the 6 months after diagnosis. Primary cutaneous lymphomas are the second most

Table 7–1. CLASSIFICATION* OF PRIMARY CUTANEOUS LYMPHOMAS	
Primary CTCL	**Primary CBCL**
Indolent	Indolent
MF	Follicular center cell lymphoma
MF+ follicular mucinosis	Immunocytoma
Pagetoid reticulosis	(marginal-zone B-cell
Large cell CTCL, CD30+	lymphoma)
Anaplastic	
Immunoblastic	
Pleomorphic	
Lymphomatoid papulosis	Intermediate
Aggressive	Large B-cell lymphoma of
SS	the leg
Large cell CTCL, CD30–	Provisional
Immunoblastic	Intravascular large
Pleomorphic	B-cell lymphoma
Provisional	Plasmocytoma
Granulomatous slack skin	
Pleomorphic small/	
medium-sized CTCL	
Subcutaneous panniculitis-	
like T-cell lymphoma	

*By the European Organization for Research and Treatment of Cancer (EORTC).
CBCL = cutaneous B-cell lymphoma; CTCL = cutaneous T-cell lymphoma; MF = mycosis fungoides; SS = Sézary syndrome.

common group of extranodal non-Hodgkin's lymphomas[4] and the most common sites for extranodal T-cell lymphomas. The vast majority of these are cutaneous T-cell lymphomas; fewer than 25 percent are of B-cell origin.[5]

It is increasingly important to consider lymphomas in the context of lymphocyte trafficking. The majority of T cells in peripheral blood are so-called naive T cells (CD45RA) and have very specific trafficking patterns.[6] All leukocytes, including T cells and B cells, exit peripheral blood into tissue through a series of adhesion and activation steps that occur in postcapillary venules. While naive T cells are efficient at migrating across postcapillary venules in a lymph node, they are unable to exit postcapillary venules in skin or other peripheral nonlymphoid tissues.[6] After antigen-mediated activation in peripheral lymph nodes, naive T cells proliferate and become memory T cells. Depending on the anatomic location of the lymph node where they undergo this naive-to-memory transition, the memory T cell expresses distinct cell surface molecules. T cells first activated in skin-draining lymph nodes express cutaneous lymphocyte antigen (CLA) and CD45RO.[7] In contrast, T cells first activated in gut-draining lymph nodes express high levels of $\alpha_4\beta_7$ integrin and CD45RO. Many of these memory cells have lost the adhesion molecules that allow them to exit into lymph nodes from blood. Extranodal T-cell lymphomas almost always express the pan-T-cell marker CD45RO, and those in skin typically express CLA.

Less is known about the specifics of B-cell extravasation into extranodal tissues, particularly the skin. However, it is reasonable to speculate that B cells that exit specifically and exclusively into skin may have lost the capacity to enter lymph nodes from blood.

Primary Cutaneous T-Cell Lymphomas

The term "cutaneous T-cell lymphoma" (CTCL) was introduced in 1979[8] as a unifying concept. It arose from Edelson's observation that in the majority of patients with cutaneous lymphoma, the neoplastic cells in the lymphoid infiltrates were predominantly T cells.[9] The most common type of CTCL is mycosis fungoides (MF); together with the less frequent Sézary syndrome, these variants account for 50 per-

cent of all cutaneous lymphomas.[3] All of these are malignancies of memory (CD45RO) skin-homing (CLA+) T cells.

Mycosis fungoides and Sézary syndrome (SS) are the most common lymphomas involving the skin. Over the last few years, the incidence rate of mycosis fungoides has stabilized, with an annual incidence rate from 1973 through 1992 of 0.3 cases per 100,000 population.[10] The incidence shows variation in race and gender: African Americans are twice as likely to be affected as Americans of European ancestry, and there is a 2:1 male-female ratio.[11] The incidence also shows some geographic variation: lower rates have been reported in China, Europe, and Australia than in the United States.[12]

Although many factors have been implicated in the pathogenesis of cutaneous lymphomas, the etiology remains unknown. Cutaneous T-cell lymphoma, particularly in the form of MF and SS, has long been suspected of being associated with long-term occupational exposure to solvents, other chemicals, and drugs.[13] This hypothesis has been impossible to prove, however. Large epidemiologic and case-control studies fail to support any of these factors.[12,14] The etiologic role of microbial agents, including human T-lymphotropic virus type 1 (HTLV-1), is still controversial. This virus, which is linked with the pathogenesis of adult T-cell leukemia/lymphoma (ATLL), has been the most investigated virus in CTCL patients. Data on the presence of HTLV-1 sequences in peripheral blood cells or lymphoma cells of CTCL patients have conflicted,[15–18] and a large study failed to support this association.[19] It has been suggested that the inconsistent findings between these reports may be partly explained by endogenous HTLV-related human sequences.[20] Histocompatibility antigen associations with MF and SS (such as increased frequency of human leukocyte antigens [HLAs] DR5 in MF patients[21] and B8 and Bw35 in SS patients)[22] have been found in a few studies.

Because it is now understood that MF and SS are malignancies of CLA+ skin-homing T cells, it is not unreasonable to suppose that the factors that induce these malignancies are encountered through the cutaneous interface with the environment. If skin-homing T cells travel from blood to skin and then back to lymph nodes via afferent lymphatics, it is plausible that they become transformed during this migration. The nature of the factors that precipitate these diseases are far from understood, but environmental factors are likely to play a role.

Epstein-Barr virus (EBV), has been reported to occasionally display an association with CTCL,[23] predominantly with three clinicopathologic subgroups: angiocentric T-cell lymphoma (lymphomatoid granulomatosis), CD30+ large T-cell lymphoma, and secondary CTCL.[24-26] The presence of the EBV viral genome has also been reported in association with cutaneous CD30+ lymphoma in immunocompromised patients.[27]

Even less is known about etiologic factors in B-cell lymphomas. The association of primary cutaneous B-cell lymphoma with infection by *Borrelia burgdorferi* has been reported in a few patients,[28,29] particularly in Europe. The recent provocative finding that a significant proportion of patients with primary cutaneous follicular center cell lymphoma have a characteristic 14:18 translocation suggests that somatic mutation plays a role in at least a subset of these patients.[30]

Mycosis Fungoides

Alibert coined the name mycosis fungoides in 1806 to describe the "mushroomlike" tumors he observed in a patient.[31] Ironically, while this name aptly describes tumor-stage disease, the vast majority of MF cases present as erythematous patches and plaques (see below).

Mycosis fungoides usually presents in adulthood, with a peak incidence in the sixth and seventh decades of life and with a slight predilection for male gender. Children are rarely affected, and young people are more likely to present with less advanced disease.[32] Patients often have a long history of nonspecific inflammatory skin lesions that tend to wax and wane over years. Repeated nondiagnostic skin biopsies are common, making it difficult to reach a correct diagnosis.

Cutaneous patches are by far the most common presentation, followed by plaque disease. Tumors may be seen in a minority of patients. Historically, these different manifestations are often described as "patch-stage," "plaque-stage," and "tumor-stage" disease. Patients may have stable patch-stage disease

Table 7–2. TUMOR-NODE-METASTASIS-BLOOD CLASSIFICATION OF CUTANEOUS T-CELL LYMPHOMA
T: Skin
T0: Clinically and/or histologically suspicious lesions
T1: Limited patch/plaque (< 10% of skin surface)
T2: Generalized patch/plaque (> 10% of skin surface)
T3: Tumors
T4: Generalized erythroderma
N: Lymph nodes
N0: No palpable lymph nodes
N1: Enlarged lymph nodes, negative pathology
N2: No palpable lymph nodes, positive pathology
N3: Enlarged lymph nodes, positive pathology
M: Visceral organs
M0: No evidence of visceral involvement
M1: Visceral involvement
B: Blood
B0: No atypical cells
B1: Atypical circulating cells > 5% of total T-cell count

for decades, or they may rapidly progress from patches to plaques and tumors. Pruritus is often a prominent feature of MF. (It is important to recall that "stage"—when used to refer to patches, plaques, and tumors—is completely independent of formal staging based on the tumor-node-metastasis [TNM] system [Tables 7–2 and 7–3] and is less closely tied to prognosis.)

Patches present as flat, well-defined, erythematous lesions that may show epidermal atrophy and fine scaling (Figure 7–1). Disease presenting in this form often has an indolent course, with slow progression over years or decades from patches to more persistent and widespread infiltrated plaques; however, recent reports indicate that most patients with limited patch or plaque lesions never progress to more advanced disease.[33,34] Plaques appear as erythematous, scaly, elevated, indurated lesions of varying size (Figure 7–2). Some regression may take place in individual plaques, giving rise to annular

Table 7–3. CLINICAL STAGING FOR MYCOSIS FUNGOIDES			
Clinical Stage	TNM Classification*		
IA	T1	N0	M0
IB	T2	N0	M0
IIA	T1–2	N1	M0
IIB	T3	N0–1	M0
IIIA/B	T4	N0–1	M0
IVA	T1–4	N2–3	M0
IVB	T1–4	N0–3	M1

*B classification does not affect the clinical stage.
TNM = tumor-node-matastasis.

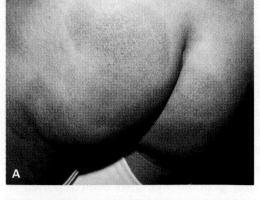

Figure 7–1. Mycosis fungoides. *A,* Erythematous flat plaque showing fine scaling on the buttocks. *B,* Established patch-stage disease. Note the perivascular infiltrate with epidermotropism. There is mild psoriasiform hyperplasia. *C,* Patch-stage disease showing atypical lymphocytes located predominantly along the basal layer of the epidermis. *D,* Compare CD4 expression (*D*) with that of CD7 (*E*).

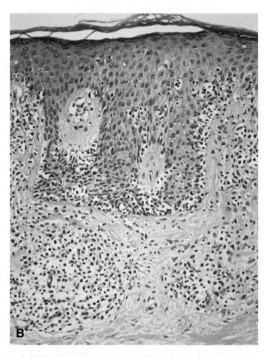

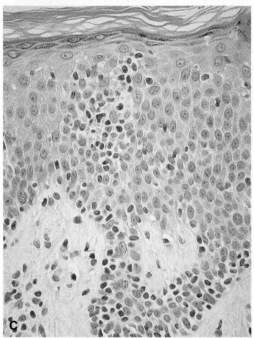

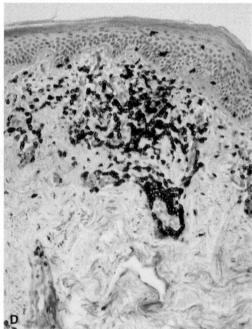

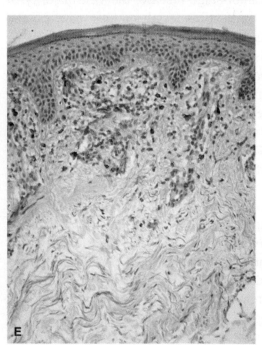

lesions with central clearing (so-called arcuate or horseshoe-shaped lesions). Tumors usually occur at sites of previous skin involvement with patches and plaques but may occur de novo (the so-called tumor d'emblee) (Figure 7–3). Those arising in pre-existing patches or plaques are thought to represent the

development of a malignant clone into a more rapid growth phase, possibly via the accumulation of an additional somatic mutation.[35] Tumors and nodules are large, raised, and red brown, and often ulcerate. Erythroderma involves most of the body surface area and may present de novo or appear after an

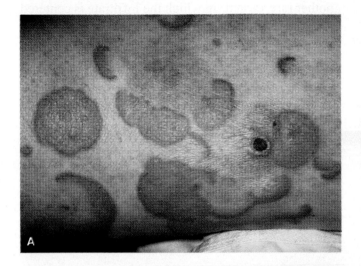

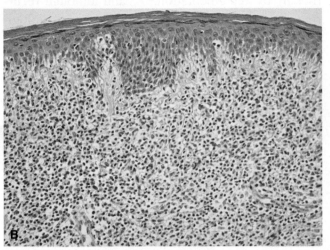

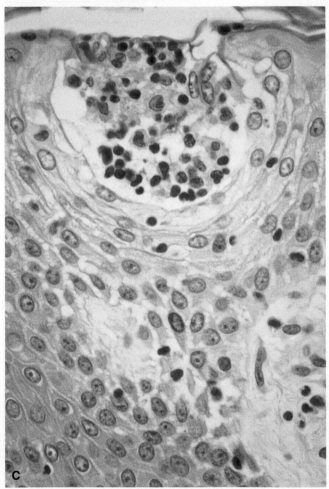

Figure 7–2. Mycosis fungoides, plaque stage. *A,* Erythematous annular and circinate plaques. *B,* Plaque-stage disease showing a heavy bandlike infiltrate. *C,* A typical Pautrier microabscess. Note the mixture of atypical lymphocytes (Sézary cells) and Langerhans' cells.

established plaque or tumor stage of disease. If peripheral blood involvement is present with transformed T cells, the affected patients are considered to have Sézary syndrome (Figure 7–4).

Less common variations have been described. The hypopigmented variant of MF is sometimes seen in dark-skinned patients. Patients respond to therapy by repigmentation,[36,37] and although recurrent diesease is common, it usually has a biologically benign course.[38] Solitary indolent lesions restricted to acral sites and that show clonal T-cell antigen receptor (TCR) gene re-arrangements and a CD8+ phenotype[39] have been termed mycosis fungoides palmaris et plantaris.[40]

The follicular variant of MF is characterized histologically by follicular lesions and pilotropism, either with or without mucinosis (see discussion of follicular mucinosis, below).[41] Clinically, alopecia is often present. Syringotropic mycosis fungoides is another rare variant, in which the infiltrate is centered on the eccrine sweat gland unit (syringotropism).[42,43]

The histologic hallmark of MF is epidermotropism, defined by the presence of atypical T cells in the epidermis and consistently seen in MF. Frank

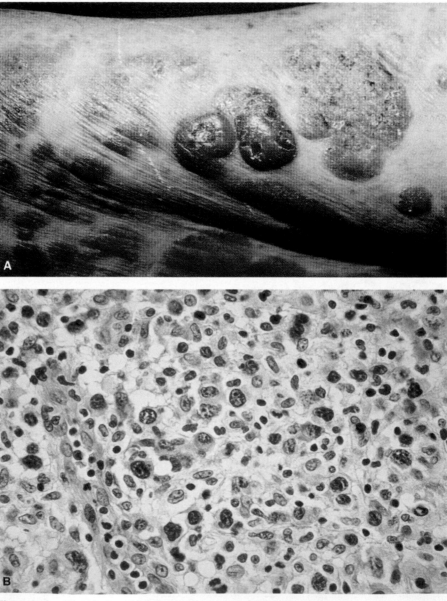

Figure 7–3.   Mycosis fungoides. Tumor-stage disease. *A,* Multiple red-brown nodules. *B,* There is marked pleomorphism, and mitoses are conspicuous.

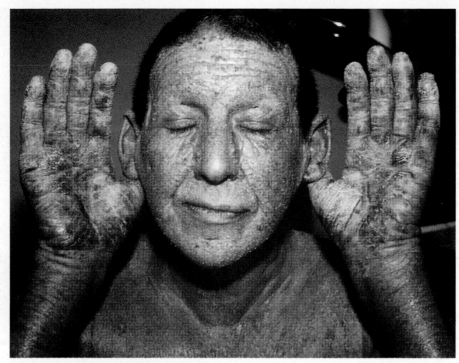

Figure 7–4. Sézary syndrome. Generalized erythema, scaling, and palmar hyperkeratosis.

epidermotropism may not always be recognized in the earliest stages of disease, making the diagnosis of patch-stage lesions more difficult. The earliest feature of CTCL is a moderate perivascular and band-like lymphocytic infiltrate of small or medium-sized lymphocytes with hyperchromatic cerebriform nuclei, within the papillary dermis. Similar cells are also usually present in the lower layers of the epidermis and at the dermal-epidermal junction (see Figure 7–1, *B, C* and *D*). Mixed in with these T cells are a variable number of inflammatory leukocytes. There may be a slight epidermal hyperplasia. With disease progression, epidermotropism may become more pronounced and the infiltrate more monomorphic, often with conspicuous atypical lymphocytes. In plaque-stage disease, infiltrates are frequently lichenoid and denser and often contain eosinophils and/or plasma cells (see Figure 7–2, *B*). The epidermal hyperplasia can be more pronounced. Pautrier's microabscesses, clusters of atypical lymphocytes in the epidermis, are a helpful finding and a diagnostic hallmark but are not always evident (presumably because of sampling error)[44] (see Figure 7–2, *C*). In advanced disease, including erythrodermic or tumor-stage MF, epidermotropism may be minimal or even lost (see Figure 7–3, *B*).

As noted above, mycosis fungoides is a malignancy of the CLA-positive skin-homing memory T cells. The transformed T cells are most commonly CD3+, CD4+, CD45RO+, and CD30– and often show reduced expression of CD7 (see Figure 7–1, *D*). Other pan-T-cell markers may also be lost, including CD2 and CD5, especially in tumor-stage disease.[45] In a small proportion of patients, infiltrating neoplastic T cells have a CD8+ phenotype; this variant has been reported to be associated with a more aggressive clinical course.[46] Similarly, rare cases of γ/δ phenotype (CD4– CD8–) are also associated with rapid progression and poor prognosis.[47,48] Expression of granzyme B (GrB) and T-cell-restricted intracellular antigen 1 (TIA-1) cytotoxic proteins by T cells have been reported to increase with progression from plaque-stage to tumor-stage disease.[49] Reports on cytokine pattern in MF T cells still conflict. In early-stage disease, a Th1-type cytokine profile has been documented that is associated with a switch to a Th2-type cytokine profile with disease progression.[50–52] Clonal T-cell antigen receptor (TCR) gene re-arrangements are detected in the majority of cases, including early patch lesions.[53] Although circulating clonal T cells are usually found in advanced stages of the disease, highly sensitive assays have detected them in the peripheral blood of many patients with early-stage MF.[54]

The most important indicators predictive of survival of patients with MF are the extent and type of skin involvement and the presence of extracutaneous disease (see Tables 7–2 and 7–3). Patients with limited patch/plaque (stage IA or T1) MF have an excellent prognosis and an overall long-term survival similar to that of a matched control population. Less than 10 percent of these patients have disease progression.[33] The median survival of patients with generalized patch/plaque (stage IB or IIA or T2) MF is more than 11 years; about 24 percent of these patients experience disease progression, and nearly 20 percent of all patients with T$_2$MF ultimately die of their disease. The presence of lymphadenopathy (stage IIA) at diagnosis does not seem to affect long-term outcome.[34]

The median survival of patients with advanced disease is significantly less favorable. Patients with tumors (stage IIB or T3) or erythroderma (stage III or T4) can expect a median survival of 3.2 and 4.6 years, respectively.[55] Important prognostic indicators in patients with erythroderma are age at presentation (< 65 years), clinical stage (III vs IV), and demonstrable peripheral blood involvement.[55] Extracutaneous disease involving lymph node effacement (stage IVA) or internal organ disease (stage IVB) is associated with a median survival of less than 1.5 years.[55]

Two diseases that are related to MF and deserve separate discussion are follicular mucinosis and pagetoid reticulosis.

Follicular mucinosis (FM) is a rare variant of CTCL, described by Pinkus[56] in 1957 under the name "alopecia mucinosa." This disease can be associated with lymphoma, in which case it may precede the development of lymphoma by years. Clinically, it is characterized by the presence of erythematous follicular papules or indurated plaques that show preferential involvement of the head and neck area (Figure 7–5, A). It can also appear as an acneiform eruption. Hair loss is often evident.[57,58]

Histologically, follicular and perifollicular infiltrates of medium-sized to large hyperchromatic cells with cerebriform nuclei (folliculotropism) associated with mucinous degeneration of the hair follicles (follicular mucinosis) and sebaceous glands are seen

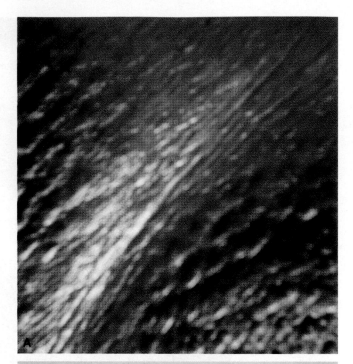

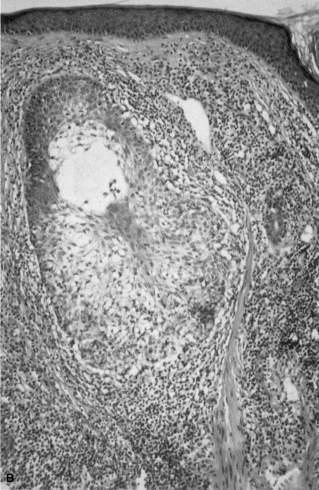

Figure 7–5. Follicular mucinosis. *A*, Follicular prominence is evident. *B*, There is a dense dermal infiltrate. Note lymphocytic infiltration and the mucinous degeneration of the hair follicle.

(see Figure 7–5, *B*). Clonal TCR gene re-arrangements are detected in the majority of cases.[59]

A 5-year survival of 70 percent has been quoted,[3] but disease hetereogeneity makes composite prognosis unhelpful. When treating this condition, it is important to remember that neither ultraviolet B (UVB) nor psoralen plus ultraviolet A (PUVA) alone are capable of reaching the deeper aspect of the hair follicle where the disease process is predominantly located. Typically, total-skin electron beam therapy (followed by maintenance PUVA therapy) is required.

Follicular mucinosis may also present as a self-limiting condition in which (a) there is no lymphocytic atypia, (b) eosinophils are sometimes numerous, and (c) polymerase chain reaction (PCR) assay is invariably negative. This latter condition is better referred to as alopecia mucinosa.

Finally, pagetoid reticulosis (Woringer-Kolopp disease)[60] is a distinct and rare variant of MF. It is characterized by a persistent but indolent solitary lesion, confined to a circumscribed region (Figure 7–6, *A*) with a distinctive histology featuring exuberant epidermotropism (Figure 7–6, *B*). A form of disseminated pagetoid reticulosis (probably an oxymoron) known as the Ketron-Goodman variant[61] runs a more aggressive clinical course. The term "pagetoid reticulosis" should be used for the localized type only.[5] Interestingly, infiltrating T cells in many cases are CD3+ CD8+.[62] Clonal TCR gene rearrangements are commonly detected.[63] The prognosis is usually excellent.

Primary CD30+ (Ki-1+) Cutaneous T-Cell Lymphoma

The hallmark of CD30+ lymphoma is proliferation of neoplastic lymphoid cells expressing the CD30 antigen. Initially, the Ki-1 (CD30) antigen was considered to be specific for the Hodgkin and Reed-Sternberg cells of Hodgkin's disease;[64] subsequently, it was

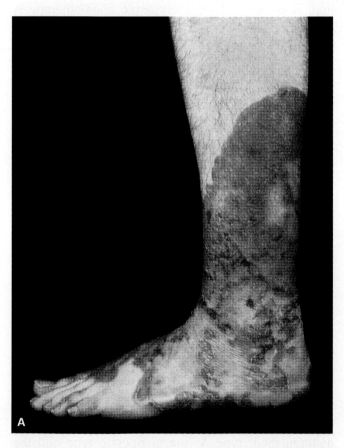

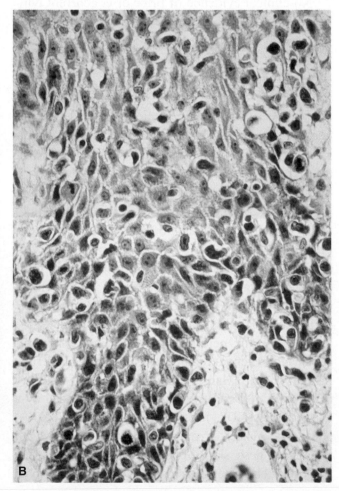

Figure 7–6. Pagetoid reticulosis. *A*, Solitary plaque, confined to the leg. *B*, In this variant of cutaneous T-cell lymphoma, there is striking epidermotropism. A CD8+ phenotype is commonly encountered.

shown to be expressed by activated lymphocytes and certain large cell lymphomas.[65] In the updated Kiel classification,[1] the National Cancer Institute working formulation,[66] and Isaacson classification[4] schemes, Ki-1+ anaplastic large cell lymphomas (ALCLs) are referred to as high-grade lymphomas since nodal CD30+ ALCLs tend to run an aggressive course. However, CD30 (Ki-1) expression in primary cutaneous large cell lymphomas has been associated with a favorable prognosis and an indolent clinical course.[67] Therefore, in the new EORTC classification scheme, primary cutaneous CD30+ lymphomas are listed in the group of low-grade non-Hodgkin's lymphomas.[3] The clinical distinction between these two is therefore critical and will guide both therapy and prognosis.

The definition of the CD30+ primary cutaneous large T-cell lymphoma by Willemze and Beljaards[68] is based on the following three criteria:

1. Predominance (> 75 percent) or large clusters of CD30+ blast cells
2. No clinical evidence of prior or concurrent lymphomatoid papulosis, MF, or other type of cutaneous lymphoma
3. Lack of extracutaneous disease at presentation (and for the following 6 months)

The disease usually affects older patients (median age, 60 years) in the form of localized solitary lesions: nodules, ulcerating tumors or papules, or (more rarely) tumors at multiple sites (multicentric). Cutaneous relapses occur frequently, but development of extracutaneous disease is unusual. Histologically, it is characterized by dermal and subcutaneous infiltrates of large non-epidermotropic clusters of CD30+ atypical lymphocytes with anaplastic morphology[69] (Figure 7–7, A). In about 20 percent of cases, the tumor consists of an almost pure infiltrate of immunoblasts or pleomorphic cells (see Figure 7–7, B). At the periphery of the lesions, normal-appearing reactive lymphocytes can be identified. Primary CD30+ large cell lymphomas of skin are most often of T-cell type and are characterized by a CD4+ (rarely CD8+) activated (CD25+, HLA-DR+) phenotype. There is occasional loss of pan-T-cell antigens. These skin-infiltrating neoplastic T cells are often characterized by a cytotoxic phenotype

defined by the expression of perforin, granzyme B, and T-cell-restricted intracellular antigen (TIA).[70] Some cells may produce Th2 cytokines.[71] Skin-infiltrating CD30+ cells are generally CLA+[72] but lack epithelial membrane antigen (EMA) and CD15 (Leu-M1) expression,[73,74] both of which may be seen in nodal variants of ALCL.[75] Molecular studies typically reveal the presence of a clonal T-cell receptor gene re-arrangement.[76] In contrast to nodal ALCL, the distinctive t(2;5)(p23;q35) translocation is not a common feature of primary cutaneous disease[77] and may be an important differentiating feature. Similarly, staining for ALK is absent.

The prognosis of primary cutaneous CD30+ large cell lymphoma (LCL) is usually very favorable, with a 5-year survival rate of more than 90 percent regardless of cell morphology (anaplastic or nonanaplastic).[78] More than 25 percent of cases of primary cutaneous ALCLs regress spontaneously; however, frequent relapses are characteristic.[30]

Local therapy, including excision or spot irradiation, is usually effective. Systemic chemotherapy is seldom required for disease truly limited to skin. Failure of CD30+ LCL to respond to conventional chemotherapy, development of extracutaneous disease, and age greater than 60 years are associated with a poor prognosis.[79] Differentiation between anaplastic and nonanaplastic (eg, CD30+ T-immunoblastic and CD30+ pleomorphic) lymphoma may sometimes be difficult.[80] The distinction is largely academic.

Lymphomatoid Papulosis

Lymphomatoid papulosis (LyP) was first described by Macaulay in 1968[81] as a chronic disease typified by a clinically benign protracted course but with histologic features suggestive of malignant lymphoma. It is characterized by remittent and relapsing reddish papules and papulonodules (in different stages) that are usually smaller than 1 cm and that often ulcerate, sometimes leaving atrophic scars (Figure 7–8, A). The lesions typically involve the trunk and extremities and tend to regress spontaneously within 3 to 4 weeks. Histologically, three major subtypes can be distinguished: type A (the histiocytic type and the most common), type B (MF-like), and type C (ALCL-like).[68] Type A is characterized by a wedge-shaped infiltrate of large atypical T cells that sometimes resemble Reed-Sternberg cells (as seen in Hodgkin's disease), frequent mitoses (including abnormal forms), and an admixture of inflammatory cells, including neutrophils and eosinophils (see Figure 7–8, *B* and *C*). Type B is less common and is characterized by a bandlike infiltrate of small atypical lymphocytes with cerebriform, hyperchromatic nuclei, and infrequent mitoses (see Figure 7–8, *D*). Epidermotropism is sometimes present. Type C is indistinguishable from ALCL, but the infiltrate is restricted to the dermis. Immunophenotypic analysis of infiltrating cells often reveals CD4+ T cells (that are CD30+ in type A lesions but not in type B lesions), variable loss of CD2 and CD5 pan-T-cell antigens, expression of activation-associated antigens (HLA-DR and CD25),[82,83] lack of EMA and CD15 expression, a Th2 cytokine profile, and interleukin-4 (IL-4) and -10 (IL-10).[71] These cells are characterized by a very high proliferative index as assessed by Ki-67 reactivity,[84] as well as a very high apoptosis index, compared to other lymphoprolifera-

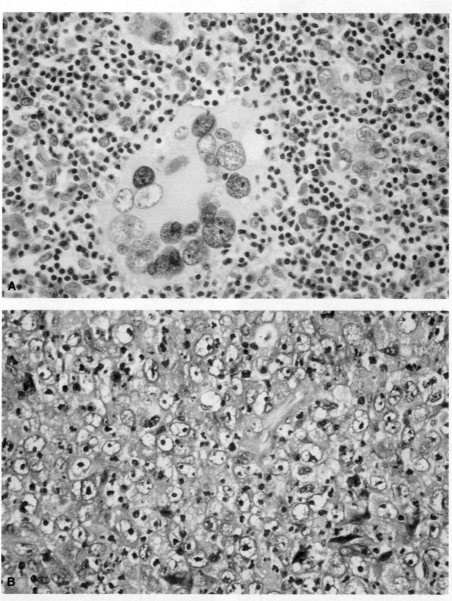

Figure 7–7. *A*, Primary cutaneous anaplastic CD30+ large cell lymphoma. In this example, the cells have abundant cytoplasm and highly irregular, vesicular nuclei. Note the bizarre giant cell. *B*, Primary cutaneous immunoblastic CD30+ lymphoma. Note the large vesicular nuclei with prominent nucleoli.

tive diseases;[85] it has been suggested that apoptosis may be a significant mechanism of regression in LyP. Clonal T-cell populations are detected in the lesions of the majority of LyP patients.[86] The t(2;5)(p23;q35) translocation is not present.

The overall prognosis of LyP patients is very good; 5-year survival is nearly 100 percent. However, LyP may be preceded by, associated with, or fol-lowed by lymphoma. There is an increased potential of developing lymphoma (MF and Ki-1+ [CD30+] LCL) and even nonlymphoid malignancies.[87–89] The risk of transformation is 5 to 20 percent, increasing up to an 80 percent cumulative risk after a 15-year follow-up period.[90] Despite this increased risk, how-ever, the overall long-term survival is only slightly decreased when compared to controls.[89]

Occasionally, it is difficult to sharply distinguish between CD30+ LCL and LyP since both have many aspects in common, show similar histologic features often,[68,69] and are best documented as CD30+ lym-phoproliferative disorders of uncertain biologic potential. Borderline cases usually have a favorable prognosis.[79] Lymphomatoid papulosis and primary cutaneous CD30+ LCL are considered to represent different poles of a common disease spectrum.

Cutaneous large cell lymphomas of the CD30+ type can develop secondarily from MF,[69,91] from

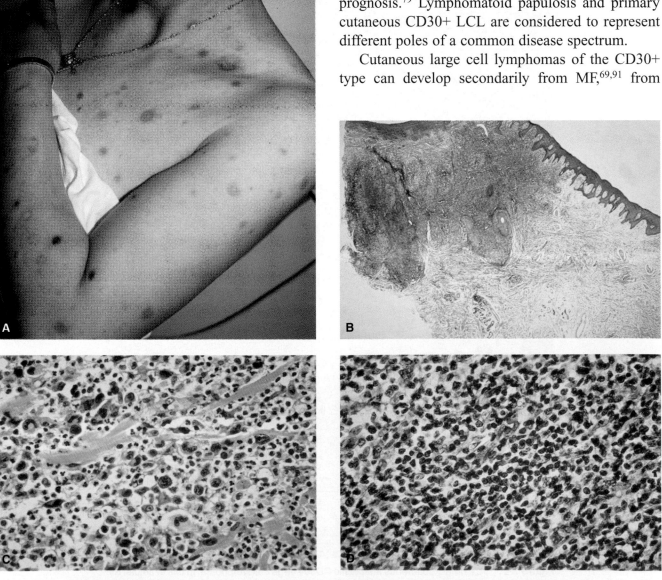

Figure 7–8. Lymphomatoid papulosis. *A*, Multiple red papules (some of which are necrotic). *B*, Note the ulceration and wedge-shaped infil-trate in this established lesion. *C*, In this type A lesion, there is marked nuclear pleomorphism, and mitoses are conspicuous. *D*, In this type B variant, the infiltrate is composed of irregular and hyperchromatic lymphocytes.

LyP,[92,93] or from primary noncutaneous (usually nodal) CD30+ LCL[94] (see "Secondary Cutaneous Lymphomas," below). In these settings, they have have a significantly worse prognosis than primary cutaneous CD30+ LCLs. The incidence of large-cell transformation of MF/SS is reportedly around 23 percent, with a cumulative probability of transformation of 39 percent.[95] The definition of large-cell transformation is the presence of > 25 percent large cells in the infiltrate[96] (Figure 7–9). Factors associated with large-cell transformation include advanced (tumor-stage) disease, increased tumor-cell CD25 expression,[97] and elevated lactate dehydrogenase (LDH) and β_2Microglobulin.[96]

Transformation of MF or LyP to a large-cell variant is associated with shortened survival and a more aggressive clinical course.[98]

Sézary Syndrome

Sézary syndrome (SS), also known as the leukemic form of MF, was first described by Sézary and Bou-

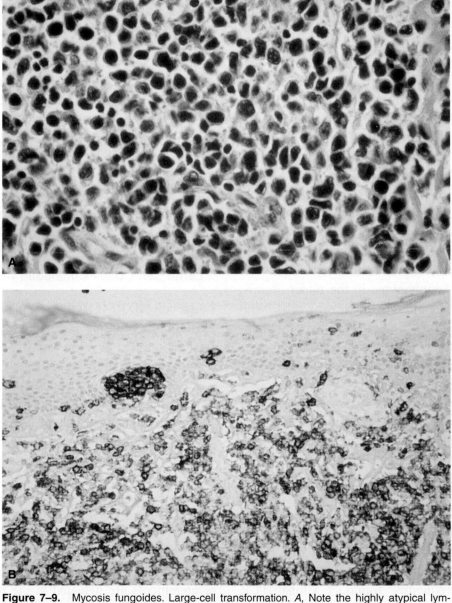

Figure 7–9. Mycosis fungoides. Large-cell transformation. *A*, Note the highly atypical lymphoid cells. *B*, Virtually all of the cells express the CD30 antigen.

vrain in 1938 as a disease characterized by generalized exfoliating erythroderma, peripheral lymphadenopathy, and "monstrous cells" in the skin and peripheral blood.[99] In 1961, Taswell and Winkelmann named this disease Sézary syndrome.[100] Patients present with a triad of generalized erythroderma, lymphadenopathy, and Sézary cells in the peripheral blood, skin, and lymph nodes.[101,102] Erythroderma appears as confluent scaling dermatitis ("red man syndrome") (see Figure 7–4) arising de novo or from pre-existent lesions and is usually accompanied by intense pruritus, atrophic or lichenified skin, scaling and fissuring of soles and palms, and constitutional symptoms including fever, chills, and weight loss.

According to a recent report, there is a high incidence of secondary malignant tumors in SS, particularly cutaneous squamous cell carcinomas and internal-organ neoplasms. In that study, these tumors were only partly due to treatment-associated immunosuppression and appear to be related to the disease itself.[103] It may be that type 2 cytokines (including IL-10) that suppress cell-mediated immunity contribute to this syndrome.

Histologically, the features are variable, and only a sparse perivascular infiltrate with few atypical lymphocytes is seen in some patients. In such patients, multiple biopsies increase the diagnostic yield. More typically, however, there is a dense diffuse infiltrate of lymphocytes in the upper dermis, along with various numbers of Sézary cells, with convoluted cerebriform nuclei. Pautrier's microabscesses containing Sézary cells are seen in a minority of cases. Indeed, epidermotropism is often less pronounced, compared with early-stage MF.

Expansion of Sézary cells (CD4+CD7–) in the peripheral blood, the skin, and lymph nodes is characteristic; however, activated T cells morphologically indistinguishable from Sézary cells are not limited to SS and can occur in a variety of inflammatory dermatoses.[104] In SS, however, neoplastic cells displaying the CD4+CD7– phenotype are larger and have been reported to exhibit diminished CD3 expression.[105] A Th2 cytokine profile (IL-4, IL-5, IL-10) associated with peripheral-blood eosinophilia is frequently found.[106] Clonal TCR gene re-arrangements are usually detected,[107] and

clonality may be present in both the CD4+CD7– and the CD4+CD7+ T-cell population.[108]

There is no agreement on diagnostic criteria; detection of at least 1,000 Sézary cells per cubic millimeter or 5 to 20 percent of the total lymphocyte count have been suggested.[109,110] Recently proposed diagnostic criteria for SS are the presence of the following: erythroderma, atypical circulating mononuclear cells, and evidence of a clonal T-cell population in the peripheral blood.[111] Flow cytometry analysis of peripheral blood can be useful; typically, an elevated CD4/CD8 ratio (> 6) and a phenotypically discrete population of CD4+CD7– cells can usually be identified.

By definition, patients with SS have at least stage IIIA disease and an overall poor prognosis. Variables associated with a poor prognosis include a previous history of MF, a high number of circulating Sézary cells, a high CD4/CD8 ratio, and elevated serum LDH levels. The reported median survival is 31 months, and the 5-year survival rate is 33.5 percent. Patients with only one adverse prognostic feature or without any such features have a more favorable prognosis with a 5-year survival of 58 percent whereas patients with two or three adverse prognostic features have an aggressive course with a 5-year survival of only 5 percent.[112]

Large Cell CD30– Cutaneous T-Cell Lymphoma

Large cell CD30– CTCL presents in elderly patients as single or multiple cutaneous nodules or tumors. Lesions tend to develop rapidly, without preceding patches and plaques.[113]

The histologic appearance may resemble MF undergoing large-cell transformation. There are diffuse or nodular infiltrates of large or medium-sized anaplastic cells that represent greater than 30 percent of the total population of neoplastic cells.[113,114] Immunoblasts may also be present; eosinophils, macrophages, and plasma cells are also sometimes seen. Epidermotropism is only rarely present. Neoplastic cells express a CD4+ phenotype, show variable loss of pan-T-cell antigens, and show minimal or absent CD30 expression.[113] Clonal TCR gene re-arrangements are detected in the majority of cases. Large cell CD30– T-cell lymphomas tend to run an aggressive course with a 5-year survival of only 15 percent.[3] Poor prognosis is associated with an increased proportion of large cells.[113] The EORTC classification includes angiocentric lymphoma with a predominance of large pleomorphic CD30– T cells in this category.

Granulomatous Slack Skin

Granulomatous slack skin (GSS) is a rare variant of CTCL, characterized by progressive skin laxity in the flexural areas due to the loss of elastic fibers. The disease usually occurs in young or middle-aged males as progressively lax skin, especially in the axillae and groin. Classic MF may be associated with GSS.[115] In a significant proportion of patients, Hodgkin's disease develops years or even decades after the initial appearance of the skin lesions.[116] Histologically, the disease is characterized by a dense infiltrate of atypical small lymphocytes in association with macrophages, multinucleated giant cells, and epithelioid cells, often forming well-developed granulomas (Figure 7–10). Dermal elastophagocytosis is typically seen, and epidermotropism may rarely be present.[117] A CD3+, CD4+, CD45RO+ phenotype has been described,[118] and a clonal T-cell population is found in the majority of the cases.[119] Granuloma-tous slack skin has an indolent clinical course although patients should be carefully screened for evidence of Hodgkin's disease.[118]

Pleomorphic Small and Medium-Sized T-Cell Lymphoma

This is a very rare variant of primary CTCL, characterized by proliferation of small and medium-sized pleomorphic T cells. It presents as nonpruritic solitary or multiple papules, nodules, or tumors,[113,120] with no preceding patches or plaques. It is also characterized by a deep and diffuse dermal infiltrate composed of mostly small to medium-sized atypical pleomorphic T cells, with large pleomorphic cells making up around 30 percent.[114] The infiltrate sometimes extends into the subcutaneous fat and shows minimal or no epidermotropism. In most cases, infiltrating tumor cells are CD4+, with variable loss of pan-T-cell antigens. Clonal TCR gene re-arrangements are usually detected.

The overall 5-year survival is about 60 percent.[3,114] Patients with pleomorphic small cell lymphomas have a more favorable prognosis.[114,120] The EORTC classification currently includes angiocentric lymphomas with a predominance of small and medium-sized pleomorphic T cells in this category.

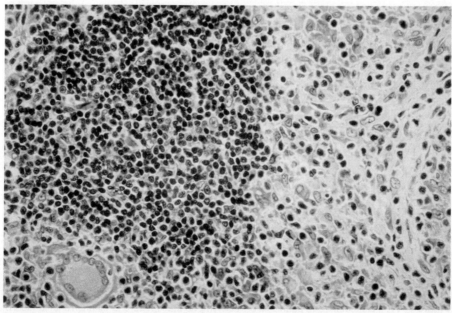

Figure 7–10.   Granulomatous slack skin. Note the admixture of atypical lymphocytes with irregular hyperchromatic nuclei and epithelioid histiocytes. A giant cell is present in the lower left field.

Subcutaneous Panniculitis-Like T-Cell Lymphoma

An uncommon variant of CTCL, subcutaneous pan-niculitis-like T-cell lymphoma is characterized by the presence of an atypical lymphocytic infiltrate predominantly within the subcutaneous fat.[121] Clinically, it presents as deep subcutaneous nodules and plaques that are preferentially localized to the lower extremities. It is often associated with a hemo-phagocytic syndrome including systemic symptoms such as fever, malaise, and weight loss. The tumor is composed of a non-epidermotropic dense and dif-fuse infiltrate of pleomorphic cells of various sizes admixed with macrophages[122,123] (Figure 7–11). Necrosis, karyorrhexis, and hemophagocytosis are commonly seen.[124]

Tumor cells in most cases exhibit a CD8+ cyto-toxic phenotype (TIA-1+ and perforin+)[125] with variable loss of pan-T-cell antigens.[121] Occasionally, CD30 or CD56 expression is present.[122,125,126] The presence of latent Epstein-Barr virus[122,127] and iso-lated cases of γ/δ-positive T-cell lymphoma have been reported and are associated with an aggressive

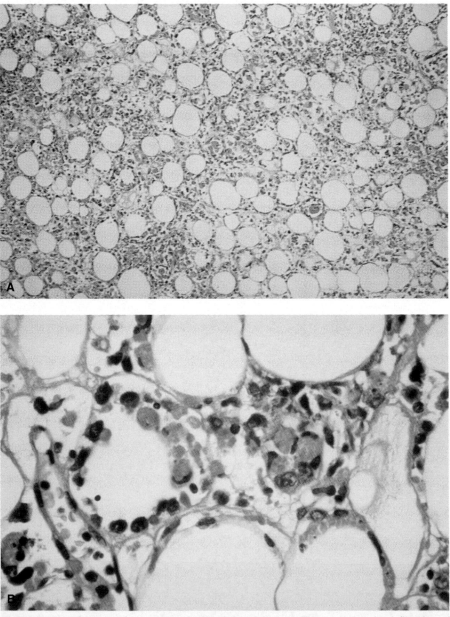

Figure 7–11. Subcutaneous panniculitic T-cell lymphoma. *A*, There is extensive infiltration of the subcutaneous fat by atypical lymphocytes and histiocytes. The lacelike pattern is character-istic. *B*, Hemophagocytosis as shown in this field is a common feature.

course.[128,129] Clonal TCR gene re-arrangements are commonly present. The prognosis is generally very poor, with a median survival of less than 3 years.

Primary Cutaneous B-Cell Lymphoma

Primary cutaneous B-cell lymphomas (PCBCLs) make up less than 25 percent of all primary cutaneous non-Hodgkin's lymphomas. While European studies cite frequencies greater than 20%, a recent paper indicates that the frequency in the US is closer to 4.5%.[130] As a result of recent progress in immunologic techniques, it has become clear that PCBCL occurs more frequently than was generally believed and that some of the conditions previously thought to be pseudolymphomas (cutaneous lymphoid hyperplasias) are in fact cutaneous lymphomas. Primary cutaneous B-cell lymphoma is defined by the presence of cutaneous involvement in the absence of extracutaneous manifestations over a period of at least 6 months. As opposed to secondary cutaneous B-cell lymphoma, there is a low risk of systemic dissemination and a very good prognosis, with a 5-year survival rate of greater than 90 percent.[3]

The classification and terminology of PCBCL is more controversial than that of CTCL.

Primary Cutaneous Follicular Center Cell Lymphoma

Primary cutaneous follicular center cell lymphoma (PCFCCL), an entity defined by the EORTC classification, accounts for approximately 40 percent of all cases of PCBCL.[131,132] Patients present with solitary or localized papules, plaques, or nodules, typically involving the head, neck, or trunk.[3,133] Histologically, a Grenz zone of sparing of the subepidermal papillary dermis is characteristic. The infiltrate, which consists of a mixture of centrocytes with a lesser number of centroblasts, may exhibit a follicular or diffuse growth pattern (Figure 7–12), and extension into the subcutaneous fat is commonly present.[3,134] Tumor cells are CD20+ CD10+ CD5–, usually bcl-2– and bcl-6–, and demonstrate monotypic light-chain expression or absence of detectable immunoglobulin (Ig). A network of CD21+ dendritic cells outlining a background fol-

licular architecture is commonly seen, and their presence is an important diagnostic criterion.

Although the earlier literature documented the chromosomal translocation t(14;18) in a very small percentage of cases,[135] a more recent publication by Yang and colleagues identified the translocation in 40 percent of PCFCCLs.[30] Monoclonal re-arrangement of Ig heavy-chain and light-chain genes[136] is often detected.

It is important to distinguish PCFCCL from nodal disease as patients with the former have a clinically benign course and an excellent prognosis. The 5-year survival is greater than 95 percent.[3]

The disease may have a tendency to recur after treatment.

Crosti's lymphoma (reticulohistiocytoma of the back) is probably synonymous with PCBCL of follicular center cell origin or with primary cutaneous marginal-zone lymphoma.[137]

Marginal-Zone B-Cell Lymphoma

Marginal-zone B-cell lymphoma (MZL) represents the second most common form of PCBCL, after follicular center cell lymphoma.[138] Marginal-zone B-cell lymphoma has been referred to as monocytoid B-cell lymphoma, primary cutaneous immunocytoma, mucosa-associated lymphoid tissue (MALT) type lymphoma, or lymphoma of skin-associated lymphoid tissue (SALT). The EORTC classifies MZL and primary cutaneous immunocytoma as a single entity since they are closely related and have overlapping histologic features.[3] However, the term "immunocytoma" is best restricted to a systemic lymphoma involving the bone marrow and lymph nodes.

Marginal zone lymphoma presents as single or multiple nodules or tumors, with a predilection for the upper extremities and trunk of middle-aged or older women.[139,140] Some cases, particularly in Europe, are associated with *Borellia burgdorferi* infection.[141]

Marginal-zone B-cell lymphoma is characterized by a dense, sometimes nodular dermal infiltrate that often extends into the subcutaneous fat. Reactive follicles with germinal centers are commonly present and are a diagnostic marker. The infiltrate consists of small centrocyte-like cells with irregular hyperchromatic nuclei (marginal-zone lymphocytes), monocytoid B cells, and lymphoplasmacy-toid cells (Figure 7–13). Eosinophils, giant cells, and epithelioid giant cells are sometimes present. The presence of germinal centers and a mixture of reactive inflammatory cells has resulted in frequent misdiagnosis of MZL as a reactive condition (eg, a persistent insect bite reaction).[139,142,143] Tumor cells express CD20 and sometimes CD43 but are negative for CD5, CD10, and CD23. Expression of mono-

typic surface Ig and cytoplasmic Ig is common. Clonal Ig gene re-arrangements are often present.[136] Marginal-zone B-cell lymphomas behave in a clinically indolent fashion, with a 5-year survival of 95 percent, but with a tendency to recur.

Due to a less favorable clinical course, primary cutaneous follicular center cell lymphoma presenting on the legs of elderly women has been classified as a separate entity in the EORTC classification

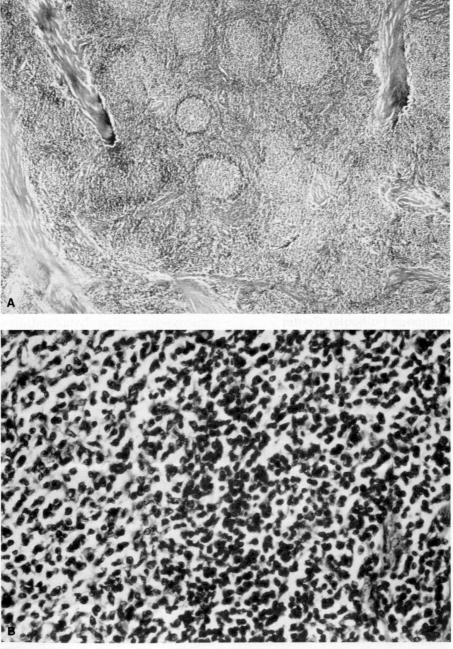

Figure 7–12.   Primary cutaneous follicular center cell lymphoma. *A*, There is widespread infiltration of the dermis by a dense lymphoid infiltrate. *B*, Note the infiltrate of centrocytes. The follicle is present on the left side of the field.

scheme.[3] However, whether this lymphoma should be considered a distinct entity is controversial. The tumor typically presents as nodules on one or both legs of elderly women (median age of 76 years). Although they respond favorably to local treatment initially, relapse occurs in a large proportion of patients.[143b] The estimated 5-year survival is 58 percent.[143b] Histologically, the majority of these represent follicular center lymphomas.[144] Neoplastic cells express CD20 and monotypic Ig.[143b] Although

t(14;18) translocation is absent, bcl-2 is expressed, as opposed to other PCFCCLs.[145] Clonal Ig gene rearrangements are usually detected.[145]

Intravascular Large B-cell Lymphoma

Cutaneous intravascular large B-cell lymphoma, originally referred to as malignant endotheliomatosis,[146] is characterized by an intravascular proliferation of neoplastic lymphocytes, particularly involving the skin and central nervous system.[147,148] It presents as

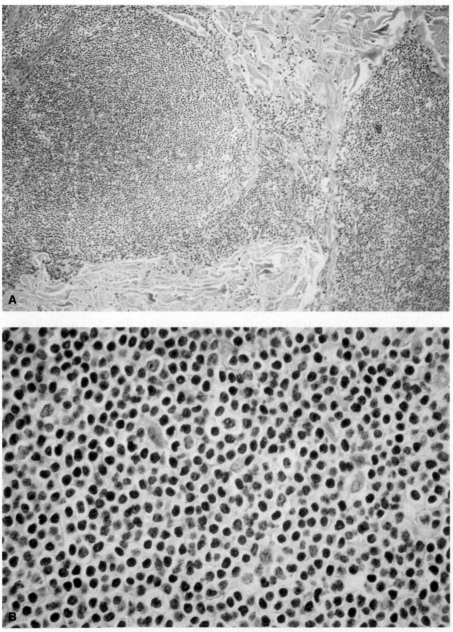

Figure 7–13. Primary cutaneous marginal-zone lymphoma. *A*, There is a dense dermal lymphoid infiltrate. Note the residual reactive follicle. *B*, In this field, there is an almost pure population of monocytoid B cells.

violaceous patches, plaques, and ulcerated tumors involving the trunk and legs.[147,149,150] It displays an aggressive clinical behavior and carries a 5-year survival rate of less than 50 percent, although primary cutaneous forms may have a more favorable course.[3] Histologically, there is a dense proliferation of large atypical B cells within the lumina of blood vessels in the dermis and subcutis, occasionally causing vascular occlusion.[153] Tumor cells express CD45RB (leukocyte common antigen), CD19, CD20, CD22, CD79a, and monotypic immunoglobulin.[152] Clonal Ig gene re-arrangements are present.[151]

Cutaneous Plasmacytoma

Cutaneous plasmacytoma is a very unusual type of cutaneous B-cell lymphoma, characterized by proliferation of plasma cells in the skin in the absence of multiple myeloma. Cutaneous plasmacytoma presents as solitary or generalized violaceous nodules.[153–155] The histologic picture shows diffuse or nodular dermal infiltrates of mature plasma cells. Expression of monotypic cytoplasmic Ig, CD79a+, CD43+, and CD38+ and lack of CD19, CD20, and CD22 expression has been reported.[153–156]

SECONDARY CUTANEOUS LYMPHOMAS

The skin is the second most commonly affected site in disseminated nodal disease.[4] "Secondary cutaneous lymphoma" is the term used to describe skin involvement as an extranodal manifestation of a primarily systemic lymphoma. This lymphoma is often associated with an aggressive clinical course and a poor prognosis. This contrast in prognosis with primary cutaneous lymphoma makes this distinction the most important one the dermatologist can make.

Adult T-Cell Leukemia/Lymphoma

Adult T-cell leukemia/lymphoma (ATLL) is a malignant T-cell lymphoma associated with infection by the human T-lymphotrophic virus type 1 (HTLV-1). It was first documented in areas where the retrovirus is endemic: Japan[157] (initially), the Caribbean basin, and the southeastern United States.[158,159] Although ATLL has a very high incidence of cutaneous involvement, it is excluded from the EORTC classification of primary cutaneous lymphomas because skin involvement is considered a manifestation of a generalized disease.[3] Characteristically, only a small proportion of infected individuals develop ATLL, usually years after exposure to HTLV-1, in the fifth decade of life. Four clinical subtypes are distinguished: smoldering, chronic, lymphoma-type, and acute.[160] Clinical findings include generalized lymphadenopathy, hepatosplenomegaly, and (frequently) leukemia. Bone marrow involvement, lytic bone lesions, hypercalcemia, and opportunistic infections may also be present. Skin involvement is seen in up to 50 percent of the patients.[161–163] Cutaneous lesions may resemble MF and appear as erythematous papules, plaques, nodules, or erythroderma. Histologically, the skin lesions consist of a usually dense infiltrate of atypical lymphocytes resembling MF. Epidermotropism and Pautrier's microabscesses are sometimes present. Blast cells may also be seen, and mitoses are often conspicuous. An admixture of inflammatory cells including plasma cells, histiocytes, and sometimes conspicuous eosinophils may also be a feature. In the peripheral blood, the tumor cells have a multilobated "clover-leaf" appearance. Neoplastic cells in the peripheral blood, lymph nodes, and skin of patients with ATLL exhibit phenotypic heterogeneity;[164] they are predominantly CD4+ (and may or may not be CD7+) but sometimes exhibit a CD8+ phenotype. High CD25 expression is detected in both the skin and peripheral blood.[165,166] Clonal TCR gene re-arrangement is commonly detected as well as integration of HTLV-1 proviral sequences in the host genome.[167] In the peripheral blood, HTLV-1 antibodies are usually detected. The disease usually has a rapidly fatal clinical course, but survival is related to the clinical subtype and the presence or absence of extracutaneous disease. Patients with acute and lymphomatous types have a poor prognosis and a median survival of under 2 years whereas the chronic and smoldering subtypes are characterized by a protracted clinical course that often progresses for more than a decade.

Secondary Cutaneous CD30+ Large Cell Lymphoma

Approximately 23 percent of primary nodal ALCL patients have secondary skin involvement.[171] Differences between primary and secondary CD30+ large cell lymphomas involve both molecular and clinical aspects. Thus, epithelial-membrane antigen (EMA) and t(2;5)(p23;q35) translocation are usually absent in primary cutaneous disease.[72,75,169] Histologically, the two conditions are indistinguishable. Systemic ALCL with secondary skin lesions is more common in children and adolescents and is associated with an unfavorable prognosis.[70,91]

Natural Killer/T-Cell Angiocentric Lymphoma

Natural killer (NK) T-cell angiocentric lymphomas most commonly involve the nasal cavity (nasal NK/T-cell lymphoma or lethal midline granuloma) but may present at other sites (they are then called nasal-type NK/T-cell lymphomas). Secondary spread of the disease often involves the skin and subcutaneous tissue. Primary cutaneous disease, which is rare, presents with (often) generalized papules, subcutaneous nodules, and ulcerated lesions. Histologically, the infiltrate is polymorphic, consisting of variably-sized pleomorphic lymphoid cells accompanied by immunoblasts. A mixed and reactive inflammatory cell infiltrate is usually present. Vascular invasion (angiocentricity) is present in many cases, and necrosis is an invariable finding (Figure 7–14). The vast majority of systemic NK lymphomas are positive for EBV. The immunophenotype characterizing NK lymphoma is CD56+ CD2+ surface CD3– (but cytoplasmic CD3+), CD16, and CD57 are usually negative.[171,172] Clonal TCR gene re-arrangements are not found. The aggressive clinical behavior that characterizes these lymphomas has been linked to the high expression of the multidrug-resistance gene.[173]

Lymphomatoid Granulomatosis

Lymphomatoid granulomatosis (LyG) is an EBV-related B-cell angiocentric and angiodestructive lymphoproliferative disorder that most often develops in the immunosuppressed.[174] In the mistaken belief that it represented a variant of T-cell lymphoma, it was formerly included within the spectrum of angiocentric immunoproliferative lesions. Lymphomatoid granulomatosis is a systemic disor-

der presenting in lungs, brain, liver, kidney, and skin.[175] Within the viscera, it is characterized by a polymorphous infiltrate of lymphocytes, histiocytes, plasma cells, and atypical B cells with pleomorphic nuclei, prominent nucleoli, and multiple mitotic figures. The majority of the mature lymphocytes are of T-cell phenotype and represent a reactive population. Vascular infiltration, destruction, and tissue necrosis are typically present. The pleomorphic cell population is CD20+, CD30+/–, and CD15–. Cutaneous lesions are common and are characterized histologically by vasculitic changes and a variably pleomorphic cellular infiltrate.

Lymphomatoid granulomatosis may sometimes be histologically confused with angiocentric NK/T-cell lymphoma. The latter shares the relationship to EBV but is of an NK/T-cell phenotype.[171]

Cutaneous Lymphoma in Human Immunodeficiency Virus Infection and Hodgkin's Disease

Cutaneous lymphomas in human immunodeficiency virus (HIV) infection are very rare. Although most nodal non-Hodgkin's lymphomas in HIV disease are of B-cell lineage, cutaneous lymphomas are usually of T-cell type. Forms of cutaneous lymphoma reported in association with HIV disease include conditions resembling MF and cases of non-epidermotropic LCLs.[176] The latter is characterized by a CD30+ phenotype, the presence of EBV, and a poor prognosis.[177]

Secondary cutaneous tumor involvement in Hodgkin's disease is very rare (incidence of 0.5 to 3.4%) and is associated with a fairly poor prognosis.[178]

APPROACHES TO DIAGNOSIS AND STAGING

Correct diagnosis may be very difficult early in the course of the disease. Frequent biopsies are often required, and ancillary techniques including immunocytochemistry and gene re-arrangement studies are usually necessary before a final conclusion can be reached.

Clinical information is necessary as many lymphomas, particularly of T-cell phenotype, share histologic features. Thus, MF, SS, ATLL, and even lymphomatoid drug reactions or actinic reticuloid may be histologically indistinguishable. Cutaneous T-cell lymphomas are usually characterized by infiltrates, typically involving the epidermis (epidermotropism) and localizing to the subepidermal papillary dermis, superficial vasculature, and periadnexal areas. A horizontal growth pattern is characteristic of early lesions.[5] In MF (the most common type of CTCL), bandlike infiltrates in the papillary dermis are frequently found. Pautrier's microabscesses (mononu-clear cells that form aggregates in the epidermis) are very specific for MF but are frequently absent. Sézary cells in biopsy specimens are identified by the characteristic increase in the nuclear contour index or increased nuclear folding and indentations; they are often localized to the lower epidermis and lie within a lacuna.

A B-cell pattern is characterized by infiltrates in the perivascular spaces of middle and deep dermis and fat separated by an infiltrate-free papillary dermis, the

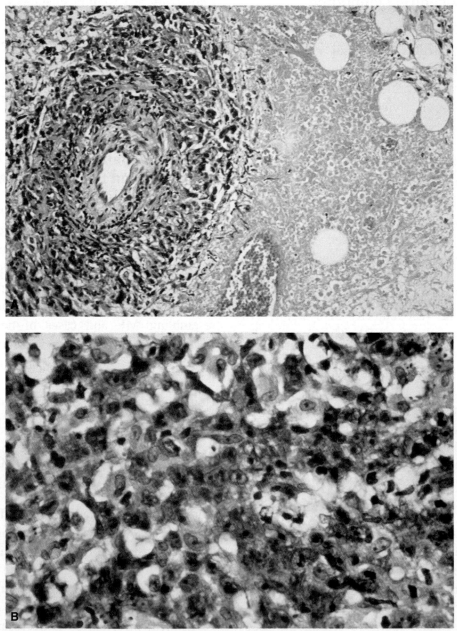

Figure 7–14.   Natural killer/T-cell angiocentric lymphoma. *A,* In this field, there is an angio-centric and angiodestructive atypical lymphoid infiltrate associated with necrosis. *B,* In addition to atypical lymphocytes, conspicuous blast forms are present.

so-called Grenz zone. B-cell infiltrates are predominantly nodular and grow in all directions.[131,179]

Although T-cell and B-cell patterns as described above usually enable an accurate prediction of cell lineage, B-cell lymphomas occasionally may show a pattern reminiscent of T-cell lymphoma (eg, B-cell epidermotropism), and conversely, T-cell lymphomas (especially non-MF CTCLs) may sometimes lack epidermotropism and resemble a B-cell lymphoma.[113,180]

Immunohistochemistry

Immunocytochemistry, in addition to identifying cellular lineage, may be of value in obtaining prognostic information. To define lineage, a range of pan-T-cell (CD2, CD3, CD5, and CD7), pan-B-cell (CD19, CD20, CD22, and CD79a) and NK (CD56, CD57, and CD16) markers are used. Additional markers may be necessary from time to time.

In the case of CTCL, the use of subset markers (CD4 and CD8), expression of the memory T-cell isoform of the leukocyte common antigen CD45RO, activation-associated antigens (such as CD25 and CD30), and cutaneous lymphocyte antigen (CLA) are also helpful in addition to pan-T-cell markers. The vast majority of CTCLs are characterized by a skin-homing memory helper T-cell (CD4+ CD45RO+ CLA+) phenotype. Reduced expression of pan-T-cell antigens, particularly CD7, is frequently observed.[181,182] Activation-associated antigens (eg, CD25) are variably present in MF but frequently present in ALCL and ATLL-associated lymphoma.[45,69,165] It is important to determine expression of CD25 because it may determine eligibility for ONTAK therapy.

Cutaneous B-cell lymphomas are characterized by expression of pan-B-cell markers (CD19, CD20, CD22, and CD79a) and frequent absence of CD5 and CD10 expression; PCBCLs may be Ig+ or Ig−. Immunohistochemistry can also be used to detect monoclonality in B-cell lymphoma by demonstrating monotypic Ig expression. Immunoglobulin-positive B-cell lymphomas are monoclonal (all tumor cells express the same Ig light chain) whereas inflammatory or reactive infiltrates (eg, cutaneous lymphoid hyperplasia) are usually polyclonal.

Antigen Receptor Gene Re-arrangements

A major feature of cutaneous lymphoma is monoclonality; therefore, identification of clonal expansion aids considerably in the diagnosis of the disease. T-cell clonality and B-cell clonality are detected by the presence of re-arrangements in the genes coding for antigen receptors in T cells (TCRs) and in B cells (Ig).

Two types of TCRs have been identified on the surface of T cells: TCRα/β, found on the majority of T cells, and TCRγ/δ, which represents a small percentage of lymphocytes. Of the four T-cell receptor genes (α, β, γ, and δ) β and γ are the most useful in detecting TCR gene re-arrangements. Analysis of clonal re-arrangements of TCRγ is commonly used. Detection of such re-arrangements in biopsy specimens are done using Southern blot (for TCRβ) or PCR (for TCRγ); PCR is more sensitive.[183,184] Amplification of the TCRγ gene re-arrangements by PCR followed by denaturing gel electrophoresis (DGGE) is a very sensitive method for detecting dominant clonality. However, due to the high sensitivity of this technique, TCRγ gene re-arrangement may be detected in some patients with chronic dermatitis who do not meet the histopathologic criteria for CTCL (so-called clonal dermatitis).[53] Also, PCR/DGGE as commonly performed has a false-negative rate of 20 percent, because rare TCRγ-gene families are not always assessed.

B cells re-arrange the immunoglobulin genes. Southern blot analysis as well as PCR/DGGE are used to detect heavy-chain (IgH) and light-chain (κ and λ) gene re-arrangements to detect clonality in B-cell lymphomas.

Although it provides strong evidence for the diagnosis of lymphoma, clonal proliferation of lymphocytes has its limitations. First, there are reports regarding TCR gene re-arrangements in B-cell lymphomas[185,186] and Ig gene (and TCR gene) re-arrangements in patients with MF.[187] Second, the presence of clonality does not necessarily mean malignancy since not all clonal populations behave in an aggressive fashion. Benign conditions such as pityriasis lichenoides et varioliformis acuta (PLEVA) and cutaneous lymphocyte hyperplasia may also demonstrate clonality.[136,188,189] Clonality is best thought of as identifying a population of lymphocytes derived from a single precursor that have a growth or survival advantage over other lymphocytes of the same class.

Flow Cytometry

Sézary cells, identified by a CD4+ CD7– phenotype[190] and a distinct forward and side scatter pattern, can be reliably detected in peripheral blood by flow cytometry. Since CD4+ CD7– cells are not restricted to Sézary syndrome but may be present in the circulation of patients with benign skin conditions,[191] detection of at least 1,000 Sézary cells per cubic millimeter (or 5 to 20% of the total lymphocyte count) has been suggested as being a diagnostic criterion.[192,193] Flow cytometry panel may also include CD3, CD4 and CD8, CD25, CD30, CD45RO, and CLA and a CD4/CD8 ratio. A CD4-CD8 ratio of > 6.0, an identifiable population of CD4+ CD7– cells (> 5%), and an absolute CD4 count of > 1,000 all suggest peripheral blood involvement. Peripheral blood involvement per se does not affect stage.

Lymph Node Biopsy

Biopsies should be performed on enlarged (> 1 cm) palpable lymph nodes although dermatopathic lymphadenopathy may be the only histologic finding in the early stages of the disease. The presence of atypical lymphocytes, with characteristic cerebriform nuclei and leading ultimately to effacement of normal nodal architecture, is characteristic of the later stages of disease. Immunohistochemistry flow cytometry, and clonality studies are also helpful.

Staging

Mycosis fungoides and Sézary syndrome (SS) patients are classified according to the tumor-node-metastasis-blood (TNMB) staging system[194,195] (see Tables 7–2 and 7–3).

The T stage refers to the extent and type of skin lesions: T1 and T2 refer to patch/plaque stages (< 10% and > 10% of total skin surface, respectively); T3 refers to tumors; and T4 refers to generalized erythroderma.

The N stage refers to lymph node involvement and is scored from N0 to N3, depending on the clinical and pathologic findings. In addition, lymph node biopsy specimens are scored from LN0 to LN4, according to the number of atypical cells in paracortical T-cell regions and the preservation or effacement of the lymph node architecture.[196] Nodes designated LN1 have a small number of atypical lymphocytes. Nodes classed as LN2 and LN3 have small and large clusters of atypical cells, respectively. Nodes scored as LN4 show effacement by atypical cells.

The M and B stages refer to the presence (M1, B1) or absence (M0, B0) of visceral and blood involvement, respectively.

Given an easy access to computed tomography (CT) scans, a baseline CT evaluation should be performed as part of the initial staging as well as a baseline for follow-up in CTCL patients.

SUMMARY OF PROGNOSIS

Cutaneous lymphomas make up a broad spectrum of neoplasias, from indolent disease associated with an unchanged life expectancy (eg, stage IA of MF) to highly aggressive types associated with an aggressive clinical course and a dismal prognosis leading to a rapidly fatal outcome (eg, SS).

There is a strong relationship between the stage of disease and the survival of CTCL patients. Skin stage and the presence or absence of extracutaneous involvement (lymph node, blood, and visceral spread) are the most important factors that predict clinical outcome.[197–199] Thus, the survival of MF patients worsens with increasing skin stage; limited skin involvement is associated with a life expectancy similar to that of a matched control population[33] whereas patients with generalized erythroderma or tumor stage have an unfavorable prognosis (see "Mycosis Fungoides" and "Sézary Syndrome," above). Peripheral blood involvement and extracutaneous spread such as lymph node and visceral involvement is associated with shortened survival.[55,198]

Clinically evident lymphadenopathy was previously thought to be associated with a worse prognosis; however, its value in the assessment of survival is controversial.[200,201] The degree of lymph node involvement correlates with prognosis. Patients with uneffaced lymph nodes (LN0–2) have a much better survival rate than patients with effaced nodes (5-year survival of 15 to 30% vs 70%).[199] The survival of patients with lymph node involvement may also be related to the cell morphology: the small cell (cerebriform) subtype is associated with a significantly better prognosis (median survival of 40 months) than other subtypes (median survival of 20 months).[202]

Sausville and colleagues[198] defined three prognostic groups among MF and SS patients. Good-risk patients are those with patch/plaque skin disease and no evidence of extracutaneous disease, (stages IA, IB, and IIA; median survival, > 12 years). Intermediate-risk patients are those who have tumors, erythroderma, or the plaque stage of the disease with lymph node or blood involvement but no visceral disease or node effacement (stages IIB and III; median survival of 5 years). Poor-risk patients have visceral disease or lymph node effacement (stage IV; median survival of 2.5 years).

Other studies have shown that (in addition to advanced disease [stages IIB or IV]) older age (> 60 years) and high LDH levels are associated with an aggressive course and poor survival.[199,203] Serum LDH is elevated in patients with lymph node involvement,[199] and serum LDH assay is probably the only laboratory test that reliably correlates with extracutaneous involvement.[204]

Several other factors have been reported to influence survival, such as (1) the presence of a monoclonal T-cell population detected by TCR gene rearrangement in lymph nodes,[205] (2) serum concentration of soluble IL-2R,[206] (3) the thickness of the skin infiltrate, (4) cytologic atypia (in T1 and T2 stages),[207] and (5) the number of skin-infiltrating CD8+ T-cells[208] and Langerhans' cells.[209]

The prognoses of non-MF/SS primary CTCLs (such as CD30-positive or CD30-negative LCL, pleomorphic CTCL, and subcutaneous T-cell lymphoma) have been less well studied. The survival data of a large number of patients have been reported by the Dutch Cutaneous Lymphoma Working Group[3] and the French Study Group of Cutaneous Lymphomas[210] and show similar survival rates. However, a major difference between these studies was the survival rate in pleomorphic small T-cell lymphomas. The Dutch analysis suggested an intermediate prognosis as opposed to the French data, which showed a more indolent clinical course (5-year survival of 62 vs 82%).[3,210]

Expression of CD30 (Ki-1) in primary cutaneous large cell lymphomas is associated with a favorable prognosis,[68] with an estimated 5-year survival of 87 to 90 percent.[3,210] However, CD30+ large cell lymphoma resulting from large-cell transformation of MF (or LyP) is associated with a significantly shortened survival, with a median survival after diagnosis of less than 2 years.[96,98,211] Patients with CD30-negative primary cutaneous large cell lymphomas often develop generalized disease and have a poor prognosis (5-year survival of 15 to 21%).[3,210]

Primary cutaneous B-cell lymphomas are usually associated with a very good prognosis (5-year survival of 88 to 97%),[3,210] showing little tendency for extracutaneous spread and having a good response to treatment. Large B-cell lymphoma of the leg is a relatively new entity, described as a separate group in the EORTC classification due to its less favorable course compared to other PCBCLs (5-year survival of 46 to 58 percent).[3,210]

Cutaneous lymphomas that develop secondarily as extranodal manifestations of systemic lymphomas are associated with widespread dissemination and a rapidly fatal outcome (eg, adult T-cell leukemia/lymphoma and NK/T-cell lymphomas).

ACKNOWLEDGMENTS

The authors would like to thank Dr. Samuel L. Moschella for providing the clinical pictures.

REFERENCES

1. Stansfeld AG, Diebold J, Noel H, et al. Updated Kiel classification for lymphomas. Lancet 1988;1(8580): 292–3.
2. Harris NL, Jaffe ES, Stein H, et al. A revised European-American classification of lymphoid neoplasms: a proposal from the International Lymphoma Study Group. Blood 1994;84(5):1361–92.
3. Willemze R, Kerl H, Sterry W, et al. EORTC classification for primary cutaneous lymphomas: a proposal from the Cutaneous Lymphoma Study Group of the European Organization for Research and Treatment of Cancer. Blood 1997;90(1):354–71.

4. Isaacson PG, Norton AJ. Extranodal lymphomas. Edinburgh: Churchill Livingstone; 1994. p. 172.

5. Burg G, Braun-Falco O. Cutaneous lymphomas, pseudolymphomas and related disorders. Berlin: Springer-Verlag; 1983.

6. Butcher EC, Picker LJ. Lymphocyte homing and homeostasis. Science 1996;272(5258):60–6.

7. Robert C, Kupper TS. Inflammatory skin diseases. T cells, and immune surveillance. N Engl J Med 1999; 341:1817–28.

8. Lamberg SI, Bunn PA Jr. Proceedings of the workshop on cutaneous T-cell lymphomas (mycosis fungoides and Sezary syndrome). Introduction. Cancer Treat Rep 1979;63(4):561–4.

9. Edelson RL, Smith RW, Frank MM, Green I. Identification of subpopulations of mononuclear cells in cutaneous infiltrates. I. Differentiation between B cells, T cells, and histiocytes. J Invest Dermatol 1973;61(2):82–9.

10. Weinstock MA, Gardstein B. Twenty-year trends in the reported incidence of mycosis fungoides and associated mortality. Am J Public Health 1999;89(8): 1240–4.

11. Weinstock MA, Horm JW. Mycosis fungoides in the United States. Increasing incidence and descriptive epidemiology. JAMA 1988;260(1):42–6.

12. Weinstock MA. Epidemiology of mycosis fungoides. Semin Dermatol 1994;13(3):154–9.

13. Fischmann AB, Bunn PA Jr, Guccion JG, et al. Exposure to chemicals, physical agents, and biologic agents in mycosis fungoides and the Sezary syndrome. Cancer Treat Rep 1979;63(4):591–6.

14. Whittemore AS, Holly EA, Lee IM, et al. Mycosis fungoides in relation to environmental exposures and immune response: a case-control study. J Natl Cancer Inst 1989;81(20):1560–7.

15. Hall WW, Liu CR, Schneewind O, et al. Deleted HTLV-I provirus in blood and cutaneous lesions of patients with mycosis fungoides. Science 1991;253(5017): 317–20.

16. Lisby G, Reitz MS Jr, Vejlsgaard GL. No detection of HTLV-I DNA in punch skin biopsies from patients with cutaneous T-cell lymphoma by the polymerase chain reaction. J Invest Dermatol 1992;98(4): 417–20.

17. Pancake BA, Zucker-Franklin D. HTLV tax and mycosis fungoides. N Engl J Med 1993;329(8):580.

18. Whittaker SJ, Luzzatto L. HTLV-1 provirus and mycosis fungoides. Science 1993;259(5100):1470–1.

19. Bazarbachi A, Soriano V, Pawson R, et al. Mycosis fungoides and Sezary syndrome are not associated with HTLV-I infection: an international study. Br J Haematol 1997;98(4):927–33.

20. Perl A, Rosenblatt JD, Chen IS, et al. Detection and cloning of new HTLV-related endogenous sequences in man. Nucleic Acids Res 1989;17(17): 6841–54.

21. Safai B, Myskowski PL, Dupont B, Pollack MS. Association of HLA-DR5 with mycosis fungoides. J Invest Dermatol 1983;80(5):395–7.

22. Rosen ST, Radvany R, Roenigk H Jr, et al. Human leukocyte antigens in cutaneous T cell lymphoma. J Am Acad Dermatol 1985;12(3):531–4.

23. Lee PY, Charley M, Tharp M, et al. Possible role of Epstein-Barr virus infection in cutaneous T-cell lymphomas. J Invest Dermatol 1990;95(3):309–12.

24. Katzenstein AL, Peiper SC. Detection of Epstein-Barr virus genomes in lymphomatoid granulomatosis: analysis of 29 cases by the polymerase chain reaction technique. Mod Pathol 1990;3(4):435–41.

25. Borisch B, Boni J, Burki K, Laissue JA. Recurrent cutaneous anaplastic large cell (CD30+) lymphoma associated with Epstein-Barr virus. A case report with 9-year follow-up. Am J Surg Pathol 1992; 16(8):796–801.

26. Su IJ, Tsai TF, Cheng AL, Chen CC. Cutaneous manifestations of Epstein-Barr virus-associated T-cell lymphoma. J Am Acad Dermatol 1993;29(5 Pt 1): 685–92.

27. Dreno B, Milpied-Homsi B, Moreau P, et al. Cutaneous anaplastic T-cell lymphoma in a patient with human immunodeficiency virus infection: detection of Epstein-Barr virus DNA. Br J Dermatol 1993; 129(1):77–81.

28. Garbe C, Stein H, Gollnick H, et al. Cutaneous B cell lymphoma in chronic *Borrelia burgdorferi* infection. Report of 2 cases and a review of the literature. Hautarzt 1988;39(11):717–26.

29. Garbe C, Stein H, Dienemann D, Orfanos CE. *Borrelia burgdorferi*-associated cutaneous B cell lymphoma: clinical and immunohistologic characterization of four cases. J Am Acad Dermatol 1991;24(4):584–90.

30. Yang B, Tubbs RR, Finn W, et al. Clinicopathologic reassessment of primary cutaneous B-cell lymphomas with immunophenotypic and molecular genetic characterization. Am J Surg Pathol 2000; 24(5):694–702.

31. Alibert JL. Description des maladies de la peau: observees a l'Hospital saint Louis, et exposition des meilleures methodes suivies pour leur traitment. Paris: Chez Barrois, l'aine et Fils; 1806. p. 167.

32. Crowley JJ, Nikko A, Varghese A, et al. Mycosis fungoides in young patients: clinical characteristics and outcome. J Am Acad Dermatol 1998;38(5 Pt 1): 696–701.

33. Kim YH, Jensen RA, Watanabe GL, et al. Clinical stage IA (limited patch and plaque) mycosis fungoides. A long-term outcome analysis. Arch Dermatol 1996;132(11):1309–13.

34. Kim YH, Chow S, Varghese A, Hoppe RT. Clinical

characteristics and long-term outcome of patients with generalized patch and/or plaque (T2) mycosis fungoides. Arch Dermatol 1999;135(1):26–32.

35. Heald PW, Edelson RL. Lymphomas, pseudolymphomas and related conditions. In: Fitzpatrick TB, Eisen AZ, Wolff K, et al. Dermatology in general medicine. New York: McGraw-Hill; 1993, p. 1285–1307.

36. Smith NP, Samman PD. Mycosis fungoides presenting with areas of cutaneous hypopigmentation. Clin Exp Dermatol 1978;3(2):213–6.

37. Breathnach SM, McKee PH, Smith NP. Hypopigmented mycosis fungoides: report of five cases with ultrastructural observations. Br J Dermatol 1982; 106(6)643–9.

38. Akaraphanth R, Douglass MC, Lim HW. Hypopigmented mycosis fungoides: treatment and a 6$\frac{1}{2}$-year follow-up of 9 patients. J Am Acad Dermatol 2000;42(1):33–9.

39. McNiff JM, Schechner JS, Crotty PL, Glusac EJ. Mycosis fungoides palmaris et plantaris or acral pagetoid reticulosis? Am J Dermatopathol 1998; 20(3):271–5.

40. Resnik KS, Kantor GR, Lessin SR, et al. Mycosis fungoides palmaris et plantaris. Arch Dermatol 1995; 131(9):1052–6.

41. Lacour JP, Castanet J, Perrin C, Ortonne JP. Follicular mycosis fungoides. A clinical and histologic variant of cutaneous T-cell lymphoma: report of two cases. J Am Acad Dermatol 1993;29:330–4.

42. Sarkany I. Patchy alopecia, anhidrosis, eccrine gland wall hypertrophy and vasculitis. Proc R Soc Med 1969;62(2):157–9.

43. Burg G, Schmockel C. Syringolymphoid hyperplasia with alopecia—a syringotropic cutaneous T-cell lymphoma? Dermatology 1992;184(4):306–7.

44. Nickoloff BJ. Light-microscopic assessment of 100 patients with patch/plaque-stage mycosis fungoides. Am J Dermatopathol 1988;10(6):469–77.

45. Ralfkiaer E. Immunohistological markers for the diagnosis of cutaneous lymphomas. Semin Diagn Pathol 1991;8(2):62–72.

46. Agnarsson BA, Vonderheid EC, Kadin ME. Cutaneous T cell lymphoma with suppressor/cytotoxic (CD8) phenotype: identification of rapidly progressive and chronic subtypes. J Am Acad Dermatol 1990;22(4):569–77.

47. Heald P, Buckley P, Gilliam A, et al. Correlations of unique clinical, immunotypic, and histologic findings in cutaneous gamma/delta T-cell lymphoma. J Am Acad Dermatol 1992;26(5 Pt 2):865–70.

48. Barzilai A, Goldberg I, Shibi R, et al. Mycosis fungoides expressing gamma/delta T-cell receptors. J Am Acad Dermatol 1996;34(2 Pt 1):301–2.

49. Vermeer MH, Geelen FA, Kummer JA, et al. Expres-sion of cytotoxic proteins by neoplastic T cells in mycosis fungoides increases with progression from plaque stage to tumor stage disease. Am J Pathol 1999;154(4):1203–10.

50. Saed G, Fivenson DP, Naidu Y, Nickoloff BJ. Mycosis fungoides exhibits a Th1-type cell-mediated cytokine profile whereas Sezary syndrome expresses a Th2-type profile. J Invest Dermatol 1994;103(1):29–33.

51. Asadullah K, Haeussler A, Sterry W, et al. Interferon gamma and tumor necrosis factor alpha mRNA expression in mycosis fungoides progression. Blood 1996;88(2)757–8.

52. Asadallah K, Docke WD, Haeussler A, et al. Progression of mycosis fungoides is associated with increasing cutaneous expression of interleukin-10 mRNA. J Invest Dermatol 1996;107(6):833–7.

53. Wood GS, Tung RM, Haeffner AC, et al. Detection of clonal T-cell receptor gamma gene rearrangements in early mycosis fungoides/Sezary syndrome by polymerase chain reaction and denaturing gradient gel electrophoresis (PCR/DGGE). J Invest Dermatol 1994;103(1):34–41.

54. Muche JM, Lukowsky A, Asadullah K, et al. Demonstration of frequent occurrence of clonal T cells in the peripheral blood of patients with primary cutaneous T-cell lymphoma. Blood 1997;90(4):1636–42.

55. Kim YH, Bishop K, Varghese A, Hoppe RT. Prognostic factors in erythrodermic mycosis fungoides and the Sezary syndrome. Arch Dermatol 1995;131(9):1003–8.

56. Pinkus H. Alopecia mucinosa: inflammatory plaques with alopecia characterized by root-sheath mucinosis. Arch Dermatol 1957;76:419–26.

57. Sentis HJ, Willemze R, Scheffer E. Alopecia mucinosa progressing into mycosis fungoides. A long-term follow-up study of two patients. Am J Dermatopathol 1988;10(6):478–86.

58. Gibson LE, Muller SA, Leiferman KM, Peters MS. Follicular mucinosis: clinical and histopathologic study. J Am Acad Dermatol 1989 Mar;20(3):441–6.

59. Zelickson BD, Peters MS, Muller SA, et al. T-cell receptor gene rearrangement analysis: cutaneous T cell lymphoma, peripheral T cell lymphoma, and premalignant and benign cutaneous lymphoproliferative disorders. J Am Acad Dermatol 1991;25 (5 Pt 1):787–96.

60. Woringer F, Kolopp P. Lesion erythemato-suameuse polycyclique de l'avant-bras evoluant depuis 6 ans chez un garconnet de 13 ans. Histologiquement infiltrat intra-epidermique d'apparance tumorale. Ann Dermatol Syph 1939;10:945.

61. Ketron LW, Goodman MH. Multiple lesions of the skin apparently of epithelial origin resembling clinically mycosis fungoides. Arch Dermatol 1931;24:758.

62. Haghighi B, Smoller BR, LeBoi PE, et al. Pagetoid retic-

ulosis (Woringer-Kolopp disease): an immunopheno-typic, molecular, and clinicopathologic study. Mod Pathol 2000;13(5):502–10.

63. Wood GS, Weiss LM, Hu CH, et al. T-cell antigen deficiencies and clonal rearrangements of T-cell receptor genes in pagetoid reticulosis (Woringer-Kolopp disease). N Engl J Med 1988;318(3):164–7.

64. Schwab U, Stein H, Gerdes J, et al. Production of a monoclonal antibody specific for Hodgkin and Sternberg-Reed cells of Hodgkin's disease and a subset of normal lymphoid cells. Nature 1982;299(5878):65–7.

65. Stein H, Mason DY, Gerdes J, et al. The expression of the Hodgkin's disease associated antigen Ki-1 in reactive and neoplastic lymphoid tissue: evidence that Reed-Sternberg cells and histiocytic malignancies are derived from activated lymphoid cells. Blood 1985;66(4):848–58.

66. Rosenberg SA, Berard CW, Brown BW Jr, et al. National Cancer Institute sponsored study of classifications of non-Hodgkin's lymphomas: summary and description of a working formulation for clinical usage. The non-Hodgkin's lymphoma pathologic classification project. Cancer 1982;49:2112–35.

67. Beljaards RC, Meijer CJ, Scheffer E, et al. Prognostic significance of CD30 (Ki-1/Ber-H2) expression in primary cutaneous large-cell lymphomas of T-cell origin. A clinicopathogic and immunohistochemical study in 20 patients. Am J Pathol 1989;135(6):1169–78.

68. Willemze R, Beljaards RC. Spectrum of primary cutaneous CD30 (Ki-1)-positive lymphoproliferative disorders. A proposal for classification and guidelines for management and treatment. J Am Acad Dermatol 1993;28(6):973–80.

69. Kaudewitz P, Stein H, Dallenbach F, et al. Primary and secondary cutaneous Ki-1+ (CD30+) anaplastic large cell lymphomas. Morphologic, immunohistologic, and clinical characteristics. Am J Pathol 1989;135(2):359–67.

70. Kummer JA, Vermeer MH, Dukers D, et al. Most primary cutaneous CD30-positive lymphoproliferative disorders have a CD4-positive cytotoxic T-cell phenotype. J Invest Dermatol 1997;109(5):636–40.

71. Vagi H, Tokura Y, Furukawa F, Takigawa M. Th2 cytokine mRNA expression in primary cutaneous CD30-positive lymphoproliferative disorders: successful treatment with recombinant interferon-gamma. J Invest Dermatol 1996;107(6):827–32.

72. Noorduyn LA, Beljaards RC, Pals ST, et al. Differential expression of the HECA-452 antigen (cutaneous lymphocyte associated antigen, CLA) in cutaneous and non-cutaneous T-cell lymphomas. Histopathology 1992;21(1):59–64.

73. Fujimoto J, Hata J, Ishii E, et al. Ki-1 lymphomas in childhood: immunohistochemical analysis and the

significance of epithelial membrane antigen (EMA) as a new marker. Virchows Arch A Pathol Anat Histopathol 1988;412(4):307–14.

74. de Bruin PC, Beljaards RC, van Heerde P, et al. Differences in clinical behaviour and immunophenotype between primary cutaneous and primary nodal anaplastic large cell lymphoma of T-cell or null cell phenotype. Histopathology 1993;23(2):127–35.

75. Delsol G, Al Saati T, Gatter KC, et al. Coexpression of epithelial membrane antigen (EMA), Ki-1, and interleukin-2 receptor by anaplastic large cell lymphomas. Diagnostic value in so-called malignant histiocytosis. Am J Pathol 1988;130(1):59–70.

76. Banerjee SS, Heald J, Harris M. Twelve cases of Ki-1 positive anaplastic large cell lymphoma of skin. J Clin Pathol 1991;44(2):119–25.

77. DeCoteau JF, Butmarc JR, Kinney MC, Kadin ME. The t(2;5) chromosomal translocation is not a common feature of primary cutaneous CD30+ lymphoproliferative disorders: comparison with anaplastic large-cell lymphoma of nodal origin. Blood 1996;87(8):3437–41.

78. Beljaards RC, Kaudewitz P, Berti E, et al. Primary cutaneous CD30-positive large cell lymphoma: definitive of a new type of cutaneous lymphoma with a favorable prognosis. A European multicenter study of 47 patients. Cancer 1993;71(6):2097–104.

79. Paulli M, Berti E, Rosso R, et al. CD30/Ki-1-positive lymphoproliferative disorders of the skin—clinicopathologic correlation and statistical analysis of 86 cases: a multicentric study from the European Organization for Research and Treatment of Cancer Cutaneous Lymphoma Project Group. J Clin Oncol 1995;13(6):1343–54.

80. Piris M, Brown DC, Gatter KC, Mason DY. CD30 expression in non-Hodgkin's lymphoma. Histopathology 1990;17(3):211–8.

81. Macaulay WL. Lymphomatoid papulosis. A continuing self-healing eruption, clinically benign—histologically malignant. Arch Dermatol 1968;97(1):23–30.

82. Willemze R, Scheffer E, Ruiter DJ, et al. Immunological, cytochemical and ultrastructural studies in lymphomatoid papulosis. Br J Dermatol 1983;108(4):381–94.

83. Kadin ME. Common activated helper-T-cell origin for lymphomatoid papulosis, mycosis fungoides, and some types of Hodgkin's disease. Lancet 1985;2(8460):864–5.

84. Wood GS, Strickler JG, Deneau DG, et al. Lymphomatoid papulosis expresses immunophenotypes associated with T cell lymphoma but not inflammation. J Am Acad Dermatol 1986;15(3):444–58.

85. Kiluchi A, Nishikawa T. Apoptotic and proliferating cells in cutaneous lymphoproliferative diseases. Arch Dermatol 1997;133(7):829–33.

86. Weiss LM, Wood GS, Trela M, et al. Clonal T-cell populations in lymphomatoid papulosis. Evidence of a lymphoproliferative origin for a clinically benign disease. N Engl J Med 1986;315(8):475–9.

87. Sanchez NP, Pittelkow MR, Muller SA, et al. The clinicopathologic spectrum of lymphomatoid papulosis: study of 31 cases. J Am Acad Dermatol 1983; 8(1):81–94.

88. Harrington DS, Braddock SW, Blocher KS, et al. Lymphomatoid papulosis and progression to T cell lymphoma: an immunophenotypic and genotypic analysis. J Am Acad Dermatol 1989;21(5 Pt 1):951–7.

89. Wang HH, Myers T, Lach LJ, et al. Increased risk of lymphoid and nonlymphoid malignancies in patients with lymphomatoid papulosis. Cancer 1999;86(7):1240–5.

90. Cabanillas F, Armitage J, Pugh WC, et al. Lymphomatoid papulosis: a T-cell dyscrasia with a propensity to transform into malignant lymphoma. Ann Intern Med 1995;122(3):210–7.

91. Sterry W, Korte B, Schubert C. Pleomorphic T-cell lymphoma and large-cell anaplastic lymphoma of the skin. A morphological, immunophenotypical, and ultrastructural study of two typical cases. Am J Dermatopathol 1989;11(2):112–23.

92. Harrington DS, Braddock SW, Blocher KS, et al. Lymphomatoid papulosis and progression to T cell lymphoma: an immunophenotypic and genotypic analysis. J Am Acad Dermatol 1989;21(5 Pt 1):951–7.

93. Chan JK, Ng CS, Hui PK, et al. Anaplastic large cell Ki-1 lymphoma. Delineation of two morphological types. Histopathology 1989;15(1):11–34.

94. Kadin ME, Sako D, Berliner N, et al. Childhood Ki-1 lymphoma presenting with skin lesions and peripheral lymphadenopathy. Blood 1896;68(5):1042–9.

95. Diamandidou E, Colome-Grimmer M, Fayad L, et al. Transformation of mycosis fungoides/Sezary syndrome: clinical characteristics and prognosis. Blood 1998 15;92(4):1150–9.

96. Salhany KE, Cousar JB, Greer JP, et al. Transformation of cutaneous T cell lymphoma to large cell lymphoma. A clinicopathologic and immunologic study. Am J Pathol 1988;132(2):265–77.

97. Stefanato CM, Tallini G, Crotty PL. Histologic and immunophenotypic features prior to transformation in patients with transformed cutaneous T-cell lymphoma: is CD25 expression in skin biopsy samples predictive of large cell transformation in cutaneous T-cell lymphoma? Am J Dermatopathol 1998;20(1): 1–6.

98. Dmitrovsky E, Matthews MJ, Bunn PA, et al. Cytologic transformation in cutaneous T cell lymphoma: a clinicopathologic entity associated with poor prognosis. J Clin Oncol 1987;5(2)208–15.

99. Sézary A, Bouvrain Y. Erythrodermie avec presence de cellules monstreuses dans le derme et le sang circulant. Bull Soc Fr Dermatol Syphil 1938;45:254.

100. Taswell HF, Winkelmann RK. Sezary syndrome—a malignant reticulemic erythroderma. JAMA 1961; 117:465–72.

101. Lutzner M, Edelson R, Schein P, et al. Cutaneous T-cell lymphomas: the Sezary syndrome, mycosis fungoides, and related disorders. Ann Intern Med 1975;83(4):534–52.

102. Fletcher V, Zackheim HS, Beckstead JH. Circulating Sezary cells. A new preparatory method for their identification and enumeration. Arch Pathol Lab Med 1984;108(12):954–8.

103. Scarisbrick JJ, Child FJ, Evans AV, et al. Secondary malignant neoplasms in 71 patients with Sezary syndrome. Arch Dermatol 1999;135(11):1381–5.

104. Duncan SC, Winkelman RK. Circulating Sezary cells in hospitalized dermatology patients. Br J Dermatol 1978;99(2):171–8.

105. Scala E, Russo G, Cadoni S, et al. Skewed expression of activation, differentiation and homing-related antigens in circulating cells from patients with cutaneous T cell lymphoma associated with CD7– T helper lymphocytes expansion. J Invest Dermatol 1999;113(4):622–7.

106. Vowels BR, Cassin M, Vonderheid EC, Rook AH. Aberrant cytokine production by Sezary syndrome patients: cytokine secretion pattern resembles murine Th2 cells. J Invest Dermatol 1992;99(1):90–4.

107. Weiss LM, Wood GS, Hu E, et al. Detection of clonal T-cell receptor gene rearrangements in the peripheral blood of patients with mycosis fungoides/Sezary syndrome. J Invest Dermatol 1989;92(4):601–4.

108. Dummer R, Nestle FO, Niederer E, et al. Genotypic, phenotypic and functional analysis of CD4+CD7+ and CD4+CD7– T lymphocyte subsets in Sezary syndrome. Arch Dermatol Res 1999;291(6):307–11.

109. Wieselthier JS, Koh HK. Sezary syndrome:diagnosis, prognosis, and critical review of treatment options. J Am Acad Dermatol 1990;22(3):381–401.

110. Vonderheid EC, Sobel EL, Nowell PC, et al. Diagnostic and prognostic significance of Sezary cells in peripheral blood smears from patients with cutaneous T cell lymphoma. Blood 1985;66(2):358–66.

111. Russell-Jones R, Whittaker S. T-cell receptor gene analysis in the diagnosis of Sezary syndrome. J Am Acad Dermatol 1999;41(2 Pt 1):254–9.

112. Bernengo MG, Quaglino P, Novelli M, et al. Prognostic factors in Sezary syndrome: a multivariate analysis of clinical, haematological and immunological features. Ann Oncol 1998;9(8):857–63.

113. Sterry W, Siebel A, Miekle V. HTLV-1-negative pleomorphic T-cell lymphoma of the skin: the clinicopathological correlations and natural history of 15 patients. Br J Dermatol 1992;126(5):456–62.

114. Beljaards RC, Meijer CJ, Van der Putte SC, et al. Primary cutaneous T-cell lymphoma: clinicopathological features and prognostic parameters of 35 cases other than mycosis fungoides and CD30-positive large cell lymphoma. J Pathol 1994;172(1):53–60.

115. Mouly F, Baccard M, Cayuela JM, et al. Cutaneous T-cell lymphoma associated with granulomatous slack skin. Dermatology 1996;192(3):288–90.

116. Noto G, Pravata G, Miceli S, Arico M. Granulomatous slack skin: report of a case associated with Hodgkin's disease and a review of the literature. Br J Dermatol 1994;131(2):275–9.

117. LeBoit PE, Zackheim HS, White CR Jr. Granulomatous variants of cutaneous T-cell lymphoma. The histopathology of granulomatous mycosis fungoides and granulomatous slack skin. Am J Surg Pathol 1988;12(2):83–95.

118. Tsang WY, Chan JK, Loo KT, et al. Granulomatous slack skin. Histopathology 1994;25(1):49–55.

119. LeBoit PE, Beckstead JH, Bond B, et al. Granulomatous slack skin: clonal rearrangement of the T-cell receptor beta gene is evidence for the lymphoproliferative nature of a cutaneous elastolytic disorder. J Invest Dermatol 1987;89(2):183–6.

120. Friedman D, Wechsler J, Delfau MH, et al. Primary cutaneous pleomorphic small T-cell lymphoma. A review of 11 cases. The French Study Group on Cutaneous Lymphomas. Arch Dermatol 1995;131(9):1009–15.

121. Gonzalez CL, Medeiros LJ, Braziel RM, Jaffe ES. T-cell lymphoma involving subcutaneous tissue. A clinicopathologic entity commonly associated with hemophagocytic syndrome. Am J Surg Pathol 1991;15(1):17–27.

122. Cho KH, Oh JK, Kim CW, et al. Peripheral T-cell lymphoma involving subcutaneous tissue. Br J Dermatol 1995;132(2):290–5.

123. Mehregan DA, Su SP, Kurtin PJ. Subcutaneous T-cell lymphoma: a clinical, histopathologic, and immunohistochemical study of six cases. J Cutan Pathol 1994;21(2):110–7.

124. Wang CY, Su WP, Jurtin PJ. Subcutaneous panniculitic T-cell lymphoma. Int J Dermatol 1996;35(1):1–8.

125. Kumar S, Krencas L, Medeiros J, et al. Subcutaneous panniculitic T-cell lymphoma is a tumor of cytotoxic T lymphocytes. Hum Pathol 1998;29(4):397–403.

126. Romero LS, Goltz RW, Nagi C, et al. Subcutaneous T-cell lymphoma with associated hemophagocytic syndrome and terminal leukemic transformation. J Am Acad Dermatol 1996;34(5 Pt 2):904–10.

127. Smith KJ, Skelton HG 3rd, Giblin WL, James WD. Cutaneous lesions of hemophagocytic syndrome in a patient with T-cell lymphoma and active Epstein-Barr infection. J Am Acad Dermatol 1991;25(5 Pt 2):919–24.

128. Burg G, Dummer R, Wilhelm M, et al. A subcutaneous delta-positive T-cell lymphoma that produces interferon gamma. N Engl J Med 1991;325(15):1078–81.

129. Avinoach I, Halevy S, Argove S, Sacks M. Gamma/delta T-cell lymphoma involving the subcutaneous tissue and associated with a hemophagocytic syndrome. Am J Dermatopathol 1994;16(4):426–33.

130. Zackheim HS, Vonderheid EC, Ramsay DL, Leboit PE, et al. Relative frequency of various forms of primary cutaneous lymphomas. J Am Acad Dermatol 2000;43:793–96.

131. Burg G, Kerl H, Przybilla B, Braun-Falco O. Some statistical data, diagnosis, and staging of cutaneous B-cell lymphomas. J Dermatol Surg Oncol 1984;10(4):256–62.

132. Rijaarsdam JU, Wilemze R. Primary cutaneous B-cell lymphomas. Leuk Lymphoma 1994;14(3–4):213–8.

133. Garcia CF, Weiss LM, Warnke RA, Wood GS. Cutaneous follicular lymphoma. Am J Surg Pathol 1986;10(7):454–63.

134. Willemze R, Meijer CJ, Sentis HJ, et al. Primary cutaneous large cell lymphomas of follicular center cell origin. A clinical follow-up study of nineteen patients. J Am Acad Dermatol 1987;16(3 Pt 1):518–26.

135. Volkenandt M, Cerroni L, Rieger E, et al. Analysis of the 14; 18 translocation in cutaneous lymphomas using the polymerase chain reaction. J Cutan Pathol 1992;19(5):353–6.

136. Rijlaarsdam U, Bakels V, van Oostveen JW, et al. Demonstration of clonal immunoglobulin gene rearrangements in cutaneous B-cell lymphomas and pseudo-B-cell lymphomas: differential diagnostic and pathogenetic aspects. J Invest Dermatol 1992;99(6):749–54.

137. Berti E, Alessi E, Caputo R, et al. Reticulohistiocytoma of the dorsum. J Am Acad Dermatol 1988;19(2 Pt 1):259–72.

138. Pimpinelli N, Santucci M, Mori M, et al. Primary cutaneous B-cell lymphoma: a clinically homogeneous entity? J Am Acad Dermatol 1997;37(6):1012–6.

139. Giannotti B, Santucci M. Skin-associated lymphoid tissue (SALT)-related B-cell lymphoma (primary cutaneous B-cell lymphoma). A concept and a clinicopathologic entity. Arch Dermatol 1993;129(3):353–5.

140. Rijlaarsdam JU, van der Putte SC, Berti E, et al. Cutaneous immunocytomas: a clinicopathologic study of 26 cases. Histopathology 1993;23(2):117–25.

141. Cerroni L, Zochling N, Putz B, Kerl H. Infection by *Borrelia burgdorferi* and cutaneous B-cell lymphoma. J Cutan Pathol 1997;24(8):457–61.

142. Harris NL. Extranodal lymphoid infiltrates and mucosa-associated lymphoid tissue (MALT). A unifying concept. Am J Surg Pathol 1991;15(9):879–84.

143a. Baldassano MF, Bailey EM, Ferry JA, et al. Cutaneous lymphoid hyperplasia and cutaneous marginal zone lymphoma: comparison of morphologic and immunophenotypic features. Am J Surg Pathol 1999;23(1):88–96.

143b. Vermeer MH, Geelen FA, van Haselen CW, et al. Primary cutaneous large B-cell lymphomas of the legs. A distinct type of cutaneous B-cell lymphoma with an intermediate prognosis. Dutch Cutaneous Lymphoma Working Group. Arch Dermatol 1996 Nov;132(11):1304–8.

144. Kerl H, Cerroni L. The morphologic spectrum of cutaneous B-cell lymphomas. Arch Dermatol 1996;132(11):1376–7.

145. Delia D, Borrella MG, Berti E, et al. Clonal immunoglobulin gene rearrangements and normal T-cell receptor, bcl-w, and c-myc genes in primary cutaneous B-cell lymphomas. Cancer Res 1989; 49(17):4901–5.

146. Pfleger L, Tappeiner J. Zur Kenntnis der systemisierten Endotheliomatose der cutanen Blutgefasse. Hautartzt 1959;10:359–63.

147. Willemze R, Kruyswijk MR, De Bruin CD, et al. Angiotropic (intravascular) large cell lymphoma of the skin previously classified as malignant angioendotheliomatosis. Br J Dermatol 1987;116(3):393–9.

148. Ferry JA, Harris NL, Picker LJ, et al. Intravascular lymphomatosis (malignant angioendotheliomatosis). A B-cell neoplasm expressing surface homing receptors. Mod Pathol 1988;1(6):444–52.

149. Wick MR, Mills SE, Scheithauer BW, et al. Reassessment of malignant "angioendotheliomatosis." Evidence in favor of its reclassification as "intravascular lymphomatosis." Am J Surg Pathol 1986;10(2): 112–23.

150. DiGiuseppe JA, Nelson WG, Seifter EJ, et al. Intravascular lymphomatosis: a clinicopathologic study of 10 cases and assessment of response to chemotherapy. J Clin Oncol 1994;12(12):2573–9.

151. Wick MR, Mills SE. Intravascular lymphomatosis: clinicopathologic features and differential diagnosis. Semin Diagn Pathol 1991;8(2):91–101.

152. Perniciaro C, Winkelmann RK, Daoud MS, Su WP. Malignant angioendotheliomatosis is an angiotropic intravascular lymphoma. Immunohistochemical, ultrastructural, and molecular genetics studies. Am J Dermatopathol 1995;17(3):242–8.

153. Torne R, Su WP, Winkelmann RK, et al. Clinicopathologic study of cutaneous plasmacytoma. Int J Dermatol 1990;29(8):562–6.

154. Llamas-Martin R, Postigo-Llorente C, Vanaclocha-Sebastian F, et al. Primary cutaneous extramedullary plasmacytoma secreting lambda IG. Clin Exp Dermatol 1993;18(4):351–5.

155. Chang YT, Wong CK. Primary cutaneous plasmacytomas. Clin Exp Dermatol 1994;19(2):177–80.

156. Walker E, Robertson AG, Boorman JG, McNicol AM. Primary cutaneous plasmacytoma: the use of in situ hybridization to detect monoclonal immunoglobulin light-chain mRNA. Histopathology 1992;20(2): 135–8.

157. Uchiyama T, Yodoi J, Sagawa K, et al. Adult T-cell leukemia: clinical and hematologic features of 16 cases. Blood 1997;50(3):481–92.

158. Jaffe ES, Blattner WA, Blayney DW, et al. The pathologic spectrum of adult T-cell leukemia/lymphoma in the United States. Human T-cell leukemia/lymphoma virus-associated lymphoid malignancies. Am J Surg Pathol 1984;8(4):263–75.

159. Swerdlow SH, Habeshaw JA, Rohatiner AZ, et al. Caribbean T-cell lymphoma/leukemia. Cancer 1984;54(4):687–96.

160. Shimoyama M. Diagnostic criteria and classification of clinical subtypes of adult T-cell leukaemia-lymphoma. A report from the Lymphoma Study Group (1984–87). Br J Haematol 1991;79(3):428–37.

161. Shimoyama M, Minato K, Saito H, et al. Comparison of clinical, morphologic and immunologic characteristics of adult T-cell leukemia/lymphoma and cutaneous T-cell lymphoma. Jpn J Clin Oncol 1979; 9 Suppl:357–72.

162. The T- and B-Cell Malignancy Study Group. Statistical analyses of clinico-pathological, virological and epidemiological data on lymphoid malignancies with special reference to adult T-cell leukemia/lymphoma: a report of the second nationwide study of Japan. Jpn J Clin Oncol 1985;15(3):517–35.

163. The T- and B-cell Malignancy Study Group. The third nation-wide study on adult T-cell leukemia/lymphoma (ATL) in Japan: characteristic patterns of HLA antigen and HTLV-I infection in ATL patients and their relatives. Int J Cancer 1988 Apr 15; 41(4):505–12.

164. Nagatani T, Miyazawa M, Matsuzaki T, et al. Adult T-cell leukemia/lymphoma (ATL)—clinical, histopathological, immunological and immunohistochemical characteristics. Exp Dermatol 1992;1(5):248–52.

165. Nagatani T, Matsuzaki T, Iemoto G, et al. Comparative study of cutaneous T-cell lymphoma and adult T-cell leukemia/lymphoma. Clinical, histopathologic, and immunohistochemical analyses. Cancer 1990;66(11):2380–6.

166. Uchiyama T, Hori T, Tsudo M, et al. Interleukin-2 receptor (Tac antigen) expressed on adult T cell leukemia cells. J Clin Invest 1985;76(2):446–53.

167. Poiesz BJ, Ruscetti FW, Gazdar AF, et al. Detection and isolation of type C retrovirus particles from fresh and cultured lymphocytes of a patient with cutaneous T-cell lymphoma. Proc Natl Acad Sci U S A 1980;77(12):7415–9.

168. Kinney MC, Greer JP, Glick AD, et al. Anaplastic large-cell Ki-1 malignant lymphomas. Recognition, biological and clinical implications. Pathol Annu 1991;26 Pt 1:1–24.

169. Bitter MA, Franklin WA, Larson RA, et al. Morphology in Ki-1(CD30)-positive non-Hodgkin's lymphoma is correlated with clinical features and the presence of a unique chromosomal abnormality, t(2;5)(p23;q35). Am J Surg Pathol 1990;14(4):305–16.

170. Walker E, Robertson AG, Boorman JG, McNicol AM. Primary cutaneous plasmacytoma: the use of situ hybridization to detect monoclonal immunoglobulin light-chain mRNA. Histopathology 1992;20(2):135–8.

171. Jaffe ES, Chan JK, Su IJ, et al. Report of the Workshop on Nasal and Related Extranodal Angiocentric T/Natural Killer Cell Lymphomas. Definitions, differential diagnosis, and epidemiology. Am J Surg Pathol 1996;20(1):103–11.

172. Chan JK, Sin VC, Wong KF, et al. Nonnasal lymphoma expressing the natural killer cell marker CD56: a clinicopathologic study of 49 cases of an uncommon aggressive neoplasm. Blood 1997;89(12):4501–13.

173. Drenou B, Lamy T, Amiot L, et al. CD3– CD56+ non-Hodgkin's lymphomas with an aggressive behavior related to multidrug resistance. Blood 1997;89(8):2966–74.

174. Jaffe ES, Wilson WH. Lymphomatoid granulomatosis: pathogenesis, pathology and clinical implications. Cancer Surv 1997;30:233–48.

175. Katzenstein AL, Carrington CB, Liebow AA. Lymphomatoid granulomatosis: a clinicopathologic study of 152 cases. Cancer 1979;43(1):360–73.

176. Beylot-Barry M, Vergier B, Masquelier B, et al. The spectrum of cutaneous lymphomas in HIV infection: a study of 21 cases. Am J Surg Pathol 1999;23(10):1208–16.

177. Kerschmann RL, Berger TG, Weiss LM, et al. Cutaneous presentations of lymphoma in human immunodeficiency virus disease. Predominance of T cell lineage. Arch Dermatol 1995;131(11):1281–8.

178. Smith JL Jr, Butler JJ. Skin involvement in Hodgkin's disease. Cancer 1980;45(2):354–61.

179. Santucci M, Pimpinelli N, Arganini L. Primary cutaneous B-cell lymphoma: a unique type of low-grade lymphoma. Clinicopathologic and immunologic study of 83 cases. Cancer 1991;67(9):2311–26.

180. Slater DN. Cutaneous lymphoproliferative disorders: an assessment of recent investigative techniques. Br J Dermatol 1991;124(4):309–23.

181. van der Putte SC, Toonstra J, van Wichen DF, et al. Aberrant immunophenotypes in mycosis fungoides. Arch Dermatol 1988;124(3):373–80.

182. Ralfkiaer E, Wantzin GL, Mason DY, et al. Phenotypic characterization of lymphocyte subsets in mycosis fungoides. Comparison with large plaque parapsoriasis and benign chronic dermatoses. Am J Clin Pathol 1985;84(5):610–9.

183. Abel EA, Wood GS, Hoppe RT, Warnke RA. Expression of Leu-8 antigen, a majority T-cell marker is uncommon in mycosis fungoides. J Invest Dermatol 1985;85(3):199–202.

184. Ashton-Key M, Diss TC, Du MQ, et al. The value of the polymerase chain reaction in the diagnosis of cutaneous T-cell infiltrates. Am J Surg Pathol 1997;21(7):743–7.

185. Park JK, McKeithan TW, Le Beau MM, et al. An (8;14)(q24;q11) translocation involving the T-cell receptor alpha-chain gene and the MYC oncogene 3' region in a B-cell lymphoma. Genes Chromosomes Cancer 1989;1(1):15–22.

186. Leber BF, Amlot P, Hoffbrand AV, Norton JD. T-cell receptor gene rearrangement in B-cell non-Hodgkin's lymphoma: correlation with methylation and expression. Leuk Res 1989;13(6):473–81.

187. Berger CL, Eisenberg A, Soper L, et al. Dual genotype in cutaneous T cell lymphoma: immunoglobulin gene rearrangement in clonal T cell malignancy. J Invest Dermatol 1988;90(1):73–7.

188. Weiss LM, Wood GS, Ellisen LW, et al. Clonal T-cell populations in pityriasis lichenoides et varioliformis acuta (Mucha-Habermann disease). Am J Pathol 1987;126(3):417–21.

189. Wood GS, Ngan BY, Tung R, et al. Clonal rearrangements of immunoglobulin genes and progression to B cell lymphoma in cutaneous lymphoid hyperplasia. Am J Pathol 1989;135(1):13–9.

190. Bogen SA, Pelley D, Charif M, et al. Immunophenotypic identification of Sezary cells in peripheral blood. Am J Clin Pathol 1996;106(6):739–48.

191. Duncan SC, Winkelmann RK. Circulating Sezary cells in hospitalized dermatology patients. Br J Dermatol 1978;99(2):171–8.

192. Wieselthier JS, Koh HK. Sezary syndrome: diagnosis, prognosis, and critical review of treatment options. J Am Acad Dermatol 1990;22(3):381–401.

193. Vonderheid EC, Sobel EL, Nowell PC, et al. Diagnostic and prognostic significance of Sezary cells in peripheral blood smears from patients with cutaneous T cell lymphoma. Blood 1985;66(2):358–66.

194. Bunn PA Jr, Lamberg SI. Report of the Committee on Staging and Classification of Cutaneous T-Cell Lymphomas. Cancer Treat Rep 1979;63(4):725–8.

195. Lamberg SI, Green SB, Byar DP, et al. Clinical staging for cutaneous T-cell lymphoma. Ann Intern Med 1984;100(2):187–92.

196. Sausville EA, Worsham GF, Matthews MJ, et al. Histologic assessment of lymph nodes in mycosis fungoides/Sezary syndrome (cutaneous T-cell lymphoma): clinical correlations and prognostic import

of a new classification system. Hum Pathol 1985; 16(11):1098–109.

197. Bunn PA Jr, Huberman MS, Whang-Peng J, et al. Prospective staging evaluation of patients with cutaneous T-cell lymphomas. Demonstration of a high frequency of extracutaneous dissemination. Ann Intern Med 1980;93(2):223–30.

198. Sausville EA, Eddy JL, Makuch RW, et al. Histopathologic staging at initial diagnosis of mycosis fungoides and the Sezary syndrome. Definition of three distinctive prognostic groups. Ann Intern Med 1988;109(5):372–82.

199. Marti RM, Estrach T, Reverter JC, Mascaro JM. Prognostic clinicopathologic factors in cutaneous T-cell lymphoma. Arch Dermatol 1991;127(10):1511–6.

200. Green SB, Byar DP, Lamberg SI. Prognostic variables in mycosis fungoides. Cancer 1981;47(11):2671–7.

201. Zackheim HS, Amin S, Kashani-Sabet M, McMillan A. Prognosis in cutaneous T-cell lymphoma by skin stage: long-term survival in 489 patients. J Am Acad Dermatol 1999;40(3):418–25.

202. Vonderheid EC, Diamond LW, Lai SM, et al. Lymph node histopathologic findings in cutaneous T-cell lymphoma. A prognostic classification system based on morphologic assessment. Am J Clin Pathol 1992;97(1):121–9.

203. Diamandidou E, Colome M, Fayad L, et al. Prognostic factor analysis in mycosis fungoides/Sezary syndrome. J Am Acad Dermatol 1999;40(6Pt1):914–24.

204. Marti RM, Estrach T, Reverter JC, et al. Utility of bone marrow and liver biopsies for staging cutaneous T-cell lymphoma. Int J Dermatol 1996; 35(6):450–4.

205. Kern DE, Kidd PG, Moe R, et al. Analysis of T-cell receptor gene rearrangement in lymph nodes of patients with mycosis fungoides. Prognostic implications. Arch Dermatol 1998;134(2):158–64.

206. Wasik MA, Vonderheid EC, Bigler RD, et al. Increased serum concentration of the soluble interleukin-2 receptor in cutaneous T-cell lymphoma. Clinical and prognostic implications. Arch Dermatol 1996;132(1):42–7.

207. Marti RM, Estrach T, Reverter JC, Mascaro JM. Prognostic clinicopathologic factors in cutaneous T-cell lymphoma. Arch Dermatol 1991;127(10):1511–6.

208. Hoppe RT, Medeiros LJ, Warnke RA, Wood GS. CD8-positive tumor-infiltrating lymphocytes influence the long-term survival of patients with mycosis fungoides. J am Acad Dermatol 1995;32(3):448–53.

209. Meissner K, Michaelis K, Rehpenning W, Loning T. Epidermal Langerhans' cell densities influence survival in mycosis fungoides and Sezary syndrome. Cancer 1990;65(9):2069–73.

210. Grange F, Hedelin G, Joly P, et al. Prognostic factors in primary cutaneous lymphomas other than mycosis fungoides and the Sezary syndrome. The French Study Group on Cutaneous Lymphomas. Blood 1999;93(11):3637–42.

211. Greer JP, Salhany KE, Cousar JB, et al. Clinical features associated with transformation of cerebriform T-cell lymphoma to a large cell process. Hematol Oncol 1990;8(4):215–27.

Uncommon Cutaneous Malignancies

DAVID A. WRONE, MD

ARTHUR J. SOBER, MD

The incidence of uncommon cutaneous malignancies is difficult to estimate as there are few population-based studies. Isolated reports of these rare tumors and a few case series provide most of the natural history. This section will discuss eight of these rare tumors: angiosarcoma, atypical fibroxanthoma, primary mucinous carcinoma, dermatofibrosarcoma protuberans, eccrine porocarcinoma, microcystic adnexal carcinoma, sebaceous carcinoma, and leiomyosarcoma.

ANGIOSARCOMA

Angiosarcoma (AS) is a malignant tumor of the vascular endothelium. The majority of angiosarcomas are diagnosed on the skin or subcutis. Cutaneous AS has three clinical presentations: face and scalp AS, AS associated with chronic lymphedema, and postradiation AS.[1] Angiosarcoma of the face and scalp presents as a rapidly growing bruiselike purple-red plaque. The border is ill defined, as seen in Figure 8.1–1, *A*. Larger tumors may contain nodular or ulcerated components (Figure 8.1–1, *B*). Although most of these tumors are diagnosed in elderly patients, no predisposing factors or causative agents are known. Sun exposure is felt to be causative in many but not all cases. Scalp AS has a very poor prognosis, with only a 12 percent 5-year survival rate.[1] Surgical excision is the preferred therapy for small tumors. Unfortunately, most patients are diagnosed with large tumors, making complete excision impossible. Wide-field electron beam therapy may provide some benefit.[2]

Angiosarcoma can also arise on the skin of patients with chronic lymphedema. The original disorder, Stewart-Treves syndrome, was described after breast cancer surgery. Today, the majority of reported cases occur in patients treated for breast cancer with mastectomy and removal of axillary

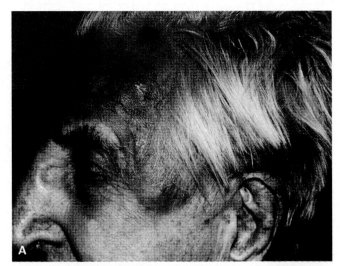
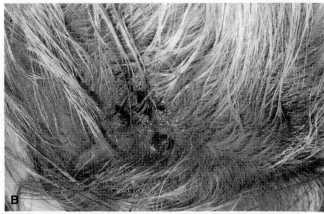

Figure 8.1–1. Angiosarcoma of the face and scalp. *A*, A bruiselike plaque is evident on this elderly man's temple. The apparent clinical margin is deceiving: biopsy proved that the tumor extended many centimeters into seemingly normal skin. *B*, The posterior frontal scalp of the same patient. Ulcerations such as this are seen in large lesions. (Courtesy of Stephen Snow, MD)

lymph nodes. Approximately 1 in 200 postmastectomy patients who survive 5 years will develop AS.[1] In addition, AS can occur in the lymphedematous tissue of patients with lymphedema from many causes. Arising within the skin of the lymphedematous extremity, it begins as a purple-red macule, papule, or nodule (Figure 8.1–2). The prognosis is similar to that of scalp AS. Long-term survival has been reported after radical surgery.

Radiation-induced AS can occur after radiation therapy for treatment of benign and malignant disorders. The average time from exposure to development of AS is 20 years. The clinical appearance and prognosis is similar to those of other forms of AS.

The histology of individual lesions varies from well differentiated to poorly differentiated, the latter sometimes showing epithelioid features, causing histologic confusion with melanoma or even carcinoma (Figure 8.1–3).

ATYPICAL FIBROXANTHOMA

Atypical fibroxanthoma (AFX) is a clinically benign tumor classically seen in two patient groups. Most AFXs occur on sun-exposed skin of the head and neck of elderly people. The second and smaller subset of tumors is found on the limbs of younger adults, but many experts feel that these are better classified as atypical fibrous histiocytomas, not as AFXs. Ultraviolet (UV) radiation is strongly sus-

pected as an etiologic agent. The growths are mobile fleshy papules or nodules that only occasionally ulcerate.[3,4] Their growth is rapid, and many tumors reach a few centimeters in size in a few months.

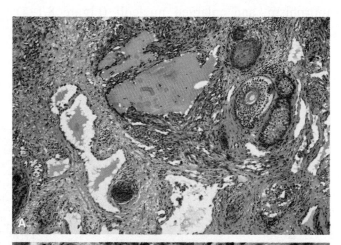
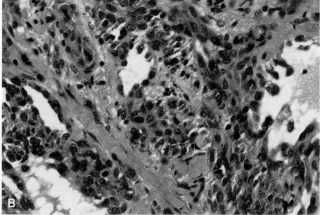
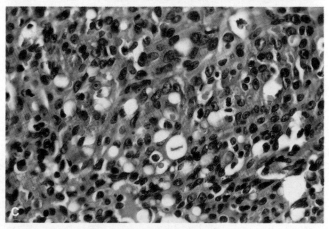

Figure 8.1–3. Angiosarcoma (AS) histopathology. *A,* A well-differentiated tumor showing vascular channels lined by atypical endothelial cells. *B,* A moderately differentiated AS showing nuclear pleomorphism. A mitosis is present in the center of the field. *C,* Some angiosarcomas have epithelioid features and are referred to as epithelioid angiosarcomas. This characteristic is present in the lesion pictured. Epithelioid endothelial cells containing intracytoplasmic lumina are seen. (Hematoxylin and eosin)

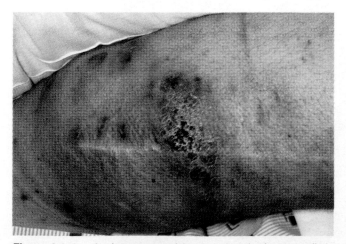

Figure 8.1–2. Angiosarcoma arising in a lymphedematous limb. This woman's arm became lymphedematous after radical mastectomy for breast cancer. The vascular papules and nodules evident on the image were the first evidence of angiosarcoma. (Courtesy of Steve Oberlender, MD, PhD)

Atypical fibroxanthoma is likely to represent a mixed cell population that includes both fibrohistiocytic and myofibroblastic cells. Microscopically, the tumor has features of malignancy, including numerous often atypical mitoses, marked cellular pleomorphism, and enlarged nucleoli (Figure 8.1–4). Features that reflect its benign nature include its circumscribed and superficial position in the dermis without extension into fat. Also, it lacks necrosis and evidence for lymphatic invasion.

The treatment of choice for AFX is surgical excision, with tissue-sparing Mohs' surgery offering an attractive option. Complete excision is curative. Metastases never occur.

PRIMARY MUCINOUS CARCINOMA

Primary mucinous carcinoma (PMC) occurs in older patients (the average patient is 61 years old), but a wide range of ages has been reported.[5] Its incidence

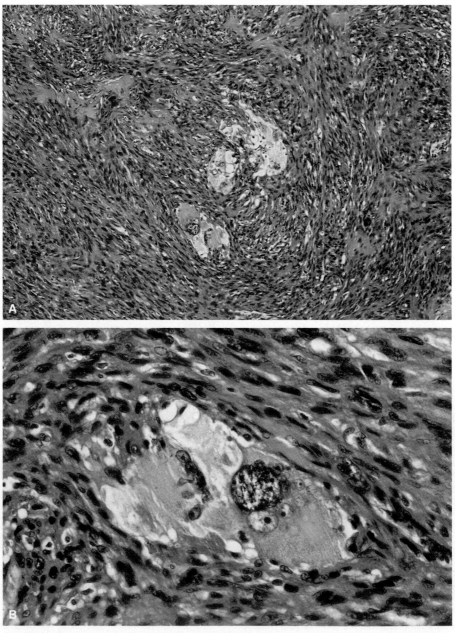

Figure 8.1–4.   Atypical fibroxanthoma histopathology. *A,* View showing spindle cells arranged in a storiform pattern. Pleomorphic giant cells are evident. *B,* A pleomorphic giant cell. (Hematoxylin and eosin)

in men is twice its incidence in women. The face (particularly the eyelid) is the most common location, but many locations have been described, including the axilla and foot. Primary mucinous carcinoma is typically a small fleshy nontender papule. The average lesion is present for 3 years before diagnosis.

On microscopic examination, PMC shows clusters of irregularly shaped cells surrounded by mucin (Figure 8.1–5, *A*). Evidence of ductal differentiation, usually in the form of intracytoplasmic lumina, is invariably present (see Figure 8.1–5, *B*). Pleomorphism is typically absent, and mitoses are sparse. Metastatic mucinous carcinoma from any location (including breast, gastrointestinal tract, and ovary) can look identical. A diagnosis of PMC can be made only if a thorough work-up for internal malignancy is performed.

Primary mucinous carcinoma can be a destructive disease, and local recurrence may be reported after excision. Local metastases occur in 10 percent

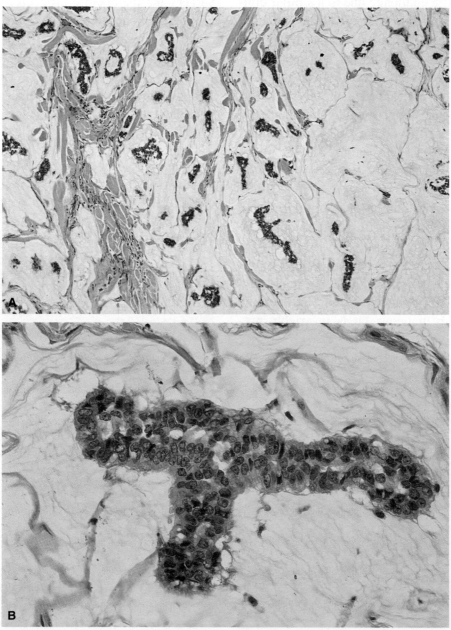

Figure 8.1–5. Primary mucinous carcinoma histopathology. *A*, Epithelial strands are seen dispersed in a mucin-rich stroma. *B*, The epithelial cells show little pleomorphism. Mitoses are sparse in this tumor. (Hematoxylin and eosin)

of cases, but distant metastases have been reported only once. Surgical excision is the best treatment available. Because some tumors express estrogen receptors, hormonal therapy has been suggested as a potential treatment.[6]

DERMATOFIBROSARCOMA PROTUBERANS

Dermatofibrosarcoma protuberans (DFSP) is a slow growing dermal tumor of possible fibroblast origin.[7] It poses a diagnostic challenge due to a similar clinical appearance to several benign growths, including dermatofibromas, epidermal inclusion cysts, and keloids. About half of the tumors are present for more than 10 years before the diagnosis is made. This tumor typically appears as a smooth flesh-colored or red plaque with irregular borders. The plaque may have a soft nodular component as pictured in Figure 8.1–6. Caucasian males are most frequently affected. The tumors occur anywhere, with the trunk being the most common location. A history of previous skin trauma such as burns and surgery has been reported as associated with some cases of DFSP.

Histologically, the tumor is a poorly circumscribed spindle cell tumor, with cells arranged in a whorled or storiform pattern within the dermis. Extension into subcutaneous fat is invariably pre-

sent; this can be seen in Figure 8.1–7, A. On the cellular level, there is usually little pleomorphism, and mitoses are often sparse (see Figure 8.1–7, B).

The recurrence rate is high after routine surgical excision. Even after wide margins are taken, recurrence rates as high as 20 percent have been reported. Head and neck tumors have a higher recurrence rate. The lesion has a 1 percent metastasis rate. The metastases are usually seen after multiple recurrences; therefore, aggressive initial treatment is usually recommended. Some dermatologists consider Mohs' surgery the therapeutic procedure of choice, but its routine use is debated and is under investigation.[8]

ECCRINE POROCARCINOMA

Eccrine porocarcinoma presents in older patients, generally in the seventh decade. While approxi-

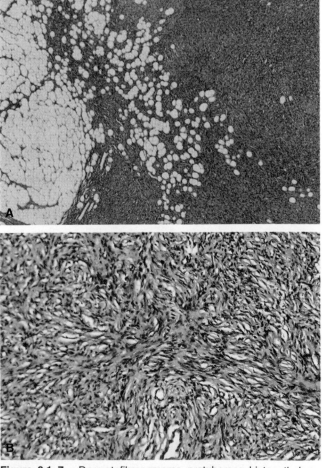

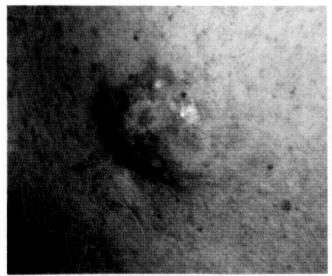

Figure 8.1–6. Dermatofibrosarcoma protuberans. A single smooth fleshy papule of the skin is seen. A cluster of papules or nodules is often seen. (Courtesy of Gregg Menaker, MD)

Figure 8.1–7. Dermatofibrosarcoma protuberans histopathology. *A*, Low-power view showing the lacelike pattern of fatty infiltration. *B*, The typical storiform pattern. (Hematoxylin and eosin)

mately half of the tumors occur on the lower extremity, many other sites have been reported.[9] Both sexes are affected equally. Clinically, the lesion can be a verrucous or ulcerated papule or nodule. The initial differential diagnosis of the lesion is broad, with lesions resembling more-common nonmelanoma skin cancers such as squamous cell and basal cell carcinoma (Figure 8.1–8).

There are too few reported cases to assess causative agents accurately. Some lesions have been reported as arising from benign eccrine poromas. Microscopic examination reveals an acanthotic epidermis with intraepithelial nests and dermal invasion by tumor cells showing evidence of eccrine differentiation (Figure 8.1–9). Pleomorphism is variable, but mitoses are usually conspicuous, and abnormal forms are present. Perineural infiltration and lymphovascular invasion are sometimes seen.

Wide local surgical excision results in about 20 percent of tumors recurring locally. About 20 percent of tumors metastasize to local lymph nodes. Prognosis for those patients with regional metastases is poor; their mortality rate is greater than 50 percent.[9] Mohs' surgery has been used; however, there are not enough data to know if it has an advantage over simple excision.[10] The role of elective lymph node dissection is also uncertain. Adjuvant radiation therapy and chemotherapy have not been shown to be effective.

MICROCYSTIC ADNEXAL CARCINOMA

Microcystic adnexal carcinoma (MAC) is a malignant adnexal tumor that occurs on the head and neck of middle-aged adults.[11] The central face is a common location; perioral or periorbital areas are the most frequent sites. This tumor presents as an asymptomatic indurated flesh-colored nodule or plaque that may have been present for several years before diagnosis (Figure 8.1–10, *A*). Occasionally, patients complain of tingling or numbness in the area of the tumor, consistent with the propensity of MAC for perineural invasion. The average tumor is 2 cm in diameter at the time of diagnosis; despite the large size, ulceration is uncommon. Microcystic adnexal carcinoma occurs almost exclusively in Caucasian patients and affects both sexes equally.

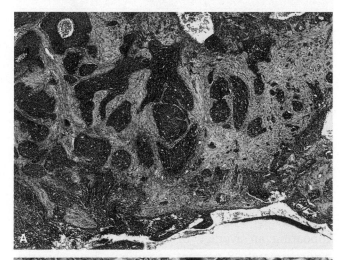

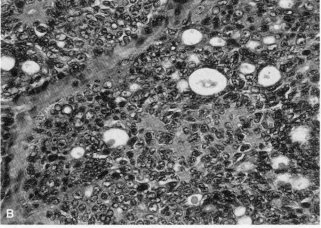

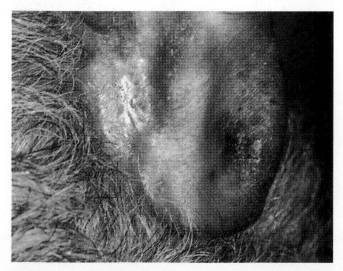

Figure 8.1–8. Eccrine porocarcinoma of the ear. This barely raised 7-mm keratotic red papule was located on the posterior helix of a middle-aged man. It could be mistaken for a squamous cell carcinoma. (Courtesy of Gregg Menaker, MD)

Figure 8.1–9. Eccrine porocarcinoma histopathology. *A*, Low-power view showing surface ulceration with widespread infiltration of the dermis by tumor. *B*, Ductal differentiation within this tumor is evident. (Hematoxylin and eosin)

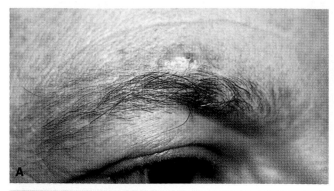

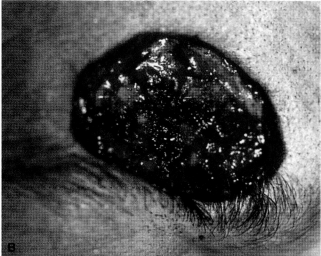

Figure 8.1–10. *A*, Microcystic adnexal carcinoma. Many tumors are similar to this one. They are nondescript flesh-colored papules occurring on the central face. *B*, The Mohs' surgery defect of the lesion seen in *A*. The defect highlights the rule that these tumors extend well beyond their clinical margins. (Courtesy of Jessica Fewkes, MD)

Radiotherapy may be a risk factor, with MACs appearing an average of 35 years after exposure. Approximately 8 percent of patients have this risk factor.[12] This tumor typically presents as a biphasic lesion (Figure 8.1–11, *A*). Superficially, it is composed of keratocysts whereas in the deeper dermis, it consists of narrow epithelial strands dispersed in a sclerotic stroma (see Figure 8.1–11, *B* and *C*). Invariably, there is evidence of ductal differentiation. Pleomorphism is mild, and the mitotic rate is low.

Microcystic adnexal carcinoma is destructive, and local recurrences are common even after extensive surgical resection. The recurrence rate of the tumor after traditional excision can be as high as 50 percent; however, no deaths have been reported from MAC. There is only 1 case report of metastasis in approximately 100 cases in the literature. Mohs' micrographic surgery is currently the recommended

treatment of choice because extensive subclinical tumor extension is frequently present (see Figure 8.1–11, *B*). A recent series showed no recurrences in 11 patients who were treated with Mohs' surgery and observed for 5 years.[12] Adjuvant radiation therapy and chemotherapy have been used, but they do not seem to alter the tumor recurrence rate.

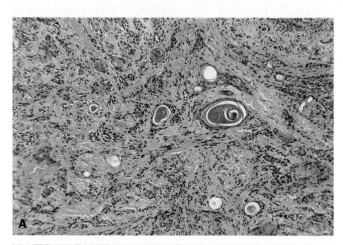

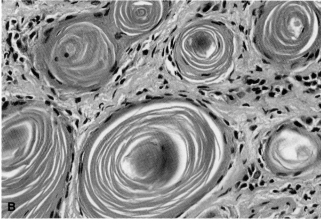

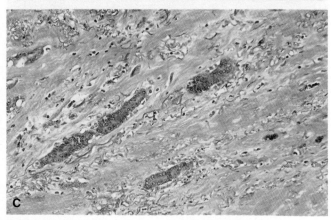

Figure 8.1–11. Microcystic adnexal carcinoma histopathology. *A*, The biphasic cell population. *B*, Keratocysts. *C*, View showing narrow epithelial strands with an associated sclerotic stroma. (Hematoxylin and eosin)

SEBACEOUS CARCINOMA

Sebaceous carcinoma (SC) is an aggressive tumor of the sebaceous glands.[13] The majority of SCs arise within the sebaceous glands of the eyelid; however, about 25 percent have been reported to occur elsewhere. Clinically, the lesion appears as a slow growing papule or nodule with a yellow or orange hue (Figure 8.1–12). It may initially be mistaken for a chalazion. Elderly patients are most likely to be affected, with women and Asians at increased risk.

Patients with a history of radiation therapy are likely to carry an increased risk for SC. A small percent of SCs are diagnosed in patients with Muir-Torre syndrome. Internal malignancies, keratoacanthomas, and sebaceous skin tumors (including SC) characterize this very rare autosomal dominant syndrome. On microscopic examination, SC consists of irregular lobules of basaloid cells showing variable sebaceous differentiation (Figure 8.1–13, *A*). Nuclear atypia (seen in Figure 8.1–13, *B*) can be striking, with many mitoses evident. Occasionally, epidermal involvement manifests as extramammary Paget's disease.

While wide excision is the treatment of choice for localized disease, even aggressive surgery can result in an approximately 30 percent local recurrence rate. Mohs' surgery may offer benefit but is associated with a high recurrence rate. Up to 25 percent of patients present with local lymph node involvement. Primary lower-lid involvement carries a better prognosis; however, bilateral lid involve-

ment is a poor prognostic factor. Radiotherapy is considered palliative.

LEIOMYOSARCOMA

Superficial leiomyosarcoma (LMS) cases can be divided into two clinical subgroups: those arising within the skin and those arising within the subcutaneous tissue.[14] Cutaneous LMS originates from the arrector pili muscles within the dermis whereas subcutaneous LMS is derived from smooth-muscle tissue within arteries and veins. Most of these tumors occur in older patients, on the lower extremity.[15] Occasionally painful, LMS presents as a solitary nodule that may be ulcerated. There are no known risk factors or causes. Histologic examination shows spindle cells with eosinophilic cytoplasm and cigar-shaped nuclei. Well-differentiated tumors

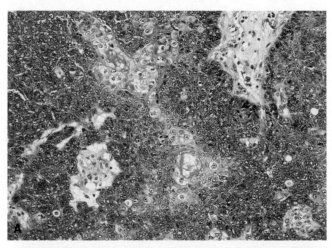

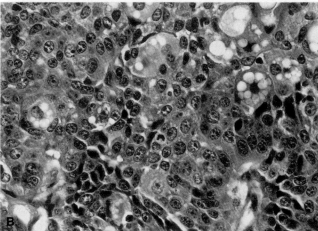

Figure 8.1–13. Sebaceous carcinoma histopathology. *A*, Basaloid cells, with focal sebaceous differentiation. *B*, Numerous mitoses are seen in this high-power view. (Hematoxylin and eosin)

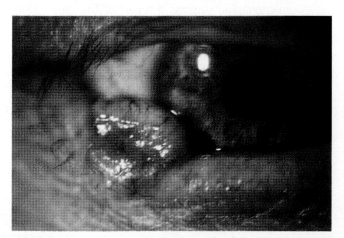

Figure 8.1–12. Sebaceous carcinoma of the lower eyelid. The yellow hue and fine fatty lobulations suggest the diagnosis, but not all tumors have these clinically suggestive features. (Courtesy of Peter Rubin, MD)

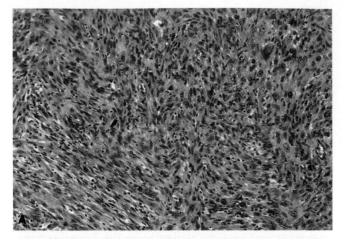

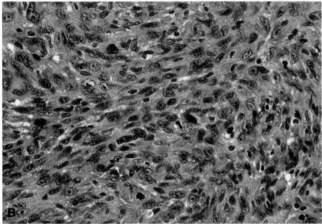

Figure 8.1–14. Cutaneous leiomyosarcoma histopathology. *A*, The pleomorphic nature of this spindle cell tumor is evident in this low-power view. *B*, Nuclear pleomorphism and mitotic activity are observed. The tumor cells have abundant eosinophilic cytoplasm. (Hematoxylin and eosin)

are arranged in fascicles, as seen in Figure 8.1–14, *A*. Sometimes a storiform pattern is evident. Mitotic activity and pleomorphism are variable, depending on the histologic grade (see Figure 8.1–14, *B*).

Treatment is wide local excision. The recurrence rate is about 50 percent for both subtypes of LMS. Very few cases of cutaneous LMS metastasize whereas subcutaneous LMS has a metastatic rate of between 30 and 60 percent and has a higher mortality. Adjuvant radiation therapy is appropriate for the latter, high-grade variants.

ACKNOWLEDGMENT

We thank Phillip H. McKee, MD, for the pathology photomicrographs.

REFERENCES

1. Requena L, Sangueza OP. Cutaneous vascular proliferation. Part III. Malignant neoplasms, other cutaneous neoplasms with significant vascular component, and disorders erroneously considered as vascular neoplasms. J Am Acad Dermatol 1998;38:143–75.
2. Bullen R, Larson PO, Landeck AE, et al. Angiosarcoma of the head and neck managed by a combination of multiple biopsies to determine tumor margin and radiation therapy. Report of three cases and review of the literature. Dermatol Surg 1998;24:1105–10.
3. Fretzin DF, Helwig EB. Atypical fibroxanthoma of the skin. A clinicopathologic study of 140 cases. Cancer 1973;31:1541–52.
4. Kuwano H, Hashimoto H, Enjoji M. Atypical fibroxanthoma distinguishable from spindle cell carcinoma in sarcoma-like skin lesions. A clinicopathologic and immunohistochemical study of 21 cases. Cancer 1985;55:172–80.
5. Karimipour DJ, Johnson TM, Kang S, et al. Mucinous carcinoma of the skin. J Am Acad Dermatol 1997; 36:323–6.
6. Hanby AM, McKee P, Jeffery M, et al. Primary mucinous carcinomas of the skin express TFF1, TFF3, estrogen receptor, and progesterone receptors. Am J Surg Pathol 1998;22:1125–31.
7. Gloster HM Jr. Dermatofibrosarcoma protuberans. J Am Acad Dermatol 1996;35:355–74.
8. Ratner D, Thomas CO, Johnson TM, et al. Mohs' micrographic surgery for the treatment of dermatofibrosarcoma protuberans. Results of a multiinstitutional series with an analysis of the extent of the microscopic spread. J Am Acad Dermatol 1997;37:600–13.
9. Snow SN, Reizner GT. Eccrine porocarcinoma of the face. J Am Acad Dermatol 1992;27:306–11.
10. Wittenberg GP, Robertson DB, Soloman AR, Washington CV. Eccrine porocarcinoma treated with Mohs' micrographic surgery: a report of five cases. Dermatol Surg 1999;25:911–3.
11. Cooper PH. Sclerosing carcinomas of sweat ducts (microcystic adnexal carcinoma). Arch Dermatol 1986;122:261–4.
12. Friedman PM, Friedman RH, Jiang SB, et al. Microcystic adnexal carcinoma: collaborative series review and update. J Am Acad Dermatol 1999;41:225–31.
13. Nelson BR, Hamlet KR, Gillard M, et al. Sebaceous carcinoma. J Am Acad Dermatol 1995;33:1–15.
14. Lange J. Leiomyosarcoma. In: Maloney ME, Miller SJ, editors. Cutaneous oncology: pathophysiology, diagnosis, and management. Malden: Blackwell Science; 1998. p. 893.
15. Landry MM, Sarma DP, Boucree JB Jr. Leiomyosarcoma of the buttock. J Am Acad Dermatol 1991; 24:618–20.

Merkel Cell (Cutaneous Neuroendocrine) Carcinoma

PAUL NGHIEM, MD, PHD

PHILLIP H. MCKEE, MD, FRCPATH

HARLEY A. HAYNES, MD

Merkel cell carcinoma (primary cutaneous neuroendocrine carcinoma, trabecular carcinoma) is a rare but often lethal tumor of uncertain histogenesis. Five cases were originally described by Toker[1] in 1972 as "trabecular carcinoma of the skin." This name was derived from the most characteristic (but least common) of three distinct histologic patterns for this tumor. Later electron microscopic analysis revealed cytoplasmic neurosecretory granules in the cells of this carcinoma and linked it to its most likely precursor, the Merkel cell. Pathologists suggest that this tumor should be called neuroendocrine carcinoma of the skin[2] because it is highly analogous to such

tumors in the lung (small cell carcinoma) and other sites, likely sharing a similar precursor cell.

The Merkel cell was initially described as a "touch" cell ("tastzellen") by the German anatomist and histopathologist Friedrich Sigmund Merkel in 1875.[3] In early studies, he found a high density of these cells in pig snout skin, and their association with cutaneous nerves suggested a role in mediating the touch sensation (Figure 8.2–1). On light microscopy, Merkel cells are difficult to differentiate from melanocytes or Langerhans' cells; however, they can be readily identified by standard electron microscopy (Figure 8.2–2) or more routinely identi-

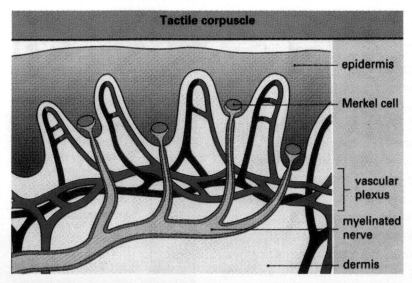

Figure 8.2–1. Schematic of the location of Merkel cells within the epidermis and association with cutaneous nerves. (Reprinted with permission from McKee. Pathology of the skin. 2nd ed. Mosby: London, 1996, pg 1.13)

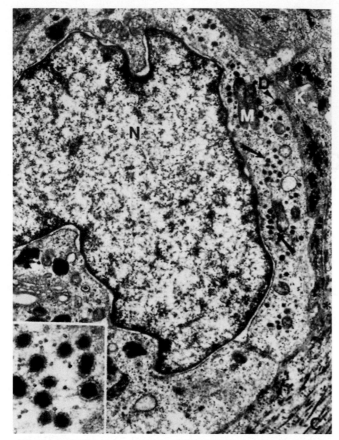

Figure 8.2–2.   Electron micrograph of a Merkel cell. *Arrows* point to specific granules of the Merkel cell. (N = nucleus of Merkel cell; M = mitochondria; D with arrowhead = desmosome between Merkel cell and keratinocyte [K]; C = collagen with cross striation.) (x20,000 original magnification) (Reproduced with permission from Lever. Histopathology of the skin. 8th ed.) Inset shows characteristic cytoplasmic Merkel granules at high magnification (x75,000 original magnification).

fied by their immunocytochemical staining profile, as discussed in the pathology section below.

With only about 400 cases per year in the United States, Merkel cell carcinoma is at least 100 times more rare than melanoma,[4,5] and with a fatality rate of about 26 percent, it is the most lethal of the skin cancers (Table 8.2–1).[5,6] There has been considerable evolution in the treatment philosophy of Merkel cell carcinoma. As recently as 1987, it was suggested that this cancer should be treated "using the same rationale as applied for the treatment of squamous cell carcinoma."[2] It is increasingly apparent that the 10-fold greater fatality rate for Merkel cell carcinoma over squamous cell carcinoma can be significantly diminished through prompt aggressive treatment involving wide excision, lymph node biopsy, and adjuvant radiation therapy.

Table 8.2–1. COMPARISON OF SKIN CANCERS: INCIDENCE AND MORTALITY IN THE UNITED STATES			
Tumor	Annual US Incidence	Deaths	Fatality Rate
Merkel cell carcinoma*	400	130	1 in 4
Melanoma	42,000	8,000	1 in 5
Squamous cell carcinoma	100,000	2,000	1 in 50
Basal cell carcinoma	850,000	< 80	< 1 in 10,000

*Figures are based on an estimated incidence of 0.16 per 100,000 and a 74 percent disease-specific survival.
Adapted from Landis SH, Murray T, Bolden S, Wingo PA. Cancer statistics, 1998. CA Cancer J Clin 1998;48:6–29.

CLINICAL PRESENTATION

Merkel cell carcinoma has a rather nonspecific appearance, usually developing on sun-exposed skin as a firm erythematous papule with occasional ulceration (Figure 8.2–3). Because of the rarity of this tumor and this nondistinctive appearance, the vast majority of these tumors are removed with a presumptive diagnosis of squamous cell carcinoma, basal cell carcinoma, keratoacanthoma, amelanotic melanoma, adnexal tumor, or lymphoma (Figures 8.2–4 to 8.2–6).[7]

The large role played by ultraviolet radiation in the development of this tumor is suggested by its presence in a sun-distribution on the body of older Caucasian individuals, many of whom already have other sun-induced skin cancers.[7] The most common primary site is the head and neck (40%), followed by the upper extremity (19%) (Figure 8.2–7).[8] In terms of gender, there is a slight male predominance (3:2). The median age for developing Merkel cell carcinoma is 66 years, with two-thirds of cases presenting in patients over 60 years of age.[8]

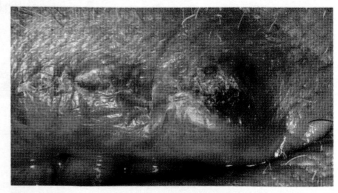

Figure 8.2–3.   A Merkel cell carcinoma on the lip of a 92-year-old man.

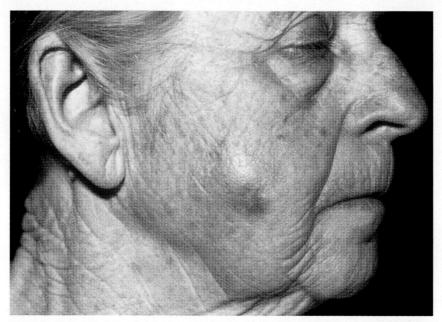

Figure 8.2–4.   Merkel cell carcinoma arising on the face. (Courtesy of Dr. Helmut Kerl)

PROGNOSIS

The outlook for patients with Merkel cell carcinoma (MCC) is partly dependent on the clinical stage of the disease although even the earliest lesion of MCC carries about a 10 percent chance of death within 2 years.[6] The staging system, the fraction of patients presenting with each stage, and survival is summarized in Figure 8.2–9. Larger primary tumors and the presence of disease in regional lymph nodes each diminish survival rates significantly. The most common sites for metastasis are listed in Table 8.2–2.[8] Several recent studies suggest that the outcomes depend on the optimal management of MCC with wide (2.5-cm margin) excision, lymphatic assessment, and radiation therapy.[9–12]

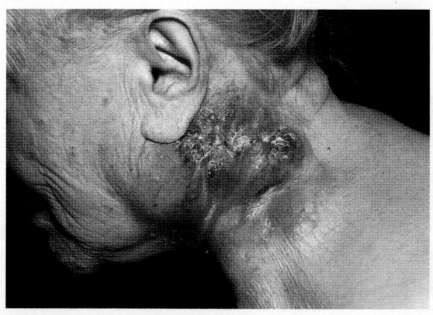

Figure 8.2–5.   An advanced Merkel cell carcinoma involving the neck. (Courtesy of Dr. Helmut Kerl)

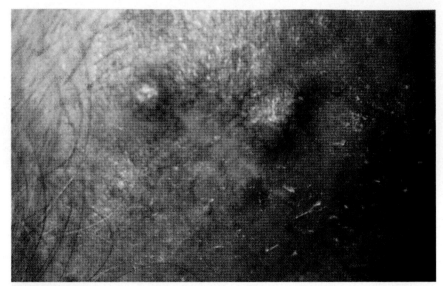

Figure 8.2–6.   Multiple small tumor nodules of Merkel cell carcinoma on the forehead. (Courtesy of Dr. R.A. Johnson)

RISK FACTORS AND ASSOCIATIONS

A history of prolonged sun exposure and age over 60 years are the major risks for MCC. Ultraviolet exposure in the form of psoralen plus ultraviolet A (PUVA) has also recently been associated with an approximately 100-fold increased MCC incidence.[13] Among 1,380 psoriasis patients treated with PUVA, 3 (0.2%) developed MCC. All 3 were elderly and had had between 4 and 60 prior non-melanoma skin cancers. In 2 patients, the MCC developed more than 20 years after PUVA therapy was initiated, and 2 patients had received more than 300 PUVA treatments.[13]

There are several recent reports of MCC associated with arsenic exposure (Figure 8.2–8).[14,15] Along the southwest coast of Taiwan prior to 1970, people drank artesian-well water containing high levels of arsenic. Elevated levels of squamous cell, basal cell, bladder, and lung carcinoma were encountered. More recently, six cases (higher than expected) of MCC were reported in this region.[15]

A role for immune surveillance in the control of MCC is suggested by several studies that document an

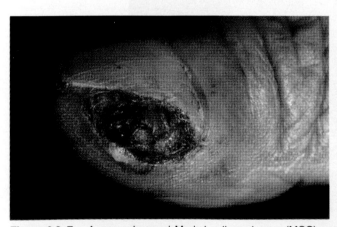

Figure 8.2–7.   A rare subungual Merkel cell carcinoma (MCC): a small fraction of MCCs arise on relatively sun-protected sites. (Courtesy of Dr. R.A. Johnson)

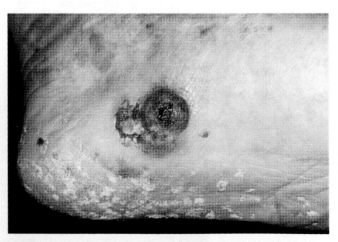

Figure 8.2–8.   A Merkel cell carcinoma arising on the foot of a Japanese man exposed to arsenic. Multiple white arsenical keratoses can also be seen in addition to the red nodule of the Merkel cell carcinoma. (Reproduced with permission from Tsuruta D, Hamada T, Mochida K, et al. Merkel cell carcinoma, Bowen's disease and chronic occupational arsenic poisoning. Br J Dermatol 1999;41:641–3.)

A

Stage	Presentation Characteristics	% of Cases
IA	Primary tumor < 2 cm	37
IB	Primary tumor > 2 cm	38
II	Spread to draining lymph nodes	23
III	Distant disease	2

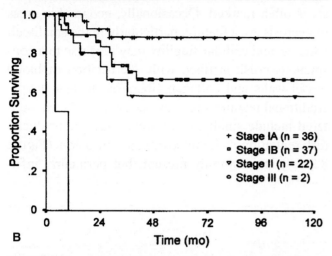

B

Figure 8.2–9. *A,* The staging classification for Merkel cell carcinoma is given with the frequency of patients presenting with each stage in 97 cases, the largest single series. *B,* Kaplan-Meier curves for 10-year disease-specific survival in patients with Merkel cell carcinoma, plotted by stage at presentation. (Reproduced with permission from Allen PJ, Zhang ZF, Coit DG. Surgical management of Merkel cell carcinoma. Ann Surg 1999;229:97–105.)

association with chronic immune suppression in organ transplant recipients. Some 52 Merkel cell carcinomas have been reported in organ transplant recipients.[16,17] Importantly, the mean age at diagnosis was younger (53 vs 66 years), and the MCC-associated death rate was more than double the death rate of MCC patients from the general population (68% vs 26%).[6,17]

A rare and welcome event in MCC management is spontaneous regression, of which 5 cases have been reported.[18] In one of these cases, a 65-year-old man was too ill to undergo treatment, and on follow-up 6 months later, the lesion had resolved.[18]

Virtually nothing is known of the molecular pathogenesis of MCC. The most commonly mutated gene in cancers in general, p53, was only targeted in a minority of MCCs (28%),[19] which suggests that it plays a minor and non-essential role in the development of this tumor. No association with clinical outcome was found after examining the expression level of proapoptotic (bax and wild-type p53) or antiapoptotic (bcl-2) genes in 25 MCCs.[20]

HISTOLOGIC FEATURES

The Merkel cell tumor belongs to the group of small "blue" cell tumors, which also includes metastatic neuroendocrine carcinoma (usually of bronchial cell origin), lymphoma, primitive peripheral neuroectodermal tumor, and small cell melanoma.

Histologically, the tumor commonly involves the full thickness of the dermis (Figure 8.2–10) and frequently extends into the subcutaneous fat and adjacent skeletal muscle.[1,21–23] While a Grenz zone of dermal sparing often separates the tumor from the overlying epidermis, epidermal changes (including ulceration) are not uncommon. Occasionally, pagetoid spread may simulate melanoma or mycosis fungoides (Figure 8.2–11), and (exceptionally rarely) the tumor may appear to be wholly intraepidermal.[24,25] The majority of neuroendocrine carcinomas arise on the sun-exposed skin of elderly individuals, and severe actinic elastosis is therefore frequently present.

Table 8.2–2. CHARACTERISTICS OF MERKEL CELL CARCINOMA IN 107 PATIENTS	
Characteristics	**% of Patients***
Gender	
Male	59
Female	36
Age (median = 66 yr)	
< 60	26
≥ 60	66
Ethnicity	
White	97
Black	1
Primary site	
Head and neck	37
Upper extremity	18
Lower extremity	17
Trunk	13
Vulva	3
Metastatic site	
Skin	28
Lymph nodes	27
Liver	13
Lung	10
Bone	10
Brain	6
Bone marrow	2
Pleura	2
Pancreas	1
Testis	1
Small bowel	1
Stomach	1

*In some cases, percentages were rounded to the nearest whole number. Reprinted with permission from Voog E, Biron P, Martin JP, Blay JY. Chemotherapy for patients with locally advanced or metastatic Merkel cell carcinoma. Cancer 1999;85:2589–95.

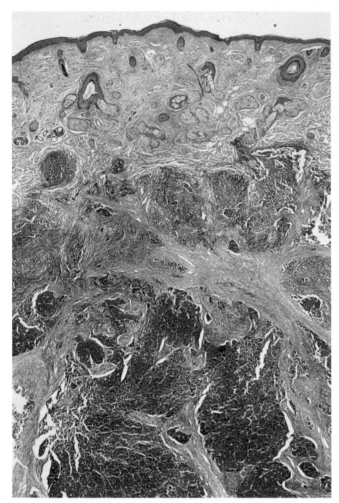

Figure 8.2–10. Scanning view shows extensive dermal infiltration by a small "blue" cell tumor.

A variety of histologic subtypes are recognized (Figures 8.2–12 to 8.2–16), including intermediate, small-cell, and trabecular.[21] Although the last conforms to the original description by Toker, it is in fact the least commonly encountered.[1] Mixed intermediate and small-cell variants are also not uncommon. Most often, the cells are present in diffuse sheets or nests sometimes showing regular borders but more often associated with an irregular infiltrating growth pattern dissecting between the collagen fibers of the adjacent dermis. In the trabecular subtype, the tumor cells are arranged in narrow strands or ribbons that are one or two cells thick, reminiscent of a carcinoid tumor.

The tumor cells have scanty indistinct amphophilic cytoplasm and generally have round or oval nuclei. The nuclei are characteristically vesicular, with pale-staining delicate chromatin (intermediate and

trabecular types), although hyperchromatic and spindle forms (small-cell type) may also be encountered (Figure 8.2–17). The latter variant often shows nuclear molding. Nucleoli are commonly present but usually not prominent. Mitoses are typically numerous, and atypical forms are frequently seen. Apoptosis is often marked. Occasionally, geographic areas of necrosis are a feature, particularly in the small-cell variants, and cellular fragility may give rise to a conspicuous crush artifact, with encrustation of blood vessel walls and collagen fibers by nuclear debris. Additional features that may occasionally be encountered include small foci of squamous and/or ductal differentiation.[26] Lymphovascular invasion (Figure 8.2–18) is commonly present, but perineural infil-

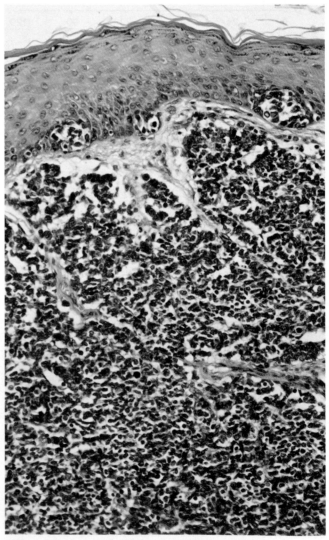

Figure 8.2–11. This view of a cutaneous neuroendocrine carcinoma shows intraepidermal involvement. The case was seen in consultation, with an initial diagnosis of cutaneous T-cell lymphoma.

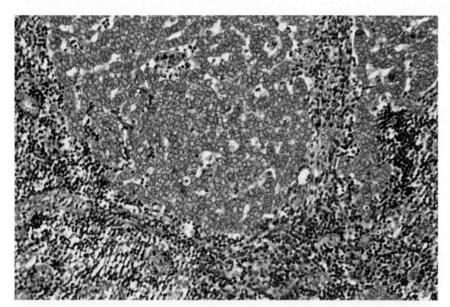

Figure 8.2–12. Intermediate neuroendocrine carcinoma. The tumor is composed of uniform small cells with minimal cytoplasm and round to oval palely staining nuclei. Lymphocytes are present in the background.

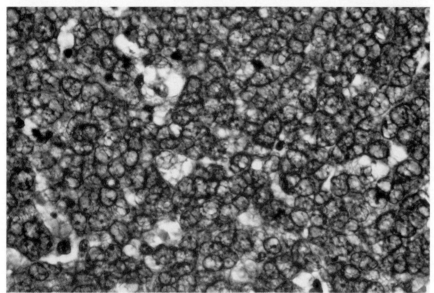

Figure 8.2–13. Intermediate neuroendocrine carcinoma; high-power view showing the characteristic nuclear morphology. There are numerous mitotic figures.

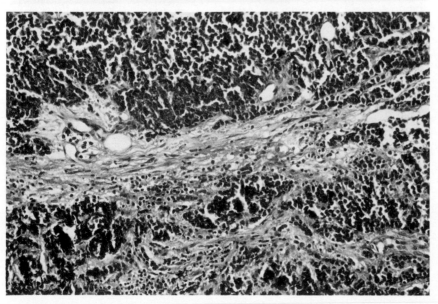

Figure 8.2–14. Small cell neuroendocrine carcinoma showing characteristic crushed nuclear debris in the lower half of the field. Such crush artifact is characteristic of neuroendocrine carcinomas, including Merkel cell carcinoma of the skin and small cell carcinoma of the bronchus.

Figure 8.2–15. Small cell neuroendocrine carcinoma composed of cells with hyperchromatic nuclei and minimal cytoplasm. An "Indian-file" distribution is seen in the center of the field. These features are indistinguishable from those of a bronchial small cell carcinoma.

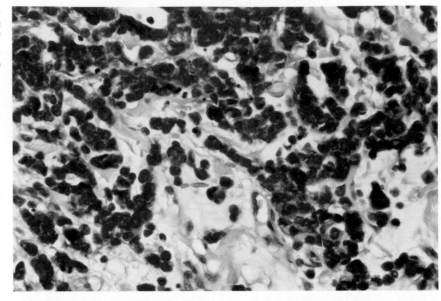

Figure 8.2–16. Primary cutaneous neuroendocrine carcinoma showing the typical appearances of the trabecular variant. This lesion may be confused with metastatic carcinoid tumor.

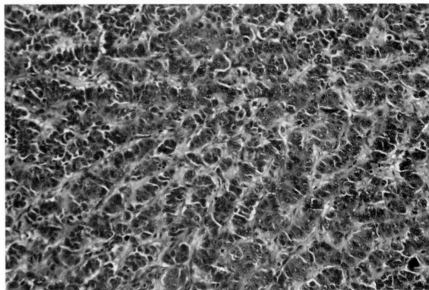

Figure 8.2–17. Small cell neuroendocrine carcinoma, showing spindle-shaped nuclei.

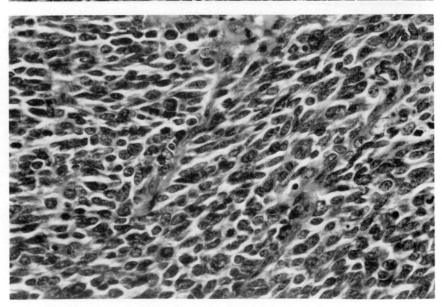

tration is rarely seen. The tumor infiltrate is usually accompanied by a lymphocytic infiltrate, and plasma cells are sometimes also present.

Occasionally, the overlying epidermis shows coexistent squamous cell carcinoma in situ although merging or continuity between the two populations is very rare. Primary cutaneous neuroendocrine carcinoma (notably the intermediate variant) may also coexist with invasive squamous cell carcinoma (Figure 8.2–19), and the two cell populations frequently appear to blend although they appear immunocytochemically distinct.[27–29] Whether this implies origin from a common stem cell is unknown. Neuroendocrine carcinoma rarely coexists with basal cell carcinoma (Figure 8.2–20) although this phenomenon likely represents a collision tumor.[30]

Immunocytochemistry (particularly in small-cell variants) plays an important role in the diagnosis of cutaneous neuroendocrine carcinoma, especially in the differentiation of cutaneous from bronchogenic neuroendocrine carcinoma (small cell carcinoma). The tumor cells express low-molecular-weight keratin (Cam 5.2, AE1/AE3, and cytokeratin 20) (Figure 8.2–21), frequently presenting as a paranuclear dot or crescent, neuron-specific enolase (Figure 8.2–22), epithelial-membrane antigen, chromogranin, synaptophysin, and PGP 9.5.[31–34] Merkel cell carcinoma is consistently negative for S-100 protein. The tumor

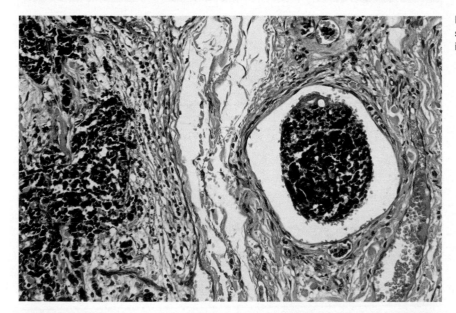

Figure 8.2–18. Lymphovascular invasion as shown in this field is an extremely common finding in cutaneous neuroendocrine carcinoma.

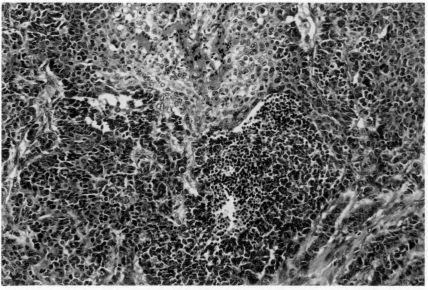

Figure 8.2–19. Occasionally, cutaneous neuroendocrine carcinoma coexists with invasive squamous cell carcinoma. This does not appear to be of any prognostic significance. Metastases are almost invariably restricted to the small-cell component.

Figure 8.2–20. Very occasionally, basal cell carcinoma (right) is seen adjacent to a neuro-endocrine carcinoma. This is almost certainly coincidental.

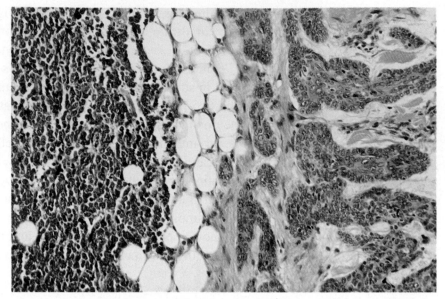

Figure 8.2–21. Cutaneous neuroendocrine carcinoma showing typical paranuclear-dot keratin positivity (Cam 5.2).

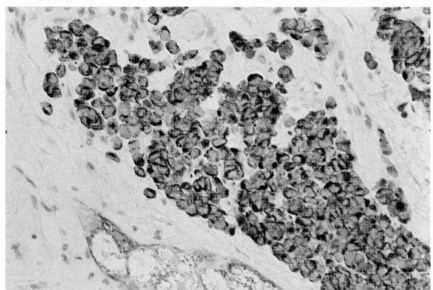

Figure 8.2–22. Cutaneous neuroendocrine carcinoma showing neuron-specific enolase expression.

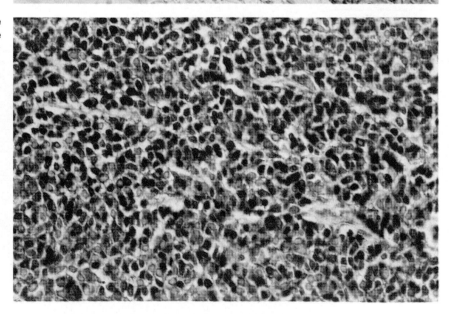

may also contain a variety of neuropeptides, including calcitonin, bombesin, somatostatin, leuenkephalin, adrenocorticotropic hormone (ACTH), and vasoactive intestinal polypeptide 2 (VIP 2).

Ultrastructurally, 100- to 250-nm membranebound neurosecretory granules are commonly seen in trabecular variants. They are sparser in intermediate variants and rare or absent in small-cell variants.[21] The presence of a paranuclear aggregate of intermediate filaments is a characteristic feature. Desmosomal cell junctions may be present in the trabecular variant.

HISTOLOGIC DIFFERENTIAL DIAGNOSIS

Although the diagnosis may seem relatively straightforward in many cases, it is always important to exclude the possibility of metastasis, particularly from small cell carcinoma of bronchial derivation.[35,36] In addition, primary cutaneous neuroendocrine carcinoma may occasionally be confused with lymphoma, peripheral primitive neuroectodermal tumor, metastatic carcinoid tumor, or amelanotic small cell melanoma.[37,38] It is the small-cell variant of cutaneous neuroendocrine carcinoma, however, that causes the most diagnostic difficulty, particularly in distinguishing it from metastatic bronchial neuroendocrine tumors. The use of cytokeratins 7 and 20 with neuro-

filament immunocytochemistry affords the distinction in the vast majority of cases. Primary cutaneous lesions are positive for both cytokeratin 20 and neurofilament and negative for cytokeratin 7 whereas in the majority of cases, bronchial tumors are positive for cytokeratin 7 and negative for cytokeratin 20. In addition, the majority (although not all) of the latter are also neurofilament negative.[25,36] Neuroendocrine (small cell) carcinomas from other sites are also usually negative for cytokeratin 20, with the exception of salivary gland lesions, which have been shown to be positive in a significant proportion of cases.[36] The use of a battery of immunoreagents (Table 8.2–3) is recommended before a diagnosis of primary cutaneous neuroendocrine carcinoma is made.

EVALUATION

This tumor's rarity and its relatively recent description (in 1972) have prevented the establishment of optimal treatment guidelines; there are only about 500 reported cases and no prospective trials of therapy. Several retrospective studies now shed light on the roles of surgery, radiation therapy, and chemotherapy in the adjuvant and recurrent-disease settings. Merkel cell carcinoma has a more aggressive behavior and different biologic responses to therapy than any of the other skin cancers. In terms

Table 8.2–3. USE OF IMMUNOREAGENTS IN DIFFERENTIAL DIAGNOSIS OF MERKEL CELL (CUTANEOUS NEUROENDOCRINE) CARCINOMA

Tumor	Immunoreagent								
	CAM 5.2/ AE1/AE3	CK 20	Neurofilament Protein	NSE	EMA	CD99	S-100 Protein	CK 7	LCA
Merkel cell carcinoma	+ve; usually dotlike	+ve; usually dotlike	+ve; dotlike	+ve	+ve	May be +ve; cytoplasmic	–ve	–ve	–ve
Neuroendocrine carcinoma of lung	+ve; usually cytoplasmic	–ve	May be +ve	+ve	+ve	May be +ve; cytoplasmic	–ve	+ve	–ve
Lymphoma	–ve	–ve	–ve	–ve	Rarely +ve; Ki-1 lymphoma	Usually –ve	–ve	–ve	+ve
Peripheral primitive neuroectodermal tumor	10% +ve	–ve	Rarely +ve	+ve	–ve	+ve; membranous	Rarely +ve	–ve	–ve
Metastatic carcinoid tumor	Often +ve	–ve	–ve	+ve	–ve	–ve	–ve	May be +ve	–ve
Small cell melanoma	5% +ve	–ve	–ve	+ve	–ve	–ve	+ve	–ve	–ve

CK = cytokeratin; NSE = neuron-specific enolase; EMA = epithelial-membrane antigen; LCA = leukocyte common antigen; +ve = positive; –ve = negative.

of its etiology and optimal management, it is not merely a variant of squamous cell carcinoma.

Upon making the diagnosis of Merkel cell carcinoma, a complete physical examination should be performed, evaluating the entire skin surface, lymph nodes, liver, and spleen. Liver function tests may help rule out spread to this organ (13% of metastatic disease is to liver). A baseline chest radiograph is important in excluding metastatic small cell carcinoma of the lung. Also useful is immunocytochemistry for cytokeratins 7 and 20, which differentiate neuroendocrine tumors of the lung from those of skin origin.[7] Computed tomography (CT) scans may be considered, especially if there is suspicion of a visceral origin of the skin lesion.

MANAGEMENT

Surgical Excision

Excision of the primary tumor mass of a Merkel cell carcinoma is essential, and several studies document the need for this excision to involve wider margins than those for squamous cell or basal cell carcinoma (Table 8.2–4). Among 38 Australian patients who had a simple excision (margins ≥ 0.5 cm), 100 percent experienced local recurrence of their Merkel cell cancers (Table 8.2–5).[11] Wide local excision with margins ≥ 2.5 cm yielded a local relapse rate of 49 percent among 41 patients in a Mayo Clinic series.[12]

The control of local recurrence is strongly linked to survival: among 35 patients in a St. Louis cohort, 2-year survival was 86 percent for those with no locoregional recurrence but only 35 percent for those with recurrence.[10] Thus, wide excision of the primary tumor with a 2.5-cm margin not only decreases the morbidity of locally recurrent MCC but also most likely improves survival.

Mohs' micrographic surgery is established for the treatment of several tumor types, including basal and squamous cell carcinoma, but its role in the treatment of Merkel cell carcinoma is unclear and doubtful. This technique has been evaluated in one small trial of 12 patients.[12] Among the patients who received Mohs' surgery alone, the local relapse rate was 50 percent, comparable to that for wide excision alone. Perhaps more important than the details of the surgical approach used to fully excise this tumor, is the

concept that lymph node biopsy and radiation treatment are essential for optimal control of local disease.

Surgical Treatment of the Draining Lymph Nodes

The critical role of adjuvant treatment with lymph node surgery is revealed by the largest cohort of MCC patients reported in the literature. Among these 102 MCC patients collected over 27 years in New York, elective lymph node dissection was the only parameter independently predictive of improved relapse-free survival.[6] This study also reported that the most common site of first recurrence is the draining lymph nodes. A separate study showed that a majority of patients with distant metastatic disease had had prior locoregional or nodal recurrence and that control of the lymph node involvement improves survival.[10]

Sentinel lymph node excision involves removing the one or two nodes shown to drain the tumor

Table 8.2–4. MERKEL CELL CARCINOMA: FACTORS INFLUENCING SURVIVAL AMONG 35 PATIENTS			
Characteristic	N	2-Year Survival (%)	p Value
Stage			
I	30	56	
II	3	33	
III	2	0	< .01
Age			
< 60 yr	8	100	
60–70 yr	8	86	
>70 yr	17	11	< .01
Surgical margin			
Wide (> 2.5 cm)	15	86	
Simple (0.5–2.5 cm)	18	28	.03
Lymph node excision			
+	11	100	
–	22	35	<.01
Radiotherapy (adjuvant)			
+	13	77	
–	20	40	.03
Chemotherapy (adjuvant)			
+	9	57	
–	24	51	NS
Locoregional recurrence			
+	20	35	
–	13	86	<.01
Distant recurrence			
+	16	17	
–	17	100	<.01

NS = not significant; N = population size.
Adapted from Kokoska ER, Kokoska MS, Collins BT, et al. Early aggressive treatment for Merkel cell carcinoma improves outcome. Am J Surg 1997;174:688–93.

Table 8.2–5. IMPORTANCE OF COMBINED SURGERY AND RADIATION THERAPY TO PREVENT LOCAL RECURRENCE OF MERKEL CELL CARCINOMA				
Treatment	Local Relapse (%)	Durability	Patients (n)	Reference
Excision (≥ 0.5 cm)	100	6 mo to relapse	38	11
Excision (≥ 0.5 cm) + RT*	30	17 mo to relapse	34	11
Wide excision (≥ 2.5 cm)	49	60 mo F/U	41	12
Mohs' surgery†	50	36 mo F/U	8	12
Mohs' surgery + RT*	0	36 mo F/U	4	12

F/U = follow-up; RT = radiation therapy.
*50 Gy of radiation delivered in 2-Gy fractions.
†Additional margins after Mohs' surgery: 0 mm in 7 cases, 5–10 mm in 6 cases. Average primary tumor size for Mohs' surgery was larger (2.98 cm) than that of the wide excision group (1.57 cm) although F/U interval was shorter for Mohs' surgery group (36 vs 60 mo).

site, using a combination of a radiotracer and a dye. This procedure is available at a growing number of centers around the country and is discussed in detail in a separate chapter in this volume. It involves much less morbidity than complete nodal dissection and has excellent sensitivity in melanoma, among other applications. Biopsy of sentinel nodes has now been investigated in two studies with Merkel cell carcinoma.[39,40] A total of 30 MCC patients were treated with the sentinel node procedure in the two studies. The 26 patients who had histologically negative sentinel nodes were followed up (mean periods of 7 or 10.5 months), and none of these patients developed recurrent disease. All four of the patients who had positive sentinel nodes had complete node excisions performed, two of which revealed additional positive nodes.[39,40] These studies suggest that the sentinel node procedure is a sensitive technique for detecting nodal involvement with MCC. With this technique, it should be possible to gain the survival benefit of lymph node dissection while sparing most patients the morbidity of a full elective lymph node dissection.

Radiation Therapy

Whether patients have received simple, wide, or Mohs' excision of their Merkel cell carcinoma, studies suggest that adjuvant radiation therapy (XRT) has an impressive additional benefit. The addition of XRT to simple excision diminished the local recurrence rate from 100 percent (of 38 patients) to 30 percent (of 34 patients).[11] For Mohs' surgery, the addition of radiation therapy cut the local recurrence rate from 50 percent (of 8 patients) to 0 percent (of

4 patients).[12] In addition to decreasing the number of patients developing local recurrence, adjuvant XRT also increased the median time to recurrence from 5.5 months to 16.5 months.[11]

Importantly, the addition of XRT was associated with a statistically significant improvement in survival: among 35 patients, the 2-year survival for XRT-treated patients was 77 percent as compared to 40 percent for those who did not receive radiation.[10] In a Massachusetts General Hospital cohort, all 9 patients who received XRT survived whereas there were 7 deaths among the 22 patients who did not receive adequate (≥ 45 Gy) radiotherapy.[9] Multiple studies suggest that the proper dose of XRT is about 50 Gy, delivered in 2-Gy fractions to the primary tumor bed and the draining node basin.[9,11,41,42]

Chemotherapy

Although Merkel cell carcinoma is partially sensitive to agents such as doxorubicin and cisplatin, there is no role for adjuvant chemotherapy in the management of Merkel cell carcinoma as multiple studies have shown that adjuvant chemotherapy has short-lived benefit,[42] does not improve survival,[8–10,42] and has significant mortality associated with its use.[8] Chemotherapy-associated deaths were significantly more common in patients over 65 years of age (16% of deaths were due to chemotoxicity) than in those less than 65 years old (3% of deaths were due to chemotoxicity).[8]

The story for chemotherapy in metastatic disease is quite different from its story in the adjuvant setting. An extensive analysis of 101 MCC patients who were treated with chemotherapy showed a response rate of 57 percent for patients with metastases and 69 percent for those with locally advanced tumors.[8] There were no survivors among patients who had MCC metastases to viscera such as liver or lung.[8] Among those with metastases to skin, lymph nodes, or bone, however, the 2-year survival rate was ~15 percent after chemotherapy.[8]

Although the optimal chemotherapeutic agents and dosing regimen for MCC is unclear, polychemotherapy was associated with a better response rate than monochemotherapy (63% versus 43%).[8] Doxorubicin plus cisplatin showed a 100 percent response rate in 7 patients while polychemotherapy including 5-fluorouracil had a 92 percent response rate in 12 patients.[8]

FOLLOW-UP

Close follow-up—every 3 months for at least a year—is warranted in monitoring Merkel cell carcinoma because most cases relapse within the 1st year.[7] This is significantly sooner on average than melanoma recurs, for example. Moreover, disease-specific survival with recurrent disease is 62 percent if recurrence is treated aggressively, so efforts to detect and treat recurrences promptly are likely to be beneficial.[6]

SUMMARY

Merkel cell carcinoma is the highest-grade variant of skin cancer; fortunately, it is at least 100 times rarer than melanoma. Its clinical appearance is nonspecific, and it typically presents as a firm nodule on sun-exposed skin. Histologically, although the trabecular variant is rather characteristic, the more

common small-cell variant can be distinguished from lymphoma and melanoma by a panel of antibodies that reveal its neuroendocrine and epithelial characteristics.

In terms of treatment, MCC is quite distinct from the other skin cancers, and it requires wide excision of the primary tumor, surgical biopsy of the draining lymph node bed, and adjuvant radiation therapy to the tumor bed and draining nodal basin (Figure 8.2–23). The role of chemotherapy is limited to metastatic disease or palliation of inoperable regional disease, because of high toxicity and the low durability of response. With optimal treatment such as this, up to 75 percent of patients can expect long-term survival.

REFERENCES

1. Toker C. Trabecular carcinoma of the skin. Arch Dermatol 1972;105:107–10.
2. Hitchcock CL, Bland KI, Laney RG 3rd, et al. Neuroendocrine (Merkel cell) carcinoma of the skin. Its natural history, diagnosis, and treatment. Ann Surg 1988;207:201–7.
3. Camisa C, Weissmann A. Friedrich Sigmund Merkel. Part II. The cell. Am J Dermatopathol 1982;4:527–35.
4. Chuang TY, Su WP, Muller SA. Incidence of cutaneous T cell lymphoma and other rare skin cancers in a defined population. J Am Acad Dermatol 1990;23:254–6.
5. Greenlee RT, Murray T, Bolden S, Wingo PA. Cancer statistics, 1998. CA Cancer J Clin 1998;50:7–33.
6. Allen PJ, Zhang ZF, Coit DG. Surgical management of Merkel cell carcinoma. Ann Surg 1999;229:97–105.
7. Ratner D, Nelson BR, Brown MD, Johnson TM. Merkel cell carcinoma. J Am Acad Dermatol 1993;29:143–56.
8. Voog E, Biron P, Martin JP, Blay JY. Chemotherapy for patients with locally advanced or metastatic Merkel cell carcinoma. Cancer 1999;85:2589–95.
9. Ott MJ, Tanabe KK, Gadd MA, et al. Multimodality management of Merkel cell carcinoma. Arch Surg 1999;134:388–93.
10. Kokoska ER, Kokoska MS, Collins BT, et al. Early aggressive treatment for Merkel cell carcinoma improves outcome. Am J Surg 1997;174:688–93.
11. Meeuwissen JA, Bourne RG, Kearsley JH. The importance of postoperative radiation therapy in the treatment of Merkel cell carcinoma. Int J Radiat Oncol Biol Phys 1995;31:325–31.
12. O'Connor WJ, Roenigk RK, Brodland DG. Merkel cell carcinoma. Comparison of Mohs' micrographic surgery and wide excision in eighty-six patients [published erratum appears in Dermatol Surg 1998 Feb;24(2):299]. Dermatol Surg 1997;23:929–33.

Surgery:
  Wide local excision (2.5 cm)
Node treatment:
  Sentinel node biopsy
  Completion adenectomy if sentinel node is positive
Radiation therapy:
  50 Gy in 2-Gy fractions to tumor bed and draining node bed
Chemotherapy:
  Not beneficial in adjuvant setting
  Metastatic disease:
    Polychemotherapy including doxorubicin or 5-FU

Figure 8.2–23. Treatment recommendations for Merkel cell carcinoma. Retrospective studies suggest that wide surgical excision, node biopsy, and radiation therapy each provide independent survival benefit in the adjuvant setting. (5-FU = fluorouracil)

13. Lunder EJ, Stern RS. Merkel-cell carcinomas in patients treated with methoxsalen and ultraviolet A radiation [letter]. N Engl J Med 1998;339:1247–8.

14. Tsuruta D, Hamada T, Mochida K, et al. Merkel cell carcinoma, Bowen's disease and chronic occupational arsenic poisoning. Br J Dermatol 1998;139:291–4.

15. Lien HC, Tsai TF, Lee YY, Hsiao CH. Merkel cell carcinoma and chronic arsenicism. J Am Acad Dermatol 1999;41:641–3.

16. Urbatsch A, Sams WM Jr, Urist MM, Sturdivant R. Merkel cell carcinoma occurring in renal transplant patients. J Am Acad Dermatol 1999;41:289–91.

17. Penn I, First MR. Merkel's cell carcinoma in organ recipients: report of 41 cases. Transplantation 1999; 68:1717–21.

18. Yanguas I, Goday JJ, Gonzalez-Guemes M, et al. Spontaneous regression of Merkel cell carcinoma of the skin. Br J Dermatol 1997;137:296–8.

19. Schmid M, Janssen K, Dockhorn-Dworniczak B, et al. p53 abnormalities are rare events in neuroendocrine (Merkel cell) carcinoma of the skin. An immuno-histochemical and SSCP analysis. Virchows Arch 1997;430:233–7.

20. Feinmesser M, Halpern M, Fenig E, et al. Expression of the apoptosis-related oncogenes bcl-2, bax, and p53 in Merkel cell carcinoma: can they predict treatment response and clinical outcome? Hum Pathol 1999;30:1367–72.

21. Gould VE, Moll R, Moll I, et al. Neuroendocrine (Merkel) cells of the skin: hyperplasias, dysplasias, and neoplasms. Lab Invest 1985;52:334–53.

22. Silva EG, Mackay B, Goepfert H, et al. Endocrine carcinoma of the skin (Merkel cell carcinoma). Pathol Annu 1984;19:1–30.

23. Schmidt U, Metz KA, Richter HJ, et al. Merkel cell carcinoma: histomorphology and immunohistochemistry of 76 cases. Am J Dermatopathol 1997;19:501.

24. Rocamora A, Badia N, Vives R, et al. Epidermotropic primary neuroendocrine (Merkel cell) carcinoma of the skin with Pautrier-like microabscesses. Report of three cases and review of the literature. J Am Acad Dermatol 1987;16:1163–8.

25. Hashimoto K, Lee MW, D'Annunzio DR, et al. Pagetoid Merkel cell carcinoma: epidermal origin of the tumor. J Cutan Pathol 1998;25:572–9.

26. Gould E, Albores-Saavedra J, Dubner B, et al. Eccrine and squamous differentiation in Merkel cell carcinoma. An immunohistochemical study. Am J Surg Pathol 1988;12:768–72.

27. Jones CS, Tyring SK, Lee PC, Fine JD. Development of neuroendocrine (Merkel cell) carcinoma mixed with squamous cell carcinoma in erythema ab igne. Arch Dermatol 1988;124:110–3.

28. Iacocca MV, Abernethy JL, Stefanato CM, et al. Mixed Merkel cell carcinoma and squamous cell carcinoma of the skin. J Am Acad Dermatol 1998;39:882–7.

29. Gomez LG, DiMaio S, Silva EG , Mackay B. Association between neuroendocrine (Merkel cell) carcinoma and squamous carcinoma of the skin. Am J Surg Pathol 1983;7:171–7.

30. Cerroni L, Kerl H. Primary cutaneous neuroendocrine (Merkel cell) carcinoma in association with squamous- and basal-cell carcinoma. Am J Dermatopathol 1997;19:610–3.

31. Heenan PJ, Cole JM, Spagnolo DV. Primary cutaneous neuroendocrine carcinoma (Merkel cell tumor). An adnexal epithelial neoplasm. Am J Dermatopathol 1990;12:7–16.

32. Shah IA, Netto D, Schlageter MO, et al. Neurofilament immunoreactivity in Merkel-cell tumors: a differentiating feature from small-cell carcinoma. Mod Pathol 1993;6:3–9.

33. Schmidt U, Muller U, Metz KA, Leder LD. Cytokeratin and neurofilament protein staining in Merkel cell carcinoma of the small cell type and small cell carcinoma of the lung. Am J Dermatopathol 1998; 20:346–51.

34. Scott MP, Helm KF. Cytokeratin 20: a marker for diagnosing Merkel cell carcinoma. Am J Dermatopathol 1999;21:16–20.

35. Johansson L, Tennvall J, Akerman M. Immunohistochemical examination of 25 cases of Merkel cell carcinoma: a comparison with small cell carcinoma of the lung and oesophagus, and a review of the literature. APMIS 1990;98:741–52.

36. Chan JK, Suster S, Wenig BM, et al. Cytokeratin 20 immunoreactivity distinguishes Merkel cell (primary cutaneous neuroendocrine) carcinomas and salivary gland small cell carcinomas from small cell carcinomas of various sites. Am J Surg Pathol 1997; 21:226–34.

37. Banerjee SS, Agbamu DA, Eyden BP, Harris M. Clinicopathological characteristics of peripheral primitive neuroectodermal tumour of skin and subcutaneous tissue. Histopathology 1997;31:355–66.

38. Hasegawa SL, Davison JM, Rutten A, et al. Primary cutaneous Ewing's sarcoma: immunophenotypic and molecular cytogenetic evaluation of five cases. Am J Surg Pathol 1998;22:310–8.

39. Messina JL, Reintgen DS, Cruse CW, et al. Selective lymphadenectomy in patients with Merkel cell (cutaneous neuroendocrine) carcinoma. Ann Surg Oncol 1997;4:389–95.

40. Hill AD, Brady MS, Coit DG. Intraoperative lymphatic mapping and sentinel lymph node biopsy for Merkel cell carcinoma. Br J Surg 1999;86:518–21.

41. Morrison WH, Peters LJ, Silva EG, et al. The essential role of radiation therapy in securing locoregional control of Merkel cell carcinoma. Int J Radiat Oncol Biol Phys 1990;19:583–91.

42. Fenig E, Brenner B, Katz A, et al. The role of radiation therapy and chemotherapy in the treatment of Merkel cell carcinoma. Cancer 1997;80:881–5.

Kaposi's Sarcoma

PATRICIA L. MYSKOWSKI, MD
SUSAN E. KROWN, MD

Kaposi's sarcoma (KS) is a multifocal and primarily cutaneous neoplasm first described by Moricz Kaposi in 1872.[1–5] He noted multiple vascular lesions on the lower extremities of elderly men, which he initially termed "idiopathisches multiples Pigmentsarkom der Haut" and later, "sarcoma idiopathicum multiplex haemorrhagicum," considering this to be a form of sarcoma. Even with the first description of what would come to be known as classic KS, Kaposi recognized the condition as a progressive and potentially fatal disease.[1,5]

INCIDENCE

Kaposi's sarcoma has been described in several clinical variants. Classic KS occurs primarily in elderly men in the United States and Europe who are of eastern European origin (Polish, Italian, Russian, or Ashkenazi Jewish)[2] or Greek origin.[6] Prior to the AIDS epidemic, KS was relatively rare in the United States, with an age-adjusted incidence of 0.29 per 100,000 in men and 0.07 per 100,000 in women[7] and a peak incidence between the sixth and eighth decades.[8] Clonic KS accounted for most of these cases. A similar pattern is seen in Greece, where the annual incidence is 0.20 per 100,000, the male-female ratio is 2.27:1, and the mean age at diagnosis is 72 years.[6]

An endemic form of KS was recognized in central Africa in the 1950s and 1960s, occurring in the same area as Burkitt's lymphoma.[9,10] The highest incidence of African KS occurs in Zaire, Burundi, Rwanda, and particularly Uganda, where KS represented 9 percent of all malignancies in the 1950s and 1960s.[11] In central Africa, the incidence of KS has increased with the human immunodeficiency virus (HIV) epidemic. In Uganda in 1989 to 1991, KS accounted for approximately 49 percent of cancers in males and 18 percent of cancers in females.[12] In Zimbabwe, KS accounted for 31.1 percent of all cancers from 1993 to 1995 and 10 percent of all childhood cancers.[13] Two major forms of endemic KS in Africa have been described.[13] The first, which occurs in adults aged 25 to 40 years, has a high male-female ratio (up to 13:1 to 17:1)[11] and includes three clinical subtypes[10,13] (nodular, florid, and infiltrative), each with varying degrees of skin, lymph node, and bone marrow involvement. The second form of endemic KS is found in children and adolescents (1 to 15 years of age; mean age, 3 years)[11] and manifests few skin lesions but has prominent lymph node and visceral involvement. In adolescents, there is a male predominance; in children less than 10 years of age, however, boys and girls are equally affected.[13]

A third form of KS was recognized in renal transplant recipients in the 1970s.[14,15] The incidence of post-transplantation KS varies among patient populations, from 0.5 to 0.6 percent in France[14,15] to 4.7 percent in Saudi Arabia.[16] Renal transplant recipients who are receiving corticosteroids or cyclosporine are at particularly high risk for KS.[15] Liver transplant recipients may be at even greater risk for KS than those receiving kidney transplants,[14] and (rarely) KS has been reported after bone marrow transplantation.[17] A slight male-female predominance has been reported in post-transplantation KS.[1,3] To a lesser extent, a higher-than-expected incidence of KS was also reported in immunosuppressed individuals, including patients with lymphoma and patients receiving immunosuppressive therapies for autoimmune diseases.[3,16]

Kaposi's sarcoma in association with HIV was the first malignancy to be recognized as part of the acquired immunodeficiency syndrome (AIDS) epidemic in 1981. In the earliest days of AIDS, 40 percent of the first 3,000 reported patients developed malignancies, and KS was the most common malignancy.[18] In homosexual men infected with human immunodeficiency virus 1 (HIV-1), the incidence of KS increased more than 73,000 times compared to the general population, but even nonhomosexual HIV-infected males have a 10,000-fold increased risk of developing KS.[19] While the incidence of KS has declined by over one-third recently with the advent of highly active anti-retroviral therapy (HAART),[20] KS continues to be the most frequently diagnosed malignancy in HIV-infected individuals.[20,21]

CLINICAL FEATURES

The four different types of KS—classic, endemic African, post-transplantation, and HIV-associated—are significantly different in clinical presentation, anatomic distribution, and biologic behavior.

Classic KS typically begins on the lower extremities of elderly men, often as erythematous or violaceous macules, patches (Figure 8.3–1), and papules on the soles (Figure 8.3–2).[4,22] Multiple papules may develop on the legs, resembling cherry angiomata (Figures 8.3–3 and 8.3–4). Lesions may become intensely red or purple nodules (Figure 8.3–5). Early lesions may be pink or red, but they become more purple or brown with time from hemosiderin deposition, particularly on the lower extremities. Hyperpigmentation and changes in cutaneous stasis, especially near the medial ankle, may make the diagnosis more difficult clinically. Lymphedema may also develop, and lymphangioma-like changes are common in long-standing KS (Figures 8.3–6 and 8.3–7). Less often, patches and plaques may involve the upper extremities (Figure 8.3–8). Ulceration of tumors may occur spontaneously or following radiation therapy or chemotherapy. Long-standing KS may develop a verrucous appearance, especially in areas where there is long-standing lymphedema. Most lesions are asymptomatic; however, KS on the sole may cause discomfort during ambulation. In the early stages of the disease, there may be some spontaneous regression while other distant lesions develop. In addition to the skin, classic KS may involve other sites, including the lymph nodes, mucous membranes (especially the palate), and glans penis. The gastrointestinal tract is one of the more common internal sites, and KS here may result in gastrointestinal bleeding or obstruction. Other visceral involvement is rare but may include the lungs, liver, spleen, and adrenal glands.[4,22]

Endemic African KS is found in adults, adolescents, or children. In adults, there are three major subtypes: nodular, florid, and infiltrative. The nodu-

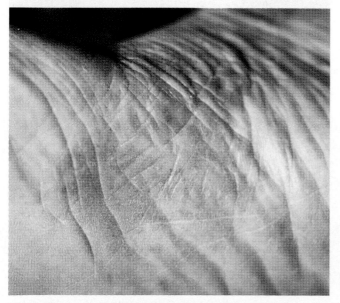

Figure 8.3–1.   Classic Kaposi's sarcoma: patch on the sole.

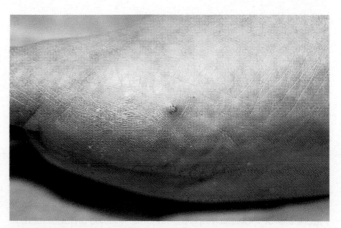

Figure 8.3–2.   Classic Kaposi's sarcoma: papules on sole.

lar subtype most closely resembles classic KS although it is more aggressive locally. In the florid subtype, the cutaneous lesions develop into fungating tumors; bone involvement is frequent. In the infiltrative subtypes, there are diffuse locally aggres-

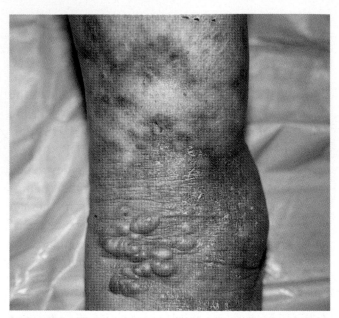

Figure 8.3–6. Classic Kaposi's sarcoma: nodules and lymphedema of ankle.

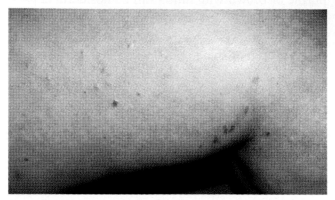

Figure 8.3–3. Classic Kaposi's sarcoma: small papules.

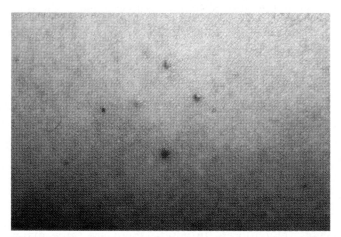

Figure 8.3–4. Classic Kaposi's sarcoma; close-up of Figure 8.3–3.

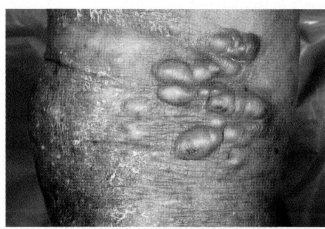

Figure 8.3–7. Classic Kaposi's sarcoma; close-up of Figure 8.3–6.

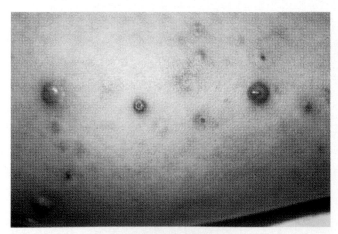

Figure 8.3–5. Classic Kaposi's sarcoma: nodules on lower extremity.

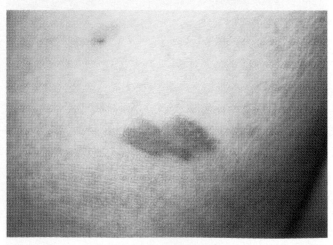

Figure 8.3–8. Classic Kaposi's sarcoma: plaque on upper extremity.

sive tumors that resemble cellulitis and that often invade soft tissues and underlying bone. Although infrequent, lymph node involvement by KS may be found in any of the adult subtypes of African KS.[11] Lymphadenopathic African KS is characterized by massive lymph node involvement in children and adolescents and is the most aggressive form of African KS. Cutaneous lesions are rare or absent. Mucous-membrane lesions and hepatosplenomegaly are common, but bone lesions are rare.[11]

Post-transplantation KS has many features similar to those of classic KS but is much more likely to be associated with widespread cutaneous or visceral involvement. Gastrointestinal lesions are common.[15,22] Perhaps the most important feature of immunosuppression-associated KS is the waxing and waning of lesions after changes in immunosuppressive therapy regimens.[16]

Human immunodeficiency virus (HIV)–associated KS is diagnosed most commonly in homosexual and bisexual men but has also been described in HIV-infected women and in men from other groups at risk for HIV transmission. Of the several clinical features that distinguish this form of KS from the classic form of KS, the distribution of lesions is particularly prominent.[23] In a study of 152 patients with HIV-associated KS and in whom the initial tumor location was known, the most frequent site was on the lower extremities (29%), followed by the upper extremities (19%), the trunk (9%), and the oral mucosa (8%). The lymph nodes were the presenting site of KS in 9 percent of patients, whereas the initial site was not known in the remainder of patients, possibly because of multiple synchronous primary lesions.[23] Thus, over 70 percent of patients did not present with lower-extremity lesions (in contrast to classic KS), and virtually all patients went on to develop KS at multiple cutaneous sites. Other studies have reported patients in whom the initial or only site of KS was in the lungs or in the gastrointestinal tract.[4,22]

Lesions of HIV-associated KS are heterogeneous in their appearance. Some lesions may resemble those of classic KS. Violaceous macules may begin on the soles and may regress and then recur, depending on the patient's concurrent (eg, anti-HIV) therapy (Figures 8.3–9 to 8.3–12). In dark-skinned individuals, the lesions may be brown (Figure 8.3–13).

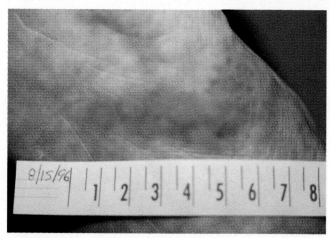

Figure 8.3–9. Human immunodeficiency virus (HIV)–associated Kaposi's sarcoma on sole.

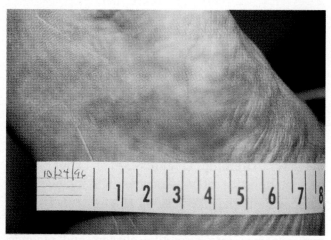

Figure 8.3–10. Human immunodeficiency virus (HIV)–associated Kaposi's sarcoma on the sole of the same patient shown in Figure 8.3–9 after highly active anti-retroviral therapy (HAART) for 2 months.

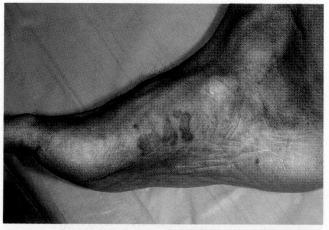

Figure 8.3–11. Human immunodeficiency virus (HIV)–associated Kaposi's sarcoma (KS) in the same patient shown in Figures 8.3–9 and 8.3–10. Minimal progression on highly active anti-retroviral therapy (HAART) but no specific anti-KS therapy.

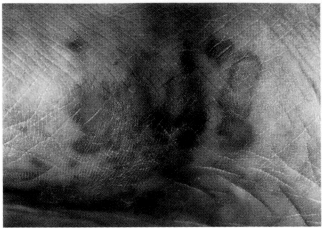

Figure 8.3–12. Human immunodeficiency virus (HIV)–associated Kaposi's sarcoma; close-up of Figure 8.3–11.

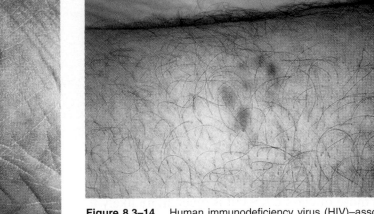

Figure 8.3–14. Human immunodeficiency virus (HIV)–associated Kaposi's sarcoma on arms. Patient had initial presentation in a lymph node (see Figure 8.3–30).

On the upper body in particular, the lesions may resemble bruises (Figure 8.3–14). On the trunk, KS lesions may follow the lines of cleavage in a pityriasis rosea-like pattern.[24] Lesions may remain papular (Figure 8.3–15) or may become confluent plaques (Figure 8.3–16). In patients with low CD4-positive T-lymphocyte counts, hyperkeratotic KS may be noted, especially in areas of lymphedema and/or on the lower extremities (Figure 8.3–17). Other clinical presentations of HIV-associated KS include pyogenic granuloma-like lesions (Figure 8.3–18) and keloidal nodules (Figure 8.3–19). Papules of KS may coalesce into grapelike clusters and plaques, especially on the trunk and back. In long-standing KS, confluent lesions may develop on the medial

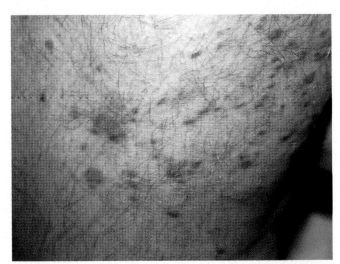

Figure 8.3–15. Diffuse human immunodeficiency virus (HIV)–associated Kaposi's sarcoma on a lower extremity.

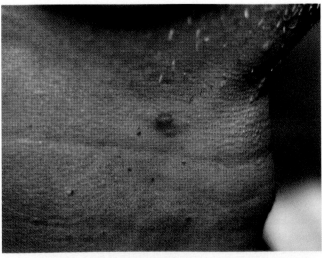

Figure 8.3–13. Human immunodeficiency virus (HIV)–associated Kaposi's sarcoma: papule in a dark-skinned patient.

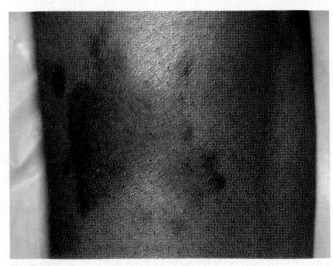

Figure 8.3–16. Human immunodeficiency virus (HIV)–associated Kaposi's sarcoma: plaque on an arm.

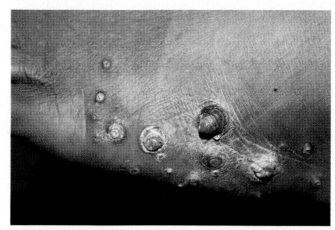

Figure 8.3–17. Hyperkeratotic nodular Kaposi's sarcoma in a patient with human immunodeficiency virus (HIV) infection.

thighs, associated with lymphedema of the thighs and scrotum. This feature is particularly difficult to manage (Figure 8.3–20). Oral mucosal KS may involve the hard palate, the buccal mucosa, and the gingivae (Figure 8.3–21).

Internal involvement may also occur in patients with HIV-associated KS; such involvement can be symptomatic or may be found incidentally at autopsy or during investigation of intestinal or pulmonary symptoms of other etiology.[4] Gastrointestinal involvement with KS is usually submucosal and often asymptomatic but may lead to pain and to fatal hemorrhage. Pulmonary KS may lead to bronchial obstruction, hemorrhage, and secondary respiratory

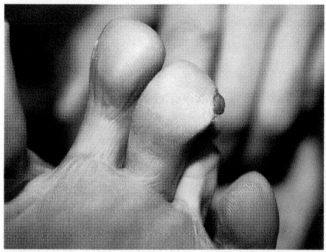

Figure 8.3–18. Human immunodeficiency virus (HIV)–associated Kaposi's sarcoma: a pyogenic granuloma-like nodule.

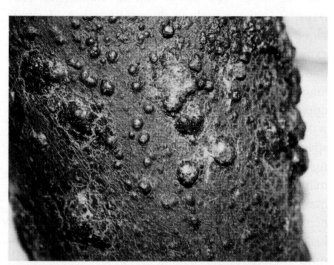

Figure 8.3–20. Confluent human immunodeficiency virus (HIV)–associated Kaposi's sarcoma and lymphedema of the thighs and scrotum.

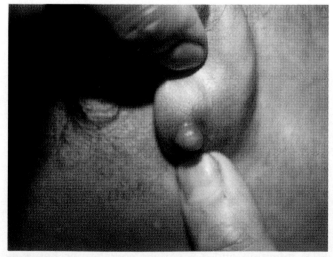

Figure 8.3–19. Human immunodeficiency virus (HIV)–associated Kaposi's sarcoma: a keloidlike nodule.

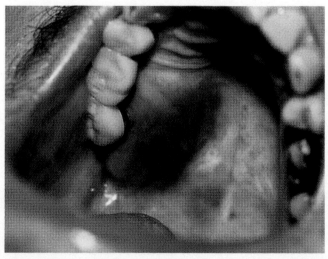

Figure 8.3–21. Human immunodeficiency virus (HIV)–associated Kaposi's sarcoma: mucosal lesions.

infections and is associated with shortened survival.[25]

The clinical differential diagnosis of KS is broad and includes a number of benign and malignant skin lesions. Dermatofibroma, stasis dermatitis (especially on the legs of older individuals), purpura, pigmented basal cell carcinoma, amelanotic melanoma, pyogenic granuloma, and angiosarcoma may all resemble KS.[4] In immunocompromised patients, especially those with HIV disease, bacillary angiomatosis and deep fungal and mycobacterial infections must also be considered.[2,4]

PATHOLOGY

All forms of KS show similar histologic features;[4,26,27] these include the proliferation of small blood vessels and spindle cells and the presence of extravasated erythrocytes. The earliest lesions of KS (patch stage) may be difficult to diagnose because many of the histologic findings are subtle. Within the upper dermis are multiple thin-walled dilated vessels with irregular outlines forming lymphatic-like spaces. Normal adnexal structures and blood vessels may be surrounded by these new vessels. An inflammatory infiltrate of lymphocytes and plasma cells may also be found. Extravasated erythrocytes with hemosiderin deposition may begin to appear as the lesions become thicker. Spindle cells are rare at this time[4,27] (Figures 8.3–22 and 8.3–23).

The plaque stage of KS shows a more diffuse infiltrate of small blood vessels involving the entire

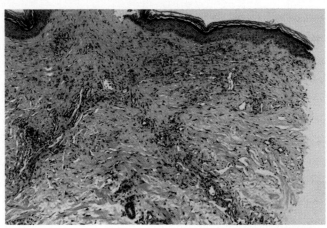

Figure 8.3–23. Histopathology close-up (hematoxylin and eosin; ×40 original magnification) of Figure 8.3–22. Irregular proliferation of small blood vessels with extravasated erythrocytes. (Courtesy of Dr. K. Busam)

dermis, with displacement of collagen bundles (Figure 8.3–24). These atypical vascular channels may vary in their morphology (Figure 8.3–25), from lymphatic-like lesions to blood-containing vasculature. Spindle cells may begin to appear, often arranged in short fascicles.[27] In nodular- or tumor-stage KS, there are well-defined nodules composed of spindle cells and vascular spaces that replace the dermal collagen and fill the dermis.[4,27] Erythrophagocytosis may be prominent. Intracytoplasmic hyalin globules (which measure 0.4 to 10 microns) are found in most cases[4] and are seen more often in patients with HIV-associated KS.[27] These globules are felt to represent the decomposition of partially phagocytosed erythrocytes. Rarely, the lesions may be ulcerated or may resemble pyogenic granulomas (Figures 8.3–26 and 8.3–27). Another finding in patients with advanced HIV disease and low CD4 lymphocyte counts is hyperkeratosis, with a markedly thickened stratum corneum overlying the nodular proliferation in the tumors (Figure 8.3–28). The histologic differential diagnosis of patch or plaque KS includes stasis dermatitis, ecchymosis, hemangioma, and angiosarcoma.[4] Nodular KS may resemble dermatofibroma, pyogenic granuloma, angiosarcoma, and bacillary angiomatosis.[4]

There is some debate about whether certain histologic parameters are specific to different types of KS. A multivariate analysis in a study of 93 patients with HIV infection and KS sought correlations between 22 histologic variables and survival.[28] Patients whose

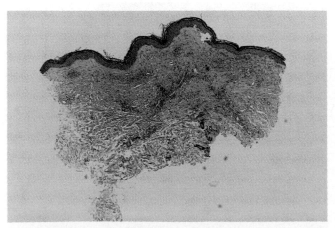

Figure 8.3–22. Histopathology of early patch-stage human immunodeficiency virus (HIV)–associated Kaposi's sarcoma in the same patient shown in Figures 8.3–9 to 8.3–12. (Hematoxylin and eosin; ×10 original magnification) (Courtesy of Dr. K. Busam)

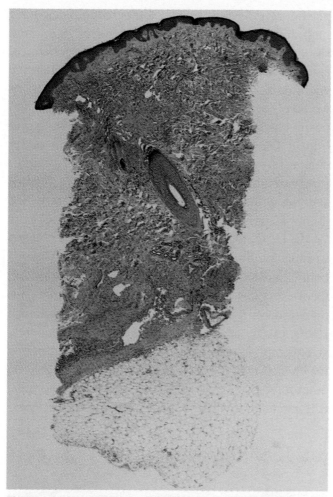

Figure 8.3–24. Plaque in human immunodeficiency virus (HIV)–associated Kaposi's sarcoma: irregular vascular spaces dissecting dermal collagen in the patient shown in Figure 8.3–15. (Hematoxylin and eosin; ×10 original magnification) (Courtesy of Dr. K. Busam)

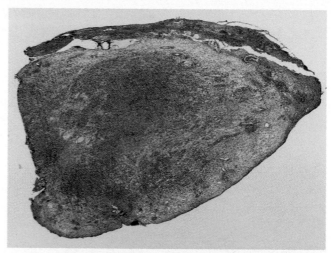

Figure 8.3–26. Human immunodeficiency virus (HIV)–associated Kaposi's sarcoma: tumor with sheets of spindle cells in inflammatory background with ulceration. (Hematoxylin and eosin; ×10 original magnification)

histologic patterns represented nodular KS tended to have the best prognosis. In a multivariate analysis, a higher ratio of helper cells to suppressor T cells was found to be the strongest predictor of longer survival, followed by initial disease on the lower extremities, the histologic presence of spindle cell nodules, and nodular histology. In addition, the presence of hemosiderin was inversely proportional to the CD4-CD8 lymphocyte ratio (a surrogate marker for CD4-positive T-lymphocyte count).[28] Other authors have also suggested that the African endemic form of KS has different histologic features from those of the other

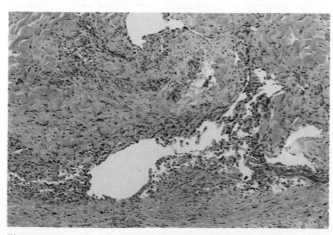

Figure 8.3–25. Plaque in human immunodeficiency virus (HIV)–associated Kaposi's sarcoma; close-up (hematoxylin and eosin; ×40 original magnification) of Figure 8.3–24: an atypical vascular channel with numerous papillary projections of endothelial cells into the vascular lumen.

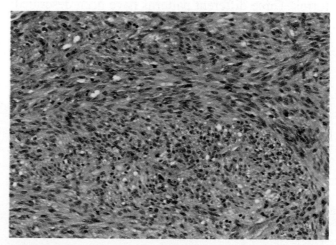

Figure 8.3–27. Human immunodeficiency virus (HIV)–associated Kaposi's sarcoma; close-up (hematoxylin and eosin; ×40 original magnification) of Figure 8.3–26: dense spindle cells, hyaline globules, and sarcomatoid changes. (Courtesy of Dr. K. Busam)

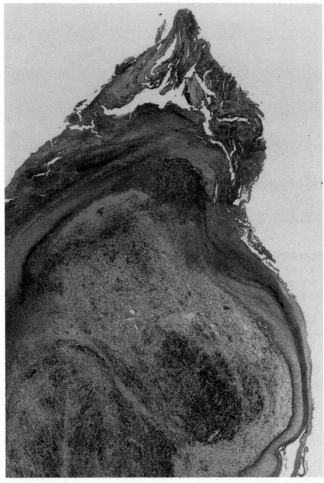

Figure 8.3–28. Hyperkeratotic human immunodeficiency virus (HIV)–associated Kaposi's sarcoma (same lesion as pictured in Figure 8.3–17): markedly thickened stratum corneum overlying a nodular proliferation of spindle cells with hemorrhage. (Hematoxylin and eosin; ×10 original magnification) (Courtesy of Dr. K. Busam)

forms. Three different patterns have been described: monocellular, mixed, and anaplastic. The anaplastic tumors may exhibit marked pleomorphism and may resemble classic angiosarcoma.[29]

In addition to involving the skin, KS may also involve lymph nodes, especially in HIV-infected individuals (Figure 8.3–30) and in those with the juvenile form of African KS. There is initial vascular proliferation of the sinuses, then proliferation of spindle cells, and finally, effacement of normal architecture (see Figure 8.3–30).

A number of aspects of the histology of KS remain controversial; among these, the cell of origin is particularly debated.[4] Some authors have suggested that an endothelial cell (whether pluripotent, lymphatic, or vascular in origin) is the primary neo-

plastic cell of this tumor. Other candidates have included pericytes, dermal dendrocytes, and smooth-muscle cells. Several immunohistochemical studies support an endothelial cell origin, in that the endothelial-like cells lining the vascular spaces, as well as (occasionally) the spindle cells in KS, stain positively for factor VIIIra, *Ulex europaeus* agglutinin-I, CD31, CD39,[27] leukocyte adhesion molecule-1, thrombomodulin, and tissue factor.[4] Support for a vascular endothelial origin comes from positive staining with the antibodies OKM2 and HCL, which do not stain lymphatic endothelium.[4]

An intriguing question is whether KS is a reactive vascular proliferation or a true malignancy. There is both clinical and laboratory evidence to support both theories. It has been suggested that the spontaneous regression of KS lesions noted in a number of clinical settings (such as the withdrawal of immunosuppressive therapy in organ transplant recipients[15]) supports the theory that KS is a reactive process. However, other tumors, such as cutaneous melanoma and renal cell carcinoma, whose malignant nature is not ques-

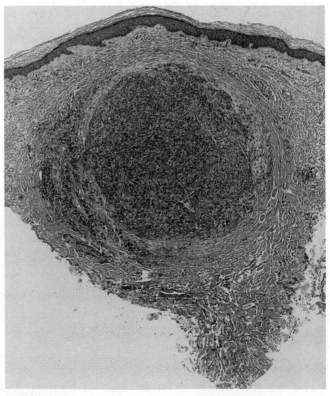

Figure 8.3–29. Classic Kaposi's sarcoma in the patient shown in Figures 8.3–3 and 8.3–4. Nodule of spindle cells in dermis. (Hematoxylin and eosin; ×10 original magnification) (Courtesy of Dr. K. Busam)

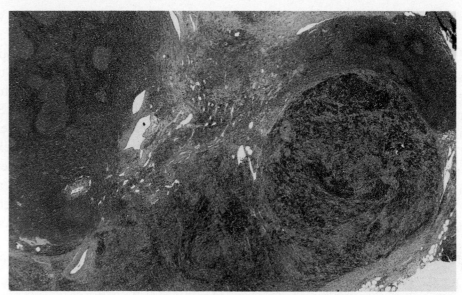

Figure 8.3–30. Human immunodeficiency virus (HIV)–associated Kaposi's sarcoma presenting in lymph node, with a hemorrhagic nodule of spindle cells. (Hematoxylin and eosin ×10 original magnification) (Courtesy of Dr. K. Busam)

tioned, may also show spontaneous regression that may be immunologically mediated. The role of immune surveillance and intact T-cell function in KS is further supported by multiple observations of the regression of HIV-associated KS after the initiation of HAART.[30,31] Gill and colleagues have shown that different KS tumors from different patients exhibit polyclonality, monoclonality, or a mixed pattern.[32] However, Rabkin and colleagues demonstrated the monoclonality of KS lesions in 28 of 32 tumors in HIV-infected women. The methylation patterns of the androgen receptor gene demonstrated a single pattern dominance in any given patient in the majority of cases.[33] Thus, it seems likely that at least some cases of KS evolve into monoclonal malignancies and may pursue an aggressive and fatal course. However, early stages of KS may be reactive and oligoclonal.

STAGING

Different staging classifications for KS have evolved over the last two decades. The staging classification system that was first proposed divided the tumor into four different stages (I to IV) and included the three major clinical variants of KS (classic, endemic African, and HIV-associated). It subtyped patients according to the presence or absence of "B" symptoms usually associated with lymphoreticular malignancies (weight loss > 10% of body weight, fever, and diarrhea).[34] However, this classification system was not useful for prognosis.

In 1988, the AIDS Clinical Trials Group attempted to address some of the problems of developing a prognostically useful staging system for patients with HIV-associated KS.[35] Patients were divided into "good-risk" and "poor-risk" groups according to the status of their immune system, the presence or absence of other systemic HIV-associated symptoms, and the extent of their tumor. Good-risk criteria included tumor lesions limited to the skin, lymph nodes, or mucous membrane lesions limited to the palate. Poor-risk criteria included tumor-associated edema, extensive oral involvement, and gastrointestinal or other visceral involvement. A CD4-positive T-lymphocyte count of ≥ 200 per microliter defined the good-risk immune-system group whereas those with CD4 counts of < 200 per microliter were considered to be in the poor-risk group. In the category of systemic illness, good-risk features included a Karnofsky performance status of ≥ 70, the absence of opportunistic infections, and B symptoms. Patients with concurrent systemic illness, B symptoms, or opportunistic infections were considered to be in the poor-risk group. This proposed classification system was evaluated prospectively and validated by the AIDS Clinical Trials Group.[35]

ETIOLOGY

Infectious Agents

The search for an infectious agent associated with KS began decades ago with the observation that endemic African KS occurred in the same geographic distributions as Epstein-Barr virus (EBV)–related Burkitt's lymphoma. In 1972, Giraldo and colleagues observed herpesvirus-like particles on electron microscopy in skin tumors from patients with both endemic African and classic KS.[36] The researchers postulated that this might be related to *Cytomegalovirus* (CMV) or an as-yet-unidentified herpesvirus. During the ensuing decade, a number of candidate viruses were proposed, including CMV, human herpesvirus 6, and *Papillomavirus*.[3] However, compelling data supporting a viral association for KS did not appear until the identification of a new human herpesvirus, the so-called Kaposi's sarcoma–associated herpesvirus (KSHV) or human herpesvirus 8 (HHV-8), by Chang and colleagues in 1994.[37] Human herpesvirus 8 is a member of the *Rhadinovirus* genus of the gammaherpesvirus subfamily and more closely resembles *Herpesvirus saimiri* (an animal rhadinovirus) than it does another human gammaherpesvirus, EBV. The viral deoxyribonucleic acid (DNA) sequences of HHV-8 were soon found in all forms of KS.[38,39] Evidence for HHV-8 infection has also been found in other tumors, specifically primary effusion lymphoma associated with HIV infection (in which 40 to 80 copies per cell are found vs one copy per cell in KS)[40] and some forms of Castleman's disease.[41] The mechanism by which HHV-8 leads to the development of KS is not clear, but it is known that the virus encodes functional homologues of human proteins that may affect cell growth and neoplastic transformation.[1,42] In addition, HHV-8 infects B lymphocytes and can infect and transform endothelial cells in vitro.[42] The presence of HHV-8 in peripheral blood mononuclear cells is much more prevalent in HIV-positive individuals with KS than in those without KS. In addition, the presence of HHV-8 in peripheral blood mononuclear cells correlated with the subsequent development of KS in patients infected with HIV. In a study by Whitby and colleagues, 6 of 11 patients who were both HHV-8- and HIV-seropositive developed KS over a median follow-up time of 30 months whereas only 12 out of 132 HIV-seropositive patients who were negative for HHV-8 developed KS.[43] In another study, 43 percent of HHV-8-seropositive HIV-seropositive patients developed KS over a 5-year follow-up.[44]

In addition to HHV-8 (which appears to be required for the development of KS but which may not be sufficient by itself to cause tumor development), a variety of other host and exogenous factors appear to promote KS development. Immunosuppressive disorders, both iatrogenic and endogenous, are associated with a higher incidence of KS, but it is not clear whether this is a consequence of faulty immune recognition of HHV-8 or a result of concomitant immune activation and release of inflammatory proangiogenic cytokines. Cultured KS-derived spindle cells secrete a variety of cytokines and growth factors (including interleukin-6 [IL-6], interleukin-1 [IL-1], basic fibroblast growth factor [bFGF], and vascular endothelial growth factor–vascular permeability factor [VEGF/VPF][45–47]) and express receptors for these factors. In addition to secreting factors with potential autocrine and paracrine activities, KS-derived spindle cells proliferate in response to exogenous cytokines and growth factors; these include tumor necrosis factor, IL-1, IL-6, interferon-γ (IFN-γ), platelet-derived growth factor, bFGF, VEGF/VPF, Oncostatin M, and granulocyte-macrophage colony–stimulating factor.[46,48–53] Many of these cytokines are also produced in excess in patients with advanced HIV infection;[54–56] can stimulate HIV expression in vitro;[48,57] and can induce normal vascular endothelial cells to acquire a spindle morphology, secrete bFGF, and express $\alpha_v\beta_3$ (a cell surface adhesion protein of the integrin family that is required for angiogenesis).[48,52,53]

Although HIV is not required for KS development, it may contribute indirectly to the development of KS and to the unusually aggressive course of KS in HIV-infected individuals. A role for HIV was originally suggested by the transient development of KS-like lesions in *tat*-transgenic mice.[58] In addition to its association with the excess production of cytokines capable of stimulating the proliferation of KS-derived spindle cells,[59] active HIV infection results in the secretion of Tat, the product of the HIV transactivator gene, *tat*.[60] Extracellular Tat binds to integrin receptors, which are strongly expressed on KS-derived spindle cells.[61] Interferon-γ, whose expression is increased in KS lesions,[51] up-regulates the expression and activation of Tat-binding integrins and induces endothelial cells to proliferate and invade the extracellular matrix in response to Tat.[52] Tat has also been shown to stimulate KS cell proliferation when combined with bFGF or inflammatory cytokines.[62] In addition, in the presence of bFGF and cytokines, normal vascular endothelial cells become responsive to the stimulatory effects of Tat on proliferation, cell migration, and angiogenic differentiation.[46,63] Tat also induces the expression in vitro of adhesion molecules, a monocyte chemoattractant protein, and IL-6 in KS-derived cells,[64] which could help recruit leukocytes to a developing KS lesion.

Host Factors

The clustering of classic KS in certain ethnic groups has long suggested a possible genetic predisposition. An increased frequency of human leukocyte antigen DR5 (HLA-DR5) has been found in classic KS patients in the United States,[65] Greece,[66] and Sardinia,[67] but not in Israel.[68] True familial classic KS is rare, however,[8] suggesting that both genetic predisposition and an environmental factor (ie, HHV-8) are required. However, the absence of HLA patterns in other KS groups suggests that host immune suppression (iatrogenic or HIV-associated) is at least as important a factor.

The male predominance in virtually all groups of KS has also been intriguing but is unexplained. Hormonal factors were suggested by the finding that a human pregnancy hormone could inhibit the growth of KS cells in vitro.[69] The discovery of this factor, originally thought to be human chorionic gonadotropin (HCG), prompted early clinical trials of intralesional HCG in KS patients.[70] However, it appears that the anti-KS activity may have been explained by an unrelated urinary protein in pregnant women.[71] Further studies will clarify what role, if any, these proteins will play in the treatment of KS.

THERAPY

Various therapeutic approaches have been used successfully to treat KS. The choice of therapy depends on the clinical variant of the disease as well as coexisting medical problems.

Treatment of Classic Kaposi's Sarcoma

Because classic KS usually progresses indolently in the lower extremities of middle-aged or elderly patients and because the tumor is highly radiosensitive, radiation therapy has been the treatment of choice for classic KS. Because of its indolent nature, classic KS is best treated by local means, thus avoiding systemic toxicity. A variety of different radiation regimens have been used, ranging from single-dose therapy at 800 rads to subtotal skin electron beam therapy of 2,400 rads over 6 weeks.[72] In a series of 20 patients with classic KS who were treated with subtotal skin electron beam therapy, 85 percent achieved complete remission with a median duration of 48 months.[72] In patients with more aggressive cutaneous disease and/or lymph node involvement, the *Vinca* alkaloids vincristine and vinblastine have been reported to be effective. Newer chemotherapeutic agents such as the liposomal anthracyclines and paclitaxel may also prove useful in this population. Intralesional or systemic interferon-α (IFN-α) has shown activity in classic KS, but some of the systemic side effects may be poorly tolerated in older patients, particularly those with pre-existing cardiac disease.[3] Subcutaneous IFN-α given at a dose of 5 million units 3 times a week for at least 6 months to 13 classic KS patients was well tolerated, and it produced major responses in most cases.[73] Cryotherapy with liquid nitrogen may also be useful for isolated lesions in selected patients.

Treatment of Endemic African Kaposi's Sarcoma

Endemic KS, which often takes a more aggressive course than the classic form, has been successfully treated with single-agent or combination chemotherapeutic drugs when there is visceral involvement or extensive local disease. Agents reported to be effective have included doxorubicin, bleomycin, *Vinca* alkaloids, and actinomycin D. Radiation therapy is not generally available to many patients with endemic African KS, and so it is difficult to evaluate its role in the treatment of this disease. Although chemotherapy frequently induces tumor regression, patients with aggressive local KS or lymphadenopathic forms of the disease have a poor prognosis, with a survival of only a few years.[11]

Treatment of Immunosuppression-Associated Kaposi's Sarcoma

Kaposi's sarcoma occurring in patients who are receiving immunosuppressive therapy to prevent the rejection of organ transplants is often treated first with the withdrawal of immunosuppressive drugs. In some cases, lowering the doses of systemic corticosteroids or cyclosporine has resulted in KS regression.[14–16] If this is impossible or ineffective, systemic chemotherapy may be useful.[1]

Treatment of Human Immunodeficiency Virus–Associated Kaposi's Sarcoma

The treatment of HIV-associated KS has presented a formidable challenge because of the frequent coexistence of severe immunosuppression, associated opportunistic infections, and other HIV-related medical problems, including wasting and cytopenia. The planning of therapy must take into account a number of parameters, including the patient's overall prognosis, immune status, and other concurrent illness.[25] Thus, a variety of approaches needs to be used.

Local therapy may be useful not only for tumor control but also for cosmetic purposes and quality of life.[74] Surgical excision may be useful in diagnosis and (rarely) may be curative; however, other modalities are more frequently employed. Cryotherapy with liquid nitrogen is effective for local tumor ablation and has virtually no systemic side effects. Patients appropriate for this approach include those with light skin and small well-circumscribed lesions, especially on the upper part of the body and face. Complete responses can be achieved in patients by using two freeze-thaw cycles with the open-spray technique and thaw times of 11 to 60 seconds. In one study, 80 percent of KS lesions treated in this way showed complete responses.[75] In dark-skinned individuals, postinflammatory hypopigmentation is usually unacceptable; thus, cryotherapy is rarely appropriate for Hispanic and African American patients.

Laser therapy has also been used to treat HIV-associated KS lesions because of the violaceous color of the lesions. When the carbon dioxide (CO_2) laser has been used, there has been concern about potential transmission of the virus within the plumes. Using pulsed dye lasers, Tappero and colleagues found that 44 percent of patients with small KS lesions had either complete or partial responses. Recurrences did occur, however.[76]

Administration of vinblastine has been the most common intralesional approach to KS. In one study, 88 percent of lesions treated by this method a had greater than 50 percent reduction in overall tumor size.[77] However, side effects included ulceration, pain, postinflammatory hyperpigmentation, and (rarely) transient neuropathy.[74] Intralesional IFN-α has also been used.[78,79] In one study of HIV-associated KS, 14 patients received either intralesional IFN-α at doses of up to 10 million units three times a week or a sterile-water placebo.[78] All patients were also being treated with the anti-retroviral drug zidovudine. Thirteen of the 14 patients showed objective tumor regression although placebo-treated lesions responded almost as often as those treated with interferon (54% vs 76%, respectively). Patients did experience some systemic side effects, including myalgia, fatigue, weakness, and fever and chills, which are commonly found with subcutaneous interferon injection.[78]

Radiation therapy (RT) is effective in HIV-associated KS. However, responses in patients with this form of KS tend to be of shorter duration than responses in patients with classic KS. In a prospectively randomized trial, Stelzer and Griffin[80] compared the results of treating individual KS skin lesions with 6 MeV electrons given as 800 cGy in a single fraction, 2,000 cGy in 10 fractions over 2 weeks, or 4,000 cGy in 20 fractions over 4 weeks. Complete resolution of the lesions was significantly better for the fractionated (2,000 and 4,000 cGy) regimens (79% and 83%) than for the single-dose regimen (50%), and complete resolution of residual pigmentation was significantly better for the 4,000-cGy regimen (43%) than for the 2,000- and 800-cGy regimens (8% for each). The 4,000-cGy regimen also led to a significantly longer median duration of lesion control (43 weeks) than the 2,000- and 800-cGy regiments (26 and 13 weeks, respectively). Acute toxicity was somewhat higher in the lesions given

4,000 cGy but was generally mild.[80] These data suggest that the type of radiotherapy should be individualized according to the intent of treatment and the overall health status of the patient.

Radiation therapy for more extensive KS usually requires larger photon fields. Severe local reactions were observed in 5 of 7 patients who received 2,000 cGy to the feet over 2 weeks. A lower incidence of high-grade local reactions was observed when a single 800-cGy fraction was used to treat KS of the foot.[81] It has been suggested, however, that lower doses per fraction and a planned rest period might allow the delivery of higher total doses without severe acute reactions and might avoid later radiation-induced edema from subcutaneous fibrosis. Although regression in KS-associated edema often occurs with radiation therapy, resolution is rarely complete.[81,82]

Although oral KS has also been treated successfully with RT, the normal tissues of patients with HIV infection have sometimes been noted to have unusual radiation sensitivity. Oral radiation (4 MeV photons at 180 cGy daily for 9 days) was reported to be associated with severe mucositis, mouth dryness, and an altered sense of taste, which were decreased (but not eliminated) by lowering the total dose to 1,400 cGy.[81] A high incidence of severe mucositis was also reported when the oropharynx was treated with high-dose fractions (180 to 400 cGy) to a total dose of 2,000 to 2,400 cGy.[82] This incidence was decreased by using 150-cGy fractions to a total dose of 1,500 cGy.[82] Tumor shrinkage is rapid with oral RT, and RT is probably the treatment of choice when very rapid relief of symptoms from bulky lesions is required. Systemic therapy is also effective for many patients with oral KS, and the decision to choose local RT or systemic therapy may depend upon whether other indications for systemic KS treatment coexist with the oral disease.

Interferon (IFN) has the potential to influence many of the complex processes involved in the growth of KS,[83,25] by both antiviral effects and effects on cell growth and function. Recombinant IFN-α2a (Roferon-A) and recombinant IFN-α2b (Intron A) were approved for the treatment of AIDS-associated KS on the basis of studies performed before the introduction of active anti-retroviral drugs. The approved doses are therefore based on the results of studies of IFN as a single agent, in which very high doses (eg, 36 million units daily or 30 million units/m^2 three times a week) were required to achieve KS regression.[84] The use of such doses was often complicated by fatigue, malaise, anorexia, and hepatotoxicity, and responses were usually observed only in patients with CD4-positive lymphocyte counts ≥ 200 per milliliter who had no history of opportunistic infection and who lacked other signs and symptoms of advanced HIV infection.

Today, IFN is generally administered in combination with anti-retroviral agents and is used at lower doses. Several phase I studies of combined IFN-α and zidovudine have demonstrated KS response rates exceeding 40 percent in patients treated with IFN-α doses ranging from 4 million to 18 million IU/day.[85–87] These high response rates were confirmed in a phase II trial of the combination, which used a daily IFN dose of 18 million IU and a zidovudine dose of 100 mg every 4 hours.[88] The combination of IFN-α and zidovudine induced KS regression in 25 to 30 percent of patients with CD4-positive lymphocyte counts below 200 per milliliter[85,88] whereas fewer than 10 percent of such patients responded to high-dose IFN-α monotherapy.[84] More recent trials are evaluating IFN in combination with less myelosuppressive anti-retroviral therapy and with anti-retroviral regimens that include protease inhibitors.

Maximal response to IFN-α alone or combined with anti-retroviral therapy often requires 6 or more months of treatment. Thus, IFN probably should not be considered for the treatment of patients with rapidly progressing KS, particularly those with symptomatic visceral involvement. Since responses to IFN may persist for several years, however, it should be considered for patients with more slowly progressing KS when rapid relief of symptoms is not urgently required.

Chemotherapy

Chemotherapy is indicated for patients with advanced or rapidly progressing KS that causes medical or functional impairment. A wide variety of single chemotherapeutic agents and drug combinations have shown activity against AIDS-related KS. However, only three agents (liposomal daunorubicin [Dauno-Xome], liposomal doxorubicin [Doxil], and paclitaxel

[Taxol]) have been approved specifically for KS by the US Food and Drug Administration. Other single agents with reported activity include etoposide,[89–93] vinblastine,[94] vincristine,[95] bleomycin,[96–98] and doxorubicin,[99–101] each of which has been studied in several clinical trials or has been shown to be effective as part of combination regimens. In addition, single clinical trials have indicated anti-KS activity for teniposide,[102] vinorelbine,[103] and epirubicin.[104] Despite demonstrated activity, disease control by these agents has often been limited by toxicities that include alopecia, mucositis, neutropenia, and peripheral neuropathy. High cumulative doses of doxorubicin are also associated with cardiac toxicity.

Before the introduction of liposomal anthracyclines and paclitaxel, combination chemotherapy was generally considered to induce higher response rates than single-agent therapy but at the expense of somewhat increased toxicity. The ABV regimen,[100] which included doxorubicin (Adriamycin), bleomycin, and vincristine, was long considered the standard of care. Other frequently used combinations have included bleomycin and vincristine[105–107] (more widely used in Europe than in the United States) and a regimen that alternates vinblastine with vincristine on a weekly schedule.[108] These combinations have largely been supplanted by the liposomal anthracyclines and, to some extent, by paclitaxel.

Liposomal encapsulation prolongs the circulating half-life of the anthracyclines (hours vs minutes for the unencapsulated drugs), increases drug concentrations within tumor tissue, and modifies toxicity.[109–111] Neutropenia is common,[112–115] but alopecia, nausea, and vomiting (which are common after the administration of free doxorubicin) are uncommon with the liposomal agents.[113,116,117] Anthracycline-induced cardiac toxicity has been observed rarely after administration of high cumulative doses of liposomal anthracyclines to patients with KS.[110,118,119] Treatment with Doxil has sometimes been associated with hand-foot syndrome (palmar-plantar erythrodysesthesia), characterized by pain, swelling, erythema, and peeling of the hands and feet, sometimes accompanied by digital ulceration. This syndrome, which has also been seen with other agents (eg, 5-fluorouracil, doxorubicin) given by continuous infusion, is probably a consequence of the markedly increased serum half-life

(approximately 48 hours) associated with the polyethylene glycol-coated liposome used to formulate Doxil.

Several prospective randomized studies have compared liposomal anthracyclines with conventional combination chemotherapy. One study compared Doxil, 20 mg/m^2, to ABV every 2 weeks. A significantly higher response rate was observed with Doxil (43%) than with ABV (25%).[115] A comparison of Dauno-Xome, 40 mg/m^2, to ABV every 2 weeks yielded equivalent response rates of 25 and 28 percent, respectively.[113] A third study compared Doxil, 20 mg/m^2, to the combination of bleomycin (15 U/m^2) and vincristine (2 mg);[121] each regimen was given every 3 weeks. A significantly higher response rate was observed among patients who received Doxil (59%) than among those who received bleomycin and vincristine (23%).[121] In each of the three studies, patients who received the liposomal anthracycline showed a significantly lower incidence of peripheral neuropathy and nausea and vomiting than those who received combination therapy. Doxil induced more neutropenia than bleomycin and vincristine induced. More mucositis was induced by Doxil than by ABV, but Doxil was less likely than ABV to cause significant alopecia and neutropenia.

Several studies have indicated that paclitaxel is highly active against KS. Two studies that used different doses and schedules of paclitaxel administration but similar planned-dose intensities were performed in patients with advanced symptomatic KS, many of whom had visceral disease, tumor-associated edema, prior chemotherapy, and low CD4 T-lymphocyte counts.[122,123] Doses of either 135 mg/m^2 every 3 weeks or 100 mg/m^2 every 2 weeks, administered as 3-hour infusions, induced objective response rates of 69 and 59 percent, respectively, in a total of 85 patients, with median-response durations of 7 to 10 months from the start of treatment. Lesion regression was accompanied by improvements in KS-associated edema, pain, and performance status, but treatment was complicated by myalgia, neutropenia, and alopecia. Neutropenia responded to the administration of granulocyte colony–stimulating factor (G-CSF).

Investigational Therapy

Various agents are under evaluation as treatment for KS or are potential candidates for future study.

Angiogenesis is a characteristic histologic feature of KS lesions, and various agents may inhibit this complex process. Among these agents are synthetic retinoids,[124–126] angiostatin,[127] endostatin,[128] and inhibitors of matrix metalloproteinases (enzymes that facilitate capillary budding and invasion by disrupting the integrity of the extracellular matrix). Other potential approaches include the administration of agents that interfere with tyrosine kinase–mediated transmembrane receptor signals for angiogenic growth factors, antisense oligonucleotides directed against these growth factors,[129] and agents directed against endothelial cell surface molecules expressed preferentially on proliferating vasculature.[130] There is also interest in evaluating the role of antiherpesvirus drugs in the treatment of KS. Anecdotal reports that established KS regressed after treatment with foscarnet,[131] along with several studies that showed a decreased incidence of subsequent KS in patients treated with antiherpesvirus agents,[132,133] suggest that inhibition of HHV-8 may also be of therapeutic or prophylactic value under some circumstances. The role of more effective anti-HIV therapy in the treatment and prevention of KS also requires better definition.

PROGNOSIS

The prognosis of classic KS tends to be good, with an indolent course being most common. Most patients survive for a decade or more and die from unrelated medical causes. Because of the chronic but progressive nature of classic KS, patients may develop serious complications related to lymphedema of the lower extremities, ulcerated tumors, and the late effects of radiation therapy. Recurrent cellulitis of the legs as well as osteomyelitis may ensue and may necessitate amputation. Rarely, as in other areas of radiation dermatitis, secondary squamous cell carcinoma may develop (Figure 8.3–31). While an increase in secondary malignancies (particularly lymphomas) was suggested in an early study of classic KS,[134] later studies either have not supported this finding[135,136] or have suggested only a minimal increase in the incidence of Hodgkin's lymphoma.[137] The median survival of 204 Italian patients with classic KS was 9.4 years and was not significantly

different from an age- and sex-matched population.[135] Specific KS-related mortality is usually low (eg, 4%).[137] However, in one study, 8 of 70 patients with classic KS died from causes directly attributable to their tumor.

The prognosis of endemic African KS is much poorer than that of classic KS although precise data are not available. In the childhood lymphadenopathic form, survival rarely exceeds 3 years, even with aggressive chemotherapy and radiation.[1,11]

Post-transplantation KS has a variable prognosis although it is generally more aggressive than classic KS. In their review of 35 patients with KS (of a total of 730 renal transplant recipients), al-Sulaiman and al-Khader noted that reduction of immunosuppression is the mainstay of therapy.[16] Twenty-eight of the 35 affected patients showed complete regression of KS, but 13 of the 28 lost their grafts. Progressive KS was the cause of death in 4 of the 35 patients.

The prognosis of HIV-related KS depends on a number of factors, including associated opportunistic infections and the degree of immunosuppression. In one study of 187 patients who had KS as their AIDS-defining illness and who were diagnosed between January 1980 and January 1985, a median survival of 15 months was noted.[23] In another series, AIDS patients with KS who were diagnosed after 1987 had a 65 percent reduction in mortality over those first seen between 1981 and 1983.[138] However, both studies[23,138] antedate the widespread use of effective antiretroviral therapy, especially the use of HAART, which has had positive effects for KS patients[30,31] and for overall survival in AIDS patients.[139]

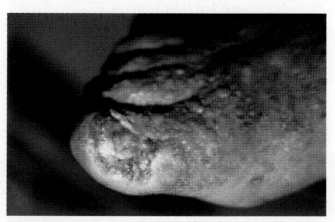

Figure 8.3–31. Classic Kaposi's sarcoma: a long-standing ulcer, with secondary fatal squamous cell carcinoma on the toe.

FUTURE DIRECTIONS

While major advances have been made recently toward the understanding of Kaposi's sarcoma, many questions remain unanswered. These include the precise role of HHV-8 in tumor pathogenesis, the nature of the KS cell of origin, and the status of KS as a reactive neoplastic process versus a true malignancy. Future challenges include the incorporation of HAART into specific antitumor regimens for HIV-associated KS and the development of HHV-8 antiviral therapy.[140,141] With the identification of high-risk patients (eg, transplant recipients infected with HHV-8, and HIV-infected individuals) and the use of safe and effective antiviral agents, prophylaxis of KS may eventually prove possible.[1]

REFERENCES

1. Antman K, Chang Y. Kaposi's sarcoma. N Engl J Med 2000;324:1027–38.
2. Myskowski PL, Ahkami R. Advances in Kaposi's sarcoma. Dermatol Clin 1997;15(1):177–88.
3. Myskowski PL. Kaposi's sarcoma: where do we go from here? Arch Dermatol 1993;129:1320–3.
4. Prieto VG, Myskowski PL, Rosai J. Kaposi's sarcoma. In: Joseph D, Demis, editor. Clinical dermatology. Vol. 2. Philadelphia: Lippincott-Raven; 1998. pp. 1–17.
5. Yarchoan R. Therapy for Kaposi's sarcoma: recent advances and experimental approaches. J Acquir Immune Defic Syndr 1999;21 Suppl 1:S66–73.
6. Stratigos JD, Potouridou I, Katoulis AC, et al. Classic Kaposi's sarcoma in Greece: a clinico-epidemiological profile. Int J Dermatol 1997;36:735–40.
7. Biggar RJ, Horn J, Fraumeni JF Jr, et al. Incidence of Kaposi's sarcoma and mycosis fungoides in the United States including Puerto Rico, 1973–1981. J Natl Cancer Inst 1984;73:89–94.
8. DiGiovanna JJ, Safai B. Kaposi's sarcoma. Retrospective study of 90 cases with particular emphasis on the familial occurrence, ethnic background and prevalence of other diseases. Am J Med 1981;7:779–83.
9. Taylor JF, Templeton AC, Vogel CL, et al. Kaposi's sarcoma in Uganda: a clinico-pathological study. Int J Cancer 1971;8:122–35.
10. Kyalwazi SK. Kaposi's sarcoma: clinical features, experience in Uganda. Antibiot Chemother 1981;29:59–69.
11. Friedman-Kien AE, Saltzman BR. Clinical manifestations of classical, endemic African and epidemic AIDS-associated Kaposi's sarcoma. J Am Acad Dermatol 1990;22:1237–50.
12. Wabinga HR, Parkin DM, Wabwire-Mangen F, Mugerwa JW. Cancer in Kampala, Uganda in 1989–91: changes in incidence in the era of AIDS. Int J Cancer 1993;54:26–36.
13. Chokunonga E, Levy LM, Bassett MT, et al. Cancer incidence in the African population of Harare, Zimbabwe: second results from the cancer registry 1993–1995. Int J Cancer 2000;85(1):54–9.
14. Farge D, the Collaborative Transplantation Research Group of Isle de France. Kaposi's sarcoma in organ transplant recipients. Eur J Med 1993;2:339–43.
15. Hiesse C, Kriaa F, Rieu P, et al. Incidence and type of malignancies occurring after renal transplantation in conventionally and cyclosporine treated recipients: analysis of a 20 year period in 1600 patients. Transplant Proc 1995;27:972–4.
16. al-Sulaiman MH, al-Khader AA. Kaposi's sarcoma in renal transplant recipients. Transplant Sci 1994;4:46–60.
17. Helg C, Adatto M, Salomon D, et al. Kaposi's sarcoma following allogeneic bone marrow transplantation. Bone Marrow Transplant 1994;14:999–1001.
18. Fauci AS, Macher AM, Longo DL, et al. Acquired immunodeficiency syndrome: epidemiologic, clinical, immunologic, and therapeutic considerations. Ann Intern Med 1984;100:92–106.
19. Biggar RJ, Rabkin CS. The epidemiology of AIDS-related neoplasms. Hematol Oncol Clin North Am 1996;10:997–1010.
20. Ledergerber B, Eggar M, Erard V, et al. AIDS-related opportunistic illness after initiation of potent antiretroviral therapy. The Swiss HIV cohort study. JAMA 1999;282:2220–6.
21. Shulz TF, Boxhoff CH, Weiss RA. HIV infection and neoplasia. Lancet 1997;348:587–91.
22. Tappero JW, Conant MA, Wolfe SF, et al. Kaposi's sarcoma. J Am Acad Dermatol 1991;28:371–95.
23. Myskowski PL, Niedzwiecki D, Shurgot BA, et al. AIDS-associated Kaposi's sarcoma: variables associated with survival. J Am Acad Dermatol 1988;18:1299–306.
24. Myskowski PL, Romano JF, Safai B. Kaposi's sarcoma in young homosexual men. Cutis 1983;29:31–4.
25. Krown SE. Acquired immunodeficiency syndrome associated Kaposi's sarcoma. Biology and management. Med Clin North Am 1997;81(2):471–94.
26. Templeton AC. Pathology. In: Ziegler JL, Dorfman RF, editors. Kaposi's sarcoma: pathophysiology and clinical management. New York: Marcel Dekker; 1988. p. 40.
27. Calonje E, Wilson-Jones E. Vascular tumors and tumor like conditions of blood vessels and lymphatics. In: Elder R, Elenitsas C, Jaworsky B, Johnson J, editors. Lever's histopathology of the skin. Philadelphia: Lippincott-Raven; 1997. p. 889–932.
28. Niedt CW, Myskowski PL, Urmachker C, et al. Histologic predictors of survival in acquired immunodeficiency syndrome–associated Kaposi's sarcoma. Hum Pathol 1992;23:1419–26.

29. Ziegler JL, Templeton AC, Vogel CL. Kaposi's sarcoma: a comparison of classical, endemic and epidemic forms. Semin Oncol 1984;11:47–52.

30. Murphy M, Armstrong D, Sepkowitz K, et al. Regression of AIDS-related Kaposi's sarcoma following treatment with an HIV-1 protease inhibitor. AIDS 1997;11:261–2.

31. Krischer J, Rutschmann O, Hirschel B, et al. Regression of Kaposi's sarcoma during therapy with HIV-I protease inhibitors. J Am Acad Dermatol 1998;38: 594–8.

32. Gill PS, Tsai YC, Rao AP, et al. Evidence for multiclonality in multicentric Kaposi's sarcoma. Proc Natl Acad Sci U S A 1998;95:8257–61.

33. Rabkin CS, Janz S, Lash S, et al. Monoclonal origin of multicentric Kaposi's sarcoma lesion. N Engl J Med 1997;336:988–93.

34. Krigel RL, Lauberstein LJ, Muggia FM. Kaposi's sarcoma: a new staging classification. Cancer Treat Rep 1983;67:531–4.

35. Krown SE, Testa MA, Huang J. AIDS-related Kaposi's sarcoma: prospective validation of the AIDS Clinical Trials Group staging classification. AIDS Clinical Trials Group Oncology Committee. J Clin Oncol 1997;9:3085–92.

36. Giraldo G, Beth E, Haguenau F, et al. Herpes-type virus particles in tissue culture of Kaposi's sarcoma from different geographic regions. J Natl Cancer Inst 1972;49:1509–26.

37. Chang Y, Cesarman E, Pessin MS, et al. Identification of herpesvirus-like DNA sequences in AIDS-associated Kaposi's sarcoma. Science 1994;266:1866–9.

38. Huang YQ, Li JJ, Kaplan MH, et al. Human herpes virus-like nucleic acid in various forms of Kaposi's sarcoma. Lancet 1995;345:768–9.

39. Dupin N, Grandadam M, Calvez V, et al. Herpes virus-like DNA sequences in patients with Mediterranean Kaposi's sarcoma. Lancet 1995;345:761–2.

40. Cesarman E, Chang Y, Moore PS, et al. Kaposi's sarcoma-associated herpes virus-like DNA sequence in AIDS-related body-cavity-based lymphomas. N Engl J Med 1995;332:1186–91.

41. Dupin N, Gorin I, Delcuze J, et al. Herpes-like DNA sequences, AIDS-related tumors and Castleman's disease. N Engl J Med 1995;333:798–9.

42. Reitz MS, Nerurkar LS, Gallo RC. Perspectives of Kaposi's sarcoma: facts, concepts and conjectures. J Natl Cancer Inst 1999;91:1453–8.

43. Whitby D, Howard MR, Tenant-Flowers M, et al. Detection of Kaposi's sarcoma associated herpesvirus in peripheral blood of HIV-infected individuals and progression to Kaposi's sarcoma. Lancet 1995;346:799–802.

44. Lin J-C, Lin S-C, Mar E-C, et al. Is Kaposi's sarcoma associated herpesvirus detectable in semen of HIV-infected homosexual men? Lancet 1995;346:1601–2.

45. Ensoli B, Nakamura S, Salahuddin SZ, et al. AIDS Kaposi's sarcoma derived cells express cytokines with autocrine and paracrine growth effects. Science 1989;243:223–6.

46. Miles SA, Rezai AR, Salazar-Gonzales JF, et al. AIDS Kaposi's sarcoma–derived cells produce and respond to interleukin 6. Proc Natl Acad Sci U S A 1990;87:4068–72.

47. Weindel K, Marme D, Weich HA. AIDS-associated Kaposi's sarcoma cells in culture express vascular endothelial growth factor. Biochem Biophys Res Commun 1992;183:1167–74.

48. Barillari G, Bunoaguro L, Fiorelli V, et al. Effects of cytokines from activated immune cells on vascular cell growth and HIV-1 gene expression. J Immunol 1992:149:3727–34.

49. Miles SA, Martinez-Maza O, Rezai A, et al. Oncostatin M as a potent mitogen for AIDS–Kaposi's sarcoma derived cells. Science 1992:225:1432–4.

50. Nair BC, DeVico AL, Nakamura S, et al. Identification of a major growth factor for AIDS–Kaposi's sarcoma cells as Oncostatin M. Science 1992;255:1430–2.

51. Sirianni MC, Vincenzi L, Fiorelli V, et al. γ-Interferon production in peripheral blood mononuclear cells and tumor infiltrating lymphocytes from Kaposi's sarcoma patients: correlation with the presence of human herpesvirus-8 in peripheral blood mononuclear cells and lesional macrophages. Blood 1998;91:1165–70.

52. Fiorelli V, Barillari G, Toschi E, et al. IFN-γ indices endothelial cells to proliferate and invade the extracellular matrix in response to HIV-1 Tat protein: implications for AIDS–Kaposi's sarcoma pathogenesis. J Immunol 1999;162:1165–70.

53. Samaniego F, Markham PD, Gendleman R, et al. Vascular endothelial growth factor and basic fibroblast growth factor present in Kaposi's sarcoma (KS) are induced by inflammatory cytokines and synergize to promote vascular permeability and KS lesion development. Am J Pathol 1998;152:1433–43.

54. Roux-Lombard P, Modoux C, Cruchaud A, Dayer JM. Purified blood monocytes from HIV 1–infected patients produce high levels of TNF alpha and IL-1. Clin Immunol Immunopathol 1989;50:374–84.

55. Jassoy C, Harrer T, Rosenthal T, et al. Human immunodeficiency virus type 1–specific cytotoxic T lymphocytes release gamma interferon, tumor necrosis factor alpha (TNF-alpha), and TNF-beta when they encounter their target antigens. J Virol 1993;67: 2844–52.

56. Graziosi C, Grant KR, Vaccarezza M, et al. Kinetics of cytokine expression during primary human immunodeficiency virus type 1 infection. Proc Natl Acad Sci U S A 1996;93:4386–91.

57. Poli G, Fauci AS. The effect of cytokines and pharmacologic agents on chronic HIV infection. AIDS Res Hum Retroviruses 1992;8:191–7.

58. Vogel J, Hinrichs SH, Reynalds RK, et al. The HIV *tat* gene induces dermal lesions resembling Kaposi's sarcoma in transgenic mice. Nature 1988;335:606–11.

59. Ensoli B, Barillari G, Salahuddin SZ, et al. Tat protein of HIV-1 stimulates growth of cells derived from Kaposi's sarcoma lesions of AIDS patients. Nature 1990;345:84–6.

60. Ensoli B, Buonaguro L, Barillari G, et al. Release, uptake and effects of extracellular human immuno-deficiency virus type one Tat protein on cell growth and viral transactivation. J Virol 1993;67:277–87.

61. Barillari G, Gendelman R, Gallo RC, et al. The Tat protein of human immunodeficiency virus type 1, a growth factor for AIDS Kaposi's sarcoma and cytokine-activated vascular cells, induces adhesion of the same cell types by using integrin receptors recognizing the RGD amino acid sequence. Proc Natl Acad Sci U S A 1993;90:7941–5.

62. Ensoli B, Gendelman R, Markham P, et al. Synergy between basic fibroblast growth factor and HIV-1 Tat protein in induction of Kaposi's sarcoma. Nature 1994;371:674–80.

63. Fiorelli V, Gendelman R, Samaniego F, et al. Cytokines from activated T cells induce normal endothelial cells to acquire the phenotypic and functional features of AIDS–Kaposi's sarcoma spindle cells. J Clin Invest 1995;95:1723–34.

64. Kelly GD, Ensoli B, Gunthel CJ, Offermann MK. Purified Tat induces inflammatory response genes in Kaposi's sarcoma cells. AIDS 1998;12:1753–61.

65. Pollack MS, Safai B, Myskowski PL, et al. Frequencies of HLA and GM immunogenetic markers in Kaposi's sarcoma. Tissue Antigens 1983;21:1–8.

66. Papasteriades C, Kaloterakis A, Filiotou A, et al. Histocompatibility antigens HLA-A, -B, -DR in Greek patients with Kaposi's sarcoma. Tissue Antigens 1984;24:313–5.

67. Contu L, Cerimele D, Carcassi C, et al. Immuno-genetic and immunological studies on classical Kaposi's sarcoma. IRCS Med Sci 1984;12:891.

68. Tzfoni EE, Scherman L, Battat S, et al. No HLA antigen is significant in classic Kaposi's sarcoma. J Am Acad Dermatol 1993;28:118–9.

69. Lunardi-Iskandar Y, Bryant JL, Zeman RA, et al. Tumorigenesis and metastasis of neoplastic Kaposi's sarcoma cell line in immunodeficient mice blocked by a human pregnancy hormone. Nature 1995;375:64–8.

70. Gill PS, Lunardi-Iskandar Y, Louie S, et al. The effects of preparations of human chorionic gonadotropin on AIDS-related Kaposi's sarcoma. N Engl J Med 1996;335:1261–9.

71. Lunardi-Iskandar Y, Bryant JL, Blattner WA, et al. Effects of a urinary factor from women in early pregancy on HIV-1, SIV and associated disease. Nat Med 1998;4:428–34.

72. Nisce LZ, Safai B, Poussin-Rosill H. Once weekly total and subtotal skin electron beam therapy for Kaposi's sarcoma. Cancer 1981;47:640–4.

73. Costada Cunha CS, Lebbé C, Rybojad M, et al. Long-term follow-up of non-HIV Kaposi's sarcoma treated with low-dose recombinant interferon alfa 2-b. Arch Dermatol 1996;132:285–90.

74. Webster GF. Local therapy for mucocutaneous Kaposi's sarcoma in patients with acquired immunodeficiency syndrome. Dermatol Surg 1995;21:205–8.

75. Tappero JW, Berger TG, Kaplan LD, et al. Cryother-apy for cutaneous Kaposi's sarcoma (KS) associated with acquired immune deficiency syndrome (AIDS): a phase II trial. J Acquir Immune Defic Syndr 1991;4:829–46.

76. Tappero JW, Grekin RC, Zanelli GA, et al. Pulsed-dye laser therapy for cutaneous Kaposi's sarcoma associated with acquired immune deficiency syndrome. J Am Acad Dermatol 1993;27:526–30.

77. Boudreaux AA, Smith LL, Cosby CD, et al. Intra-lesional vinblastine for cutaneous Kaposi's sarcoma associated with acquired immunodeficiency syndrome. J Am Acad Dermatol 1993;28:61–5.

78. Dupuy J, Price M, Lynch G, et al. Intralesional interferon-alfa and zidovudine in epidemic Kaposi's sarcoma. J Am Acad Dermatol 1993;28:966–72.

79. Sulis E, Floris C, Sulis ML, et al. Interferon administered intralesionally in skin and oral cavity lesions in heterosexual drug addicted patients with AIDS-related Kaposi's sarcoma. Eur J Cancer Clin Oncol 1988;25:759–61.

80. Stelzer KJ, Griffin TW. A randomized prospective trial of radiation therapy for AIDS-associated Kaposi's sarcoma. Int J Radiat Oncol Biol Phys 1993;27:1057–61.

81. Chak LY, Gill PS, Levine AM, et al. Radiation therapy for acquired immunodeficiency syndrome-related Kaposi's sarcoma. J Clin Oncol 1988;6:863–7.

82. Berson AM, Quivey JM, Harris JW, Wara WM. Radiation therapy for AIDS-related Kaposi's sarcoma. Int J Radiat Oncol Biol Phys 1990;19:569–75.

83. Karp JE, Pluda JM, Yarchoan R. AIDS-related Kaposi's sarcoma: a template for the translation of molecular pathogenesis into targeted therapeutic approaches. Hematol Oncol Clin North Am 1996;10:1031–49.

84. Krown SE, Real FX, Cunningham-Rundles S, et al. Preliminary observations on the effect of recombinant leukocyte A interferon in homosexual men with Kaposi's sarcoma. N Engl J Med 1983;308:1071–6.

85. Krown SE, Gold JWM, Niedzwiecki D, et al. Interferon-α with zidovudine: safety, tolerance and clinical and virologic effects in patients with Kaposi's sarcoma associated with the acquired immunodeficiency syndrome (AIDS). Ann Intern Med 1980;112:812–21.

86. Fischl MA, Uttamchandani R, Resnick L, et al. A phase I study of recombinant human interferon-alpha 2a or human lymphoblastoid interferon-alpha

n1 and concomitant zidovudine in patients with AIDS-related Kaposi's sarcoma. J Acquir Immune Defic Syndr 1991;4:1–10.

87. Kovacs JA, Deyton L, Davey R, et al. Combined zidovudine and interferon-α therapy in patients with Kaposi's sarcoma and the acquired immunodeficiency syndrome (AIDS). Ann Intern Med 1989; 111:280–7.

88. Fischl MA, Finkelstein DM, He W, et al. A phase II study of recombinant human interferon-2a and zidovudine in patients with AIDS-related Kaposi's sarcoma. J Acquir Immune Defic Syndr Hum Retrovirol 1996;11:379–84.

89. Laubenstein LJ, Krigel RL, Odajnyk CM, et al. Treatment of epidemic Kaposi's sarcoma with etoposide or a combination of doxorubicin, bleomycin and vinblastine. J Clin Oncol 1984;2:1115–20.

90. Bakker PJM, Danner SA, Lange JMA, Veenhof KHN. Etoposide for epidemic Kaposi's sarcoma: a phase II study. Eur J Cancer Clin Oncol 1988;24:1047–8.

91. Paredes J, Kahn JO, Tong WP, et al. Weekly oral etoposide in patients with Kaposi's sarcoma associated with human immunodeficiency virus infection: a phase I multicenter trial of the AIDS Clinical Trials Group. J Acquir Immune Defic Syndr Hum Retrovirol 1995;9:138–44.

92. Sander E, Zampese M, Prolla G, et al. Phase II trial of low-dose oral etoposide in AIDS-related Kaposi's sarcoma [abstract]. Proc Am Soc Clin Oncol; 1992; 11:54.

93. Bufill JA, Grace WR, Astrow AB. Phase II trial of prolonged, low-dose, oral VP-16 in AIDS-related Kaposi's sarcoma (KS) [abstract]. Proc Am Soc Clin Oncol 1992;11:47.

94. Volberding PA, Abrams DI, Conant M, et al. Vinblastine therapy for Kaposi's sarcoma in the acquired immunodeficiency syndrome. Ann Intern Med 1985;103:335–58.

95. Mintzer DM, Real FX, Jovino L, et al. Treatment of Kaposi's sarcoma and thrombocytopenia with vincristine in patients with acquired immunodeficiency syndrome. Ann Intern Med 1985;102:200–2.

96. Caumes E, Guermonprez G, Katlama C, et al. AIDS-associated mucocutaneous Kaposi's sarcoma treated with bleomycin. AIDS 1992;6:1483–7.

97. Lassoused K, Clauvel JP, Katlama C, et al. Treatment of acquired immune deficiency syndrome-related Kaposi's sarcoma with bleomycin as a single agent. Cancer 1990;66:1869–72.

98. Remick SC, Reddy M, Herman D, et al. Continuous infusion bleomycin in AIDS-related Kaposi's sarcoma. J Clin Oncol 1994;12:1130–6.

99. Fischl MA, Krown SE, O'Boyle KP, et al. Weekly doxorubicin in the treatment of patients with AIDS-related Kaposi's sarcoma. J Acquir Immune Defic Syndr 1993;6:259–64.

100. Gill PS, Rarick M, McCutchan JA, et al. Systemic treatment of AIDS-related Kaposi's sarcoma: results of a randomized trial. Am J Med 1991;90:427–33.

101. Gill PS, Akil B, Colletti P, et al. Pulmonary Kaposi's sarcoma: clinical findings and results of therapy. Am J Med 1989;87:57–61.

102. Schwartzmann G, Sprinz E, Kronfeld M, et al. Phase II study of teniposide in patients with AIDS-related Kaposi's sarcoma. Eur J Cancer 1991;27:1637–9.

103. Errante D, Spina M, Nasti G, et al. Evidence of activity of vinorelbine (VNR) in patients (pts) with previously treated epidemic Kaposi's sarcoma (KS). (Abstracts of the National AIDS Malignancy Conference, Bethesda, MD, April 28–30, 1997, abstract 79.) J Acquir Immune Defic Syndr Hum Retrovirol 1997;14(4):A36.

104. Shepherd FA, Burkes RL, Paul KE, Gross, PE. A phase II study of 4'-epirubicin in the treatment of poor-risk Kaposi's sarcoma and AIDS. AIDS 1991;5:305–9.

105. Gompels MM, Hill A, Jenkins P, et al. Kaposi's sarcoma in HIV infection treated with vincristine and bleomycin. AIDS 1992;6:1175–80.

106. Gill PS, Rarick M, Berstein-Singer M. Treatment of advanced Kaposi's sarcoma using a combination of bleomycin and vincristine. Am J Clin Oncol 1990; 13:315–9.

107. Rizzardini G, Pastecchia C, Vigevani GM, et al. Stealth liposomal doxorubicin or bleomycin/vincristine for the treatment of AIDS-related Kaposi's sarcoma. (Abstracts of the National AIDS Malignancy Conference, Bethesda, MD, April 28–30, 1997, abstract 17.) J Acquir Immune Defic Syndr Hum Retrovirol 1997;14(4):A20.

108. Kaplan L, Abrams D, Volberding P. Treatment of Kaposi's sarcoma in acquired immunodeficiency syndrome with an alternating vincristine-vinblastine regimen. Cancer Treat Rep 1989;70:1121–2.

109. Brenner DC. Liposomal encapsulation: making old and new drugs do new tricks. J Natl Cancer Inst 1989;81:13–5.

110. Gill PS, Espina BM, Muggia F, et al. Phase I/II clinical and pharmacokinetic evaluation of liposomal daunorubicin. J Clin Oncol 1995;13:996–1003.

111. Northfelt DW, Martin FJ, Kaplan LD, et al. Pharmacokinetic (PK) tumor localization (TL) and safety of Doxil (liposomal doxorubicin) in AIDS patients with Kaposi's sarcoma (AIDS-KS) [abstract]. Proc Am Clin Oncol 1993;12:51.

112. Bogner JR, Kronawitter U, Rolinski B, et al. Liposomal doxorubicin in the treatment of advanced AIDS-related Kaposi's sarcoma. J Acquir Immune Defic Syndr 1994;7:463–8.

113. Gill PS, Wernz J, Scadden DT, et al. Randomized phase III trial of liposomal daunorubicin versus doxorubicin, bleomycin, vincristine (ABV) in AIDS-related Kaposi's sarcoma. J Clin Oncol 1996; 14:2353–64.

114. Harrison M, Tomlinson D, Stewart S. Liposomal-entrapped doxorubicin: an active agent in AIDS-related Kaposi's sarcoma. J Clin Oncol 1995; 13:914–20.

115. Northfelt DW, Dezube B, Miller B, et al. Randomized comparative trial of Doxil vs Adriamycin, bleomycin and vincristine (ABV) in the treatment of severe AIDS-related Kaposi's sarcoma [abstract]. Blood 1995;86:382a.

116. Cowens JW, Creaven PJ, Brenner DE, et al. Phase I study of doxorubicin encapsulated in liposomes [abstract]. Proc Am Soc Oncol 1990;9:87.

117. Wagner D, Kern WV, Kern P. Liposomal doxorubicin in AIDS-related Kaposi's sarcoma: long term experiences. Clin Invest 1994;72:417–23.

118. Berry G, Billingham M, Alderman E, et al. Reduced cardiotoxicity of Doxil (pegylated liposomal doxorubicin) in AIDS Kaposi's sarcoma patients compared to a matched control group of cancer patients given doxorubicin [abstract]. Proc Am Soc Clin Oncol 1996;15:303.

119. Ross M, Gill PS, Espina BM, et al. Liposomal daunorubicin (DaunoXome) in the treatment of advanced AIDS-related Kaposi's sarcoma: results of a phase II study [abstract PoB 3123]. Int Conf AIDS 1992;8:B107.

120. Gordon KB, Tajuddin A, Guitart J, et al. Hand-foot syndrome associated with liposome-encapsulated doxorubicin therapy. Cancer 1995;75:2169–73.

121. Stewart JSW, Jablonowski H, Goebel FD, et al. A randomized comparative trial of Doxil® versus bleomycin and vincristine (BV) in the treatment of AIDS-related Kaposi's sarcoma [abstract 190]. Proc ASCO 1997;16:55a.

122. Saville MW, Lietzau J, Pluda JM, et al. Treatment of HIV-associated Kaposi's sarcoma with paclitaxel. Lancet 1995;346:26–8.

123. Gill PS, Tulpule A, Espina BM, et al. Paclitaxel is safe and effective in the treatment of advanced AIDS-related Kaposi's sarcoma. J Clin Oncol 1999; 17:1876–83.

124. Duvic M, Friedman Kien AE, Miles SA, et al. Phase I-II evaluation of Panretin™ (ALRT1057; LGD1057; AGN192013; 9-cis-retinoic acid) topical gel for AIDS-related cutaneous Kaposi's sarcoma [abstract 160]. Proc Am Soc Clin Oncol 1997;16:46a.

125. Bonhomme L, Fredj G, Averous S, et al. Topical treatment of epidemic Kaposi's sarcoma with all-trans retinoic acid. Ann Oncol 1991;2:234–5.

126. Bernstein ZP, Cohen P, Rios A, et al. A multicenter, phase II/III study of Atragen™ (tretinoin liposomal) in patients with AIDS-related Kaposi's sarcoma. (Abstracts of the National AIDS Malignancy Conference, Bethesda, MD, April 28–30, 1997, abstract 14.) J Acquir Immune Defic Syndr Hum Retrovirol 1997;4(14):A19.

127. O'Reilly MS, Boehm T, Shing Y, et al. Angiostatin: a novel angiogenesis inhibitor that mediates the suppression of metastases by a Lewis lung carcinoma. Cell 1994;70:315–28.

128. O'Reilly MS, Boehm T, Shing Y, et al. Endostatin: an endogenous inhibitor of angiogenesis and tumor growth. Cell 1997;88:277–85.

129. Ensoli B, Markham P, Kao V, et al. Block of AIDS-Kaposi's sarcoma (KS) cell growth, angiogenesis and lesion formation in nude mice by antisense oligonucleotide targeting basic fibroblast growth factor. J Clin Invest 1994;94:1736–46.

130. Brooks PC, Montgomery AMP, Rosenfelt M, et al. Integrin a_vb_3 antagonists promote tumor regression by inducing apoptosis of angiogenic blood vessels. Cell 1994;79:1157–64.

131. Morfeldt L, Torssander J. Long-term remission of Kaposi's sarcoma following foscarnet treatment of HIV-infected patients. Scand J Infect Dis 1994;26: 749–52.

132. Jones JL, Hanson DL, Chu SY, et al. AIDS-associated Kaposi's sarcoma [letter]. Science 1995;267:1078–9.

133. Mocroft A, Youle M, Gazzard B, et al. Anti-herpesvirus treatment and risk of Kaposi's sarcoma in HIV infection. Royal Free/Chelsea and Westminster Hospitals collaborative group. AIDS 1996;10:1101–5.

134. Safai B, Mike E, Giraldo G, et al. Association of Kaposi's sarcoma with second primary malignancies. Possible etiopathogenetic implications. Cancer 1980;45:1472–6.

135. Franceschi S, Arniani S, Balzi D, Geddes M. Survival of classic Kaposi's sarcoma and risk of second cancer. Br J Cancer 1996;74:1812–4.

136. Hjalgrim H, Frisch M, Pukkala E, et al. Risk of second cancers in classical Kaposi's sarcoma. Int J Cancer 1997;73:840–3.

137. Iscovich J, Boffetta P, Brennan P. Classic Kaposi's sarcoma as a first primary neoplasm. Int J Cancer 1999;80:173–7.

138. Miles SA, Wang H, Elashoff R, Mitsuyasu RT. Improved survival for patients with AIDS-related Kaposi's sarcoma. J Clin Oncol 1994;12(9):1910–6.

139. Palella FJ Jr, Delaney KM, Moorman AC, et al. Declining morbidity and mortality with advance human immunodeficiency virus infection. HIV Outpatient Study Investigators. N Engl J Med 1998;338(13):853–60.

140. Kedes DH, Ganem D. Sensitivity of Kaposi's sarcoma-associated herpesvirus replication to antiviral drugs: implications for potential therapy. J Clin Invest 1997;99:2082–6.

141. Neyts J, De Clercq E. Antiviral drugs susceptibility of human herpesvirus 8. Antimicrob Agents Chermother 1997;41:2754–46.

9

Melanoma: Biopsy Techniques

MARNI C. WISEMAN, MD
VINCENT C. HO, MD

Any patient who presents with a lesion that is clinically suspect for melanoma should undergo a biopsy. The early diagnosis of melanoma is important to minimize the morbidity and mortality associated with advanced disease. The choice of biopsy technique employed to obtain tissue for evaluation depends on the location, size, and shape of the lesion in question. This chapter will review the application of biopsy techniques commonly used in the diagnosis of melanoma.

An adequate biopsy must provide sufficient tissue for a histologic evaluation that includes assessment of depth of invasion. The most common techniques are excisional biopsy and incisional biopsy.[1-4] Alternative tissue-sampling techniques include shave biopsy, scissors biopsy, curettage, electrocutting knife or laser biopsy, and needle biopsy.[2] Since melanoma prognostication depends upon the depth of invasion, the removal of a superficial skin lesion with scissors biopsy, shave biopsy, or curettage is not recommended. Excision by electrocutting knife or laser does not offer an advantage over scalpel excision and may create artifact in the surgical margin. A needle biopsy may be useful in the diagnosis of metastatic melanoma but has no role in the diagnosis of primary cutaneous melanoma.

EXCISIONAL AND INCISIONAL BIOPSY

An excisional biopsy for suspected melanoma is the removal of the entire lesion suspect for melanoma, down to and including the subcutaneous fat. An elliptical excision is most commonly employed; however, punch biopsy, saucerization, or wedge excision are occasionally used.[1-4] The excisional

biopsy is planned and oriented with future treatment or investigation in mind, such as re-excision or sentinel node biopsy. It is also planned to maximize cosmetic and functional outcomes (Figure 9–1). Preoperatively, a Wood's lamp may facilitate the delineation of the borders of the lesion,[1] and a surgical marking pen is used to draw a line 1 to 2 mm outside the clinically apparent lesion on normal skin.[2] A margin of 1 to 2 mm is selected since smaller margins may be insufficient and because larger margins are excessive for benign lesions yet insufficient for a melanoma.[5-7] The technique of excisional biopsy is illustrated in Figure 9–1. A full-thickness biopsy including the subcutaneous fat should be performed. An orientation suture or paint should be placed on the excisional specimen and detailed on the pathology requisition to facilitate the mapping of surgical margins and aid in the planning of wider excisions that may be required in the future.

An incisional biopsy is the partial removal of a lesion. There is good evidence that the performance of an incisional biopsy does not negatively affect ultimate patient prognosis or survival.[8-13] In general, the portion of the lesion that is the darkest or most elevated should be selected as the biopsy site, in an attempt to clinically identify the portion with the most worrisome histologic findings.[1] Occasionally, multiple incisional biopsies may be required, especially if the lesion is large and morphologically varied. The incisional biopsy can be performed with a scalpel (saucerization; wedge or elliptical resection) or punch.[1-4] The surgical technique is identical to that of the excisional biopsy. The technique of punch biopsy is outlined in Figure 9–2. A punch of 3 to 6 mm in diameter is selected. Gentle pressure is applied as the punch is rotated through the dermis into the subcutaneous tissue. The specimen is gently grasped to avoid crush artifact and is divided at the level of the subcutis with a scalpel or scissors.

Biopsy of the Nail Bed

It is preferable to perform a biopsy of a nail bed lesion suspect for melanoma under direct visualization. This is accomplished through partial or total nail plate avulsion. Using local anesthetic without epinephrine, a digital block is performed or the area is locally infiltrated. The nail plate is avulsed from its two points of

attachment at the proximal nail fold and nail bed with a Freer periosteal elevator and hemostat.

Biopsy of the lesion in question may be either incisional or excisional, depending on the size of the lesion. For lesions located in the nail matrix, the incision is oriented transversely to minimize scarring. Biopsies of lesions located in the nail bed are performed with a longitudinal orientation. Alternatively, a punch biopsy may be performed. Following biopsy, primary closure is achieved with a fine absorbable suture. The avulsed nail plate should also be submitted for histologic evaluation because it often contains a portion of the nail bed

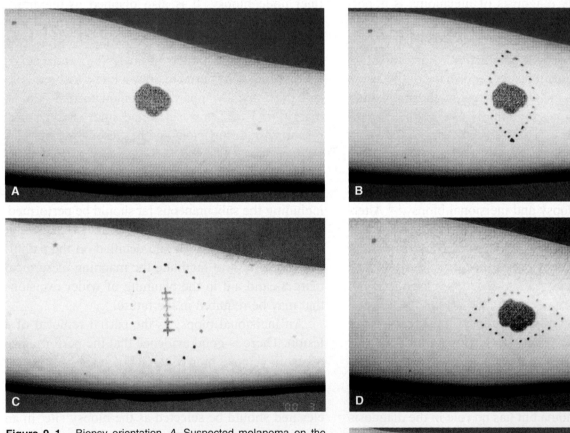

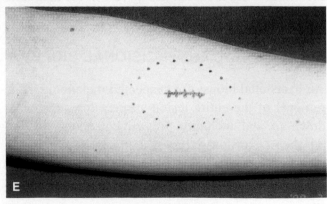

Figure 9–1. Biopsy orientation. *A,* Suspected melanoma on the volar aspect of the forearm. *B,* An incorrect excisional biopsy orientation. *C,* Re-excision after biopsy will likely necessitate skin grafting rather than primary closure. *D,* A correct excisional biopsy orientation, parallel to lymphatic drainage and maximum skin tension lines. *E,* This orientation will usually allow for primary closure of the postsurgical defect, after re-excision with appropriate margins.

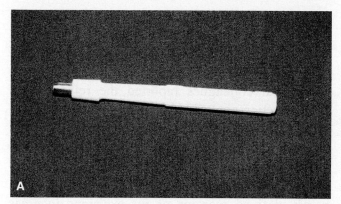 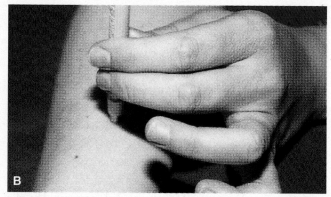

Figure 9–2. Incisional biopsy for melanoma, using a punch biopsy technique. *A,* An example of a 4-mm biopsy punch. *B,* The surgical site is first cleaned, and the lesion is anesthetized. A biopsy punch is placed over the darkest or most-raised portion of the lesion, and gentle pressure is applied as the punch is rotated through the dermis into the subcutaneous tissue. The specimen is transected at the base, using fine-tip scissors or a scalpel. Care must be taken to avoid crushing the tissue.

epithelium and may contain a portion of the lesion suspect for melanoma.[14]

Biopsy of Mucosal Lesions

The same biopsy techniques are used for both mucosal and cutaneous lesions. It is important to pay particular attention to proper lighting and exposure. A headlight may help to provide acceptable lighting when working in a cavity. Mucous membranes, lacking a stratified squamous epithelium, are ideal sites for topical anesthesia prior to intralesional anesthetic infiltration. Additionally, mucosa may bleed more than skin because of greater vascularity. Hemostasis can be achieved with instrumentation, manual pressure, chemicals (such as ferrous subsulfate), or sutures.

NEEDLE BIOPSY

A needle biopsy is performed with a fine needle and with negative pressure generated by a syringe attached to a Cameco handle. This technique provides information only about cell cytology. It is appropriate for the diagnosis of metastatic melanoma but should not be used for diagnosis of a primary cutaneous lesion. The cytologic criteria for the diagnosis of metastatic disease include epithelioid and spindled tumor cells; melanin within neoplastic cells; lack of cohesion between malignant cells; multinucleate and binucleate cells, macronucleoli, and intranuclear vacuolation; and malig-

nant cells with regular nuclei and evenly dispersed chromatin. Although intracellular melanin within malignant cells is diagnostic, melanin may be absent in up to 60 percent of cases.[15–17] Absence of visible melanin in the needle biopsy specimen should not preclude a diagnosis of metastatic melanoma. Comparison with the primary melanoma and/or immunocytochemical stains for HMB-45 and S-100 antigen are often helpful in diagnosis of metastatic amelanotic melanomas. Because a needle biopsy samples only a small portion of tumor cells and because a sampling error may produce a false-negative result, any clinically suspicious lesion with a negative result should be confirmed with an open biopsy.

FROZEN-SECTION BIOPSY

Following the biopsy of a lesion suspect for melanoma, the tissue obtained is submitted to pathology, processed, embedded in paraffin, and sectioned. Because of this processing, a pathologic diagnosis may not be generated until days after the biopsy was performed. In some instances, this delay in diagnosis is undesirable because it postpones definitive management. Under such circumstances, a frozen-section biopsy may be performed, and a pathologic diagnosis can be generated as early as 1 hour after the biopsy procedure. The tissue obtained is oriented and embedded in a cutting compound, frozen to –70°C, oriented, sectioned at –20°C in a cryostat machine, mounted, stained, and then examined.

Some of the characteristic pathologic features of melanoma are altered by the frozen-section processing technique. In a series of 158 subjects, Braun-Falco and colleagues put forth six diagnostic histologic criteria that can be applied to the frozen-section diagnosis of melanoma. These criteria were pleomorphic melanocytes, mitosis, pagetoid spread, adnexal involvement, infiltrative pattern, and the presence of ulceration or erosion. The presence of three or more of these criteria successfully identified all melanomas. Because this study did not specify the type of melanoma examined, it is unclear whether or not these results can be extrapolated to the various types of melanoma (such as regressing or desmoplastic melanoma).[18]

Davis and Little examined 233 frozen sections of pigmented lesions and determined a diagnostic accuracy of 98.8 percent. Although two patients received a false-positive diagnosis of melanoma and underwent unnecessary surgery, false-negative diagnoses were not established.[19] A further study examined 84 pigmented lesions by frozen section and accurately diagnosed melanoma in 30 of 31 cases. (The misdiagnosed lesion was a regressing melanoma.) This study cautioned against the routine use of frozen sections in the diagnosis of melanoma and recommended that this technique be used in experienced centers and in conjunction with confirmation of the diagnosis by routine paraffin-embedded sections.[20]

In addition to the ability to correctly identify the pathologic features of melanoma, another important consideration of the frozen-section biopsy is its ability to accurately reflect tumor thickness, the cornerstone of prognostication. Shafir and colleagues determined that frozen-section tumor thicknesses were slightly greater than the thicknesses of paraffin-embedded sections but were unable to determine a constant relationship.[20] In a further series of 20 patients, significant differences were indentified when comparing tumor thicknesses obtained by frozen and paraffin section. A relationship between these differing values was not found.[21] In contrast, Kiehl and colleagues examined 112 melanocytic lesions, including 33 melanomas, and determined no significant difference between Breslow levels on paraffin and frozen sections. However, greater dif-

ferences in Breslow levels were observed among thicker lesions in 7 subjects (6.25%).[22]

Despite these issues regarding the diagnosis and depth analysis of melanoma by frozen section, Zitelli and colleagues reported the reliability of frozen-section analysis in the evaluation of surgical margins for melanoma. They determined a sensitivity of 100 percent and a specificity of 90 percent in 221 specimens analyzed by frozen section and suggested its clinical applicability for melanomas with poorly defined margins or for excisions in areas where tissue conservation is desirable for cosmetic or functional reasons.[23]

Overall, it appears that frozen-section biopsy specimens are not as reliable as paraffin sections but may have a role in the diagnosis of melanoma in the setting of experienced centers and in conjunction with concomitant routine paraffin sections.

SELECTION OF BIOPSY TECHNIQUE

An excisional biopsy is recommended as the technique of choice in the biopsy of melanoma. To establish a diagnosis, the pathologist must be supplied with adequate tissue to assess lesion breadth, depth, symmetry, and circumscription.[24] The excisional biopsy can usually be performed for lesions up to 2 cm in diameter and when excision is desirable, regardless of final diagnosis.[1] The biopsy should include the lesion and a 1- to 2-mm peripheral zone of clinically normal skin, and it should extend into the subcutaneous fat.[25] An elliptical excision is usually the technique of choice because it most consistently provides adequate tissue for examination.[24] An excisional biopsy can also be performed with a saucerization technique or punch method. Because the saucerization technique is more superficial, the biopsy bed and the base of the biopsy specimen should be examined for pigmentation. If pigmentation is present at the base of the specimen, a deeper tissue specimen should be obtained.[25]

An incisional biopsy is considered suboptimal because it does not provide the entire lesion for analysis. An incisional biopsy may be considered when the lesion is too large for complete excision, when the suspicion for melanoma is low, if the lesion is situated in a cosmetically sensitive location, or when it is impractical to perform an excisional biopsy.[1,25] Although it was previously believed that incisional biopsy promoted tumor dissemination, several studies have demonstrated that biopsy technique does not adversely influence patient survival, rate of metastatic disease, or overall patient outcome.[8–13] Immunohistochemical studies have also demonstrated that atypical cells are not seeded into the dermis with a punch biopsy technique.[13] A sampling error—the removal of tissue not pathologically representative of the whole lesion—is a major limitation of the incisional biopsy technique. Such an error can lead to the misdiagnosis of a melanoma. Although the most clinically suspicious area of the tumor is sampled, a repeat biopsy should be undertaken if the histologic features do not correlate with the clinical impression or if the index of suspicion for melanoma is high. This is particularly applicable to acral-lentiginous melanoma and lentigo maligna melanoma as both may be difficult to diagnose with a small specimen that may not be representative of the whole lesion. Another limitation of the incisional biopsy technique is that it may not provide a final determination of tumor thickness, and prognostication may need to be deferred until a definitive excision is undertaken. Despite these limitations, the incisional biopsy is a practical technique by which rapid diagnosis can be established for large or potentially cosmetically disfiguring tumors.

A superficial shave or curettage technique should not be used in the diagnosis of a suspected melanoma because it does not provide adequate tissue for either pathologic analysis or the determination of depth of invasion. Although a needle biopsy plays an important role in the diagnosis of metastatic melanoma, needle biopsy should not be used in the diagnosis of primary cutaneous melanoma because it allows for only cytologic analysis and not for a histologic diagnosis or the determination of Breslow thickness.

The role of the frozen section in the diagnosis of melanoma remains controversial. Overall, frozen-section analysis is suboptimal and should not be performed in situations where paraffin-embedded sections are practical and feasible. Frozen sections may fail to identify subtle histopathologic features of melanoma (such as regression) and are not always reliable in the determination of depth of invasion. When tumor tissue is submitted for a frozen-section analysis, a portion of the tissue should concurrently be submitted for future paraffin-embedding. In addition, the frozen-section technique should only be performed in centers experienced in the proper processing and pathologic analysis. However, the frozen-section technique may be useful in the examination of surgical margins for melanoma.

REFERENCES

1. National Institutes of Health Consensus Development Conference statement on diagnosis and treatment of early melanoma, January 27–29, 1992. Am J Dermatopathol 1993;15(1):34–43.
2. Bart RS, Kopf AW. Techniques of biopsy of cutaneous neoplasms. J Dermatol Surg Oncol 1979;5:979–83.
3. Harris MN, Gumport SL. Biopsy technique for malignant melanoma. J Dermatol Surg 1975;1:24–7.
4. Urist MM, Balch CM, Milton GW. Surgical management of the primary melanoma. In: Balch CM, Milton GW, Shaw HM, Soong SJ, editors. Cutaneous melanoma: clinical management and treatment results worldwide. Philadelphia: J B Lippincott; 1992. p. 71.
5. Ledwig PA, Robinson JK. Should the excisional biopsy of clinically probable melanomas include a margin that might also serve as adequate for treatment? Arch Dermatol 1990;126:877–88.
6. Lederman JS, Sober AJ. Does wide excision as the initial diagnostic procedure improve prognosis in patients with cutaneous melanoma? J Dermatol Surg 1986;12:697–9.
7. Landthaler M, Braun-Falco O, Leitl A, et al. Excisional biopsy as the first therapeutic procedure versus primary wide excision of malignant melanoma. Cancer 1989;64:1612–6.
8. Sondergaard K, Schou G. Biopsy and optimal size of margins of resection of primary cutaneous malignant melanomas. Am J Dermatopathol 1985;7 Suppl:127–9.
9. Lees VC, Briggs JC. Effect of initial biopsy procedure on prognosis in stage 1 invasive cutaneous malignant melanoma: review of 1086 patients. Br J Surg 1991;78:1108–10.
10. Bagley FH, Cady B, Lee A, Legg AM. Changes in clinical presentation and management of malignant melanoma. Cancer 1981;47:2126–34.
11. Drzewiecki KT, Ladefoged C, Christensen HE. Biopsy and prognosis for cutaneous malignant melanomas in clinical stage I. Scand J Plast Reconstr Surg 1980;14:141–4.

12. Lederman JS, Sober AJ. Does biopsy type influence survival in clinical stage I cutaneous melanoma? J Am Acad Dermatol 1985;13:983–7.
13. Penneys NS. Excision of melanoma after initial biopsy. An immunohistochemical study. J Am Acad Dermatol 1985;13:995–8.
14. MacFarlane D, Scher RK. Nail surgery. In: Ratz JL, Geronemus RG, Goldman MP, et al, editors. Textbook of dermatologic surgery. Philadelphia: Lippincott-Raven; 1998. p. 621.
15. Perry MD, Gore M, Seigler HF, Johnston WW. Fine needle aspiration biopsy of metastatic melanoma. A morphologic analysis of 174 cases. Acta Cytol 1986;30:385–96.
16. Woyke S, Domagaa W, Czerniak B, Strokowska M. Fine needle aspiration cytology of malignant melanoma of the skin. Acta Cytol 1980;24:529–38.
17. Daskalopoulou D, Gourgiotou K, Thodou E, et al. Rapid cytological diagnosis of primary skin tumors and tumor-like conditions. Acta Derm Venereol 1997;77:292–5.
18. Braun-Falco O, Korting HC, Konz B. Histological and cytological criteria in the diagnosis of malignant melanoma by cryostat sections. Virchows Arch Pathol Anat Histol 1981;393:115–21.
19. Davis NC, Little JH. The role of frozen sections in the diagnosis and management of malignant melanoma. Br J Surg 1974;61:505–8.
20. Shafir R, Hiss J, Tsur H, Bubis JJ. Pitfalls in frozen section diagnosis of malignant melanoma. Cancer 1983;51:1168–70.
21. Nield DV, Saad MN, Khoo CTK, et al. Tumor thickness in malignant melanoma: the limitations of frozen section. Br J Plast Surg 1988;41:403–7.
22. Kiehl P, Matthies B, Ehrich K, et al. Accuracy of frozen section measurements for the determination of Breslow tumor thickness in primary malignant melanoma. Histopathology 1999;34:257–61.
23. Zitelli JA, Moy RL, Abell E. The reliability of frozen sections in the evaluation of surgical margins for melanoma. J Am Acad Dermatol 1991;24:102–6.
24. Macy-Roberts E, Ackerman AB. A critique of techniques for biopsy of clinically suspected malignant melanomas. Am J Dermatopathol 1992;4:791–8.
25. Salopek TG, Slade J, Marghoob AA, et al. Management of cutaneous malignant melanoma by dermatologists of the American Academy of Dermatology. I. Survey of biopsy practices of pigmented lesions suspected as melanoma. J Am Acad Dermatol 1995;22:441–50.

10

Surgical Management of Cutaneous Melanoma

A. BENEDICT COSIMI, MD

It is generally agreed that the treatment of cutaneous melanoma—whether one is considering the primary site, spread to regional nodes, or even distant metastases—is primarily surgical. Nevertheless, controversy continues regarding the exact type and extent of the surgical procedure that should be performed in individual patients. Fortunately, the identification of the important prognostic characteristics of primary lesions (see Chapter 3), the completion of several prospectively randomized therapeutic trials (see below), and the validation of the concept and technology of sentinel lymph node (SLN) mapping and biopsy (see Chapter 11) have now combined to resolve much of the controversy. The following discussion will review and illustrate current surgical recommendations and the rationale upon which they are based.

CLINICAL DIAGNOSIS

Once a suspicious lesion has been identified, tissue for definitive histopathologic examination can be obtained by several biopsy techniques (as detailed in Chapter 9). Immediate complete excision of the entire lesion with minimal margins of surrounding normal skin (Figure 10–1) should be the preferred approach whenever technically feasible. Exceptions include lesions that are so large or so anatomically situated that total removal could not be accomplished by simple primary suture.

There are two major reasons for favoring total excision. The most important for the surgeon is the fact that recommendations for each patient's definitive surgical management are entirely dependent

upon the histologic analysis of the primary melanoma site. In some instances, this analysis may not accurately characterize the extent of invasion or the degree of risk of the primary lesion if only a part of the tumor is available for pathologic examination.

Of comparable importance to many patients is the concern, despite reassurances to the contrary, that a surgical incision into a tumor increases the risks of dissemination. They almost invariably express a sense of greater mental comfort if the entire lesion has been absent during the typical 1 to 2 weeks that elapse between the initial biopsy and the definitive surgical procedure.

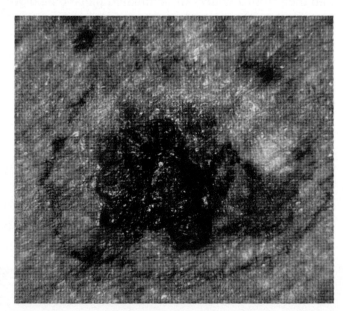

Figure 10–1. Proposed excisional biopsy of probable superficial spreading cutaneous melanoma, with minimal margins of grossly normal skin.

MANAGEMENT OF THE PRIMARY SITE

Historical Approaches

For decades, the traditional surgical treatment of cutaneous melanoma was justified by anatomic studies of the mode of spread of these tumors, initially detailed by Handley in 1907.[1] His dissections identified "permeation of lymphatics" as the principal agent in the centrifugal spread of the primary neoplasm. His original suggestion that the primary lesion be excised with 1-inch (2.5-cm) margins of normal skin and underlying subcutaneous tissue gradually evolved to recommendations that margins as great as 6 cm beyond the initial lesion had to be removed if local recurrences at the primary excision site were to be prevented (Figure 10–2). As a result, most surgical reviews and textbooks advised that complete excision required skin grafting or flap rotation for wound closure in essentially every instance, and warned that primary skin approximation of the melanoma excision site suggested that inadequate tissue had been resected.[2,3]

An interesting aspect of Handley's influence on surgical practice is the little-appreciated fact that his observations were not actually of primary cutaneous melanoma sites but were derived from an autopsy dissection of the thigh and groin of a woman who had died from a widely disseminated melanoma that had originated on the foot. Interestingly, there had been no recurrence at the primary excision site in that patient, and Handley's description was clearly

that of in-transit and inguinal node metastases. Nevertheless, his detailed dissections and illustrations convincingly supported his deduction that similar lymphatic "permeation" occurs as the initial process of dissemination around the primary site. This valid but overly simplified conclusion continued to dominate surgical guidelines for patients with cutaneous melanoma until the late 1970s.

By that time, more precise histopathologic microstaging of melanoma had developed, and it had become increasingly apparent that the risk of recurrence for individual cutaneous lesions could be quite accurately predicted, particularly by the depth of invasion at the primary site.[4,5] Because of the low probability of recurrence following removal of superficially invasive lesions, the concept of radical surgical therapy for all patients began to be challenged.[6–10] These and other reports from uncontrolled retrospective clinical studies strongly suggested that local recurrences rarely (< 1%) developed in patients with thin primary lesions even if definitive resection margins of less than 1 cm had been achieved (Table 10–1).[6–13] However, since some reports continued to caution that narrow excision could be associated with an increased rate of local recurrence,[14] it was obvious that prospectively randomized trials would have to be designed before definitive surgical guidelines for the optimal management of the primary lesion site could be established.

Controlled Clinical Trials

Randomized prospective studies designed to compare the efficacy of narrower excision margins to traditional more-radical surgery have now been completed for patients with primary cutaneous melanomas up to 4 mm thick. In a World Health Organization (WHO) international study, 687 patients with lesions ≤ 2 mm thick were randomly assigned to definitive surgical resection encompassing the primary lesion (or initial excision site) plus radial margins of normal skin of either 1 or 3 cm.[15] Seventy-five patients were excluded from the final analysis, mostly because of retrospective changes in pathologic diagnoses. After a follow-up period of 8 years for the remaining 612 patients, the disease-free and overall survival rates were found to be

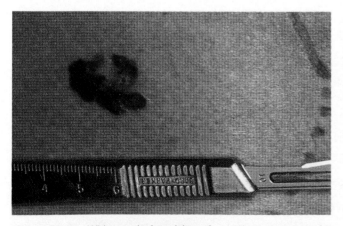

Figure 10–2. Wide surgical excision of a melanoma proven by punch biopsy. Definitive therapeutic guidelines historically advised 5- to 6-cm margins of surrounding skin.

Table 10–1. RETROSPECTIVE STUDIES OF NARROW-EXCISION MARGINS FOR THIN CUTANEOUS MELANOMA				
No. of Patients	Thickness (mm)	Margin (cm)	Local Recurrences	Reference
62	< 0.76	0.1–2.0	0	6
36	< 0.76	0.5–5.0	0	7
16	< 0.75	< 2.0	0	9
49	< 1.20	0.7–4.0	0	10
346	< 1.00	0.1–5.0	4	11
571	< 1.00	< 2.0	0	12
73	< 0.76	1.0–1.5	1	13
1,153			5 (0.43%)	

essentially identical in the two treatment groups.[16] No local recurrences had developed in any patient whose primary melanoma was thinner than 1 mm. There were six local recurrences in patients with primary lesions between 1.1 and 2 mm in thickness, five of which had been treated by narrow excision. The investigators concluded that a 1-cm excision is safe for primary lesions not thicker than 1 mm and that the risk of local recurrence is only 3.3 percent after similarly narrow excision of lesions that are between 1.1 and 2 mm in thickness.

This study thus established optimal surgical management as excision with 1-cm margins for primary lesions less than 1 mm thick and suggested that wider resection margins should probably be obtained for thicker lesions.

The issue has been further clarified by a second multi-institutional randomized surgical trial that prospectively studied cutaneous melanomas that were more deeply invasive.[17] In this study, 486 patients whose primary lesions were between 1 and 4 mm in thickness were randomly assigned to definitive surgical resection with margins of either 2 or 4 cm. Sixteen patients were subsequently excluded from analysis because of pathologic criteria, violation of surgical protocol, or loss to follow-up. At a mean follow-up of 92 months, local recurrence had been observed in 2.1 percent of the patients who had

been treated with 2-cm excision margins and in 2.6 percent of those treated with a 4-cm margin.[18] The 5-year disease-free survival was similar in the two groups of patients (79 to 80%).

Another prospectively randomized trial, conducted by the Swedish Melanoma Study Group, has confirmed the efficacy of conservative surgical margins for primary lesions that are not deeply invasive.[19] In this study, 769 patients whose melanomas were between 0.8 and 2.0 mm in thickness were randomly assigned to surgical resection with margins of either 2 or 5 cm. With a mean follow-up of 5.8 years, no differences in local recurrence or survival rates have become evident.

These studies have thus established 2-cm surgical margins as adequate local therapy for primary cutaneous melanomas that are 1 to 4 mm in thickness.

The optimal surgical margins for lesions more than 4 mm in thickness have not been defined by prospective studies. Based on the theoretically higher likelihood of microscopic satellite lesions in such patients, a margin of more than 2 cm appears appropriate. Nevertheless, in a recently reported retrospective study of 278 patients with thick primary melanomas (4.1 to 35 mm), the width of the excision margins did not appear to affect either the incidence of local recurrence or disease-free survival.[20] Although the authors suggest that 2-cm margins are therefore adequate for these thicker lesions, many centers continue to recommend wider excision if anatomically feasible. The current surgical guidelines defined by these trials and experiences are summarized in Table 10–2.

Surgical Techniques

The Trunk and Extremities

Essentially all primary cutaneous melanomas less than 4 mm in thickness and arising on the trunk or

Table 10–2. CURRENTLY RECOMMENDED EXCISION MARGINS				
Primary Tumor	Thickness (mm)	Excision Margin (cm)	Clinical Studies	References
Shallow	< 1	1	WHO* Melanoma Group	15,16
Intermediate	1–4	2	Intergroup and Swedish Melanoma Study Group	17–19
Thick	> 4	2–3	Retrospective only	20

* World Health Organization.

extremities can be surgically excised and closed primarily using local anesthesia. Split or full-thickness skin grafts are occasionally required for lesions on a distal extremity; but even here, reconstruction by advancement of full-thickness skin flaps can often be comfortably achieved (Figures 10–3 and 10–4). The width of the definitive surgical excision (1-cm margins for lesions < 1 mm thick and 2 cm for lesions 1 to 4 mm thick) is measured from the edge of the previous excisional biopsy wound (or intact tumor if a punch or incisional biopsy was performed). The excision should be elliptical, with the long axis approximately three times the width and oriented to follow natural skin creases or "lines of minimal tension" whenever possible. The entire specimen, including skin and subcutaneous tissue down to but not including the underlying fascia, is removed en bloc. The consequences of removing the muscle fascia with the excised specimen have been controversial, with some reports suggesting a worsened prognosis for patients following such deeper resections.[21] However, subsequent experience has not established any correlation between either beneficial or detrimental effects and fascia excision.[22] Since the cosmetic result is usually improved in wounds with intact fascia (particularly for lower-extremity lesions, where fascial disruption allows localized herniation of underlying muscle), most surgeons recommend limiting the depth of the defin-

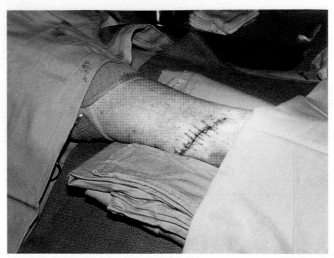

Figure 10–4.   The same patient as shown in Figure 10–3, with primary skin closure of the re-excised wound above the lateral malleolus. Mobilization and advancement of skin flaps was aided by centrally placed "pulley" sutures that reduce the tension on the wound edges.

itive excision to the skin and subcutaneous tissues. It is important for the surgeon to place a marking stitch, typically at "12 o'clock," on the excised specimen to orient it for the pathologist.

For the large majority of excision sites, the skin margins can be undermined just above the retained muscle fascia until the flaps can be advanced to close the soft-tissue defect without undue tension. The subcutaneous tissues are usually approximated with interrupted absorbable sutures to provide a smoother contour of the wound than that achieved with continuous suturing. For wounds with limited mobility of the skin flap edges, the skin is closed with interrupted fine nonabsorbable sutures incorporating several larger "pulley" sutures (placed near-far, far-near) at the center of the wound to relieve the tension (see Figure 10–4). For most other primarily closed wounds, subcuticular closure with a continuous absorbable suture will provide a better cosmetic result and will also avoid the need for an early postoperative visit merely for suture removal.

For the few trunk and extremity wounds that cannot be closed by these simple measures, split or full-thickness grafts must be applied. This author prefers to use defatted, full-thickness grafts that (1) allow primary closure (and thus more cosmetic and less painful healing) of the donor sites; (2) cover the defect with a graft that more closely resembles normal skin in color, texture, and flexibility; and (3)

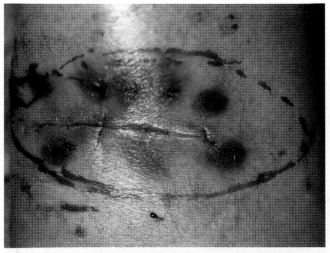

Figure 10–3.   Re-excision and sentinel lymph node (SLN) biopsy of a local resection site for a 1.3-cm-thick melanoma above the ankle. Lymphazurin dye has been injected intradermally within the planned 2-cm skin margins.

avoid the contracture, instability, and late breakdown that sometimes occur in the thin epithelialized scar tissues of wounds closed by split-thickness grafts, particularly if placed on weight-bearing areas or sites of constant mobility and recurrent trauma. The advantages of full-thickness grafts must be measured in light of the more exacting requirements for their survival. Nevertheless, with meticulous hemostasis of the excision site, complete removal of the graft subcutaneous fat, and careful immobilization of the graft site, one can anticipate primary healing for most wounds closed with full-thickness skin grafts.

The Digits and Subungual Sites

The functional requirements of these body parts, together with the difficulty of obtaining convention-ally recommended margins, make treatment of melanomas in the digits and subungual locations par-ticularly challenging for the surgeon. Reports from most earlier series advised that melanomas of all dig-its are best treated by amputation. For toe lesions, ray amputation has been felt to be most appropriate. This approach continues to provide the best functional and cosmetic results for primary melanomas of the small toes. However, most surgeons discourage the use of ray amputation of the great toe, preferring to retain the first metatarsal head, which improves foot stabil-ity and allows more normal ambulation.

Complete amputation of the thumb or fingers is a much more disabling procedure. In the attempt to improve local tumor control for hand lesions, some investigators have added isolated limb perfusion with melphalan to more-distal amputation,[23] but this approach has not been shown to provide a significant benefit over surgery alone. However, a number of reports do indicate that there is no difference in local recurrence or survival rates following amputation for subungual melanoma, whether the amputation was of just the distal phalanx or was at a more proximal level.[24–26] Thus, the current treatment recommenda-tion for subungual melanoma of the thumb or fingers is amputation of the distal phalanx only (Figures 10–5 and 10–6). More-proximal melanomas of the thumb or fingers are managed by soft-tissue excision with conventional margins (Table 10–3) and closure with full-thickness skin grafts or tissue flaps.

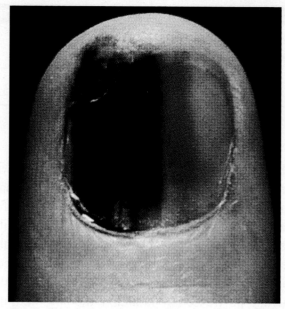

Figure 10–5. Subungual melanoma of the third finger.

The Head and Neck

Special therapeutic considerations are required for melanomas of the head and neck region because of their distinct biologic properties, their proximity to adjacent nonresectable vital structures, and the highly visible anatomic location of the resultant sur-gical reconstruction. A number of studies have indi-cated that patients with lesions of the scalp fare worse than patients with comparably invasive lesions of the non-hair-bearing skin of the head and neck.[27,28] Multifactorial analysis in some reports also implicates the neck subsite as an independent

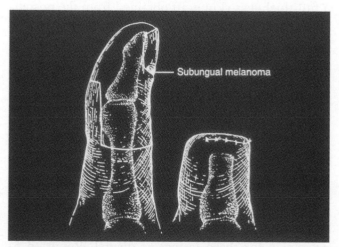

Figure 10–6. Amputation of the distal phalanx just proximal to the interphalangeal joint for definitive treatment of subungual melanoma.

	Table 10–3. SURGICAL TREATMENT OF HAND MELANOMAS		
	Location of Melanoma		
Thickness (mm)	Subungual	Digital	Dorsum/Palm
≤ 1.0	Distal phalanx amputation	1-cm excision	1-cm excision
> 1.0	Distal phalanx amputation plus SLN	2-cm excision plus SLN	2-cm excision plus SLN

SLN = sentinel lymph node mapping and biopsy.

higher risk factor.[29] As a result, wider excisions with more frequent use of skin grafts for closure have been suggested, particularly for scalp lesions. Unfortunately, such wide resections are often not possible where margins of more than 1 to 2 cm unacceptably interfere with the function or appearance of adjacent facial structures. One approach to this constraint is adjuvant postresection radiation therapy, administered to the reconstructed area to reduce the risk of local recurrences. The author frequently advises this following the resection of deeper lesions located over branches of the facial nerve. Fortunately, advancement and rotation skin flaps can be used, with highly acceptable cosmetic results, for reconstruction of even extensive resections of the neck area (Figures 10–7 and 10–8).

Most primary melanomas of the external ear occur on the helix and can be treated by wedge resection and primary reconstruction. If possible, the superior portion of the helix should be preserved to support eyeglasses or an ear prosthesis. Lesions on the tragus or antitragus can usually be resected with margins of 1 to 2 cm that extend either anteriorly or into the external canal. Reconstruction using a full-thickness skin graft obtained from the postauricular area provides excellent cosmetic results.

The Anorectum

Melanomas arising at the anorectal site are rare and constitute only 1 to 2 percent of all primary lesions. These tumors arise primarily from or near the anoderm. As a result, patients with these tumors often note abnormal sensations related to the area, but the most common presenting complaint is bleeding. Unfortunately, the correct diagnosis often is not made until the tumors are quite advanced; thus, the prognosis for these lesions is dismal. Reported 5-year survival rates have ranged from 0 to 20 percent.

Because of its success in the treatment of adenocarcinoma of the rectum, abdominoperineal resection (APR) has been recommended for the surgical treatment of anorectal melanoma as well,[30,31] and some authors have even advocated simultaneous groin node dissection.[32]

More recent reviews, however, have seriously questioned the usefulness of such radical approaches.[33–37] All of these reports concluded that conservative sphincter-saving excision of anorectal melanoma confers comparable survival rates to those achieved with APR. Most anorectal melanoma patients succumb to distant metastases regardless of the surgical approach, but those treated by APR will

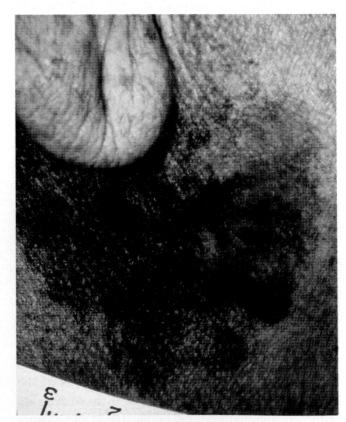

Figure 10–7. Extensive cutaneous melanoma of the preauricular and upper neck areas.

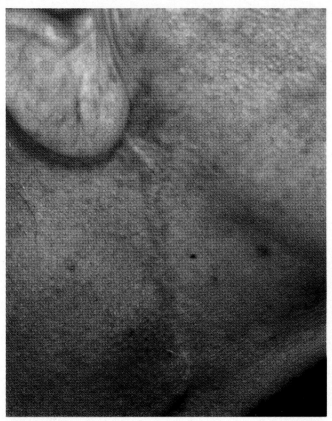

Figure 10–8. Same patient as shown in Figure 10–7, after wide excision. Primary closure was achieved by rotation of local skin flaps.

have suffered significantly greater perioperative morbidity. One review does suggest a survival benefit for patients treated with APR, but this did not reach statistical significance.[38] Nevertheless, these authors continue to recommend this procedure for anorectal melanoma because most of their long-term surviving patients were treated with APR.

The majority of surgical groups, however, currently advise sphincter-sparing excision with tumor-free margins of at least 1 cm as the initial treatment of choice for these patients. Abdominoperineal resection should be reserved for large melanomas not amenable to this approach, or for palliation of obstructing lesions, or for salvage therapy in selected patients with local recurrences.

The Vulva

The vulva has also been considered an unfavorable location for melanoma. Based upon therapy guidelines for squamous cell lesions, most early clinical reviews of vulvar melanoma concluded that radical vulvectomy and bilateral groin dissection (including deep pelvic nodes) were required for adequate surgical treatment.[39] However, on the basis of retrospective observations mainly from individual small clinical reports, surgeons subsequently have largely abandoned such extensive and mutilating resections. In a prospective study of 81 patients, the Gynecologic Oncology Group concluded that the biologic behavior of vulvar melanoma is similar to that of nongenital cutaneous melanoma.[40] Although the study was not designed to evaluate various surgical approaches, it suggested that the more conservative guidelines that had been developed for cutaneous lesions could probably be safely extended to patients with vulvar melanoma. Two subsequent reviews of more than forty separate clinical reports increased the suspicion that radical vulvectomy does not improve survival when compared to more limited resection.[41,42] The largest clinical series reported to date has confirmed the fact that treatment modality is not a significant predictor of survival.[43]

As with the management of cutaneous melanoma, therefore, current guidelines for definitive surgical treatment of primary vulvar melanoma include local excision with 1-cm margins for lesions ≤ 1 mm thick and 2-cm margins for those 1 to 4 mm thick.[44] Simultaneous elective lymphadenectomy is not indicated, and the need for lymph node dissection is determined by SLN mapping and biopsy (see Chapter 11).

MANAGEMENT OF REGIONAL LYMPH NODES

Historical Perspectives

Whether or not elective (prophylactic) resection of the lymph nodes that drain the primary melanoma site should be recommended as part of the initial surgical procedure has been the most controversial issue surrounding the treatment of this malignancy for years. The major argument favoring elective lymph node dissection (ELND) was based upon retrospective observations indicating that survival of patients whose ELND revealed microscopically positive nodes consistently exceeded, by 20 to 40 percent, the survival of patients whose nodes were not removed until they had become clinically suspicious (Table 10–4).[45–50] These clinical reviews seemed to indicate that deferring removal of the nodes until the micrometastatic deposits became clinically evident significantly diminished the possibility of cure for patients who had harbored undetectable nodal disease when they initially presented for treatment. Proponents of the divergent viewpoint emphasized the unreliability of retrospective clinical studies, in which surgical bias in patient selection is difficult to assess. After decades of such disagreement, definitive surgical recommendations were expected to finally result from four prospective randomized trials that were eventually conducted.

Controlled Clinical Trials

The first report, reviewing 553 patients in the WHO Melanoma Group Study, concluded that delayed removal of involved lymph nodes (ie, after they become clinically detectable) is as effective for disease control as immediate dissection.[51] The preliminary results of the Mayo Clinical Trial seemed to confirm this conclusion.[52] However, both of these trials were immediately challenged as having troubling flaws. The major criticism of the Mayo Clinical Trial was that it included patients with minimally invasive primary lesions (two-thirds were < 1.5 mm thick). As a result, only 6.4 percent of patients undergoing ELND had microscopically positive nodes, in contrast to the 20 to 25 percent incidence in most other reports. Issues raised regarding the WHO study included (1) the unavailability of pathologic material suitable for thickness measurements in 44 percent of

the patients, (2) the disproportionate ratio (4.5:1) of female to male patients, (3) the unusually high proportion (1:1) of nodular to superficial spreading melanoma, and (4) the unexpectedly low 5-year survival rate (37%) for patients with microscopic disease discovered at the time of ELND.[53,54]

A subsequent WHO-sponsored surgical trial randomly assigned 252 patients with trunk lesions thicker than 1.5 mm to wide local excision (WLE) alone or WLE plus ELND.[55] Overall patient survival at 5 years was not significantly different in the two groups (51.3 vs 61.7 percent, respectively). However, as in the earlier retrospective studies (see Table 10–4), the removal of node metastases only after they became clinically evident was found to result in a significant disadvantage as compared to the outcome in patients with histopathologically positive nodes removed at ELND (5-year survival was 26.6 and 48.2 percent, respectively). The authors concluded that earlier node dissection does offer a survival benefit but (not unexpectedly) only for patients with metastases. Thus, diagnostic approaches more sensitive than clinical examination for detecting occult nodal metastases are required. As discussed elsewhere in this volume, such approaches have become available with the development of SLN mapping (see Chapter 11) and more extensive histopathologic, immunopathologic, and even molecular assessment of the biopsied nodal material.[56,57]

The recently updated Intergroup Melanoma Trial included 740 patients with melanomas between 1 and 4 mm thick who had been randomly assigned to either WLE or WLE plus ELND.[58] With a 10- to 15-year follow-up available, there was again no significant overall survival difference between the two groups. However, the investigators now report that for each of the stratified variables studied (eg, ulcerated primary lesion), a significant improvement in survival was provided by ELND. They therefore concluded that the benefits of early surgical removal of nodal micrometastases had been conclusively demonstrated for these subgroups of patients. This suggests that the pendulum had again moved back in favor of ELND, at least for high-risk patients selected on the basis of pathologic criteria. However, even this more selective approach would require complete lymphadenectomy in a significant propor-

Table 10–4. RETROSPECTIVE STUDIES OF 5-YEAR SURVIVAL: ELECTIVE VERSUS THERAPEUTIC NODE DISSECTION

Patients Reviewed	ELND* (%)	Therapeutic† (%)	Reference
87	60	10	45
335	52	19	46
243	59	22	47
306	30	10	48
150	62	20	49
482	38	17	50

ELND = elective lymph node dissection.
*Pathologically positive.
†Clinically positive.

tion of patients who prove to have no micrometas-tases (eg, 65 to 70 percent of patients with primary tumor ulceration).

Fortunately, SLN biopsy has changed the stan-dard of care for melanoma patients, so that the entire controversy regarding ELND can finally be dis-missed. Only "early therapeutic" node dissection for metastatic disease documented by SLN biopsy is currently recommended.[59] Although there continues to be some disagreement regarding the minimal thickness of the primary lesion for which SLN biopsy is appropriate, the most widely accepted cur-rent surgical guidelines advise this procedure for primary lesions > 1 mm thick. Most centers now rec-ommend that complete lymphadenectomy be per-formed in all patients with micrometastases in the pathologically examined SLN. With further experi-ence, this recommendation could change as some reviews are beginning to indicate that the micrometastatic disease may be confined to the SLN in patients with thin primary lesions.[60]

Surgical Techniques

Detailed descriptions of the surgical procedures required for complete regional lymphadenectomy are beyond the scope of this text but are available in a number of excellent reviews.[61] The following brief comments outline some important guidelines and considerations for each of the nodal basins that typ-ically require resection. In every case, the SLN biopsy incision should be placed in the same line as that required for definitive node dissection, so that the previous surgical wound plus the underlying nodes can be removed en bloc without entering the SLN dissection field.

Head and Neck Dissections

The major morbidity of nodal resection in the head and neck region results from the cosmetic and func-tional consequences of removing nonlymphatic struc-tures that are normally sacrificed in a radical neck dissection. Since the micrometastases of melanoma (identified by SLN biopsy) are presumed to be con-fined to the lymph nodes, radical neck dissection is seldom if ever indicated in the primary surgical man-

agement of these patients. Therefore, the most com-monly recommended procedures are either a modi-fied (functional) neck dissection or a selective dissec-tion. The former, as in the radical procedure, includes removal of the nodes from all five neck levels (com-prehensive dissection) but preserves important struc-tures such as the sternocleidomastoid muscle, the internal jugular vein, and the spinal accessory nerve. In contrast, selective dissection excludes node removal from one or more of the five neck levels. For example, since primary lesions of the anterior face or neck seldom drain to the posterior cervical triangle, the surgical resection would include parotidectomy plus dissection of only the submental, the upper, and the middle jugular node groups. In the case of poste-rior head and neck lesions, on the other hand, all jugu-lar nodes plus the posterior triangle and occipital groups should be removed, with preservation of the spinal accessory nerve and with no need for parotid and submental dissection.[62]

Axillary Dissection

It must be emphasized that the rationale and thus the technique of axillary node dissection for breast can-cer patients is different from that for melanoma patients with a positive SLN biopsy. The objective with breast cancer patients is to provide tissues for accurate pathologic staging, which then defines the combination of therapeutic agents that will best con-trol both local and systemic disease. In this circum-stance, only axillary sampling of level I (lateral to the pectoralis minor) and II (behind the pectoralis minor) nodes is required. In contrast, the goal with melanoma patients is to surgically eradicate the local and regional disease. Thus, complete axillary lymphadenectomy, including the level III (highest) axillary nodes, must be accomplished.

This dissection is approached through a trans-verse or gently curved incision extending between the anterior and posterior axillary folds and incorpo-rating the previous biopsy site. To limit postopera-tive disability ("winged scapula"), the long thoracic nerve should always be preserved. Similarly, at least one of the anterior thoracic nerves must be retained to prevent atrophy of the pectoralis major muscle. The intercostal brachial nerve and even the thoracodorsal nerve can be resected with little consequence. The highest axillary nodes can usually be reached by medial and anterior retraction of the intact pectoralis minor muscle while the arm is adducted over the chest. Only in particularly muscular individuals is it necessary to detach the pectoralis minor insertion from the coracoid process. Postoperative wound catheter suction drainage is continued until the daily output is less than 30 cc. This usually occurs within 10 to 14 days, but a longer period may be required, especially in older individuals. Premature removal of the drain results in subcutaneous seroma formation that often requires repeated needle aspirations.

Groin Dissection

Groin dissection can be associated with considerable immediate and long-term morbidity.[63,64] The incidence of the more commonly encountered immediate complications has been reported to be as high as 15 to 18 percent for lymphocele or lymphorrhea, 10 to 15 percent for wound infection, 8 to 10 percent for skin edge necrosis, and 5 to 30 percent for venous thromboembolic disease. Persistent lymphedema requiring chronic control measures has been observed in 5 to 10 percent of patients.

To limit this morbidity, several technical and perioperative management approaches are recommended. First, the extent of the resection should almost always be confined to the superficial (inguinal) nodes for those patients with clinically undetectable disease. The most proximal node removed (Cloquet's node) at the femoral canal can be pathologically assessed by frozen section intraoperatively; the procedure is then extended to an ilioinguinal (deep) dissection only on the rare occasions when this node contains micrometastases.

Second, the sartorius muscle can be detached from its origin at the anterior iliac spine and transposed medially to prevent exposure of the femoral vessels should subsequent necrosis of the overlying skin flaps occur.

Third, approximately 1 to 2 cm of both skin flaps at the central portion of the incision should be excised during wound closure to remove any traumatized or ischemic tissue that is marginally viable.

Fourth, although the value of routine anticoagulation remains controversial, with some studies suggesting a benefit[65] and others suggesting no benefit or even an increased risk of complications,[63] many surgeons recommend perioperative low-dose subcutaneous heparin prophylaxis for these patients. In this author's experience, heparin has been safely administered, and no clinically detected thromboembolic episodes have occurred in over 150 consecutive patients undergoing groin dissection since this practice was instituted.

Finally, preventive measures should be taken against chronic lymphedema, perhaps the most dreaded nonmalignant complication of groin dissection and (even) SLN biopsy[66] (Figure 10–9). Patients with chronic lymphedema must deal with a variety of special problems ranging from the annoying (different shoe size, decreased exercise tolerance, increased swelling during air travel) to the more serious (skin breakdown) and even life-threatening episodes (recurrent cellulitis). Preventive measures should be instituted in the immediate postoperative period. These include aggressive treatment of wound complications to limit the development of fibrosis, elevation of the extremity, and soft-tissue compression (usually with preoperatively fitted elastic garments).

For patients who had already developed significant chronic swelling (as depicted in Figure 10–9), Ko and colleagues have found pneumatic pumping devices and surgical procedures to be ineffective and even harmful.[67] An aggressive noninterventional program of physical therapy, nocturnal bandaging, daytime stocking compression, and meticulous skin care, however, can provide significant long-term improvement in over 80 percent of these individuals (Figure 10–10).

Aberrant Nodal Basins

Interestingly, nodal metastases from distal-extremity primary melanomas present infrequently in the popliteal or epitrochlear basins. Although one report suggested that as many as 18 percent of patients with upper-extremity lesions develop epitrochlear nodal metastases,[68] this is not the common experience. A review of 801 Australian patients with upper-extremity lesions defined an incidence of 1.1

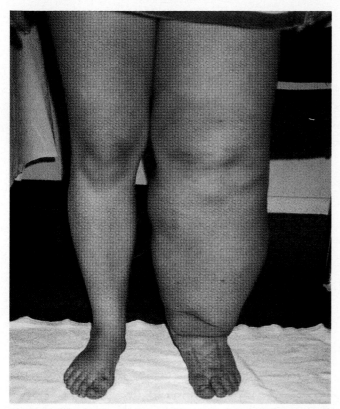

Figure 10–9. Secondary lymphedema of the leg after previous femoral and deep iliac lymph node dissection for a level III melanoma of the foot.

percent for epitrochlear nodal metastases,[69] and popliteal node involvement (except in patients with extensive lower-limb recurrences) remains anecdotal in usual reports. Most surgeons, therefore, advise that routine clearance of these nodal regions at the time of axillary or groin dissection is not indicated.

RECURRENT MELANOMA

Approximately 30 to 35 percent of patients treated for primary melanoma will eventually develop recurrent disease. Most treatment failures appear within the first 10 years following the initial diagnosis, but 1 to 6 percent of patients develop their first recurrence even later,[70–72] thus emphasizing the need for prolonged follow-up. In a review co-written by the author, 77 percent of the patients with metastatic melanomas initially presented with recurrences in lymph nodes or nonvisceral soft tissues.[73] This emphasizes that regularly scheduled physical examination is the most effective follow-up for patients after treatment for primary cutaneous melanoma. In

practice, most recurrences are symptomatic or patient detected; thus, these individuals must be instructed on the importance of promptly bringing any newly observed masses, pigmented lesions, or symptoms to the attention of their physician. Multiple laboratory studies and radiologic examinations are less likely to be useful in detecting recurrent melanoma in asymptomatic patients. In addition to sequential physical examinations, the Massachusetts General Pigmented Lesion Clinic routinely recommends only annual chest radiography; more extensive radiologic evaluations are reserved for unexplained symptoms.

With aggressive treatment, a significant proportion of these patients can achieve long-term disease-free survival, sometimes even after multiple recurrences at distant sites. When feasible, complete surgical excision of all resectable metastases offers the greatest likelihood for cure or prolonged palliation.[73–76] Recognition of the natural history of metastatic melanoma is therefore essential if the surgeon is to provide appropriate recommendations for the ongoing care of these patients.

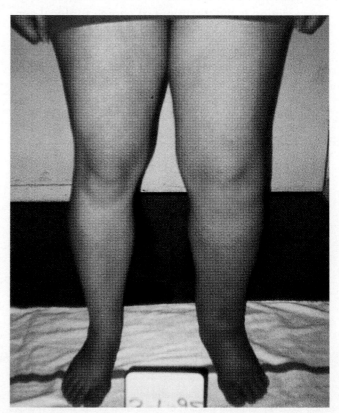

Figure 10–10. Same patient as shown in Figure 10–9, after decongestive physiotherapy and compressive bandaging.

The site of first recurrence is influenced by the stage of disease and the extent of surgery at the time of primary treatment. In a review of 231 patients with metastatic melanoma, recurrence first appeared in regional nodes in 41 percent, in nonvisceral soft tissues in 36 percent, and in viscera in 23 percent of those studied.[73] Obviously, the likelihood of regional node recurrence depends partly upon whether or not complete lymphadenectomy has been performed as part of the original melanoma treatment.

The overall risk for local recurrence (ie, within 3 to 4 cm of the definitive excision site) is quite low, such recurrences being reported in less than 5 percent of patients.[18] The majority of these recurrences appear during the first 5 years following the initial surgical excision although later recurrences are not uncommon, particularly for thinner primary lesions. If the recurrence is truly local (contiguous with the previous surgical site), wide surgical resection can be expected to provide highly effective control in the majority of patients.[77] The prognosis for other "local" recurrences is more grave, since the appearance of these true satellite metastases is strongly associated with regional and distant disease.[73] Surgical resection is the treatment of choice for local control unless the extent of the disease (Figures 10–11 and 10–12) requires a more complex approach, such as isolated regional perfusion.

Treatment by Regional Chemotherapy

Chemotherapy by isolated hyperthermic regional perfusion to control cancer of the limbs was first

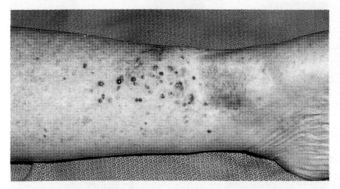

Figure 10–11. Extensive intracutaneous metastases 3 years after wide excision and skin grafting of melanoma of the ankle. Multiple previous recurrences had been treated by resection, intralesional bacille Calmette-Guérin (BCG), and local irradiation.

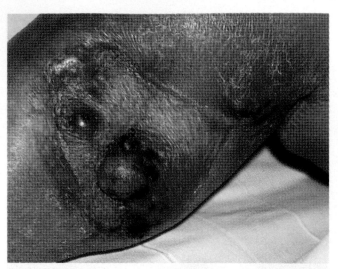

Figure 10–12. Bulky local recurrences of melanoma of the calf after radical resection and skin grafting for a level V melanoma.

described more than 40 years ago.[78] This approach was devised to obtain the maximum tumoricidal effect with minimal systemic toxicity. The procedure requires surgical isolation of the major artery and the venous drainage supplying the area, so that an oxygenated, heated, extracorporeal circuit can deliver the therapeutic agent to the tumor-bearing region (Figure 10–13).

The most commonly used chemotherapeutic agent is L-phenylalanine mustard (L-PAM, or melphalan), which is typically infused over a period of 60 to 90 minutes for control of nonresectable metastases that are clinically limited to an extremity. Dacarbazine (DTIC), cisplatin, nitrogen mustard, and thiotepa, alone or in combination, have proved to be less effective than melphalan.[79] Some trials show that a combination of high-dose cytokines (such as tumor necrosis factor and interferon-γ) plus melphalan may be even more effective than melphalan alone.[80]

Retrospective studies have documented objective response rates of up to 80 percent in measurable lesions[81] (Figures 10–14 and 10–15). Five-year survival rates as high as 55 percent and 15-year survival rates of over 20 percent have been reported even in patients with the worst prognosis—that is, those with extensive nodal and soft-tissue involvement.[81,82]

Despite careful efforts to isolate the perfusion to the extremity, there is inevitable systemic leakage, so that these patients usually experience 12 to 24 hours of postoperative nausea, vomiting, and fever.

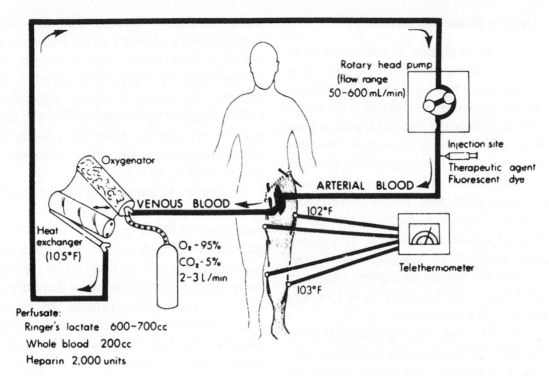

Figure 10–13. Flow diagram for isolated hyperthermic regional chemotherapy of lower-limb melanoma. The femoral or iliac artery and vein are surgically cannulated. A tourniquet is held around the root of the limb by Steinmann pins inserted at the iliac crest and pubic ramus. The limb is perfused with oxygenated heated blood by the arterial and venous cannulas connected to a heart-lung bypass circuit. Thermistor probes continuously monitor the subcutaneous temperature. Fluorescent dye is added to the circuit to confirm that there is no significant systemic leakage from the isolated limb. The perfusion is terminated by flushing the extremity with Ringer's lactate solution.

Leukopenia ($< 1,000$ neutrophils/mm^3) and thrombocytopenia ($< 100,000$ platelets/mm^3) typically reach a nadir at 10 to 12 days; patients then recover without treatment. Patients may also experience transient or persistent lymphedema, nerve dysfunction, lymph fistula, or venous/arterial thrombosis, which has been reported to lead to limb amputation in rare cases. Most important, inadequate isolation of the extremity can cause hypotension or shock, fatal leukopenia, or thrombocytopenia. Nevertheless, in the author's experience, isolated perfusion has been well tolerated and provides a method of local tumor control with limb preservation in most patients. Some studies suggest that the procedure also has a positive impact on overall survival by "sterilizing" the treated extremity and thereby limiting systemic metastases.[82]

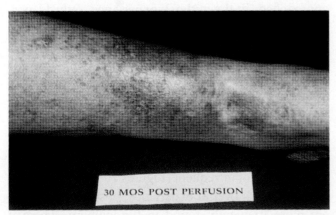

Figure 10–14. Same patient as shown in Figure 10–11, 30 months after hyperthermic regional perfusion with melphalan.

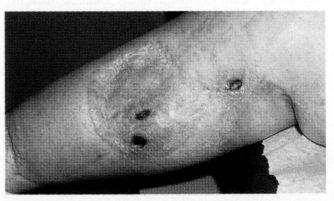

Figure 10–15. Same patient as shown in Figure 10–12, 3 months after hyperthermic regional perfusion. Even such massive recurrences can usually be controlled locally, so that amputation is rarely indicated.

Lymph Node Metastases

Approximately 10 to 30 percent of patients develop nodal recurrence in the regional drainage basin after a previous therapeutic lymphadenectomy.[83,84] Historically, the risk has been primarily related to the tumor burden in the nodes originally dissected, with an incidence as high as 33 percent if more than 10 nodes were positive.[84] As noted above, surgical guidelines have since evolved so that earlier therapeutic dissection is now being performed for micrometastatic node disease that has been detected by SLN biopsy at the time of initial melanoma treatment. It is hoped that the tumor burden in the resected tissues from these patients and the risk of subsequent relapse in the same nodal basin will thus prove to be less than that observed in earlier experience.

The risk of failure within the mapped nodal basin after negative SLN biopsy alone has not been established. After a relatively short-term follow-up (median, 24 to 36 months), 4 to 7 percent of patients have been reported to develop their first recurrence in a previously mapped negative SLN basin.[85,86] Retrospective re-examination by further serial sectioning or immunohistochemical staining of the SLN has revealed occult metastases in a significant proportion of these patients. With the routine use of these more sensitive pathologic studies, the incidence of "false-negatives" and thus of treatment failure in the sampled regional node basin is expected to be lower in future series.[57]

Since patients with nodal failure are at high risk for other metastases, they should undergo further radiologic staging, including a computed tomography (CT) scan or magnetic resonance imaging (MRI) of the brain, lungs, and abdomen. Primary lymphadenectomy or a more radical redissection of the basin is then indicated unless detection of other disease mandates systemic therapy. Some groups have recommended the addition of high-dose external beam radiation therapy to improve local control in patients with recurrent nodal metastases.[87]

Nodal Metastases with an Unknown Primary Lesion

Melanoma can occasionally become manifest as nodal metastases without any identifiable primary lesion or history of tumor removal although such manifestation is unusual. In the Massachusetts General Pigmented Lesion Clinic experience, this occurs in approximately 4 percent of all newly presenting patients. The axilla is most frequently involved (47%), followed by the neck (29%) and groin (24%) nodes.[88] Presumably, either the primary lesion has regressed spontaneously or the melanoma has arisen de novo within the lymph node.

In addition to undergoing careful clinical examination for a possible primary lesion or for a site of previous "mole" regression or excision, these patients should undergo radiologic staging. In most instances, systemic disease is not identified, and complete lymphadenectomy is therefore indicated. Survival rates for these patients are the same as, or even somewhat better than, those observed in patients with clinically positive nodes and a known primary site.[89,90] Therefore, the surgical guidelines and anticipated outcome for patients presenting with nodal metastases without an identifiable primary lesion should be the same as those outlined above for the more commonly seen patients with lymph node metastases and known primary lesions.

Visceral Metastases

Melanoma can metastasize to virtually any organ or tissue. The median survival for patients with visceral metastases is only 7 to 9 months.[73] Nevertheless, many individuals present with symptomatic metastases well before the terminal stages of their disease, and they deserve aggressive attempts to excise all identified metastases that can be reasonably approached. In the author's experience, only 11 percent of these patients achieved long-term survival; however, for the subset in whom complete surgical excision of visceral lesions was possible, a 5-year survival rate of 25 percent was noted.[73] Others have reported similar observations.[91,92]

Gastrointestinal metastases, typically presenting with anemia and occult bleeding (Figure 10–16) or symptoms of intermittent obstruction due to intussusception, are not infrequent (Figures 10–17 and 10–18). In the author's overall experience, obstructing lesions are more frequently found in the jejunum, where it may be necessary to resect one or more bulky lesions

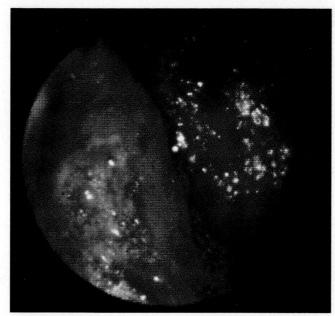

Figure 10–16. Endoscopic view of gastric mucosal metastasis from previously treated cutaneous melanoma of the back. The patient presented with chronic anemia and guaiac-positive stools but negative radiologic studies.

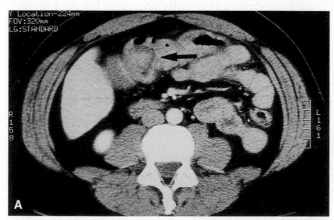
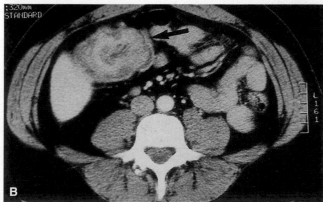

Figure 10–17. Computed body tomography of abdomen performed for the evaluation of symptoms of intermittent bowel obstruction in a patient with previously resected cutaneous melanoma. Intussusception of a right colonic lesion at the hepatic flexure (*black arrows*) is evident.

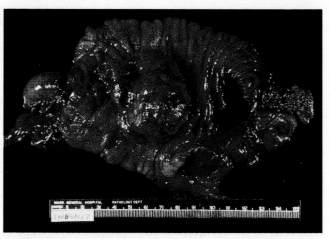

Figure 10–18. Resected right-colon mucosal metastasis from the same patient shown in Figure 10–17. The patient remains alive and well more than 2 years after this surgery.

(that serve as the lead point of the intussusceptum) together with adjacent mesenteric nodes (Figure 10–19). The operative morbidity and mortality rates are generally very low, and the complete resection of gross disease is associated with prolonged survival in approximately 20 percent of patients.[93,94]

Extended survival can similarly be achieved after aggressive resection of stage IV melanoma deposits in the adrenal gland,[95,96] lung,[97,98] and even brain.[99,100] However, patients with hepatic metas-

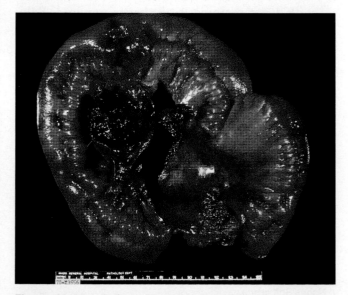

Figure 10–19. Excised jejunum, containing multiple mucosal lesions and extensive nodal metastases from melanoma of the scalp. The patient presented with melena and symptoms of partial bowel obstruction. Excellent palliation of the gastrointestinal symptoms was achieved for almost 2 years before the patient expired with multiple intracranial metastases.

Table 10–5. SURGICAL GUIDELINES FOR INITIAL MANAGEMENT OF CUTANEOUS MELANOMA

Depth of Primary Lesion (mm)	Surgical Margin (cm)	Perform SLN Biopsy	Perform Lymphadenectomy	Expected 5-yr Survival (%)
≤ 1.0	1.0	No	No	98
1.0–4.0	2.0	Yes		
		Negative	No	70–85
		Positive	Yes	30–55
> 4.0	> 2.0	Yes		
		Negative	No	25–50
		Positive	Yes	10–30

SLN = sentinal lymph node.

tases continue to have a dismal prognosis. Except in rare cases in which a solitary lesion is detected, surgical resection of liver metastases is not beneficial and should not be considered.

SUMMARY

The current guidelines for the surgical management of cutaneous melanoma (summarized in Tables 10–5 and 10–6) are as follows:

1. Excisional biopsy of the suspicious lesion, with minimal margins of surrounding normal skin, is the preferred approach for definitive diagnosis.
2. For patients with biopsy-proven melanoma less than 1 mm thick, re-excision of the biopsy site with 1-cm margins is all that is required. Excision of the muscle fascia beneath the primary site is unnecessary.
3. For lesions between 1 and 4 mm in thickness, a 2-cm re-excision is adequate. Intraoperative SLN mapping and biopsy should also be performed.
4. For patients with lesions more than 4 mm thick, a re-excision margin of more than 2 cm is appropriate if anatomically feasible. Intraoperative SLN mapping and biopsy should also be performed.
5. Completion lymphadenectomy of the nodal basin where biopsy was performed is indicated for patients with micrometastases identified in the SLN. The dissection at this early stage should be less extensive than that required for later recurrences. Modified (functional) dissection or selective dissection is usually adequate for neck nodes, as is superficial groin dissection for ileofemoral nodes. Iliac dissection should be reserved for patients with metastases in Cloquet's node.[101]
6. Local recurrences should be excised if possible. Extensive in-transit metastases limited to an extremity can be effectively managed with isolated limb perfusion.
7. Lymph node metastases that become clinically evident after primary treatment or whose primary site is unknown should be resected by radical lymphadenectomy.
8. Limited distant metastatic disease in almost any organ except the liver should be considered for surgical resection.

Table 10–6. SURGICAL GUIDELINES FOR MANAGEMENT OF RECURRENT MELANOMA

Metastasis	Therapy	Reported 5-yr Survival (%)
Local		
Resectable	Excision	30–80
Unresectable	Isolated perfusion	15–55
Nodes/Soft tissue		
Resectable	Excision	10–45
Unresectable	Biochemo Rx ± irradiation	5–15
Visceral		
Resectable	Excision (except if hepatic)	5–25
Unresectable	Biochemo Rx	< 5

REFERENCES

1. Handley WS. The pathology of melanotic growths in relation to their operative treatment. Lancet 1907; 1:927–33, 996–1003.
2. Lee YTN. Diagnosis, treatment and prognosis of early melanoma: the importance of depth of microinvasion. Ann Surg 1980;191:87–96.
3. Adam YG, Efron G. Cutaneous malignant melanoma: current views on pathogenesis, diagnosis, and surgical management. Surgery 1983;93:481–94.
4. Clark WH, From L, Bernardino EA, Mihm MC. The

histogenesis and biologic behavior of primary human malignant melanoma of the skin. Cancer Res 1969;29:705–26.

5. Breslow A. Tumor thickness, level of invasion, and node dissection in stage I cutaneous melanoma. Ann Surg 1975;182:572–5.

6. Breslow A, Macht SD. Optimal size of resection margin for thin cutaneous melanoma. Surg Gynecol Obstet 1977;145:691–2.

7. Balch CM, Murad TM, Soong S-J, et al. Tumor thickness as a guide to surgical management of clinical stage I melanoma patients. Cancer 1979;43:833–8.

8. Stehlin JS. Treatment of the primary lesion in melanoma. Surg Gynecol Obstet 1981;152(4):499–500.

9. Elder DE, Guerry DIV, Heiberger RM, et al. Optimal resection margin for cutaneous malignant melanoma. Plast Reconstr Surg 1983;71:66–72.

10. Cosimi AB, Sober AJ, Mihm MC, Fitzpatrick TB. Conservative surgical management of superficially invasive cutaneous melanoma. Cancer 1984;53:1256–9.

11. Kelly JW, Sagebiel RW, Calderon W, et al. The frequency of local recurrence and microsatellites as a guide to reexcision margins for cutaneous malignant melanoma. Ann Surg 1984;200:759–63.

12. Urist MM, Balch CM, Soong SJ, et al. The influence of surgical margins and prognostic factors predicting the risk of local recurrence in 3445 patients with primary cutaneous melanoma. Cancer 1985;65:1398–1402.

13. O'Rourke MGE, Altmann CR. Melanoma recurrence after excision: is a wide margin justified? Ann Surg 1993;217:2–5.

14. Milton GW, Shaw HM, McCarthy WH. Resection margins of melanoma. Aust N Z J Surg 1985;55:255–6.

15. Veronesi U, Cascinelli N, Adamus J, et al. Thin stage I primary cutaneous malignant melanoma: comparison of excision with margins of 1 or 3 cm. N Engl J Med 1988;318:1159–62.

16. Veronesi U, Cascinelli N. Narrow excision (1-cm margin): a safe procedure for thin cutaneous melanoma. Arch Surg 1991;126:438–41.

17. Balch CM, Urist MM, Karakousis CP, et al. Efficacy of 2-cm surgical margins for intermediate-thickness melanomas (1 to 4 mm). Ann Surg 1993;218:262–9.

18. Karakousis CP, Balch CM, Urist MM, et al. Local recurrence in malignant melanoma: long-term results of the multiinstitutional randomized surgical trial. Ann Surg Oncol 1996;3:446–52.

19. Ringborg U, Andersson R, Eldh J, et al. Resection margins of 2 versus 5 cm for cutaneous malignant melanoma with a tumor thickness of 0.8 to 2.0 mm: randomized study by the Swedish Melanoma Study Group. Cancer 1996;77:1809–14.

20. Heaton KM, Sussman JJ, Gershenwald JE, et al. Surgical margins and prognostic factors in patients with thick (> 4 mm) primary melanoma. Ann Surg Oncol 1998;5:322–8.

21. Olsen G. Removal of fascia—cause of more frequent metastases of malignant melanomas of the skin to regional lymph nodes? Cancer 1964;17:1159–64.

22. Kenady DE, Brown BW, McBridge CM. Excision of underlying fascia with a primary malignant melanoma: effect on recurrence and survival rates. Surgery 1982;92:615–8.

23. Lingam MK, McKay AJ, Mackie RM, Aitchison T. Single-centre prospective study of isolated limb perfusion with melphalan in the treatment of subungual malignant melanoma. Br J Surg 1995;82:1343–5.

24. Finley RK, Quinn MJ, Thompson JE, et al. Subungual melanoma of the hand. J Hand Surg [Am] 1996; 21:506–11.

25. Finley RK, Driscoll DL, Blumenson LE, Karakousis CP. Subungual melanoma: an eighteen year review. Surgery 1994;116:96–100.

26. Tseng JF, Tanabe KK, Gadd MA, et al. Surgical management of primary cutaneous melanomas of the hands and feet. Ann Surg 1997;225:544–53.

27. Close LG, Goepfert H, Ballantyne AJ, Jesse RH. Malignant melanoma of the scalp. Laryngoscope 1979;89:1189–96.

28. Garbe C, Buttner P, Bertz J, et al. Primary cutaneous melanoma: prognostic classification of anatomic location. Cancer 1995;75:2492–8.

29. Urist MM, Balch CM, Soong SJ, et al. Head and neck melanoma in 534 clinical stage I patients: a prognostic factors analysis and results of surgical treatment. Ann Surg 1984;200:769–75.

30. Quan SHQ. Anal and para-anal tumors. Surg Clin North Am 1978;58:591–603.

31. Abaas JS, Karakousis CP, Holyoke DE. Anorectal melanoma: clinical features, recurrence and patient survival. Int Surg 1980;65:423–6.

32. Pack GT, Oropeza R. A comparative study of melanoma and epidermoid carcinoma of the anal canal: a review of 200 melanomas and 29 epidermoid carcinomas (1930 to 1965). Dis Colon Rectum 1967;10:161–75.

33. Ross M, Pezzi C, Pezzi T, et al. Patterns of failure in anorectal melanoma. A guide to surgical therapy. Arch Surg 1990;125:313–6.

34. Slingluff CL, Vollmer RT, Seigler HF. Anorectal melanoma: clinical characteristics and results of surgical management in twenty-four patients. Surgery 1990;107:1–9.

35. Frank W, Kurban RS, Hoover HC Jr, Sober AJ. Anorectal melanoma. A case report and brief review of the literature. J Dermatol Surg Oncol 1992;18:333–6.

36. Roumen RM. Anorectal melanoma in the Netherlands. Eur J Surg Oncol 1996;22:598–601.

37. Thibault C, Sagar P, Nivatvongs S, et al. Anorectal

melanoma—an incurable disease? Dis Colon Rectum 1997;40:661–8.

38. Brady MS, Kavolius JP, Quan SH. Anorectal melanoma. A 64 year experience at Memorial Sloan-Kettering Cancer Center. Dis Colon Rectum 1995; 38:146–51.

39. Chung AF, Woodruff JM, Lewis JL. Malignant melanoma of the vulva. A report of 44 cases. Obstet Gynecol 1975;45:638–46.

40. Phillips GL, Bundy BN, Okagaki T, et al. Malignant melanoma of the vulva treated by radical hemivulvectomy. A prospective study of the Gynecologic Oncology Group. Cancer 1994;73:2626–32.

41. Dunton CJ, Kautzky M, Hanau C. Malignant melanoma of the vulva: a review. Obstet Gynecol Surv 1995;50:739–46.

42. Paniyzon RG. Vulvar melanoma. Semin Dermatol 1996;15:67–70.

43. Ragnarsson-Olding BK, Nilsson BR, Kanter-Lewensohn LR, et al. Malignant melanoma of the vulva in a nationwide, 25 year study of 219 Swedish females: predictors of survival. Cancer 1999;86:1285–93.

44. Trimble EL. Melanomas of the vulva and vagina. Oncology (Hungt) 1996;10:1017–23.

45. Lane N, Lattes R, Malm J. Clinicopathological correlations in a series of 117 malignant melanomas of the skin of adults. Cancer 1958;11:1025–43.

46. McNeer G, Das Gupta T. Prognosis in malignant melanoma. Surgery 1964;56:512–8.

47. Mundth ED, Guralnick EA, Raker JW. Malignant melanoma: a clinical study of 427 cases. Ann Surg 1965;162:15–28.

48. Gumport SL, Harris MN. Results of regional lymph node dissection for melanoma. Ann Surg 1974;179: 105–8.

49. Das Gupta TK. Results of treatment of 269 patients with primary cutaneous melanoma: a five-year prospective study. Ann Surg 1977;186:201–9.

50. Fortner JG, Woodruff J, Schottenfeld D, Maclean B. Biostatistical basis of elective node dissection for malignant melanoma. Ann Surg 1977;186:101–8.

51. Veronesi U, Adamus J, Bandiera DC, et al. Inefficacy of immediate node dissection in stage 1 melanoma of the limb. N Engl J Med 1977;297:627–30.

52. Sim FH, Taylor WF, Ivins JC, et al. A prospective randomized study of the efficacy of routine elective lymphadenectomy in management of malignant melanoma. Cancer 1978;41:948–56.

53. Goldsmith HS. The debate over immediate lymph node dissection in melanoma. Surg Gynecol Obstet 1979;149:403–5.

54. Balch CM. Surgical management of melanoma: results of prospective randomized trials. Ann Surg Oncol 1998;5:301–9.

55. Cascinelli N, Morabito A, Santinami M, et al. Immediate or delayed dissection of regional nodes in patients with melanoma of the trunk: a randomized trial. Lancet 1998;351:793–6.

56. Blaheta HJ, Ellwanger U, Schittek B, et al. Examination of regional lymph nodes by sentinel node biopsy and molecular analysis provides new staging facilities in primary cutaneous melanoma. J Invest Dermatol 2000;114:637–42.

57. Yu LL, Flotte TJ, Tanabe KK, et al. Detection of microscopic melanoma metastases in sentinel lymph nodes. Cancer 1999;86:617–27.

58. Balch CM, Soong S, Ross MI, et al. Long-term results of a multi-institutional randomized trial comparing prognostic factors and surgical results for intermediate thickness melanomas (1.0 to 4.0 mm). Ann Surg 2000;7:87–97.

59. Cascinelli N. WHO declares lymphatic mapping to be the standard of care for melanoma. Oncology 1999;13:288–90.

60. Joseph E, Brobeil A, Glass F, et al. Results of complete lymph node dissection in 83 melanoma patients with positive sentinel nodes. Ann Surg Oncol 1998;5:119–25.

61. Karakousis CP. Therapeutic node dissections in malignant melanoma. Ann Surg Oncol 1998;5:473–82.

62. Shah JP, Andersen PE. The impact of patterns of nodal metastasis on modifications of neck dissection. Ann Surg Oncol 1994;1:521–32.

63. Arbeit JM, Lowry SF, Line BR, et al. Deep venous thromboembolism in patients undergoing inguinal lymph node dissection for melanoma. Ann Surg 1981;194:648–55.

64. Karakousis CP, Driscoll DL, Rose B, Walsh DL. Groin dissection in malignant melanoma. Ann Surg Oncol 1994;1:271–7.

65. Kakkar VV, Corrigan TP, Fossard DP, et al. Prevention of fatal postoperative pulmonary embolism by low doses of heparin. Lancet 1977;1:567–9.

66. Wrone DA, Tanabe KK, Cosimi AB, et al. Lymphedema after sentinel lymph node biopsy for cutaneous melanoma. Arch Dermatol 2000;136:511–4.

67. Ko DSC, Lerner R, Klose G, Cosimi AB. Effective treatment of lymphedema of the extremities. Arch Surg 1998;133:452–8.

68. Smith TJ, Sloan GM, Baker AR. Epitrochlear node involvement in melanoma of the upper extremity. Cancer 1983;51:756–60.

69. Hunt JA, Thompson JF, Uren RF, et al. Epitrochlear lymph nodes as a site of melanoma metastasis. Ann Surg Oncol 1998;5:248–52.

70. Briele HA, Beattie CW, Ronan SG, et al. Late recurrence of cutaneous melanoma. Arch Surg 1983;118: 800–3.

71. Crowley NJ, Seigler HF. Late recurrence of malignant melanoma: analysis of 168 patients. Ann Surg 1990;212:173–7.

72. Tsao H, Cosimi AB, Sober AJ. Ultra-late recurrence

(15 years or longer) of cutaneous melanoma. Cancer 1997;79:2361–70.

73. Markowitz JS, Cosimi LA, Carey RW, et al. Prognosis after initial recurrence of cutaneous melanoma. Arch Surg 1991;126:703–8.

74. Overett TK, Shiu MH. Surgical treatment of distant metastatic melanoma: indications and results. Cancer 1985;56:1222–30.

75. Karakousis CP, Velez A, Driscoll BA. Metastasectomy in malignant melanoma. Surgery 1994;115:295–302.

76. Wong JH, Skinner KA, Kim KA, et al. The role of surgery in the treatment of nonregionally recurrent melanoma. Surgery 1993;113:389–94.

77. Brown CD, Zitelli JA. The prognosis and treatment of true local cutaneous recurrent malignant melanoma. Dermatol Surg 1995;21:285–90.

78. Creech O, Krementz ET, Ryan RF, Winblad JN. Chemotherapy of cancer: regional perfusion utilizing an extra-corporeal circuit. Ann Surg 1958;148: 616–32.

79. Thompson JF, Gianoutsos MP. Isolated limb perfusion for melanoma: effectiveness and toxicity of cisplatin compared with that of melphalan and other drugs. World J Surg 1992;16:227–33.

80. Bartlett DL, Ma G, Alexander HR, et al. Isolated limb reperfusion with tumor necrosis factor and melphalan in patients with extremity melanoma after failure of perfusion with chemotherapeutics. Cancer 1997;80:2084–90.

81. Krementz ET. Regional perfusion: current sophistication, what next? Cancer 1986;57:416–32.

82. Brobeil A, Breman C, Cruse CW, et al. Efficacy of hyperthermic isolated limb perfusion for extremity-confined recurrent melanoma. Ann Surg Oncol 1998;5:376–83.

83. Gadd MA, Coit DG. Recurrence patterns and outcome in 1019 patients undergoing axillary or inguinal lymphadenectomy for melanoma. Arch Surg 1992; 127:1412–6.

84. Calabro A, Singletary SE, Balch CM. Patterns of relapse in 1001 consecutive patients with melanoma nodal metastases. Arch Surg 1989;124:1051–5.

85. Gershenwald JE, Colome MI, Lee JE, et al. Patterns of recurrence following a negative SLN biopsy in 243 patients with stage I or II melanoma. J Clin Oncol 1989;16:2253–60.

86. Gadd MA, Cosimi AB, Yu J, et al. Outcome of patients with melanoma and histologically negative sentinel lymph nodes. Arch Surg 1999;134:381–7.

87. Strom EA, Ross MI. Adjuvant radiation therapy after axillary lymphadenectomy for metastatic melanoma: toxicity and local control. Ann Surg Oncol 1995; 2:455–9.

88. Evans GRD, Manson PN. Review and current perspectives of cutaneous malignant melanoma. J Am Coll Surg 1994;178:523–5.

89. Chang P, Knapper WH. Metastatic melanoma of unknown primary. Cancer 1982;49:1106–11.

90. Santini H, Byers RM, Wolf PF. Melanoma metastatic to cervical and parotid nodes from an unknown primary site. Am J Surg 1985;150:510–2.

91. Balch CM. Palliative surgery for stage IV melanoma: is it a primary treatment? Ann Surg Oncol 1999;6:623–4.

92. Barth A, Wanek LAS, Morton DL. Prognostic factors in 1,521 melanoma patients with distant metastases. J Am Coll Surg 1995;181:193–201.

93. Agrawal S, Yao TJ, Coit DG. Surgery for melanoma metastatic to the gastrointestinal tract. Ann Surg Oncol 1999;6:336–44.

94. Berger AC, Buell JF, Venzon D, et al. Management of symptomatic malignant melanoma of the gastrointestinal tract. Ann Surg Oncol 1999;6:155–60.

95. Branum GD, Epstein RE, Leight GS, Seigler HF. The role of resection in the management of melanoma metastatic to the adrenal gland. Surgery 1991;109: 127–31.

96. Haigh PI, Essner R, Wardlaw JC, et al. Long-term survival after complete resection of melanoma metastatic to the adrenal gland. Ann Surg Oncol 1999;6:633–9.

97. Gorenstein LA, Putnam JB, Balch CM, Roth J. Improved survival following resection of pulmonary metastases from malignant melanoma. Ann Thorac Surg 1991;52:204–10.

98. Tafra L, Dale PS, Wanek LA, et al. Resection and adjuvant immunotherapy for melanoma metastatic to the lung and thorax. J Thorac Cardiovasc Surg 1995;110:119–28.

99. Stevens G, Firth I, Coates A. Cerebral metastases from malignant melanoma. Radiother Oncol 1992;23: 185–91.

100. Patchell RA, Tibbs P, Walsh JW, et al. A randomized trial of surgery in the treatment of single metastases to the brain. N Engl J Med 1990;322:494–500.

101. Balch CM, Ross MI. Melanoma patients with iliac nodal metastases can be cured. Ann Surg Oncol 1999;6:230–1.

11

Lymphatic Mapping and Sentinel Lymph Node Biopsy

MICHELE A. GADD, MD
JENNIFER F. TSENG, MD
KENNETH K. TANABE, MD

HISTORY

Lymphatic mapping and sentinel lymph node biopsy are recent milestones in a lengthy evolution in cancer treatment. In general, therapeutic lymphadenectomy is performed in patients with melanoma when there is either high clinical suspicion or pathologic evidence for metastases in regional lymph nodes. Elective lymph node dissection (ELND) in the absence of clinically apparent metastases has been promoted since the nineteenth century;[1] a lively debate has ensued since then. Elective lymph node dissection has been advocated both as a staging procedure and as a possible therapeutic maneuver to prevent the stepwise progression of primary melanoma to distant disease via regional nodes. Although retrospective studies have demonstrated a survival benefit in patients managed with ELND compared to delayed therapeutic lymph node dissection,[2] prospective randomized trials have not been as convincing.[3]

Donald Morton and his colleagues at the John Wayne Cancer Institute first proposed lymphatic mapping as a procedure with lower morbidity than ELND for the treatment of patients with melanoma. Lymphatic mapping is based on the premise that primary melanoma will spread via lymphatic channels to the sentinel node or nodes before reaching the other lymph nodes in the nodal basin. In 1977, Morton's group used lymphoscintigraphy to identify the nodal basin to which truncal skin melanoma might spread.[4] Subsequently, Morton and colleagues used blue dye to identify the sentinel node, the first lymph node in the lymphatic channel from primary tumor to nodal basin.[5] They reported successful sentinel node identification in 82 percent of reported cases and a 4 percent false-negative sentinel node biopsy rate.

Incorporation of radioisotope into the lymphatic mapping procedure further improved the rate of successful identification of the sentinel node. Krag and others introduced the use of gamma-probe-guided localization to identify the sentinel node in melanoma patients.[6,7] In a 1999 summary of clinical trials performed to date, Morton and colleagues found that sentinel nodes were identified in 82 to 100 percent of cases, the identified nodes being positive for tumor 15 to 26 percent of the time. The false-negative rate ranged from 0 to 2 percent in these studies.[8] Analysis of melanoma patient data collected by the John Wayne Cancer Institute demonstrated that an average patient with a tumor-positive sentinel node had tumor present in 30 percent of resected nonsentinel lymph nodes.[8]

The development of lymphatic mapping and sentinel lymphadenectomy has fostered a concurrent growth in the methods used for pathologic analysis. Complete lymph node dissection specimens are subject to pathologic understaging; when these relatively large specimens are analyzed by representative sectioning and hematoxylin-eosin staining, small or microscopic foci of tumor may be missed. The compact sentinel node specimens are amenable to complete examination by serial thin sectioning. Finally, the molecular analysis of specimens has increased the sensitivity of sentinel node biopsy.

Specific immunohistochemical stains for melanoma antigens have been developed, including stains for S-100[9] and HMB-45.[10]

At present, lymphatic mapping and sentinel lymphadenectomy are the subjects of intense interest and investigation for use in melanoma and other malignancies. The available data suggest that sentinel node biopsy, when performed by experienced operators with appropriate support, is a potent tool for identifying lymph node metastases in patients with melanoma.

PATIENT SELECTION AND INDICATIONS

The decision whether or not to recommend lymphatic mapping and sentinel lymph node biopsy to patients with melanoma cannot be summarized by a set of rules and guidelines. The decision for each and every patient is an individual one that reflects the balance between potential benefits and potential risks. There are at least five theoretic benefits from lymphatic mapping (Table 11–1): (1) elective lymph node dissection may enhance survival in a subset of patients with melanoma;[3] (2) more accurate staging allows therapy to be matched more accurately to stage of disease; (3) sentinel lymph node information provides patients, family, and physicians with a better understanding of the risk for recurrence;[11] (4) lymphatic mapping allows more rigorous evaluation techniques to be applied to one or two sentinel lymph nodes whereas it is not feasible or cost-effective to apply these techniques to all of the lymph nodes in a regional basin;[12] and (5) because sentinel lymph node analysis provides valuable prognostic information, this procedure improves the quality of many clinical trials for melanoma patients by reducing heterogeneity in the population of enrolled patients.

Balanced against these potential benefits are the costs and potential risks of the procedure. The cost of the procedure in monetary terms has not been well studied. The risks of the procedure are minimal

---

Table 11–1. BENEFITS OF LYMPHATIC MAPPING

1. Enhanced survival
2. More accurate staging
3. Better understanding of prognosis
4. Rigorous pathologic evaluation of the sentinel node
5. Improved quality of clinical trials

---

but present. A very small percentage of patients will experience minor complications, including wound infection, seroma, postoperative bleeding, neuropathic pain, or extremity edema.[11,13] Many melanoma excisions can be performed under local anesthesia. However, the addition of lymphatic mapping and sentinel lymph node biopsy to the procedure nearly always requires either intravenous sedation or general anesthesia. Nonetheless, nearly all lymphatic mapping and lymph node biopsy procedures can be performed in the outpatient setting.

At Massachusetts General Hospital, we recommend lymphatic mapping for patients who would be candidates for adjuvant therapy if they were diagnosed with American Joint Commission on Cancer (AJCC) stage III melanoma and who have at least a 5 percent statistical risk for occult regional lymph node metastases. This risk is calculated on the basis of tumor thickness, anatomic site, and the presence or absence of ulceration.[14] Accordingly, we recommend lymphatic mapping to patients whose primary melanomas are thicker than 1.0 mm although we also will recommend mapping to male patients whose melanomas are slightly thinner but are located on the trunk or are ulcerated. In rare situations, we recommend sentinel lymph node biopsy for patients whose primary tumors are of indeterminate biologic behavior, in which case the identification of metastatic melanoma in sentinel lymph nodes provides useful prognostic information (Table 11–2). We do not recommend lymphatic mapping and sentinel lymph node biopsy for patients who have already undergone definitive wide excision of their primary melanoma. It has recently been demonstrated that lymphatic mapping in patients who have undergone wide excision is less accurate than in those who have undergone only a biopsy of their melanoma, but that it can be applied cautiously in select circumstances.[15] Patients who have had a recent surgical procedure in the regional lymph node basin or in an anatomic site between the primary melanoma and regional lymph node basin are excluded from lymphatic mapping because the lymphatic pathways may have been altered. However, the accuracy of lymphatic mapping is probably not adversely affected when a surgical procedure affecting the lymphatic channels clearly predates the development of the melanoma. Finally,

Table 11–2. INDICATIONS FOR LYMPHATIC MAPPING			
Indications*			
Thickness	Sex	Site	Other
> 1 mm	M/F	Any	—
< 1 mm	M/F	Any	Ulcerated
< 1 mm	M/F	Any	Clark level IV
0.75 mm	M	Axial	—
	M/F	Any	Indeterminate biology

*No evidence of metastatic melanoma in regional lymph nodes or distant sites

Relative Contraindications
Age > 70 yr
Comorbidity
Previous wide local excision
Previous surgery in regional lymph node basin
Scar between primary tumor and lymph node basin

Absolute Contraindications
Pregnancy
Ocular melanoma
Mucous membrane melanoma
Allergy to isosulfan blue or technetium

the teratogenicity of vital blue dyes is unknown, and we therefore do not recommend lymphatic mapping, with or without isotope, to patients who are pregnant.

PREOPERATIVE LYMPHOSCINTIGRAPHY

Lymphoscintigraphy is performed to demonstrate primary lymphatic drainage. Lymphoscintigraphic images are particularly helpful for defining lymphatic drainage from melanomas located in axial (head, neck, trunk) sites with ambiguous lymphatic drainage. These images are also helpful for defining in-transit sentinel lymph nodes and sentinel lymph nodes residing in aberrant anatomic locations.

The radioisotope currently used in the United States for lymphatic mapping is technetium 99m–labeled sulfur colloid. Although technetium 99m–labeled antimony sulfide produces better lymphoscintigraphic images, it is not available in the United States (Table 11–3).[16] Technetium 99m has a short half-life (approximately 6 hours) and is a weak gamma emitter. Because of these properties, patients, staff, and family members receive only a negligible dose of radiation that poses no health risk.

Technetium 99m–labeled sulfur colloid should be freshly prepared; it is typically filtered prior to administration to restrict the range of particle sizes. If the

isotope is stored for more than 2 hours following preparation, it begins to clump, resulting in a larger particle size that may affect migration into the lymphatic system. The average dose is 9 to 18 MBq but may vary depending on the proximity of the lesion to the draining lymph node basin, to minimize background from the injection site. The isotope is typically prepared in a volume of 1.0 mL and injected intradermally through a 25-gauge needle around the center of the melanoma. When the lymphatic drainage from a small scar left from a biopsy of the melanoma is being mapped, the isotope is typically divided into four portions and injected into the dermis in four quadrants surrounding the scar. When mapping the lymphatic drainage of larger areas, it may be necessary to divide the total dose of isotope into more than four portions to permit a greater number of injections. To map the dermal lymphatics, it is important that the isotope be injected into the dermis instead of the subcutaneous tissue. Inadvertent injection into the subcutaneous tissue may result in the identification of an incorrect sentinel node or in the complete absence of isotope migration. The application of a topical anesthetic called EMLA (lidocaine/prilocaine) reduces the discomfort associated with this procedure and does not seem to affect the diffusion or migration of the isotope.

The patient is placed under a gamma camera immediately after the injection. The radioisotopically labeled colloid is rapidly transported to the regional lymph node basin by cutaneous lymphatics. Lymphoscintigraphic images are acquired sequentially to identify the primary drainage channels and sentinel lymph node locations. Multiple lymphatic channels may coalesce to a single channel and lead to a single lymph node (Figure 11–1). Alternatively, several

Table 11–3. REAGENTS FOR LYMPHATIC MAPPING		
Reagent	**Advantages**	**Disadvantages**
Isosulfan blue (lymphazurin 1%) Patent blue dye	Selectively picked up by lymphatic vessels	Stains skin 1.5% allergic reaction
Technetium 99m sulfur colloid	Filtered to 20-nm particles	Variable transit time
Technetium antimony trisulfide	Particle size 3–30 nm; optimal transit time	Not available in US
Human serum albumin	Uniform particle size	Rapid pass through

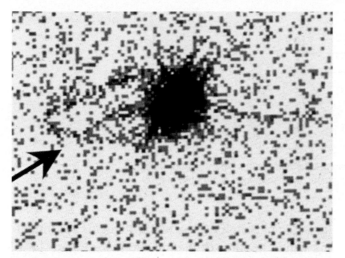

Figure 11-1. Lymphoscintigram of a patient with a melanoma of the leg, demonstrating lymphatic channels coalescing to a single channel leading to a sentinel lymph node.

channels may lead to separate individual lymph nodes in either a single basin or in multiple basins (Figure 11–2). If multiple nodes are identified in a single basin, it is usually not possible to determine whether some of the lymph nodes represent "secondary" lymph nodes rather than sentinel lymph nodes. In some patients, true "flow through" of the radiolabeled colloid from sentinel nodes to secondary nodes may occur. In other patients, an afferent lymphatic channel directs lymph flow to two separate lymph nodes that appear linked in "series" but are actually linked in "parallel." Lymphoscintigraphy cannot accurately distinguish between these two scenarios, even with the acquisition of multiple high-

resolution images sequentially. It is therefore prudent to assume that each of the radioactive lymph nodes identified on preoperative lymphoscintigraphic images represents a sentinel lymph node.

Because aberrant routes of lymphatic drainage exist with moderate frequency,[17–19] it is important to image all areas of the body. For example, the entire arm, axilla, and neck should be imaged following injection into an upper-extremity site[20] (Figure 11–3); the entire leg, pelvis, and trunk should be imaged followed injection into a lower-extremity site (Figure 11–4); and the entire neck and trunk should be imaged following injection into a truncal site (Figure 11–5). The patient should be scanned in multiple projections to accurately localize sentinel lymph nodes. Lateral views are important for the trunk and neck areas, to determine if the node is located in anterior or posterior cervical triangle, as well as in the groin, to determine if the node is in the superficial inguinal fossa or deep iliac fossa. If the basins are in different locations, more than one imaging session may be necessary, but this is unusual. Imaging the patient on a cobalt flood source nicely outlines the body contour and improves preoperative anatomic localization of sentinel lymph nodes.

OPERATIVE TECHNIQUE

Lymphatic mapping and sentinel lymph node biopsy are routinely performed as outpatient procedures. While the procedures can be performed under local

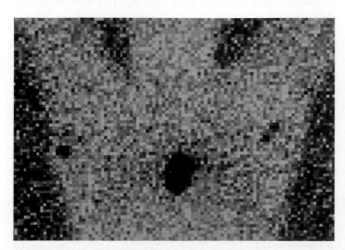

Figure 11-2. Lymphoscintigram of a patient with a melanoma located on the trunk, demonstrating lymphatic channels draining to both axilla, where the sentinel lymph nodes are visualized.

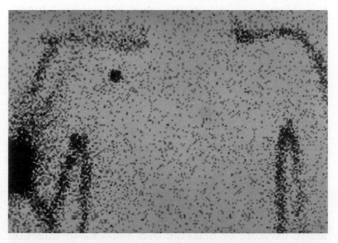

Figure 11-3. Lymphoscintigram of a patient with an upper extremity melanoma, demonstrating drainage to a sentinel node that is not in the axilla but was identified intraoperatively in the deltopectoral groove.

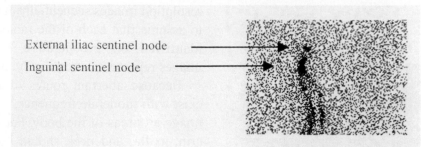

Figure 11–4.   Lymphoscintigram of a patient with a melanoma of the posterior thigh, demonstrating drainage to both superficial inguinal and deep inguinal lymph nodes.

anesthesia alone, patients are likely to be more comfortable if intravenous sedation is used in addition to local anesthesia. When lymphatic mapping requires dissection in the neck or dissection in more than one lymph node basin, patients are generally more comfortable under general anesthesia. A wide local excision of the primary melanoma and lymphatic mapping are generally performed during the same operation. Of importance, lymphatic mapping may not be accurate in patients who have already undergone a wide excision (≥ 1 cm of surgical margin) since lymphatic drainage patterns may be altered by definitive melanoma surgery.

Although some surgeons perform lymphoscintigraphy 1 day prior to the operation,[21] the radioisotope injection and lymphoscintigraphy can be performed on the same day as the operative procedure for patient convenience. The interval between isotope injection and sentinel lymph node biopsy can range from 30 minutes to 24 hours although the vast majority of surgeons perform the operation on the same day as the lymphoscintigraphy. In the operating room, 0.5 to 2.0 mL of lymphazurin is injected intradermally around the lesion in the same locations as the isotope (Figure 11–6, *A*). A Luer-Lok syringe with a 25- to 30-gauge needle is recommended for this injection. Use of a syringe with this type of lock rather than one with a sliplock reduces the chance of a disconnection between the needle hub and syringe during the injection, which can create relatively high pressures in the syringe. If treated immediately, isosulfan blue dye inadvertently spilled onto the skin can be easily removed with 70 percent ethanol. A few minutes of active exercise or massage over the area of injection enhances movement of the dye to the sentinel lymph node. The isosulfan blue dye is rapidly transported to

the sentinel lymph nodes, where it begins accumulating within minutes of the injection (see Figure 11–6, *B*). The dye begins to wash through the lymph nodes and fades within 20 to 40 minutes. In contrast, the radioactive signal in the sentinel lymph nodes remains for hours following the injection.

A handheld gamma probe (United States Surgical Corporation, Norwalk, CT; Care Wise Medical Product Corporation, Morgan Hill, CA; Neoprobe Corporation, Dublin, OH) is used to identify the location of the radioactive sentinel lymph nodes (Figure 11–7). A "hot spot" is defined as the area of skin through which the sentinel lymph node can be detected, using a handheld gamma probe. More than a single hot spot may be identified. When searching for radioactive lymph nodes, it is important not to direct the handheld probe directly toward the primary injection site. Gamma radiation penetrates through tissue, and radiation from the injection sites surrounding the primary melanoma will "shine through" and appear as a hot spot if the probe is directed toward the primary melanoma. A common

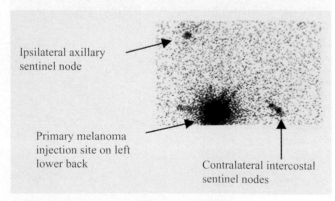

Figure 11–5.   Lymphoscintigram of a patient with a melanoma of the lower back, demonstrating drainage across the midline to an intercostal lymph node as well as to the ipsilateral axilla.

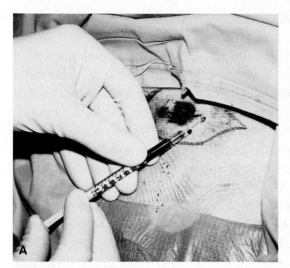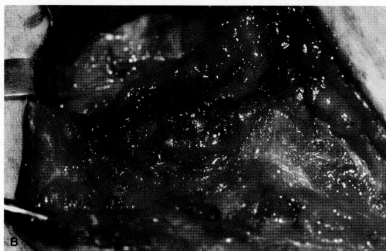

Figure 11–6. *A,* Intradermal injection of isosulfan blue in four quadrants around a scar left from an excisional biopsy of a melanoma. *B,* The dye begins to accumulate within minutes in the sentinel lymph node.

example of this error occurs when scanning the axilla in search of hot spots in a patient with a melanoma on the upper back. If the probe is inadvertently angled toward the primary melanoma, the radioactivity detected by the probe will simulate a hot spot. Shine-through from the primary tumor injection site can also obscure the sentinel node if the draining lymph node basin is very close to the injection site. If shine-through complicates accurate identification of the sentinel lymph node, it may be necessary to perform a wide local excision of the primary melanoma before searching for the sentinel lymph node. In such a case, the sentinel lymph nodes will no longer be stained blue when the time comes to identify them because of the relatively short retention time of isosulfan blue dye in sentinel lymph nodes. In most cases, fortunately, it is possible to identify the sentinel lymph node without first excising the primary injection site.

After the hot spot is identified, an incision is made over the sentinel lymph node, and the hand-held probe is used to direct dissection toward the radioactive sentinel lymph node. Avoiding extensive dissection and mobilization of flaps decreases postoperative pain and seroma formation and may also decrease the incidence of lymphedema. In most cases, surgical dissection is guided by both the gamma probe and the visualization of blue-stained lymphatic channels. With careful and bloodless dissection, blue lymphatic channels are identified and

followed to the sentinel lymph nodes. Sentinel lymph nodes have been defined as lymph nodes stained with blue dye or containing radioactivity. Most blue lymph nodes are radioactive; however, some radioactive lymph nodes are not stained blue.[22] Debate continues over the best definition of a sentinel lymph node[23] although most investigators treat all blue or radioactive lymph nodes as sentinel lymph nodes. During the dissection, lymphatic channels should be clipped or tied to reduce the risk of postoperative seroma formation. The sentinel node is dissected free from the surrounding tissues, and the level of radioactivity in the sentinel lymph

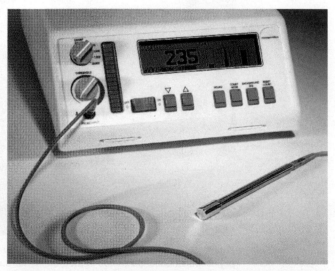

Figure 11–7. A handheld gamma probe manufactured by Neoprobe Corporation (Dublin, OH), together with a signal analyzer.

node is measured and recorded along with the level of radioactivity in the dissection bed following removal of the sentinel lymph node. Persistent radioactivity in the basin indicates that at least one additional sentinel lymph node is in the basin. In general, if the level of radioactivity in the dissection bed is at least 10 percent of the most radioactive sentinel lymph node, further dissection is recommended to search for an additional sentinel node. Since the level of radioactivity should return to background level following successful removal of all sentinel lymph nodes, one of the benefits of using the isotope is being able to verify that all of the sentinel nodes have been removed. Often, the sentinel node is adherent to another lymph node (sentinel or nonsentinel), and it may be easier to remove both nodes than to dissect the sentinel node free. The number of sentinel nodes removed typically ranges from 1 to 3 per lymph node basin.[7,11] The wound is then closed in layers without a drain, and a wide excision of the primary melanoma is performed (Figure 11–8).

If the sentinel lymph node is found to contain metastatic melanoma, it is reasonable to subsequently resect the remaining lymph nodes in the basin. Approximately 20 percent of patients with a sentinel lymph node that contains metastatic melanoma will harbor additional lymph nodes that contain metastatic melanoma in the same basin.[11] When an interval sentinel lymph node contains metastatic melanoma, the lymph node basin to which the interval node drains should be completely dissected. Axillary dissections can be limited to level 1 and level 2 lymph nodes; it is not necessary to resect level 3 lymph nodes unless gross metastatic disease is identified in the basin. For positive inguinal sentinel lymph nodes, a superficial groin dissection should be performed; further dissection of the iliac lymph nodes can be based on the results of intraoperative frozen-section analysis of Cloquet's node. If an iliac sentinel lymph node contains metastatic melanoma, it is reasonable to perform both superficial and deep (iliac) lymph node dissections. A complete functional neck dissection should be performed when sentinel nodes in the neck are found to contain

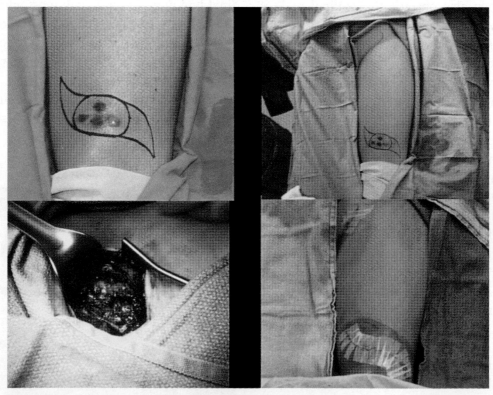

Figure 11–8. This patient has a melanoma just above the knee. After preoperative lymphoscintigraphy, isosulfan blue is injected intradermally, surrounding the scar from the melanoma biopsy. After harvesting the sentinel lymph node, the primary melanoma is widely excised, and the resulting defect is closed primarily.

metastatic melanoma. Although theoretic concern exists over the seeding of melanoma cells into the wound following resection of a sentinel lymph node, studies have demonstrated that the risk of a recurrence in a completely dissected basin is no greater when preceded by a sentinel lymph node biopsy.

ABERRANT PATTERNS OF LYMPHATIC DRAINAGE

Historically, the discussion of cutaneous lymphatic drainage patterns has been dominated by the tenets set forth by Sappey in the mid-nineteenth century[24] (Figure 11–9, *top*). Sappey's dictum that lymphatic drainage never crossed the midline was later amended to postulate 5-cm midline zones in which lymphatics could drain to either or both sides.[25] The relatively recent development of lymphatic mapping has necessitated a dramatic revision of these traditional views of lymphatic drainage, as lymphoscintigraphy in large numbers of patients has demonstrated significant differences from these previously described lymphatic drainage patterns[17,18,26] (Figure 11–9, *bottom*). Although a complete discussion of lymphatic drainage patterns revealed by lymphatic mapping is beyond the scope of this text, prominent findings are summarized below by anatomic location.

The Head and Neck

A substantial group of patients with head and neck melanoma will have aberrant lymphatic drainage. In 1994, Wells and colleagues reported that 84 percent of patients undergoing lymphoscintigraphy had lymphatic drainage inconsistent with clinical impression and historical anatomic patterns.[27] Using more liberal guidelines, O'Brien and colleagues found that 34 percent of lymphoscintigrams were discordant with clinical predications.[28] For example, patients with facial or anterior scalp lesions often showed unexpected drainage to postauricular, low cervical, and supraclavicular sentinel nodes. Thompson and colleagues from the Sydney Melanoma Unit emphasized this variability in their study of 261 patients with head and neck melanomas.[18] Drainage crossing the midline was observed in 15 percent of patients with scalp and face melanomas. Melanomas of the

base of the neck had exceptionally diverse drainage: lymphoscintigraphy demonstrated drainage to supraclavicular, cervical, axillary, triangular-intermuscular-space, interval, and suboccipital nodes.

The Trunk

Using lymphoscintigraphy, investigators from the Sydney Melanoma Unit reported novel patterns of

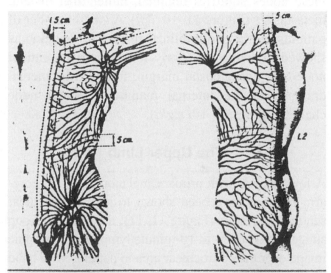

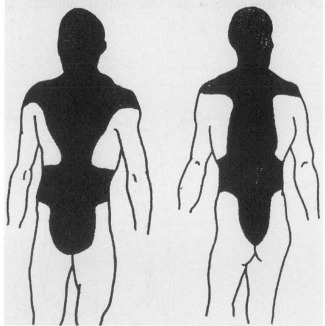

Figure 11–9. *Top*, Sappey's classic anatomic description of the cutaneous lymphatic flow. *Bottom*, Areas of ambiguous lymphatic flow as mapped by lymphoscintigraphy; note the expanded area of ambiguous lymphatic flow, including the entire head, neck, and shoulder (in black), compared with the anatomic drawing. (Reproduced with permission from Hung JC, Wiseman GA, Wahner HW, et al. Filtered technetium-99m-sulfur colloid evaluated for lymphoscintigraphy. J Nucl Med 1995;36:1895–901.)

lymphatic drainage of truncal melanomas. For some lesions of the posterior trunk, nonclassic drainage to lymph nodes in the triangular intermuscular space was noted; this drainage passed subsequently to second-tier nodes in the axilla.[29] Posterior trunk lesions were also found to drain anteriorly through the posterior thoracic or abdominal wall to paravertebral, para-aortic, or retroperitoneal nodes, with the clinical correlation that the presence of melanoma in these nodes signifies regional, rather than distant, metastasis[18] (Figure 11–10, *left*). A small number of patients with periumbilical primary melanomas showed drainage superiorly to an interval sentinel node over either costal margin, followed by medial drainage to the internal mammary lymph node chain[30] (Figure 11–10, *right*).

The Upper Limb

A few patients with primary melanomas on the forearm or hand have been shown to have epitrochlear sentinel nodes[31,32] (Figure 11–11); the Sydney group suggested that a 5- to 10-minute lymphoscintigraphic image over the epitrochlear area in patients with hand or forearm lesions may demonstrate drainage to epitrochlear sentinel nodes in 21 percent of patients.[18] Direct drainage from the forearm to interpectoral or supraclavicular nodes and to axillary nodes has been documented. Another patient had drainage from a lateral elbow lesion to an interval node on the medial arm; this was the only patient with an arm melanoma without a sentinel node in the axilla noted by Thompson and colleagues in their series. One patient with a melanoma located on the ipsilateral upper limb and who had previously undergone an axillary dissection for breast cancer was found to have a sentinel node in the contralateral axilla. A number of patients with upper-limb melanomas had direct drainage to neck or supraclavicular sentinel nodes.

The Lower Limb

Up to 20 percent of patients with lower-extremity melanomas studied by lymphoscintigraphy have aberrant lymphatic drainage, most commonly to sentinel nodes found in the popliteal fossa.[18,33] The Sydney group recommended a 5- to 10-minute scan over the popliteal fossa in all patients with leg melanomas; in the authors' own experience, however, sentinel lymph nodes are only rarely located in the popliteal fossa.

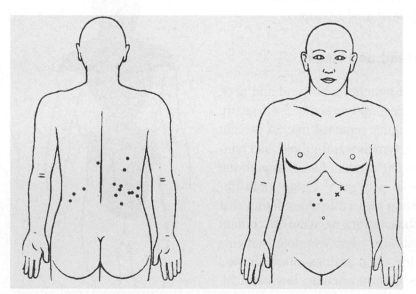

Figure 11–10.   *Left*, Posterior trunk melanoma sites that drained through the posterior body wall directly to retroperitoneal and paravertebral nodes. The majority of these sites also showed drainage to a groin or axillary node field, but there were three patients whose drainage was exclusively to such intra-abdominal nodes. *Right*, Anterior trunk melanoma sites that drained from periumbilical skin to interval nodes over the costal margin. (Reproduced with permission from Norman J, Cruse CW, Wells K, et al. A redefinition of skin lymphatic drainage by lymphoscintigraphy for malignant melanoma. Am J Surg 1991;162:432–7.)

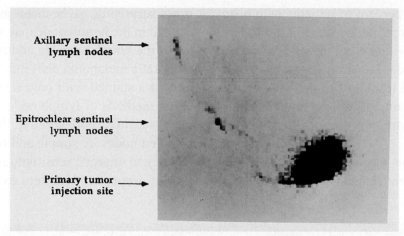

Figure 11–11. Lymphoscintigram of a patient with a melanoma of the forearm, demonstrating drainage to both epitrochlear and axillary lymph nodes.

Moreover, this site represents an extremely rare site of clinically apparent metastases. In contrast, many patients with lower-extremity melanomas will have sentinel lymph nodes located along the external iliac artery and vein in the pelvis (Figure 11–4). In a series from the Sydney Melanoma Unit, one patient who had a lower-extremity melanoma and who had undergone a previous ipsilateral node biopsy was found to have metastatic disease in a contralateral sentinel node.[18] This supports the notion that surgical intervention may cause further deviation of lymphatic anatomy from historically described patterns.

Interval nodes, while rare, provide a strong argument for systematic lymphatic mapping. These particular sentinel nodes can be identified in the deep subcutaneous fat layer at any location between a primary melanoma and a lymphatic basin. Frequent locations for interval nodes include the upper back, the upper arm, the midaxillary line on the lateral chest, the costal margin, and the posterior loin (Figure 11–5). Thompson and colleagues caution that the existence of interval nodes signifies that "hot" nodes located in traditional lymph node basins on occasion may in fact be second-tier nodes receiving drainage from the true interval sentinel nodes.[18]

In summary, lymphatic drainage patterns in patients with primary cutaneous melanomas show a remarkable diversity in a substantial number of patients. Knowledge of common variations is essential to perform accurate lymphatic mapping for melanoma staging and treatment.

ANALYSIS OF SENTINEL LYMPH NODES FOR OCCULT METASTASES

The frequency with which metastatic melanoma is identified in a lymph node is a function of the rigor of the analytic method used. The most commonly used technique involves bisection of the lymph node along its long axis, embedding of the two halves of the bivalved node, and hematoxylin-eosin (H+E) staining of a single section obtained from each half. Substantial data suggest that this technique fails to identify metastatic melanomas present in lymph nodes with relative frequency. For example, results of clinical trials in which patients were prospectively randomized to elective dissection versus observation of regional lymph node basins provided a group of patients in whom the accuracy of lymph node examination could be evaluated. In these trials, metastatic melanoma was identified in only about 20 percent of patients who were randomized to elective lymph node dissection, yet 22 to 37 percent of patients who were randomized to observation ultimately developed clinical evidence of regional lymph node metastases.[34,35] The magnitude of this discrepancy represents the fraction of patients that may be understaged using simple techniques of lymph node examination. Cell culture techniques have been used to improve the sensitivity of metastatic melanoma identification in regional lymph nodes.[36] Results from these studies also point out the inadequacies of the routine bivalve approach; 31 percent of patients with histologically negative lymph nodes were found to have melanoma cells in primary cultures derived from half of the lymph node. However, establishing primary cultures derived from half of the lymph nodes of sentinel lymph nodes to detect metastatic melanoma is an extremely labor-intensive and expensive technique.

The notion that the simple bivalve technique of lymph node assessment understages many patients is not surprising, given that a small metastatic tumor deposit in the lymph node may not straddle the equator of the lymph node. In addition, clusters of a few metastatic melanoma cells may easily be overlooked on slides stained with only H+E (Figure 11–12, A). Other methods of lymph node analysis appear to be more sensitive and specific than H+E staining of bivalved nodes. A simple and relatively inexpensive strategy to improve sensitivity involves the examination of deeper sections into each cut surface of the

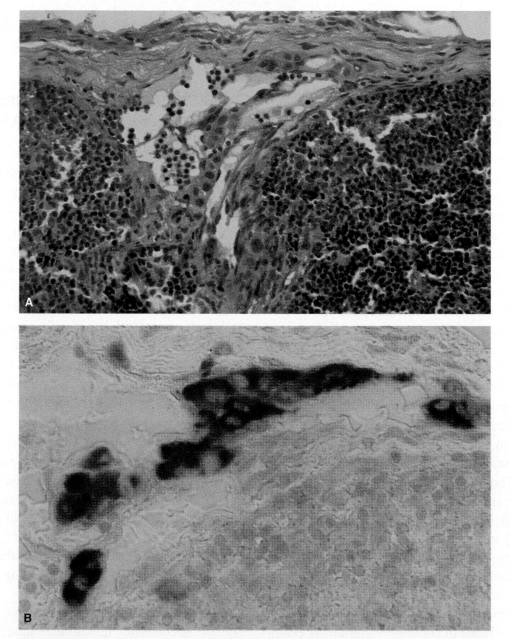

Figure 11–12.   A, Analysis of a sentinel lymph node by routine hematoxylin-eosin (H+E) staining. B, Analysis of the same sentinel lymph node by serial section and immunohistochemistry more clearly identifies occult nodal micrometastases.

node stained by H+E.[12] This approach increases the odds of detecting small metastatic tumor foci that do not straddle the equator of the node (Figure 11–12, *B*). This technique of sectioning can be combined with the use of immunoperoxidase stains for S-100, HMB-45, NK1C3, or MART-1 to enhance sensitivity. In a study of patients whose sentinel lymph nodes were reported as negative on the basis of routine histologic methods, 12 percent were found to have lymph node metastases through the use of serial sections and immunohistochemical stains.[12] Pathologists at the Massachusetts General Hospital process sentinel lymph nodes according to the algorithm in Figure 11–13.

Another technique for analyzing sentinel lymph nodes to determine the presence of metastatic melanoma involves polymerase chain reaction (PCR) amplification for detection of tyrosinase messenger ribonucleic acid (mRNA).[37] Tyrosinase is a key enzyme during melanin synthesis in melanocytes and melanoma cells. One melanoma cell in a background of one million normal lymphocytes can be detected using this technique (Figure 11–14).[38] In patients with histologically negative regional lymph nodes, this technique detects evidence of tyrosinase mRNA in the lymph nodes in as much as 52 percent of patients.[38] Detection of tyrosinase mRNA with PCR in lymph nodes does correlate with survival.[38] In

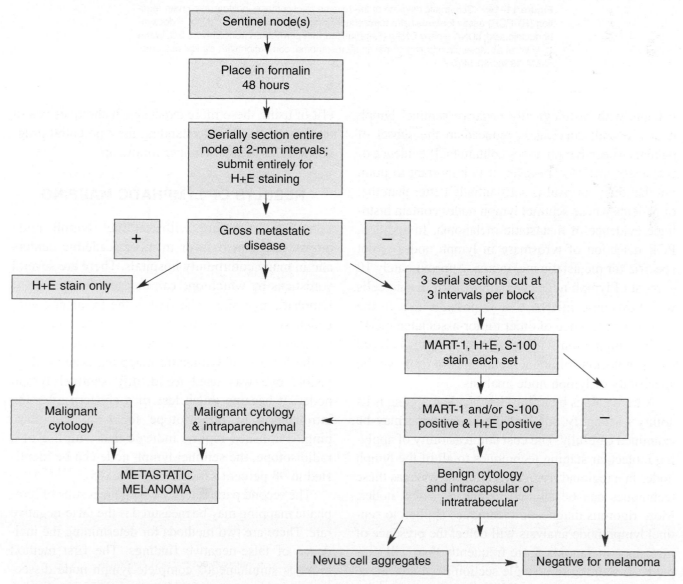

Figure 11–13. Algorithm for the pathologic evaluation of sentinel lymph nodes. (H+E = hematoxylin-eosin)

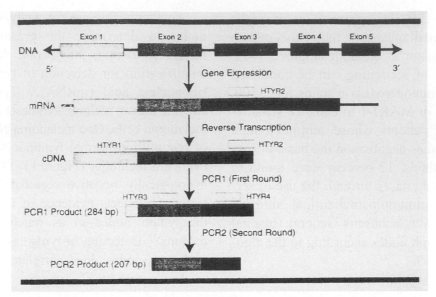

Figure 11–14.   Schematic diagram of the reverse transcriptase–polymerase chain reaction (RT-PCR) assay for tyrosinase messenger ribonucleic acid (mRNA). (DNA = deoxyribonucleic acid; cDNA = copy DNA.) (Reproduced with permission from Shivers SC, Wang X, Li W, et al. Molecular staging of malignant melanoma: correlation with clinical outcome. JAMA 1998;280:1410–5.)

patients with histologically negative sentinel lymph nodes, overall survival is reduced in the subset of patients whose lymph nodes contain PCR evidence of tyrosinase mRNA. However, it is important to point out that their survival is substantially better than that of patients whose sentinel lymph nodes contain histologic evidence of metastatic melanoma. In addition, PCR detection of tyrosinase in lymph nodes is not specific for metastatic melanoma. Approximately 10 percent of lymph nodes contain rests of nevoid cells with tyrosinase mRNA.[12] It is possible that in the future, the presence of other tumor-associated markers in combination with tyrosinase will be analyzed using molecular biologic techniques to improve the specificity of lymph node analysis.

A tremendous benefit of lymphatic mapping is its ability to identify one or a few nodes that may be examined carefully. The cost and feasibility of applying molecular staging techniques to all of the lymph nodes in a regional basin is prohibitive whereas these techniques can be applied to one or a few nodes. More-rigorous diagnostic techniques applied to sentinel lymph node analysis will detect the presence of metastatic melanoma more frequently than will simple H+E staining of a single section from a bivalved lymph node (Table 11–4).[12,36,38–43] However, the ben-

efit of using these more expensive techniques is still under study, and understanding their potential prognostic value requires longer follow-up.

RESULTS OF LYMPHATIC MAPPING

Lymphatic mapping with sentinel lymph node biopsy has gained favor in most academic centers and in many community hospitals. There are several yardsticks by which one can measure the results of lymphatic mapping. The first is the frequency with which surgeons are able to successfully locate the sentinel node. While this issue was of concern early in the history of lymphatic mapping, when only a visible dye was used to identify sentinel lymph nodes, it became much less of a concern after the introduction of radioisotope for lymphatic mapping.[7] Published reports indicate that with use of a radioisotope, the sentinel lymph node can be identified in 98 percent of cases (Table 11–5).[5,7,11,44–46]

The second parameter by which the results of lymphatic mapping may be measured is the false-negative rate. There are two methods for determining the incidence of false-negative findings. The first method requires simultaneous complete lymph node dissection at the time of sentinel lymph node biopsy, to per-

Table 11-4. DIAGNOSTIC TECHNIQUES USED TO ANALYZE THE SENTINEL LYMPH NODE

| Author | Date | Pathologic Examination of SLN | | | |
		H+E	IHC	RT-PCR	Cell Culture
Yu et al[12]	1999	—	12%*	—	—
Goscin et al[39]	1999	12% (48/405)	5% (22/405)	—	—
Shivers et al[38]	1998	20%*	—	52% (47/91)	—
Blaheta et al[40]	1998	—	39% (31/79)	44% (21/48)	—
Van der Veld-Zimmerman et al[41]	1996	—	25%* (4/16)	50% (6/12)	—
Wang et al[42]	1994	38% (11/29)	—	44% (8/18)	—
Heller et al[36]	1991	39% (12/41)	—	—	31% (9/29)
Cochran et al[43]	1984	10%	29%	—	—

SLN = sentinel lymph node; H+E = hematoxylin-eosin; IHC = immunohistochemical; RT-PCR = reverse transcriptase–polymerase chain reaction.
*Serial sections.

mit comparison of the histologic status of the sentinel lymph node with that of the remaining nodes in the basin; published reports demonstrate that the false-negative rate as assessed by this method is approximately 4 percent.[5] The other method is performance of sentinel lymph node biopsy alone and determination of the clinical outcome with long-term follow-up. At least two such studies demonstrate that as many as 11 percent of patients with histologically negative sentinel lymph nodes will experience recurrence with melanoma[13,47] (see "Patterns of Recurrence," below).

The third parameter by which the results of lymphatic mapping may be measured is the accuracy of the prognostic information it provides. Given that the most significant prognostic factor for survival is the presence or absence of lymph node metastases, it follows that the histologic status of a sentinel lymph node should accurately stratify patient risk for recurrence. Indeed, the risk of recurrence in patients with histologically positive sentinel lymph nodes is greater than that in patients with negative sentinel lymph nodes (Figure 11–15).[11] Sentinel lymph nodes that are found histologically negative by routine analysis can be divided into those that are positive by PCR analysis for tyrosinase mRNA and those that are negative. Patients with negative nodes by PCR analysis have a reduced risk for recurrence compared to those with positive nodes.[38] Nonetheless, patients with sentinel nodes that are negative by routine analysis but positive only by PCR analysis still have a relatively good prognosis and survival rates of 90 percent at 4 years (Figure 11–16).

A fourth parameter by which the results of lymphatic mapping may be measured is the safety of the procedure. No detailed reports concerning the prospective analysis of complications resulting from lymphatic mapping have been published. Although the complication rate is low and the types of complications are minor, it is expected that a small percentage of patients will experience wound infection, seroma, postoperative bleeding, allergy to the vital blue dye, or minor extremity edema.

Table 11-5. RESULTS OF SENTINEL LYMPH NODE MAPPING SERIES

Author	Year	Marker	Number	Detection Rate (%)	SN Positivity	False-Negative Rate
Morton et al[5]	1992	D	237*	82	12% H+E 9% IHC only	< 1%
Reintgen et al[44]	1995	D/I	42	90	19% H+E	0
Krag et al[7]	1995	D/I	121	98	12% H+E	ND
Albertini et al[45]	1996	D/I	129*	96	15% H+E	ND
Gershenwald et al[11]	1999	D/I	6/2	95	15% H+E	ND
Morton et al[46]	1999	D ± I				ND
JWCI			610	96	23% SS/IHC	
MSLT			681	97	19% SS/IHC	

SN = sentinel node; SS = serial sections; ND = not done; D = dye; I = isosulfan blue; H+E = hematoxylin-eosin; IHC = immunohistochemical; JWCI = John Wayne Cancer Institute; MSLT = Multicenter Selective Lymphadenectomy Trial.
*Number of lymph node basins.

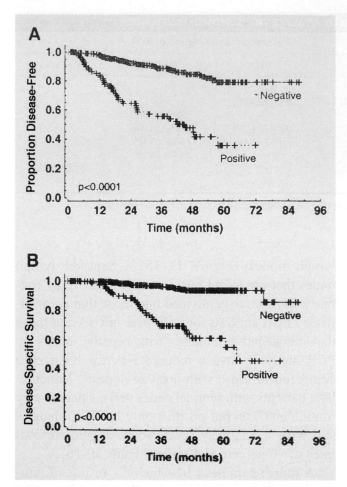

Figure 11–15. Influence of reverse transcriptase–polymerase chain reaction (RT-PCR) status of the sentinel lymph node on disease-free survival and overall survival. (Reproduced with permission from Gershenwald JE, Thompson WP, Mansfield PF, et al. Multi-institutional melanoma lymphatic mapping experience: the prognostic value of sentinel lymph node status in stage I or II melanoma patients. J Clin Oncol 1999;17:976–83.)

Finally, the results of lymphatic mapping should be assessed according to its ability to affect patient outcome whether by enhancing survival or by reducing the morbidity of therapy. Certainly, in comparison to elective lymph node dissection, the morbidity associated with lymphatic mapping and sentinel lymph node biopsy is minimal. However, it is unclear whether a strategy of lymphatic mapping leads to less morbidity than a strategy of observation of the regional lymph nodes (with subsequent therapeutic lymph node dissection for patients who develop clinical evidence of lymph node metastases). Nonetheless, lymphatic mapping with sentinel lymph node biopsy may lead to a reduction in risk for recurrence by allowing those with metastatic melanoma in the

regional lymph nodes to undergo a complete regional lymph node dissection.[3,35] Prospective randomized trials of elective lymph node dissection have not conclusively demonstrated that this procedure enhances survival. Given that the technique of elective lymph node dissection is now outdated, another trial has been initiated that asks the same survival question but that instead stages patients with lymphatic mapping.[46] In this trial, patients are prospectively randomized to undergo observation of the regional lymph node basin or sentinel lymph node mapping, with complete dissection of the lymph node basin in those patients who have histologic evidence of metastatic melanoma in the sentinel lymph node. It is hoped that the results of this trial will determine whether lymphatic mapping and sentinel lymph node biopsy enhance survival compared to the observation of regional lymph nodes.

Another plausible way in which lymphatic mapping may enhance survival is by identifying patients who harbor occult lymph node metastases so that

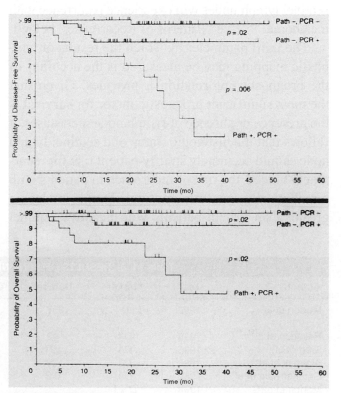

Figure 11–16. *Top,* Disease-free survival based on sentinel lymph node status. *Bottom,* Overall survival based on sentinel lymph node status. (PCR = polymerase chain reaction.) (Reproduced with permission from Shivers SC, Wang X, Li W, et al. Molecular staging of malignant melanoma: correlation with clinical outcome. JAMA 1998;280:1410–5.)

they may be treated with adjuvant therapy. Although initial reports from a randomized clinical trial suggest that administration of high-dose interferon to patients with AJCC stage III melanoma reduces their risk for recurrence, most of the patients in this trial had clinical evidence of regional lymph node metastases.[48] It remains to be proven whether the same benefit of high-dose interferon is afforded to patients with occult regional lymph node metastases determined by sentinel lymph node biopsy.

PATTERNS OF RECURRENCE

The accuracy of the sentinel lymph node mapping technique was initially evaluated by complete lymphadenectomy performed immediately after the sentinel lymph node biopsy.[5] In these studies, the histologic status of the sentinel lymph node was compared with that of the other lymph nodes in the basin. The false-negative rate was approximately 4 percent, and the predictive value of the absence of metastatic melanoma in a sentinel lymph node was approximately 99 percent. However, data from prospective randomized trials designed to evaluate lymph node dissection suggest that the false-negative rate as assessed by histopathologic evaluation of lymph nodes may be lower than the false-negative rate as assessed by clinical observation. Recently, several reports have provided information on the accuracy of sentinel lymph node mapping as assessed by clinical follow-up. In the largest study reported to date,[47] 11 percent of 243 patients with histologically negative sentinel lymph nodes followed on average for 35 months developed recurrences. Ten patients (4.1%) developed a recurrence in the previously mapped regional lymph node basin. In a report from Massachusetts General Hospital, 12 percent of 89 patients with histologically negative sentinel lymph nodes followed on average for 23 months developed a recurrence.[13] The previously mapped lymph node basin was the site of recurrence in 7 (8%) of these patients. The risk of recurrence following excision of a histologically negative sentinel lymph node rises with increasing primary-tumor thickness and the presence of ulceration. Approximately 7 percent of patients with histologically negative sentinel lymph nodes will develop distant metastases.

The possible explanations for false-negative results of lymphatic mapping (Table 11–6) can be divided into three general mechanisms. The first mechanism involves technical aspects of lymphatic mapping. There are several technical errors that can lead to a false-negative result. Failure to correctly identify and retrieve all sentinel lymph nodes from a basin may lead to recurrence of melanoma in an unresected sentinel lymph node. For example, in the case of a patient who undergoes lymphatic mapping without the intraoperative use of a handheld gamma detector, the surgeon may believe that all of the sentinel lymph nodes have been resected, when in reality an additional sentinel lymph node remains undetected. It is equally important to note that the accuracy of lymphatic mapping has been most clearly demonstrated in individuals who have undergone excisional biopsy of the primary melanoma without disruption of intervening lymphatic channels. Attempts to perform lymphatic mapping on patients who have already undergone wide excision of their primary melanoma or whose intervening lymphatic channels are disrupted may lead to mapping of irrelevant lymphatic channels. Another important factor is the experience of the surgeon. Surgeons early in their experience of lymphatic mapping are more likely to miss sentinel nodes.[5]

The biology of melanoma progression accounts for the second general mechanism leading to false-negative results. Some patients may have melanoma cells in transit in the lymphatic pathways at the time of lymphatic mapping, without metastases in the sentinel lymph node. Subsequent migration of melanoma cells to regional lymph nodes may lead to a recurrence in the previously mapped basin. Changes in the anatomic routes of lymph flow over time may also lead to false-negative results. Yet

Table 11–6. REASONS FOR FALSE-NEGATIVE RESULTS IN LYMPHATIC MAPPING	
Technical	Surgeon failure to correctly identify sentinel node or remove true sentinel node
	Isotope or dye fails to accumulate in a sentinel node
Biologic	Local or in-transit disease not removed by wide local excision
	Altered lymphatic drainage pattern (biopsy, inflammation, infection)
	Immune-induced regression
Pathologic	H+E examination only (sampling error)

H+E = hematoxylin-eosin.

another sequence of events that could lead to a false-negative result involves the spread of melanoma beyond sentinel lymph nodes into second-tier (non-sentinel) lymph nodes, followed by immune-induced complete regression in the sentinel nodes.

The third general mechanism that may lead to false-negative results involves the degree of scrutiny with which sentinel lymph nodes are analyzed for metastatic disease. In some patients, metastatic melanoma may be present but undetected in sentinel (and nonsentinel) lymph nodes. Of patients with histologically negative sentinel lymph nodes, 80 percent of those who have recurrences in the lymph node basin show evidence of metastatic melanoma in their sentinel nodes when the lymph nodes are examined again, using serial sectioning and immunohisto-chemical staining.[47]

Several approaches are being examined as possible methods to improve the prognostic accuracy of lymphatic mapping and sentinel lymph node biopsy. For now, it must be recognized that even patients with sentinel lymph nodes that do not harbor metastatic melanoma must be observed for recurrence.

SUMMARY

The ability to accurately determine the site of the first draining lymph node(s) for cutaneous melanomas and to surgically resect these sentinel lymph nodes has greatly improved the ability to identify regional lymph node metastases with simple lymph node biopsy. Modern techniques of lymphatic mapping have provided significant insights into the lymphatic drainage of the skin. The application of sentinel lymph node biopsy to melanoma patients has also fostered the simultaneous development of more sensitive techniques of lymph node analysis. Taken together, these developments have provided physicians with a powerful investigative tool with which to optimize therapy for melanoma patients.

REFERENCES

1. Snow H. Melanotic cancerous disease. Cancer 1892;2: 828–75.
2. Morton DL, Wanek L, Nizze JA, et al. Improved long-term survival after lymphadenectomy of melanoma metastatic to regional nodes. Analysis of prognostic factors in 1134 patients from the John Wayne Cancer Clinic. Ann Surg 1991;214:491–9.
3. Balch CM, Soong S-J, Bartolucci AA, et al. Efficacy of an elective regional lymph node dissection of 1 to 4 mm thick melanomas for patients 60 years of age and younger. Ann Surg 1996;224:255–66.
4. Robinson DS, Sample WF, Fee HJ, et al. Regional lymphatic drainage in primary malignant melanoma of the trunk determined by colloidal gold scanning. Surg Forum 1977;28:147–8.
5. Morton DL, Wen D-R, Wong JH, et al. Technical details of intraoperative lymphatic mapping for early stage melanoma. Arch Surg 1992;127:392–9.
6. Alex JC, Weaver DL, Fairbank JT, et al. Gamma-probe-guided lymph node localization in malignant melanoma. Surg Oncol 1993;2:303–8.
7. Krag DN, Meijer SJ, Weaver DL, et al. Minimal-access surgery for staging of malignant melanoma. Arch Surg 1995;130:654–8.
8. Morton DL, Chan AD. Current status of intraoperative lymphatic mapping and sentinel lymphadenectomy for melanoma: is it standard of care? J Am Coll Surg 1999;189:214–23.
9. Gaynor R, Herschman HR, Irie R, et al. S100 protein: a marker for human malignant melanomas? Lancet 1981;1:869–71.
10. Ordonez NG, Ji XL, Hickey RC. Comparison of HMB-45 monoclonal antibody and S-100 protein in the immunohistochemical diagnosis of melanoma. Am J Clin Pathol 1988;90:385–90.
11. Gershenwald JE, Thompson W, Mansfield PF, et al. Multi-institutional melanoma lymphatic mapping experience: the prognostic value of sentinel lymph node status in 612 stage I or II melanoma patients. J Clin Oncol 1999;17:976–83.
12. Yu LL, Flotte TJ, Tanabe KK, et al. Detection of microscopic melanoma metastases in sentinel lymph nodes. Cancer 1999;86:617–27.
13. Gadd MA, Cosimi AB, Yu J, et al. Outcome of patients with melanoma and histologically negative sentinel lymph nodes. Arch Surg 1999;134:381–7.
14. Soong S-J, Weiss HL. Predicting outcome in patients with localized melanoma. In: Balch CM, Houghton AN, Sober AJ, Soong S-J, editors. Cutaneous melanoma. St. Louis: Quality Medical Publishing, Inc.; 1998. p. 51–61.
15. Kelemen PR, Essner R, Foshag LJ, Morton DL. Lymphatic mapping and sentinel lymphadenectomy after wide local excision of primary melanoma. J Am Coll Surg 1999;189:247–52.
16. Hung JC, Wiseman GA, Wahner HW, et al. Filtered technetium-99m-sulfur colloid evaluated for lymphoscintigraphy. J Nucl Med 1995;36:1895–901.
17. Norman J, Cruse CW, Wells K, et al. A redefinition of skin lymphatic drainage by lymphoscintigraphy for malignant melanoma. Am J Surg 1991;162:432–7.
18. Thompson JF, Uren RF, Shaw HM, et al. Location of sentinel lymph nodes in patients with cutaneous melanoma: new insights into lymphatic anatomy. J Am Coll Surg 1999;189:195–204.

19. Uren RF, Howman-Giles R, Thompson JF. Direct lymphatic drainage from a melanoma on the back to paravertebral lymph nodes in the thorax. Clin Nucl Med 1999;24:388–9.

20. Uren RF, Howman-Giles R, Thompson JF, Quinn MJ. Direct lymphatic drainage from the skin of the forearm to a supraclavicular node. Clin Nucl Med 1996;21:387–9.

21. White DC, Schuler FR, Pruitt SK, et al. Timing of sentinel lymph node mapping after lymphoscintigraphy. Surgery 1999;126:156–61.

22. Gershenwald JE, Tseng C-H, Thompson W, et al. Improved sentinel lymph node localization in primary melanoma patients with use of radiolabeled colloid. Surgery 1998;124:203–10.

23. Morton DL, Bostick PJ. Will the true sentinel node please stand [editorial; comment]? Ann Surg Oncol 1999;6:12–4.

24. Sappey MPC. Anatomie, physiologie, pathologie des vaisseaux lymphatiques consideres chez l'homme et les vertebres. In: Paris: A Delahaye et E Lacrosnier; 1874–1885.

25. Sugerbaker EV, McBride CM. Melanoma of the trunk: the results of surgical excision and anatomic guidelines for predicting nodal metastasis. Surgery 1976;80:22–30.

26. Norman J, Wells K, Kearney R, et al. Identification of lymphatic drainage basins in patients with cutaneous melanoma. Semin Surg Oncol 1993;9:224–7.

27. Wells KE, Cruse CW, Daniels S, et al. The use of lymphoscintigraphy in melanoma of the head and neck. Plast Reconstr Surg 1994;93:757–61.

28. O'Brien CJ, Uren RF, Thompson JF, et al. Prediction of potential metastatic sites in cutaneous head and neck melanoma using lymphoscintigraphy. Am J Surg 1995;170:461–6.

29. Uren RF, Howman-Giles R, Thompson JF, et al. Lymphatic drainage to triangular intermuscular space lymph nodes in melanoma on the back. J Nucl Med 1996;37:964–6.

30. Uren RF, Howman-Giles RB, Thompson JF, et al. Lymphatic drainage from peri-umbilical skin to internal mammary nodes. Clin Nucl Med 1995;20:254–5.

31. Tanabe KK. Lymphatic mapping and epitrochlear lymph node dissection for melanoma. Surgery 1997;121:102–4.

32. Hunt JA, Thompson JF, Uren RF, et al. Epitrochlear lymph nodes as a site of melanoma metastasis. Ann Surg Oncol 1998;5:248–52.

33. Lieber KA, Standiford SB, Kuvshinoff BW, Ota DM. Surgical management of aberrant sentinel lymph node drainage in cutaneous melanoma. Surgery 1998;124:757–61.

34. Veronesi U, Adamus J, Bandiera DC, et al. Delayed regional lymph node dissection in stage I melanoma of the skin of the lower extremities. Cancer 1982; 49:2420–30.

35. Cascinelli N, Morabito A, Santinami M, et al. Immediate or delayed dissection of regional nodes in patients with melanoma of the trunk: a randomised trial. WHO Melanoma Programme. Lancet 1998;351:793–6.

36. Heller R, Becker J, Wassalle J, et al. Detection of submicroscopic lymph node metastases in patients with malignant melanoma. Arch Surg 1991;126:1455–60.

37. Reintgen DS, Conrad AJ. Detection of occult melanoma cells in sentinel lymph nodes and blood. Semin Oncol 1997;24:S11–5.

38. Shivers SC, Wang X, Li W, et al. Molecular staging of malignant melanoma: correlation with clinical outcome. JAMA 1998;280:1410–5.

39. Goscin C, Glass LF, Messina JL. Pathologic examination of the sentinel lymph node in melanoma. In: Cady B, editor. Surgical Oncology Clinics of North America; 1999. p. 427–34.

40. Blaheta H-J, Schittek B, Breuninger H, et al. Lymph node micrometastases of cutaneous melanoma: increased sensitivity of molecular diagnosis in comparison to immunohistochemistry. Int J Cancer 1998;79:318–23.

41. Van der Velde-Zimmerman D, Roijers JFM, Bouwens-Rombouts A, et al. Molecular test for the detection of tumor cells in blood and sentinel nodes of melanoma patients. Am J Pathol 1996;149:759–64.

42. Wang X, Heller R, VanVoorhis N, et al. Detection of submicroscopic lymph node metastases with polymerase chain reaction in patients with malignant melanoma. Ann Surg 1994;220:768–74.

43. Cochran AJ, Wen D-R, Herschman HR. Occult melanoma in lymph nodes detected by antiserum to S-100 protein. Int J Cancer 1984;34:159–63.

44. Reintgen D, Albertini J, Berman C, et al. Accurate nodal staging of malignant melanoma. Cancer Control 1995; Sept/Oct: 405–14.

45. Albertini J, Cruse CW, Rappaport D, et al. Intraoperative radiolymphoscintigraphy improves sentinel lymph node identification for patients with melanoma. Ann Surg 1996;223:217–24.

46. Morton DL, Thompson JF, Essner R, et al. Validation of the accuracy of intraoperative lymphatic mapping and sentinel lymphadenectomy for early-stage melanoma: a multicenter trial. Multicenter Selective Lymphadenectomy Trial Group. Ann Surg 1999; 230:453–63.

47. Gershenwald JE, Colome MI, Lee JE, et al. Patterns of recurrence following a negative sentinel lymph node biopsy in 243 patients with stage I or II melanoma. J Clin Oncol 1998;16:2253–60.

48. Kirkwood JM, Strawderman MH, Ernstoff MS, et al. Interferon alfa-2b adjuvant therapy of high-risk resected cutaneous melanoma: the Eastern Cooperative Oncology Groups trial EST 1684. J Clin Oncol 1996;14:7–17.

12

Adjuvant Therapy for Melanoma

C. KOMEN BROWN, MD, PhD

JOHN M. KIRKWOOD, MD

BACKGROUND

Melanoma incidence in the United States has been increasing steadily over this century. In 1935, the documented incidence of malignant melanoma in the population was 1 in 1,500. The incidence increased to 1 in 250 by 1980, and it was estimated that it would be approximately 1 in 75 by the year 2000 (Figure 12–1).[1] During this period, there has been much progress in the understanding of basic melanoma biology and the natural history of this disease process. Despite these advances, effective treatment for recurrent melanoma remains lacking.

Currently, the 5-year survival for metastatic melanoma is approximately 5 to 10 percent, and median survival is less than 1 year.[2,3] The majority of melanoma patients present with resectable disease at the time of diagnosis. However, those with thick or ulcerated lesions and those with metastatic disease residing in the regional draining lymph nodes are at high risk of recurrence. Current tumor-node-metastasis (TNM) staging for melanoma is depicted in Table 12–1. Stage I and II patients harbor localized disease, and stage III patients have extension of disease to the local draining lymph nodes. Stage IV patients have distant metastatic disease.[4] Figure

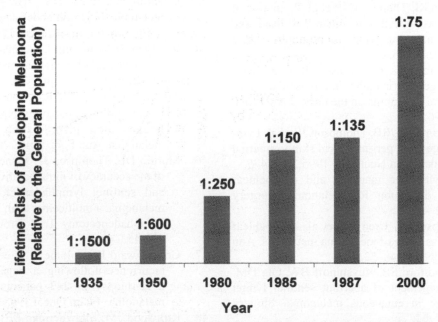

Figure 12–1. Lifetime risk of developing melanoma for an individual in the United States. The number for the year 2000 is a projected risk. The figure depicts the increasing trend over the past century. (Reproduced with permission from Rigel DS, Kopf AW, Friedman RJ. The rate of malignant melanoma in the US: are we making an impact? J Am Acad Dermatol 1987;17:1050.)

Table 12–1. CURRENT STAGING FOR CUTANEOUS MELANOMA*

Disease Stage	TNM Staging	Description
IA	T1N0M0	Localized disease; T ≤ 0.75 mm
IB	T2N0M0	Localized disease; 0.75 < T ≤ 1.50 mm
IIA	T3N0M0	Localized disease; 1.50 < T ≤ 1.50 mm
IIB	T4N0M0	Localized disease; T > 4.00 mm
III	any T, N1M0	Regional nodal metastases and/or in-transit disease. N1: regional nodes ≤ 3 cm; N2: regional nodes > 3 cm
IV	any T, any N, M1	Systemic metastases (M1)

T = primary tumor; N = regional node; M = metastasis; TNM = tumor-node-metastasis.
*American Joint Committee on Cancer (AJCC) classification.
Reprinted with permission from International Union against Cancer. Malignant melanoma of skin. In: Sobin LH, Wittekind C, editors. TNM classification of malignant tumors. 5th ed. New York: John Wiley and Sons; 1997. p. 118.

12–2 depicts the survival of melanoma patients over a 15-year period, stratified according to stage, and clearly shows the high mortality associated with stage IV disease. The subsets of individuals who are at high risk of recurrence are those with stage IIB and III disease. The recurrence rates for stage IIB and III patients are 40 to 50 percent, and 50 to 80 percent, respectively.[2] Recurrence at any site portends a poor prognosis, and distant (M1) recurrence is closely associated with death from this disease. It is the poor outcome associated with metastatic disease that has prompted investigations into adjuvant therapy to prevent relapse in patients resected of disease who can be projected to have a poor prognosis for disease-free and overall survival.

As primary melanomas grow, the phenotype of each tumor becomes more heterogeneous, judged by a variety of analytic techniques including routine histopathology, immunohistochemical staining for markers associated with pigmentation, and analysis of the expression of markers such as the major histocompatibility (MHC) antigens class I and II. Cells within the tumor accumulate mutations secondary to an inherent genetic instability, leading to an increased phenotypic heterogeneity. Some of these phenotypes are believed to be responsible for the therapeutic resistance of tumor cells. Adjuvant therapy with cytotoxic chemotherapeutic drugs is predicated on the notion that smaller numbers of cells are likely to be more vulnerable to therapeutic intervention following surgical extirpation of the primary

disease. Similarly, adjuvant immunotherapy is predicated upon the greater susceptibility of low-burden tumors to a variety of immunologic interventions in experimental animals. Such mechanisms as accumulated MHC class I or II antigen loss as well as loss of cellular antigen expression in tumors may partially explain the increased susceptibility of early disease to immune interventions designed to augment antitumor responses against melanoma and other cancers. Many clinical trials for the adjuvant treatment of melanoma have been performed over the past two decades. However, only interferon-α (IFN-α) has been shown to be efficacious in phase III randomized controlled settings and replicated for confirmation.[5,6]

ADJUVANT INTERFERON-α THERAPY

Isaac and Lindenmann initially discovered interferons in 1957.[7] Interferons were found to make up a family of naturally occurring cytokines that are produced by cells in response to viral infection, antigen stimulation, and mitogen activation. Interferons were named such because of their ability to "interfere" with viral infection and induce an antiviral state. Since their discovery, interferons have also been found to be important in immunoregulation, proliferation and differentiation of both immune and nonimmune cells, and antiangiogenesis. They also play a

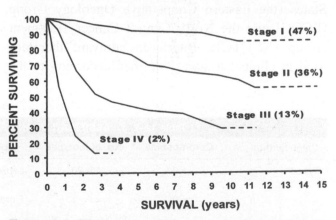

Figure 12–2. Fifteen-year survival curves of melanoma patients, grouped according to the current American Joint Committee on Cancer (AJCC) classification of cutaneous melanomas. The distribution in each group is shown in parentheses. (Reprinted with permission from Ketcham AS, Balch CM. Classification and staging systems. In: Balch CM, Milton GW, editors. Cutaneous melanoma: clinical management and treatment results worldwide. Philadelphia: J.B. Lippincott; 1985. p. 55.)

broad role in infectious disease, cancer therapeutics, and even the treatment of other disorders such as hemangiomas.[8-17] According to their biochemical properties, interferons are classified into a number of types known as IFN-α, IFN-β, IFN-ω, and IFN-γ. In practice, only three major species have reached clinical application (Table 12–2). There are at least 14 closely related genes and several pseudogenes for IFN-α that most likely arise from gene duplication.[18] Interferon-β is encoded by a single gene and is structurally related to the IFN-α gene family. Collectively, IFN-α and IFN-β are also referred to as type I interferons. Interferon-γ is a type II interferon and has little homology to the type I family. Type II interferons are produced by T cells and natural killer cells during antigen activation whereas type I interferons are produced by fibroblasts and most leukocytes during viral infections.[19-27]

The selection of IFN-α in the adjuvant setting was based on early experiences of this cytokine in treating metastatic melanoma. Studies done at Yale in the early 1980s showed that IFN-α has an objective response rate of approximately 20 percent and some complete responses of years in duration, much as has been observed with interleukin-2.[28] Although other chemotherapeutic agents gave similar response rates, none gave similar long-term responses. These early studies led to the introduction of IFN-α into the adjuvant treatment of melanoma in trials that were begun in the cooperative groups in the United States (the Eastern Cooperative Oncology Group [ECOG] and the North Central Cancer Treatment Group [NCCTG]). Interferon adjuvant therapies used in clinical trials are defined according to the dosages delivered and are listed in Table 12–3. The range varies from 20 mU/m² in high-dose interferon (HDI) therapy to 3 mU/m² in low-dose interferon (LDI) therapy. Essentially, the only significant impact on survival and relapse-free interval has been identified in trials of adjuvant HDI, which was shown to improve disease-free interval and overall survival in a phase III randomized ECOG protocol known as E1684. Based on the results of E1684, IFN-α2b was approved by the US Food and Drug Administration (USFDA) in 1995 and has been evaluated in two subsequent trials showing data consistent with E1684 for relapse interval benefits in the intergroup setting.

High-Dose Interferon Therapy

The first trial to show the efficacy of IFN-α2b in the adjuvant setting was E1684, a two-arm study in which patients with stage IIB and III disease were assigned at random to receive either IFN-α2b therapy (experimental arm) or observation alone (control arm) following surgical resection.[5] Two hundred eighty-seven patients were randomized into the study. The HDI regimen is notable because it used a 1-month intravenous induction consisting of 20 mU/m² for 5 days per week for 4 weeks. Following this induction regimen, IFN-α2b was administered subcutaneously (SQ) at 10 mU/m² three times per week for 48 weeks. At a median follow-up duration of 7 years, a significant prolongation of relapse-free survival and overall survival was demonstrated. Median time to relapse increased from 0.98 years in the observation group to 1.7 years in the group treated with IFN-α ($p_2 = .005$),

Table 12–2. CLASSIFICATION AND FUNCTION OF VARIOUS INTERFERONS				
Classification	Chromosome	No. of Isotypes	Source	Function
Type I* α	9	> 20	Leukocytes	Antiviral activity Induces MHC class I expression
β	9	1	Fibroblasts	Stimulates NK cell activity Antiproliferative and antiangiogenic
Type II γ	12	1	T cells	Induces MHC class I and II expression Activates macrophages, endothelial cells, and NK cells Antiviral activity

MHC = major histocompatibility complex; NK = natural killer.
*The proximity and similarity of interferon-α and interferon-β genes on chromosome 9 indicates a common origin for both and their classification as type I interferons.
Reprinted with permission from Kurzrock R, Talpaz M, Gutterman JU. Interferons—α, β, γ: basic principles and preclinical studies. In: DeVita VT Jr, Hellman S, Rosenberg SA, editors. Biologic therapy of cancer. Philadelphia: J.B. Lippincott; 1991. p. 247.

Table 12–3. INTERFERON REGIMENS IN CLINICAL TRIALS

Regimen	Dose and Schedule
High	
Induction	20 mU/m², intravenous, 5 times per week for 4 weeks
Maintenance	10 mU/m², subcutaneous, 3 times per week for 48 weeks
Intermediate	
Induction	10 mU, subcutaneous, 5 times per week for 4 weeks
Maintenance	10 mU, subcutaneous, 3 times per week for 12–24 months
Low	3 mU, subcutaneous, 3 times per week for 1.5–3 years

and the respective median survival increased from 2.8 years to 3.8 years ($p2 = .047$). Five-year continuous relapse-free survival was 26 percent in the observation group and 37 percent in the treatment group. Overall 5-year survival also increased to 47 percent with treatment as compared to the 36 percent in the control group (Figure 12–3). The respective survival curves are depicted in Figure 12–4. Based on the results of this pivotal study, the USFDA approved IFN-α2b for adjuvant treatment of melanoma in patients who are at high risk of disease recurrence, including both deep-primary (T4) patients and node-positive (N1) patients.

The North Central Cancer Treatment Group (NCCTG study 83-7052) also evaluated the efficacy of IFN-α in the adjuvant treatment of melanoma.[29] Patients with lesions greater than 1.69 mm in Breslow thickness or with lymph-node positive disease (subset of stage IIA, IIB, and III patients) were randomized to receive IFN-α2a given at 20 mU intramuscularly three times weekly for 3 months versus observation. This study evaluated 260 patients and demonstrated no significant prolongation of relapse-free survival or overall survival between the two patient groups. However, the Cox analysis of patients with nodal metastasis (n = 162) in this trial demonstrated a relapse-free interval benefit (with $p = .03$) and a benefit resembling that seen in the larger and more homogeneously node-positive E1684 trial.

Significant toxicity associated with IFN-α therapy was encountered in E1684. The acute and chronic toxicity, chiefly manifest as flulike symptoms, only allowed 75 percent of the patients to complete the 1-year regimen.[5] Dose delays or adjustments were necessary in approximately 50 percent of the patients in the 1st month and in a similar fraction of patients during the subsequent maintenance therapy, predominantly in the initial 3 to 4 of 11 months. Thus, an intergroup sequel study led by ECOG (E1690/S9111/C9190) was initiated to test whether or not a lower-dosage interferon regimen might be as effective in improving disease-free survival and overall survival while lessening the side effects associated with HDI.[30] This study consisted of three arms. Patients were assigned at random to

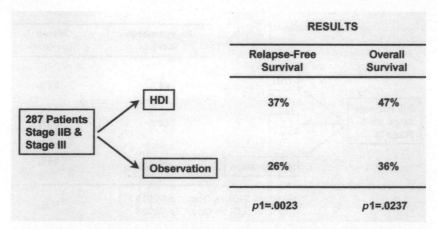

Figure 12–3. Trial design and outcome of Eastern Cooperative Oncology Group (ECOG) trial E1684, the pivotal trial that led the US Food and Drug Administration (FDA) to approve interferon-α2b (IFN-α2b) for adjuvant therapy in melanoma. Both the relapse-free survival and overall survival in the HDI group are significantly improved over the observation group. The patient number signifies the number of eligible patients analyzed in the study. (HDI = high-dose IFN-α2b therapy.) (Reproduced with permission from Kirkwood JM, Strawderman MH, Ernstoff MS, et al. Adjuvant therapy of high-risk resected cutaneous melanoma: the Eastern Cooperative Oncology Group trial EST 1684. J Clin Oncol 1996;14:7.)

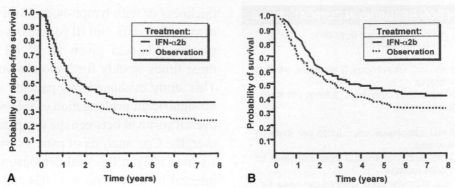

Figure 12–4. Relapse-free and overall survival curves from trial E1684. Panel *A* depicts the relapse-free survival while panel *B* depicts the overall survival of trial E1684. There is a statistically significant improvement of relapse-free survival and overall survival in the group treated with high-dose interferon-α2b (IFN-α2b) (solid line) versus survival in the observation group (dotted line).

receive high-dose IFN-α2b (as in E1684), low-dose IFN-α2b (3 mU SQ three times per week for 2 years), or observation. An observation arm was included because E1690 was designed and partly conducted before the significant benefit of HDI upon overall survival was known. The inclusion of an observation arm and an HDI arm also served as a confirmatory trial for E1684. A total of 642 patients were enrolled, with 608 patients eligible. At a median follow-up of 52 months, HDI demonstrated an improved relapse-free survival as compared to the LDI group or to the observation group (Figure 12–5). The relapse-free survival at 5 years in this

trial was 44 percent for the HDI arm, 40 percent for the LDI arm, and 35 percent for the observation arm. No overall survival impact was evident when the HDI or LDI arm was compared to the observation arm, however. A notable difference between E1690 and E1684 is the much improved median overall survival (6 years vs 2.8 years, respectively). The failure of E1690 to corroborate improvement in overall survival from E1684 may be due to several factors. One such factor may be the availability of interferon salvage therapy for patients in the observation arm following relapse of disease. This salvage therapy was unavailable to patients during

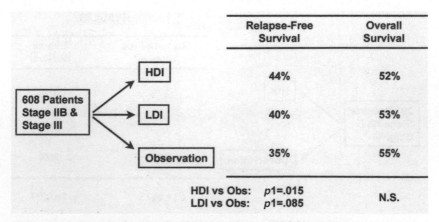

Figure 12–5. Eastern Cooperative Oncology Group (ECOG) trial E1690, a three-arm trial randomizing patients to receive high-dose interferon (HDI) therapy, to receive low-dose interferon (LDI) therapy, or to be observed following surgery for stage IIB or III melanoma. This study showed a significant prolongation of relapse-free survival in the HDI group as compared to the observation group. Patient number signifies the number of eligible patients analyzed in the study. (Obs = observation; N.S. = not significant.) (Reproduced with permission from Kirkwood JM, Ibrahim JG, Sondak VK, et al. High- and low-dose interferon alfa-2a in high-risk melanoma: first analysis of intergroup trial E1690/S9111/C9190. J Clin Oncol 2000;18:2444.)

E1684. As a result, approximately one-third of patients who relapsed in the observation arm of E1690 received salvage therapy following disease relapse. Thus, the availability of interferon salvage therapy for the observed patients in E1690 may be a confounding factor in the analysis of this data.

Confirmatory data for HDI efficacy in the adjuvant therapy of melanoma recently became available from the intergroup phase III study E1694/S9512/C509801 conducted by ECOG. This study was designed to test the efficacy of a melanoma vaccine formulated from the ganglioside GM_2 antigen. This trial employed a commercially produced preparation of the ganglioside GM_2 vaccine designated GMK (ganglioside GM_2 conjugated to the carrier molecule keyhole limpet hemocyanin [KLH], administered with the saponin adjuvant QS21 [Progenics, Inc., Tarrytown, NY]) in a randomized fashion versus high-dose interferon therapy. (This study is also discussed in the adjuvant immunotherapy section of this chapter).[6] The trial was closed in June 2000 due to the appearance of a highly significant benefit of HDI over GMK in terms of relapse-free survival (hazard ratio 1.47; $p1 = .0015$, $p2 = .003$) and overall survival (hazard ratio 1.52; $p1 = .009$, $p2 = .018$) (Figure 12–6). The relapse-free survival hazard ratio of 1.47

translates to a 47 percent higher recurrence rate in the GMK group as compared to the HDI group, and the similar overall survival hazard ratio for GMK versus interferon of 1.52 demonstrates a comparably increased risk of death among the recipients of the vaccine as compared to the HDI group. There is no evidence to suggest that GMK vaccination adversely affected the outcome in the GMK group, and it has been suggested that as the trial was closed, the effects of the vaccine may not have been fully apparent at 16 months of median follow-up. In any case, the significant improvement in overall and relapse-free survivals found with HDI in E1694 reconfirms the efficacy of HDI in the adjuvant therapy of melanoma patients originally demonstrated by E1684.[6]

Since a survival benefit of HDI has been demonstrated in two of three phase III randomized trials, it has been of great interest to define the minimal essential component of this 12-month regimen of IFN-α2b. Based on the hazard function analysis of E1684, the benefit of HDI therapy was manifest early in the year of therapy, suggesting that this benefit may be attributable to the intravenous induction component of the therapy employed in the 1st month of the regimen. Thus, it has been hypothesized that the 1-month intravenous-induction IFN-α2b therapy (20 mU 5 days a week for

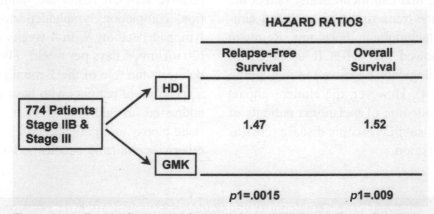

Figure 12–6. Eastern Cooperative Oncology Group (ECOG) trial E1694. Trial E1694 randomized patients to receive high-dose interferon (HDI) or GMK (GM₂ melanoma antigen conjugated to keyhole limpet hemocyanin) after surgery for patients with stage IIB or III melanoma. The GMK is given as a vaccination. Significant benefit for HDI over GMK is demonstrated. The relapse-free survival hazard ratio of 1.47 translates to a 47 percent higher rate of disease recurrence in the GMK group as compared to the HDI group. Similarly, the overall survival hazard ratio of 1.52 denotes a 52 percent higher mortality rate in the GMK group as compared to the HDI group. (Reproduced with permission from Kirkwood JM, Ibrahim J, Sondak VK, et al. Relapse-free and overall survival are significantly prolonged by high-dose IFN-alpha2b (HDI) compared to vaccine GM2-KLH with QS21 [GMK, Progenics] for high-risk resected stage IIB-III melanoma: results of the intergroup phase III study E1694/S9512/C509801. Ann Oncol 2000.)

4 weeks) may be necessary or sufficient to achieve the benefits of the full-year HDI regimen. In conjunction with the National Clinical Trials Group in Canada, the intergroup trial E1697 is being conducted by ECOG to address the issue of the role of this 1-month intravenous regimen alone. The targeted patient population consists of individuals who are at intermediate risk of recurrence of melanoma. This includes stage II (lesion larger than 1.5 mm in Breslow thickness, without lymph node disease) and stage IIIA (spread of disease to a single node) patients. The study plans to accrue 1,420 patients over a 3-year period. Its goal is to better define the role of the 1-month induction component of the 1-year HDI regimen.

The introduction of sentinel lymph node biopsy has allowed for more careful evaluation of nodal disease.[31–36] This has led to more accurate lymph node staging and to frequent identification of micrometastasis in the sentinel node.[37,38] The usual low number of sentinel lymph nodes obtained from each biopsy sample (usually 1 to 2 nodes) has made it feasible to apply substantially more intensive immunohistochemical studies on step sections, as well as molecular techniques such as reverse transcriptase polymerase chain reaction (RT-PCR), in the analysis of the sentinel node(s). Reverse transcriptase polymerase chain reaction is an exquisitely sensitive technique that can theoretically detect the presence of even one transcript in an analyzed sample. Applying this technique in melanoma, Reintgen and colleagues showed that RT-PCR upstaged 58 percent of the histologically negative sentinel lymph nodes[39] (Table 12–4). However, the clinical impact on the long-term outcome of melanoma patients of being able to detect submicroscopic disease remains incompletely understood.

A trial that may help to delineate the significance of submicroscopic disease is the Sunbelt Melanoma Trial (SMT), a multicenter trial designed to evaluate the role of adjuvant HDI and a similar derivative therapy limited to 1 month (IV induction only), in the setting of sentinel lymph node biopsy. This study focuses on an assessment of the impact of IFN-α2b in patients with microscopic regional nodal metastases whose primary melanoma is greater than 1 mm in Breslow thickness. The trial consists of two parts (Figure 12–7). The first part evaluates the role of the sentinel node mapping. All enrolled patients initially undergo a sentinel lymph node biopsy, and those individuals with a positive sentinel node must then undergo completion lymphadenectomy. Patients who are found to have only a single lymph node positive for disease are randomized to 1 year of HDI or to observation. Patients who have more than one node positive for metastatic disease are offered standard treatment with HDI for 1 year. Those patients who at the outset are found to have no sign of nodal disease following sentinel lymph node biopsy by routine pathologic analysis are entered into the second part of the study. This second portion of the SMT evaluates the role of RT-PCR in the analysis of lymph nodes that are histologically free of metastatic disease. Individuals with a negative RT-PCR result are observed whereas those with a positive RT-PCR result are randomized to observation, completion lymphadenectomy, or completion lymphadenectomy with 4 weeks of intravenous HDI ($20\ mU/m^2$, 5 days per week). Thus, this trial seeks to delineate the role of the 1-month intravenous HDI in a spectrum of patients who have not previously been addressed, in addition to issues of sentinel lymph node biopsy and patients with RT-PCR–evident (but otherwise clinically occult) nodal disease.

Table 12–4. CLINICAL CORRELATION OF NODAL STATUS WITH REVERSE TRANSCRIPTASE POLYMERASE CHAIN REACTION ASSAY				
Nodal Status	Number*	Recurrences	Locoregional[†] Recurrences	Systemic[‡] Recurrences
Histology positive, RT-PCR positive	22	14 (64%)	8 (57%)	6 (43%)
Histology negative, RT-PCR positive	59	6 (10%)	2 (33%)	4 (66%)
Histology negative, RT-PCR negative	43	1 (2%)	1	0

RT-PCR = reverse transcriptase polymerase chain reaction.
*Number of patients whose sentinel nodes were analyzed.
[†]Number of patients whose recurrences were local. Percentage is relative to number of all recurrences.
[‡]Number of patients with systemic recurrences. (Patients may have both systemic and locoregional recurrences.) Percentage is relative to number of recurrences.
Reprinted with permission from Reintgen DS, et al. Accurate nodal staging of malignant melanoma: cancer control. J Moffitt Cancer Center 1995;2:405.)

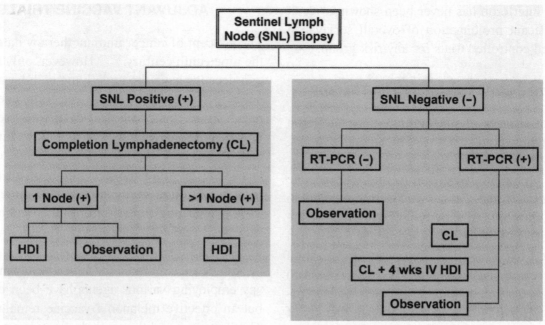

Figure 12–7. Trial design of the Sunbelt Melanoma Trial. The Sunbelt Melanoma Trial is actually two trials in one. The first portion of the trial (highlighted on the left of the figure) is designed to address the role of sentinel lymph node biopsy in the care of melanoma patients. The second portion of the trial (highlighted on the right of the figure) addresses how lymph node analysis by reverse transcriptase polymerase chain reaction (RT-PCR) will affect outcomes in melanoma patients. The targeted patient population is those individuals with melanomas greater than 1 mm. (IV = intravenous; HDI = high-dose interferon therapy.)

Low-Dose Interferon Therapy

The significant toxicity associated with high-dose interferon therapy has prompted clinicians to investigate the efficacy of LDI in the adjuvant treatment of melanoma. The World Health Organization (WHO) conducted a trial (WHO trial 16) to address this issue.[40] Interferon-α2a was given subcutaneously (3 mU three times a week for 3 years) and was tested in a randomized fashion against observation. A total of 444 patients were enrolled, and a significant fraction of the patients exhibited extracapsular nodal involvement. Analysis of the data with a median follow-up of 39 months indicated no apparent impact upon either disease-free survival or overall survival in the patient group receiving low-dose interferon. These data are consistent with the results of E1690, in which LDI (IFN-α2b, 3 mU SQ three times a week for 2 years) did not significantly improve relapse-free survival or overall survival as compared to the observed group.

The French Cooperative Group on Melanoma performed a randomized trial of LDI as adjuvant therapy in melanoma patients with primary lesions greater than 1.5 mm in thickness. These patients had resection of the primary lesion and also had no clinically detectable nodal metastasis although no sentinel node investigations were performed. Four hundred ninety-nine patients were randomized to either observation or IFN-α2a therapy (3 mU SQ three times weekly for 18 months). With 489 patients eligible, and after a median follow-up of 5 years, data analysis demonstrated a significant improvement of relapse-free interval ($p = .035$) and a trend toward an increase in overall survival that did not reach significance ($p = .059$). The authors concluded that adjuvant therapy with low-dose IFN-α2a is safe and beneficial for melanoma patients at high risk of disease recurrence but that the benefit was transient.[41] A smaller Austrian multicenter trial (n = 311) of a somewhat altered schedule at the same dosage also showed an impact only on relapse-free survival.[42] Thus, LDI has shown a durable impact on neither relapse interval nor survival in high-risk melanoma patients as tested in E1690 and WHO trial 16, and has shown an early impact on relapse interval but not on survival in intermediate-risk melanoma patients as tested in the French and Austrian multicenter trials.

Low-dose interferon has never been shown to result in a significant prolongation of overall survival in randomized controlled trials for any risk group.

Intermediate-Dose Interferon Therapy

The lack of efficacy of adjuvant low-dose interferon in prolonging overall survival of melanoma patients, coupled with the efficacy but toxicity of the HDI regimen, has prompted investigations into intermediate dosages of interferon. These investigations attempt to discover a threshold of activity that will preserve the efficacy of HDI while minimizing the associated dose-related toxicities. The European Organization for the Research and Treatment of Cancer (EORTC) has completed a trial employing an intermediate dosing strategy for IFN-α2b in the adjuvant therapy of melanoma (EORTC study 18-952). The regimen consists of an induction phase (IFN-α2b, 10 mU SQ 5 days per week for 1 month) followed by a maintenance phase of either 10 mU SQ three times a week for 12 months or 5 mU SQ three times a week for 24 months. Enrollment of 1,400 patients for this three-arm study has been completed, and results are anticipated in the next year.

Another three-arm trial investigating an intermediate-dose regimen is being conducted by the Scandinavian Melanoma Cooperative Group. There are two treatment arms, each with the same induction phase (IFN-α2b, 10 mU 5 days per week for 1 month) followed by a maintenance dose of 10 mU three times a week for 12 months (arm B) or 24 months (arm C). The two treatment arms will be compared to an observation group (arm A). Overall, the role of intermediate-dose interferon therapy in the adjuvant treatment of melanoma is unknown; the completion of the two trials mentioned above will help to clarify whether there is a role for lower dosages. The underlying issue in dose-response analysis for the interferons is whether it is the peak dose effects (maximum concentration [CMax] for 20 mU/m^2 reaching 10,000 U/mL) or the total dose delivered that is correlated with the durable antitumor effects and survival benefits of the high-dose regimen. Unfortunately, the lack of a high-dose arm in the EORTC 18-952 and Scandinavian trials will make it more difficult to know how to interpret survival benefit that may be observed.

ADJUVANT VACCINE TRIALS

The concept of cancer immunotherapy dates back to the nineteenth century.[43–46] However, only in the last two decades have the underlying cellular and molecular mechanisms of tumor rejection been illuminated. From this preclinical data, we have come to understand somewhat the concept of the tumor-associated antigen (TAA).[47–49] The presence of a TAA has made possible the generation of an antitumor response through immune reactivity directed at the TAA. Benefiting directly from this preclinical data, improved cancer vaccine strategies have been devised and tested in clinical trials.

Tumor vaccine trials for adjuvant melanoma therapy employing various agents have been conducted, but an effective melanoma vaccine remains elusive. The tested modalities include peptide vaccines,[49,50] intact melanoma cells and/or cell extracts,[51–53] recombinant viruses,[54] genetically modified cells,[51,55] and melanoma-specific and anti-idiotype antibodies.[56] In general, vaccinations against melanoma using various tumor vaccine preparations have been able to generate immunologic responses. However, these immune responses, which include generation of melanoma-specific cellular and humoral reactivities, have not been directly correlated with clinical response in metastatic disease or with disease-free and overall survival in the adjuvant setting. Curiously, with even the most refined peptide vaccine approaches, trials that have been associated with some of the most striking clinical responses have shown no identifiable T-cell response to the vaccine antigen[57] whereas others in which immune responses have been recorded have shown negligible clinical impact.[49–56,58]

The first randomized controlled trial in adjuvant melanoma vaccines used a Newcastle disease viral oncolysate preparation and was reported in 1995.[58] This prospective study enrolled 250 patients with resected melanomas who were at moderate to high risk of disease recurrence (stage II). Vaccination with this approach did not confer any therapeutic benefit to the treated group.

A second double-blinded phase III randomized trial of active specific immunotherapy using vaccinia melanoma oncolysate (VMO) was performed in patients with stage III melanoma and reported in

1998.[59] The goal of this study was to determine the efficacy of VMO in increasing the disease-free interval or overall survival in these patients. The study randomized 250 patients to treatment with either VMO (2 mg of total protein derived from 5×10^6 melanoma cells and vaccinia virus) or vaccinia (V) alone once a week for 13 weeks and then once every 2 weeks for 12 months or until recurrence. Analysis of 217 eligible patients showed no statistically significant improvement in disease-free interval or overall survival in all patients given VMO. Relapse-free survivals at 2-, 3-, and 5-year intervals were 47.8, 43.8, and 41.7 percent, respectively, for the VMO arm and 51.2, 44.8, and 40.4 percent, respectively, for the V arm. The overall survivals at 2-, 3-, and 5-year intervals were 70.0, 60.0, and 48.6 percent, respectively, for the VMO arm and 65.4, 55.6, and 48.2 percent, respectively, for the V arm.

A substantially larger study of VMO (n = 800) is being conducted in Australia by Hersey, but this has been reported only in preliminary form to date (Proceedings of the World Congress on Melanoma, 1997), and a full report is anticipated in the next year.

Ganglioside GM_2 is a well-defined melanoma antigen.[60,61] Prior studies have shown a favorable prognosis associated with the generation of anti-GM_2 antibodies following vaccination with ganglioside GM_2.[50,62,63] This observation suggests that antibody induction may confer protection from melanoma relapse. A single-institution study carried out at Memorial Sloan-Kettering Cancer Center between 1987 and 1988 evaluated ganglioside GM_2 and bacillus Calmette-Guérin (BCG) in stage III melanoma patients following surgery.[63] This phase III study enrolled 122 patients and randomized them to receive GM_2/BCG vaccination or observation. At more than 5 years of follow-up, the study demonstrated that vaccination was associated with a prolonged relapse-free survival in all vaccinated patients (compared to the observation group) that was not statistically significant. This result was confounded by the occurrence of native anti-GM_2 antibody response in 6 patients, 5 of whom were randomized into the control group. Analysis of patients who were seronegative at the time of enrollment demonstrated a significant improvement in relapse-free survival following GM_2/BCG vaccination ($p = .02$).

Conjugation of ganglioside GM_2 to KLH has resulted in improved antibody response following GM_2/BCG vaccination.[64,65] An improvement in titer and duration of immunoglobulin M (IgM) response, as well as the induction of an immunoglobulin G (IgG) response was observed. In the absence of KLH, only IgM response was demonstrable in prior studies.[66] An intergroup trial evaluating GM_2/KLH vaccine with the QS21 saponin adjuvant (commercially prepared by Progenics, Inc., and designated as GMK) was initiated by ECOG in 1994 (E1694/S9512/C509801).[6] The study accrued 880 patients; 774 were eligible. Patients were randomized to receive either GMK vaccination, given weekly (for 4 weeks) and then every 12 weeks ($\times$8), or high-dose IFN-α2b (same regimen as E1684). The trial was closed in June 2000 as a consequence of a significant benefit of HDI over GMK in terms of both relapse-free survival and overall survival for the eligible population. There is no evidence to suggest that the GMK group was adversely affected by vaccination. Thus, from the results of appropriately conducted and rigorously controlled phase III studies, the standard of adjuvant therapy for melanoma remains HDI.

ADJUVANT RADIOTHERAPY TRIALS

Radiotherapy (RT) has an important role in the adjuvant care of certain malignancies, notably carcinoma of the breast.[67-74] However, its role in the adjuvant treatment of melanoma remains undefined. As a modality, there has been no appropriately controlled randomized trial to evaluate treatment outcomes of adjuvant RT in melanoma patients. There has been one study, conducted by Ang and colleagues at the M.D. Anderson Cancer Center, for head and neck melanomas.[75] This nonrandomized study was initiated in 1983 to evaluate the role of RT in the treatment of clinically node-negative patients at high risk of nodal metastases or as an adjuvant in patients following therapeutic nodal dissection. Two hundred twenty-four patients were recruited, and patients were divided into three groups. Group I consisted of patients with Clark level IV or V lesions or with lesions greater than 1.5 mm in Breslow thickness and no palpable lymphadenopathy. Radiotherapy was administered to the tumor bed and to at least two echelons of proximally draining nodes. After a median follow-up of 38 months, the 5-year actuarial rate of local control for this group was 86 percent, and the 5-year survival was 63 percent.

Group II consisted of patients with clinically positive lymphadenopathy. Most of the patients in this group received postoperative radiation therapy. A few patients received preoperative RT. Analysis of this group demonstrated a 5-year actuarial local control rate of 92 percent and a 5-year survival of 41 percent. Group III consisted of patients with recurrent local or regional disease and without distant metastases. Patients received adjuvant RT after resection of their recurrent disease. The 5-year local control rate was 88 percent, and survival was 45 percent for this group. Following adjuvant RT, the number of positive nodes did not influence the locoregional control rates in patients in groups II and III.

Overall, the results of this nonrandomized study suggest that adjuvant RT may have a role in the locoregional control of melanoma, but the absence of randomized data makes it impossible to exclude selection bias, and the evaluation of this issue awaits phase III trial results.

ADJUVANT CHEMOTHERAPY TRIALS

No chemotherapeutic agent has been shown to significantly improve survival rates of patients with melanoma, when used in the adjuvant or advanced disease setting. Only one chemotherapeutic agent is approved for the treatment of metastatic melanoma: dacarbazine (DTIC). A randomized trial using DTIC and BCG in the adjuvant treatment of melanoma was conducted by the World Health Organization.[76] The results of the study actually showed a statistically significant decrease in survival of the treatment arm. Another randomized controlled study using DTIC and cyclophosphamide in patients with resectable melanoma was also conducted, with 136 patients enrolled. All study patients received nonspecific adjuvant immunotherapy with *Corynebacterium parvum*; half of the patients were then randomized to adjuvant chemotherapy with DTIC and cyclophosphamide while the other half was observed. Analysis of this chemoimmunotherapy trial showed that adjuvant chemotherapy did not pro-

vide any demonstrable effect, either in terms of disease-free survival or in terms of overall survival.[77] Thus, adjuvant chemotherapy for melanoma should be considered only in the setting of the clinical trial at this point and not as a standard-of-care regimen.

NEW AMERICAN JOINT COMMITTEE ON CANCER GUIDELINES

Central to the diagnosis, prognosis, and treatment of melanoma patients is the staging classification. Current (1987, old) TNM staging for cutaneous melanoma is listed in Table 12–1.[4] However, a number of key additional factors that have shown consistent predictive prognostic values and that were not incorporated into the previous system have been reported. The importance of these factors has led the American Joint Committee on Cancer (AJCC) Melanoma Task Force Committee to recommend a new staging system for primary tumor (T), regional nodal disease (N), and distant metastasis (M) (Table 12–5).[78] As melanoma staging is critical in the design and analysis of adjuvant therapeutic trials, it is a worthwhile endeavor to briefly discuss the new AJCC staging for melanoma as proposed by the committee.

Primary tumor thickness and ulceration have been shown to be the most important prognostic factors in virtually all studies of patients with localized disease.[79–86] These strong predictors of outcome are the only two criteria for T classification in the newly proposed AJCC staging of melanoma. Historically, thickness has been shown to be an independent and important prognostic factor of the primary tumor. The current (old) system divides thickness into thin (pT1, ≤ 0.75 mm), intermediate (pT2, 0.76 to 1.50 mm; pT3, 1.51 to 4.00 mm), and thick (pT4, > 4.00 mm) melanomas. However, as thickness is a continuous variable and is without natural breakpoints of prognosis, a more simplified system that divides thickness in increments of whole integers has been proposed. The relationship of survival rates and tumor thickness is depicted in Figure 12–8, which shows a worse prognosis with increasing primary tumor thickness. Another important but previously unrecognized variable is tumor ulceration. The presence of ulceration in the primary lesion portends a

Table 12–5. PROPOSED TUMOR-NODE-METASTASIS CLASSIFICATION FOR CUTANEOUS MELANOMA*	
Classification	**Description**
Thickness	**Ulceration Status**
T1 ≤ 1.0 mm	a: No ulceration b: With ulceration
T2 1.01–2.0 mm	a: No ulceration b: With ulceration
T3 2.01–4.0 mm	a: No ulceration b: With ulceration
T4 > 4.0 mm	a: No ulceration b: With ulceration
No. of Positive Nodes	**Nodal Size**
N1 1	a: Micrometastasis[†] b: Macrometastasis[‡]
N2 2–4	a: Micrometastasis[†] b: Macrometastasis[‡] c: In-transit metastasis or satellite lesions without metastatic nodes
N3 ≥ 5 nodes or matted nodes; or satellite lesions or in-transit disease and metastatic nodes	
Site	**Serum LDH**
M1a Distant skin or nodal metastasis	Normal
M1b Lung metastasis	Normal
M1c All other visceral or any distant metastases	Elevated

LDH = lactate dehydrogenase.
*Proposed by the American Joint Committee on Cancer.
[†]Diagnosed after elective or sentinel lymphadenectomy and confined within the capsule of a normal-sized lymph node.
[‡]Clinically detectable nodal metastasis diagnosed after therapeutic lymphadenectomy or with extracapsular extension.
Reprinted with permission from Balch CM, Buzaid AC, Atkins MB, et al. A new American Joint Committee on Cancer staging system for cutaneous melanoma. Cancer 2000;88:1484.

worse prognosis (in both recurrence and mortality from melanoma) than nonulcerated lesions of comparable thickness.[79–81,84,86–96] The adverse influence of primary tumor ulceration in melanoma patients with stage I to III disease is shown in Figure 12–9. Thus, the committee proposed that the absence or presence of ulceration be denoted by "a" or "b," respectively, for the secondary criteria of T classification in the new system.

The predictive value of the presence or absence of metastatic disease in the local draining lymph nodes has been verified in virtually all studies reported[84,86,97–107] (Table 12–6). Two criteria used in the proposed N classification are (1) the number of lymph nodes involved with disease and (2) whether the metastatic nodal disease is macroscopic or microscopic. The current system uses lymph node dimension as a stratification criterion. In practice, this factor has not been applied in the reporting and analysis of clinical trials. Thus, the committee has recom-

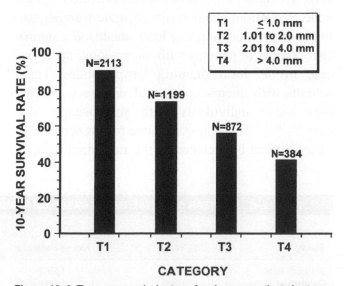

Figure 12–8. Ten-year survival rates of melanoma patients by tumor thickness, shown according to each tumor grouping. This graph depicts the inverse relationship of tumor thickness and ulceration on the overall survival of melanoma patients. (Reproduced with permission from Buzaid AC, Ross MI, Balch CM, et al. Critical analysis of the current American Joint Committee on Cancer staging system for cutaneous melanoma and proposal of a new staging system. J Clin Oncol 1997;15:1039.)

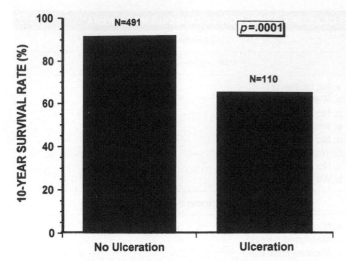

Figure 12–9. Ten-year survial rates of stage I to III melanoma patients in lesions with or without ulceration. (Reproduced with permission from Averbook BJ, Russo LJ, Mansour EG. A long term analysis of 620 patients with malignant melanoma at a major referral center. Surgery 1998;124:746.)

mended that nodal dimension be abandoned as a staging criterion. The proposed new system classifies regional nodal disease according to the number of lymph nodes involved with disease: N1, N2, and N3 for one, two to four, and greater than four lymph node involvements, respectively. Whether lymph node disease is micrometastatic or macrometastatic is the secondary criterion of N classification. Lymph node evaluations made more accurate through sentinel lymph node mapping have identified a significant number of patients with microscopic nodal disease in the local draining lymph nodes. Those patients with microscopic nodal disease fare better than those individuals with macroscopic disease.[101,104,108] Thus, the committee recommended that tumor burden be included in the new classification,

with "a" and "b" designations for micrometastatic and clinically apparent, macrometastatic diseases, respectively, in N1 and N2 classifications. The issues of satellite lesions and in-transit metastasis are also addressed in the N classification because they represent lymphatic spread of disease within the dermal lymphatics. As patients presenting with satellite lesions or in-transit disease have a very poor prognosis, the committee recommended that these criteria be included in the proposed new system. Patients with satellite lesions or in-transit disease and with no nodal disease spread will be classed as N2c while individuals with additional disease spread to the local draining nodes will be classed as N3.

The sites of metastases, the number of metastatic sites, and abnormally elevated serum lactate dehydrogenase (LDH) levels are most predictive in all studies that examine prognosis based on distant metastases by using a Cox regression analysis.[109–113] Though all distant metastases portend a poor prognosis, metastases at different sites have different prognostic imports. Patients with distant spread of disease to skin and remote lymph nodes fare better than patients with metastatic disease to any other site. Spread of disease to the lungs has an intermediate prognosis whereas metastasis to any other viscera has the worst prognosis (Figure 12–10). These metastatic diseases will be designated M1a, M1b, and M1c, respectively, as recommended by the committee. Additionally, patients with metastasis to any site and a concomitant elevated LDH (10% above the upper limits of normal) will be assigned to the M1c classification. Applying the above-discussed prognostic criteria, the committee has proposed a new stage grouping, as shown in Table 12–7.

Table 12–6. TEN-YEAR SURVIVAL RATES BASED ON NUMBER OF LYMPH NODES POSITIVE FOR METASTIC DISEASE					
			10-Year Survival (%)		
Study	Year	No. of Patients	1 Node*	2 to 4 Nodes†	≥ 5 Nodes‡
Slingluff et al	1988	1,273	38	31	18
Calabro et al	1989	1,001	43	32	18
Balch et al	1992	234	40	28	18
Buzaid et al	1995	442	55	34	25

*Corresponds to N1 of newly proposed American Joint Committee on Cancer (AJCC) melanoma guidelines.
†Corresponds to N2 of newly proposed AJCC melanoma guidelines.
‡Corresponds to N3 of newly proposed AJCC melanoma guidelines.
Reprinted with permission from Buzaid AC, Ross MI, Balch CM, et al. Critical analysis of the current American Joint Committee on Cancer staging system for cutaneous melanoma and proposal of a new staging system. J Clin Oncol 1997;15:1039.

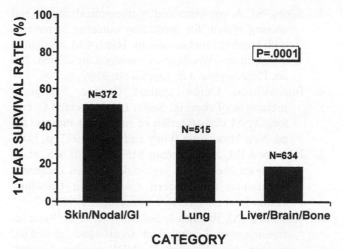

Figure 12–10. One-year survival rates of melanoma patients by metastatic category. Melanoma patients with distant metastases have very poor prognoses, as depicted by this 1-year survival graph. Patients with metastases to skin, distant nodes, and the gastrointestinal (GI) tract fare the best whereas patients with metastases to the liver, brain, and bone fare the worst. Pulmonary metastasis has an intermediate prognosis. (Reproduced with permission from Barth A, Wanek LA, Morton DL. Prognostic factors in 1,521 melanoma patients with distant metastases. J Am Coll Surg 1995;181:193.)

CONCLUSION

The incidence of melanoma has been increasing at a significant and disturbing pace since the early 1900s. It was projected that if this trend continued, the incidence of melanoma in the general population in the United States would be 1 in 75 by the year 2000.[1] Outcome following a diagnosis of metastatic disease is poor; fewer than 10 percent of patients survive at 5 years.[2,3] Individuals with stage IIB and III disease are at high risk of recurrence following resection of their primary disease, with or without resection of nodal metastasis. A significant portion of these patients will experience recurrence, presumably due to the presence of microscopic occult systemic disease. The period during which they are disease free presents a unique opportunity for eradicating residual microscopic disease through adjuvant therapy. This notion stems from the theoretic consideration that a tumor is most susceptible to therapeutic intervention when its cell number is small and the likelihood of developing therapeutic resistance is minimized. Through the rigorous and time-consuming but reproducible process of randomized controlled trials, high-dose IFN-α2b has emerged as the only effective adjuvant agent capable of prolonging relapse-free and overall survival in melanoma patients.

The advent of sentinel lymphatic mapping has allowed clinicians to identify those individuals with nodal diseases more accurately and with less morbidity. Elective lymph node dissection has significant morbidity; prior to sentinel lymph node biopsy, it

Table 12–7. PROPOSED STAGE GROUPING FOR CUTANEOUS MELANOMA							
Clinical Staging*				**Pathologic Staging†**			
0	Tis	N0	0	Tis	N0	M0	
IA	T1a	N0	M0	IA	T1a	N0	M0
IB	T1b	N0	M0	IB	T1b	N0	M0
	T2a	N0	M0		T2a	N0	M0
IIA	T2b	N0	M0	IIA	T2b	N0	M0
	T3a	N0	M0		T3a	N0	M0
IIB	T3b	N0	M0	IIB	T3b	N0	M0
	T4a	N0	M0		T4a	N0	M0
IIIA	T4b	N0	M0	IIIA	T4b	N0	M0
	Any	N1	M0		T1–4a	N1	M0
IIIB	Any	N2	M0	IIIB	T4b	N1	M0
	Any	N3	M0		Any	N2	M0
					Any	N3	M0
IVA	Any	Any	M1a	IVA	Any	Any	M1a
IVB	Any	Any	M1b	IVB	Any	Any	M1b
IVC	Any	Any	M1c	IVC	Any	Any	M1c

*Clinical staging includes microstaging of the primary melanoma and clinical/radiologic evaluation for metastases; by convention, it should be used after definitive management of the primary melanoma with clinical assessment for regional and distant metastases.
†Pathologic staging includes microstaging of the primary melanoma and pathologic information about the regional nodes after partial or complete lymphadenectomy, except for pathologic stage 0 or stage 1A patients who do not need pathologic evaluation of their lymph nodes.
Reprinted with permission from Balch CM, Buzaid AC, Atkins MB, et al. A new American Joint Committee on Cancer staging system for cutaneous melanoma. Cancer 2000;88:1484.

was the only reliable technique allowing for the identification of lymph node disease in clinically node-negative patients. However, elective lymph node dissection remains a controversial procedure as conclusive evidence for its improving overall survival is still lacking. The advent of sentinel lymph node biopsy has allowed lymph node evaluation in individuals who normally would not undergo elective lymph node dissection because of the inherent morbidity of the procedure. Data on how sentinel lymph node mapping will affect disease-free survival and overall survival in patients undergoing sentinel lymph node biopsy will be available pending a randomized protocol being performed by the SMT.

Overall, a much greater understanding of the natural history and biology of melanoma has been gained from both clinical and preclinical data. Although there remains much to address in this disease, the biologic relevance of micrometastasis stands as one of the most intriguing questions in the evolution of melanoma therapy. The increasing precision available in the diagnosis of regional nodal micrometastasis in the current practice of oncology is no accident. Technologic advances in electronics and instrumentation alone have increased the sensitivity and accuracy of detecting and diagnosing small-volume disease. Additionally, advances in molecular biology can only be expected to further push back this "detection envelope." The molecular understanding of the basis of effective therapies like IFNα-2b and IL-2 will allow clinicians to better identify those individuals who are most likely to benefit from adjuvant therapy to increase the therapeutic index. The ability to address micrometastasis in melanoma patients has positioned melanoma as a disease model for evaluating immunologic therapies uniquely in cancer therapy.

REFERENCES

1. Rigel DS, Kopf AW, Friedman RJ. The rate of malignant melanoma in the US: are we making an impact? J Am Acad Dermatol 1987;17:1050.
2. Balch CM, Soong SJ, Shaw HM, et al. An analysis of prognostic factors in 8500 patients with cutaneous melanoma. In: Balch CM, Houghton AN, Milton GW, editors. Cutaneous melanoma. 2nd ed. Philadelphia: J.B. Lippincott; 1992. p. 165.
3. Soong SJ. A computerized mathematical model and scoring system for predicting outcome in patients with localized melanoma. In: Balch CM, Houghton AN, Milton GW, editors. Cutaneous melanoma. 2nd ed. Philadelphia: J.B. Lippincott; 1992. p. 200.
4. International Union against Cancer. Malignant melanoma of skin. In: Sobin LH, Wittekind C, editors. TNM classification of malignant tumors. 5th ed. New York: John Wiley and Sons; 1997. p. 118.
5. Kirkwood JM, Strawderman MH, Ernstoff MS, et al. Adjuvant therapy of high-risk resected cutaneous melanoma: the Eastern Cooperative Oncology Group Trial EST 1684. J Clin Oncol 1996;14:7.
6. Kirkwood JM, Ibrahim J, Sondak VK, et al. Relapse-free and overall survival are significantly prolonged by high-dose IFN-alpha2b (HDI) compared to vaccine GM2-KLH with QS21 (GMK, Progenics) for high-risk resected stage IIB-III melanoma: results of the intergroup phase III study E1694/S9512/C509801. Ann Oncol 2000. [In press]
7. Lindenmann IA. Virus interference: I. The interferon. Proc R Soc Lond (Biol) 1957;147:258.
8. Talpaz M, Kantarjian HM, McCredie K, et al. Hematologic remission and cytogenetic improvement induced by recombinant human interferon alpha A in chronic myelogenous leukemia. N Engl J Med 1986;314:1065.
9. Kurzrock R, Gutterman JU, Kantarjian HM, et al. Therapy of chronic myelogenous leukemia with interferon. Cancer Invest 1989;7:83.
10. Quesada JR, Reuben J, Manning JT, et al. Alpha interferon for induction of remission in hairy cell leukemia. N Engl J Med 1984;310:15.
11. Bunn PA, Ihde DC, Foon K. The role of recombinant interferon-alfa-2a in the therapy of cutaneous T-cell lymphomas. Cancer 1986;57:1689.
12. Talpaz M, Kurzrock R, Kantarjian H, et al. Recent advances in the therapy of chronic myelogenous leukemia. In: DeVita V, editor. Important advances in oncology. Philadelphia: J.B. Lippincott; 1988. p. 297.
13. Ludwig H, Linkesch W, Gisslinger H, et al. Interferon-alfa corrects thrombocytosis in patients with myeloproliferative disorders. Cancer Immunol Immunother 1987;25:266.
14. Foon Ka, Sherwin SA, Abrams PG, et al. Treatment of advanced non-Hodgkin's lymphoma with recombinant leukocyte A interferon. N Engl J Med 1984;311:1148.
15. Quesada JR, Alexanian R, Hawkins M, et al. Treatment of multiple myeloma with recombinant alpha-interferon. Blood 1986;67:275.
16. Gutterman JU, Blumenschein GR, Alexanian R, et al. Leukocyte interferon-induced tumor regression in human metastatic breast cancer, multiple myeloma, and malignant lymphoma. Ann Intern Med 1980;93:399.

17. Talpaz M, Kurzrock R, Kantarjian H, et al. Recombinant interferon-alpha therapy of Philadelphia chromosome-negative myeloproliferative disorder with thrombocytosis. Am J Med 1989;86:554.

18. Zoo KC. Human interferons: structure and function. In: Gresser I, editor. Interferon 9. New York: New York Academic Press; 1987. p. 1.

19. Epstein LB, Gupta S. Human T-lymphocyte subset production of immune (gamma) interferon. J Clin Immunol 1981;1:186.

20. O'Malley J, Nussbaum-Blumenson A, Sheedy D, et al. Identification of the T cell subset that produces human gamma-interferon. J Immunol 1982;128:2522.

21. Chang J, Testa D, Kung PC, et al. Cellular origin and interactions involved in gamma-interferon production induced by OKT3 monoclonal antibody. J Immunol 1982;128:585.

22. Kasahara T, Hooks JJ, Dougherty SF, et al. Interleukin 2-mediated immune interferon (IFN-gamma) production by human T cells and T cell subsets. J Immunol 1983;130:1784.

23. Handa K, Suzuki R, Matsui H, et al. Natural killer (NK) cells as a responder to interleukin 2 (IL 2): II IL 2-induced interferon-gamma production. J Immunol 1983;130:988.

24. Kasahara T, Djeu JY, Dougherty SF, et al. Capacity of human large granular lymphocytes (LGL) to produce multiple lymphokines: interleukin 2, interferon, and colony stimulating factor. J Immunol 1983;131:2379.

25. Trinchieri G, Matsumoto-Kobayashi M, Clark SC, et al. Response of resting human peripheral blood natural killer cells to interleukin 2. J Exp Med 1984;160:1147.

26. Ortaldo JR, Mason AT, Gerard JP, et al. Effects of natural and recombinant IL-2 on regulation of IFN-gamma production and natural killer activity: lack of involvement of the Tac antigen for these immunoregulatory effects. J Immunol 1984;133:779.

27. Kelly CD, Welte K, Murray HW. Antigen-induced human interferon-gamma production: differential dependence on interleukin 2 and its receptor. J Immunol 1987; 139:2325.

28. Kirkwood JM, Ernstoff M. Melanoma: therapeutic options with recombinant interferons. Semin Oncol 1985;12(Suppl 5):7.

29. Creagan ET, Dalton RJ, Ahmann DL, et al. Randomized, surgical adjuvant clinical trial of recombinant interferon alfa-2a in selected patients with malignant melanoma. J Clin Oncol 1995;13:2776.

30. Kirkwood JM, Ibrahim JG, Sondak VK, et al. High- and low-dose interferon alfa-2a in high-risk melanoma: first analysis of intergroup trial E1690/S9111/C9190. J Clin Oncol 2000;18:2444.

31. Morton DL, Wen DR, Wong JH, et al. Technical details of intraoperative lymphatic mapping for early stage melanoma. Arch Surg 1992;127:392.

32. Morton DL, Wen DR, Cochran AJ. Management of early-stage melanoma by intraoperative lymphatic mapping and selective lymphadenectomy or "watch and wait." Surg Oncol Clin N Am 1992;1:247.

33. Reintgen DS, Cruse CW, Berman C, et al. An orderly progression of melanoma nodal metastases. Ann Surg 1994;220:759.

34. Ross M, Reintgen DS, Balch C. Selective lymphadenectomy: emerging role of lymphatic mapping and sentinel node biopsy in the management of early stage melanoma. Semin Surg Oncol 1993;9:219.

35. Thompson JF, McCarthy WH, Robinson E, et al. Sentinel node biopsy in 102 patients with clinical stage I melanoma undergoing elective lymph node dissection [abstract]. Proceedings of the 47th Cancer Symposium, Society of Surgical Oncology; 1994; Houston (TX).

36. Krag DN, Meijer SJ, Weaver DL, et al. Minimal-access surgery for staging of malignant melanoma. Arch Surg 1995;130:65.

37. Albertini JJ, Cruse CW, Rapaport D, et al. Intraoperative radiolymphoscintigraphy improves sentinel node identification in melanoma patients. Ann Surg 1996;223:217.

38. Gershenwald J, Thompson W, Manfield P, et al. Pattern of failure in melanoma patients after successful lymphatic mapping and negative sentinel node biopsy [abstract]. Proceedings of the 49th Annual Cancer Symposium, Society of Surgical Oncology; 1996; Atlanta (GA).

39. Wang X, Heller R, VanVoorhis N, et al. Detection of submicroscopic metastases with polymerase chain reaction in patients with malignant melanoma. Ann Surg 1994;220:768.

40. Cascinelli N. Evaluation of efficacy of adjuvant rIFN alpha-2a in melanoma patients with regional node metastases [abstract]. Proc Am Soc Clin Oncol 1995;14:410.

41. Grob JJ, Dreno B, de la Salmoniere P, et al. Randomised trial of interferon alpha-2a as adjuvant therapy in resected primary melanoma thicker than 1.5 mm without clinically detectable node metastases. French Cooperative Group on Melanoma. Lancet 1998;351:1905.

42. Pehamberger H, Soyer HP, Steiner A, et al. Adjuvant interferon alfa-2a treatment in resected primary stage II cutaneous melanoma. Austrian Malignant Melanoma Cooperative Group. J Clin Oncol 1998; 16:1425.

43. Hericourt J, Richet C. Physiologie pathologique de la serotherapie dans le traitement du cancer. Compte rend Seanc Acad Sci 1895;121:567.

44. Dor L. Premiers assays de cytolyse des cancers. Gaz hebd de med et de chir. Nouvelle serie 1901;6:73.

45. Vidal E. Les serotherapies des tumeurs malignes. In: Alcan F, editor. 2° Conference Internationale pour l'Etude du Cancer; 1910; Paris. p. 210.

46. Berkeley WN. Results of three years' observation on a new form of cancer treatment. Am J Obstet 1914; 69:1060.

47. Roth JA, editor. Monoclonal antibodies for the diagnosis and therapy of cancer. Mount Kisco (NY): Futura Publishing; 1986.

48. Hellstrom KE, Hellstrom I. Oncogene-associated tumor antigens as targets for immunotherapy. FASEB J 1989;3:1715.

49. Hellstrom KE, Hellstrom I. Principles of tumor immunity: tumor antigens. In: DeVita VT Jr, Hellman S, Rosenberg SA, editors. Biologic therapy of cancer. Philadelphia: J.B. Lippincott; 1991. p. 35.

50. Livingston PO. The basis for ganglioside vaccines in melanoma. In: Metzgar RS, Mitchell MS, editors. Human tumor antigens and specific tumor therapy. UCLA symposia on molecular and cellular biology. Vol. 99. New York: Alan R. Liss; 1989.

51. Berd D, Maguire HC Jr, Mastrangelo MJ. Treatment of human melanoma with a hapten-modified autologous vaccine. Ann N Y Acad Sci 1993;690:147.

52. Bystryn J-C, Oratz R, Harris MN, et al. Immunogenicity of a polyvalent melanoma antigen vaccine in humans. Cancer 1988;61:1065.

53. Livingston PO, Takeyama H, Pollack MS, et al. Serological responses of melanoma patients to vaccines derived from allogeneic cultured melanoma cells. Int J Cancer 1983;31:567.

54. Hersey P, Edwards A, Coates A, et al. Evidence that treatment with vaccinia melanoma cell lysate (VMCL) may improve survival of patients with stage II melanoma. Cancer Immunol Immunother 1987;25:257.

55. Morton DL, Davtyan DG, Wanek LA, et al. Multivariate analysis of the relationship between survival and the microstage of primary melanoma by Clark level and Breslow thickness. Cancer 1993;71:3737.

56. Livingston PO. Approaches to augmenting the immunogenicity of tumor antigens. Monoclonal antibodies and cancer therapy. UCLA symposia on molecular and cellular biology, new series. New York: Alan R. Liss; 1985.

57. Stoute JA, Slaoui M, Heppner DG, et al. A preliminary evaluation of a recombinant circumsporozoite protein vaccine against Plasmodium falciparum malaria. RTS,S Malaria Vaccine Evaluation Group. N Engl J Med 1997;336:86.

58. Wallack MK, Sivanandham M, Balch CM, et al. A phase III randomized, doubled-blind, multiinstitutional trial of vaccinia melanoma oncolysate—active specific immunotherapy for patients with stage II melanoma. Cancer 1995;75:34.

59. Wallack MK, Sivanandham M, Balch CM, et al. Surgical adjuvant active specific immunotherapy for patients with stage III melanoma: the final analysis of data from a phase III, randomized, double-blind, multicenter vaccinia melanoma oncolysate trial. J Am Coll Surg 1998;187:69.

60. Morton DL, Nizze RJ, Gupta RK, et al. Active specific immunotherapy of malignant melanoma. In: Kim JP, Jim BS, Park J-G, editors. Current status of cancer control and immunobiology. Seoul, Korea; 1987. p. 152.

61. Livingston PO, Natoli EJ, Calves MJ, et al. Vaccines containing purified GM2 ganglioside elicit GM2 antibodies in melanoma patients. Proc Natl Acad Sci U S A 1987;84:2911.

62. Livingston PO, Watanabe T, Shiku H, et al. Serological response of melanoma patients receiving melanoma cell vaccines. I. Autologous cultured melanoma cells. Int J Cancer 1982;30:413.

63. Jones PC, Sze LL, Liu PY, et al. Prolonged survival for melanoma patients with elevated IgM antibody to oncofetal antigen. J Natl Cancer Inst 1981;66:249.

64. Helling F, Shang A, Calves M, et al. GD3 vaccines for melanoma: superior immunogenicity of keyhole limpet hemocyanin conjugate vaccines. Cancer Res 1994;54:197.

65. Livingston PO. Approaches to augmenting the immunogenicity of melanoma gangliosides: from whole cells to ganglioside-KLH conjugate vaccines. Immunol Rev 1995;145:147.

66. Livingston PO, Calves Mj, Natoli EJ Jr. Approaches to augmenting the immunogenicity of the ganglioside GM2 in mice: purified GM2 is superior to whole cells. J Immunol 1987;138:1524.

67. Veronesi U, Saccozzi R, Del Vecchio M, et al. Comparing radical mastectomy with quadrantectomy, axillary dissection, and radiotherapy in patients with small cancers of the breast. N Engl J Med 1981;305:6.

68. Veronesi U, Banfi A, Salvadori B, et al. Breast conservation is the treatment of choice in small breast cancer: long term results of a randomized clinical trial. Eur J Cancer 1990;26:668.

69. Fisher B, Redmond C, for the National Surgical Adjuvant Breast and Bowel Project. Lumpectomy for breast cancer: an update of the NSABP experience. J Natl Cancer Inst Monogr 1992;11:7.

70. Fisher B, Anderson S, Redmond C, et al. Reanalysis and results after 12 years of follow-up in a randomized clinical trial comparing total mastectomy with lumpectomy with and without irradiation in the treatment of breast cancer. N Engl J Med 1995;333: 1456.

71. Van Dongen J, Bartelink H, Fentimen I, et al. Randomized clinical trial to assess the value of breast-conserving therapy in stage I and II breast cancer, EORTC 10801 trial. J Natl Cancer Inst Monogr 1992;11:15.

72. Blichert-Toft M, Brincker H, Andersen, J, et al. A Danish randomized trial comparing breast preserving therapy with mastectomy in mammary carcinoma. Acta Oncol 1988;27:671.

73. Lichter A, Lippman M, Danforth D, et al. Mastectomy versus breast conserving therapy in the treatment of stage I and II carcinoma of the breast: a randomized trial at the National Cancer Institute. J Clin Oncol 1992;10:976.

74. Sarrazin D, Le M, Arriagada R, et al. Ten-year results of a randomized trial comparing a conservative treatment to mastectomy in early breast cancer. Radiother Oncol 1989;14:177.

75. Ang KK, Byers RM, Peters LJ, et al. Regional radiotherapy as adjuvant treatment for head and neck malignant melanoma. Arch Otolaryngol Head Neck Surg 1990;116:169.

76. Randomized controlled trial of adjuvant chemoimmunotherapy with DTIC and BCG after complete excision of primary melanoma with a poor prognosis or melanoma metastases. Can Med Assoc J 1983;128:929.

77. Balch CM, Murray D, Presant C, Bartolucci AA. Ineffectiveness of adjuvant chemotherapy using DTIC and cyclophosphamide in patients with resectable metastatic melanoma. Surgery 1984;95:454.

78. Balch CM, Buzaid AC, Atkins MB, et al. A new American Joint Committee on Cancer staging system for cutaneous melanoma. Cancer 2000;88:1484.

79. Balch CM, Murad TM, Soong SJ, et al. A multifactorial analysis of melanoma: prognostic histopathological features comparing Clark's and Breslow's staging methods. Ann Surg 1978;188:732.

80. Balch CM, Soong SJ, Murad TM, et al. A multifactorial analysis of melanoma. II. Prognostic factors in patients with stage I (localized) melanoma. Surgery 1979;86(2):343.

81. Balch CM, Soong SJ, Milton GW, et al. A comparison of prognostic factors and surgical results in 1,786 patients with localized (stage I) melanoma treated in Alabama, USA, and New South Wales, Australia. Ann Surg 1982;196:677.

82. Buttner P, Garbe C, Bertz J, et al. Primary cutaneous melanoma. Optimized cutoff points of tumor thickness and importance of Clark's level for prognostic classification. Cancer 1995;75:2499.

83. Sondergaard K. Depth of invasion and tumor thickness in primary cutaneous malignant melanoma. A study of 2012 cases. Acta Pathol Microbiol Immunol Scand [A] 1985;93(2):49.

84. Buzaid AC, Ross MI, Balch CM, et al. Critical analysis of the current American Joint Committee on Cancer staging system for cutaneous melanoma and proposal of a new staging system. J Clin Oncol 1997;15:1039.

85. Schuchter L, Schultz DJ, Synnestvedt M, et al. A prognostic model for predicting 1-year survival in patients with primary melanoma. Ann Intern Med 1996;125:369.

86. Balch CM. Cutaneous melanoma: prognosis and treatment results worldwide. Semin Surg Oncol 1992;8 (6):400.

87. Averbook BJ, Russo LJ, Mansour EG. A long-term analysis of 620 patients with malignant melanoma at a major referral center. Surgery 1998;124(4):746.

88. Kuehnl-Petzoldt C, Wiebelt H, Berger H. Prognostic groups of patients with stage I melanoma. Arch Dermatol 1983;119:816.

89. Thorn M, Ponten F, Bergstrom R, et al. Clinical and histopathologic predictors of survival in patients with malignant melanoma: a population-based study in Sweden. J Natl Cancer Inst 1994;86:761.

90. Gershenwald JE, Thompson W, Mansfield PF, et al. Multi-institutional melanoma lymphatic mapping experience: the prognostic value of sentinel lymph node status in 612 stage I or II melanoma patients. J Clin Oncol 1999;17:976.

91. Urist MM, Balch CM, Soong SJ, et al. Head and neck melanoma in 534 clinical stage I patients. A prognostic factors analysis and results of surgical treatment. Ann Surg 1984;200(6):769.

92. Balch CM, Wilkerson JA, Murad TM, et al. The prognostic significance of ulceration of cutaneous melanoma. Cancer 1980;45(12):3012.

93. Cascinelli N, Marubini E, Morabito A, Bufalino R. Prognostic factors for stage I melanoma of the skin: a review. Stat Med 1985;4:265.

94. Soong SJ, Shaw HM, Balch CM, et al. Predicting survival and recurrence in localized melanoma: a multivariate approach. World J Surg 1992;16(2):191.

95. Ostmeier H, Fuchs B, Friedrich O, et al. Can immuno-histochemical markers and mitotic rate improve prognostic precision in patients with primary melanoma? Cancer 1999;85:2391.

96. Day CL Jr, Lew RA, Harrist TJ. Malignant melanoma prognostic factors 4: ulceration width. J Dermatol Surg Oncol 1984;10:23.

97. Balch CM, Soong SJ, Murad TM, et al. A multifactorial analysis of melanoma: III. Prognostic factors in melanoma patients with lymph node metastases (stage II). Ann Surg 1981;193(3):377.

98. Buzaid AC, Tinoco LA, Jendiroba D, et al. Prognostic value of size of lymph node metastases in patients with cutaneous melanoma. J Clin Oncol 1995;13 (9):2361.

99. Slingluff CL Jr, Vollmer R, Seigler HF. Stage II malignant melanoma: presentation of a prognostic model and an assessment of specific active immunotherapy in 1,273 patients. J Surg Oncol 1988;39:139.

100. Drepper H, Bieb B, Hofherr B, et al. The prognosis of patients with stage III melanoma. Cancer 1993; 71:1239.

101. Coit DG, Rogatko A, Brennan MF. Prognostic factors in patients with melanoma metastatic to axillary or inguinal lymph nodes. A multivariate analysis. Ann Surg 1991;214:627.

102. Kissin MW, Simpson DA, Easton D, et al. Prognostic factors related to survival and groin recurrence following therapeutic lymph node dissection for lower limb malignant melanoma. Br J Surg 1987;74:1023.

103. Karakousis CP, Hena MA, Emrich LJ, Driscoll DL. Axillary node dissection in malignant melanoma: results and complications. Surgery 1990;108:10.

104. Roses DF, Provet JA, Harris MN, et al. Prognosis of patients with pathologic stage II cutaneous malignant melanoma. Ann Surg 1985;201:103.

105. Cascinelli N, Vaglini M, Nava M, et al. Prognosis of skin melanoma with regional node metastases (stage II). Surg Oncol 1984;25:240.

106. Koh HK, Sober AJ, Day CL Jr, et al. Prognosis of clinical stage I melanoma patients with positive elective regional node dissection. J Clin Oncol 1986;4(8):1238.

107. Morton DL, Wanek L, Nizze JA, et al. Improved long-term survival after lymphadenectomy of melanoma metastatic to regional nodes. Ann Surg 1991;214:491.

108. Cascinelli N, Morabito A, Santinami M, et al. Immediate or delayed dissection of regional nodes in patients with melanoma of the trunk: a randomised trial. Lancet 1998;351:793.

109. Keilholz U, Conradt C, Legha SS, et al. Results of interleukin-2-based treatment in advanced melanoma: a case record-based analysis of 631 patients. J Clin Oncol 1998;16(9):2921.

110. Eton O, Legha SS, Moon TE, et al. Prognostic factors for survival of patients treated systemically for disseminated melanoma. J Clin Oncol 1998;16(3):1103.

111. Balch CM, Soong SJ, Murad TM, et al. A multifactorial analysis of melanoma. IV. Prognostic factors in 200 melanoma patients with distant metastases (stage III). J Clin Oncol 1983;1(2):126.

112. Barth A, Wanek LA, Morton DL. Prognostic factors in 1,521 melanoma patients with distant metastases. J Am Coll Surg 1995;181:193.

113. Brand CU, Ellwanger U, Stroebel W, et al. Prolonged survival of 2 years or longer for patients with disseminated melanoma. Cancer 1997;79:2345.

13

Immunotherapy for Melanoma

SIXUN YANG, MD, PhD

FRANK G. HALUSKA, MD, PhD

RATIONALE FOR IMMUNOTHERAPY

The application of immunology to the problem of cancer has fascinated immunologists since the beginning of the twentieth century, and the concept of experimentally triggering the human immune system in an attempt to eliminate cancers can be traced to studies initiated over 100 years ago. During the 1890s, William Coley, a general surgeon from New York City, observed tumor regression in a patient with a systemic bacterial infection. He surmised that the host immune response to the bacterial infection somehow extended to an antitumor response; so he deliberately infected cancer patients with live and heat-killed bacteria in an attempt to eliminate the tumor cells by stimulating the patients' own immune systems. Although complete tumor regression was seen in some patients, his results overall were inconsistent, and the approach was eventually discontinued.[1] Subsequent developments in cancer immunology were driven by laboratory advances. Indeed, after the development of inbred mouse strains, tumor transplantation studies in the 1950s and '60s demonstrated that mice could be immunized against transplants of chemically or ultraviolet (UV)-induced cancers that arose in the same inbred mouse strains. These studies, providing the first evidence for the existence of "tumor-specific antigens" that could be perceived by the immune system, initiated the modern era of tumor immunology.

Increasing evidence has accumulated that tumor-specific antigens also exist in human cancers. Melanoma has been the type of solid tumor most intensively studied from the immunologic perspective, and many patients with melanoma exhibit phenomena that suggest that the immune system recognizes the tumor. The following section reviews some of the principles that underlie the tumor immunology of melanoma and summarizes the development of specific experimental antimelanoma vaccines.

CLINICAL IMMUNOLOGIC PHENOMENA ASSOCIATED WITH MELANOMA

Four clinical observations noted in melanoma cases suggest that the host immune system recognizes and responds to the malignancy. The first is lymphocytic infiltration of tumors, evident on examination of both primary and metastatic lesions. The second is halo phenomena (depigmentation immediately adjacent to pigmented lesions). The third is vitiligo, a regional or generalized loss of melanocytes through immunologic mechanisms. The last and most compelling is spontaneous regression. This is manifest both clinically and histologically, in which case it has prognostic significance.

Lymphocytic Infiltration of Tumors

Primary lesions frequently exhibit histologic evidence of lymphocyte recognition (Figure 13–1). Lymphocytic infiltration can be localized or generalized and can be characterized pathologically by the location and extent of the infiltrate. Infiltrating lymphocytes have been characterized; usually they are CD4 and CD8 T cells. Data suggest that brisk lymphocytic infiltration is correlated with an improved prognosis.

Metastatic lesions are also often infiltrated by lymphocytes. These are termed "tumor-infiltrating lymphocytes" (TILs) and have been used both as

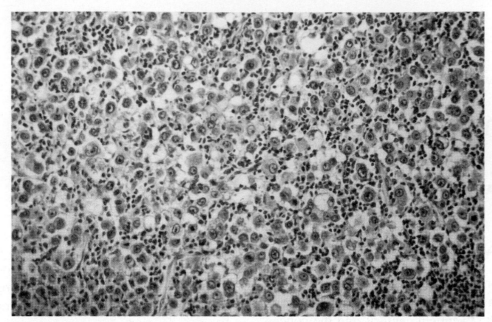

Figure 13–1. Histology of a melanoma infiltrated by tumor-infiltrating lymphocytes. The region is diffusely involved with lymphocytic infiltration.

laboratory reagents by which to isolate stimulating antigens and as therapeutic agents after ex vivo expansion. Both of these uses are discussed below.

Halo Phenomena and Vitiligo

Halos and vitiligo are thought to be examples of similar biologic mechanisms. The infiltrating lympho-

cytes described above recognize antigenic epitopes on the melanoma cell surface; these determinants are also expressed on normal melanocytes. As a consequence, immunologic recognition of melanoma can also lead to the recognition and destruction of normal melanocytes.[2] When this occurs locally, an areola of depigmentation may surround either a nevus or a frank melanoma (Figures 13–2 and 13–3). Evidence

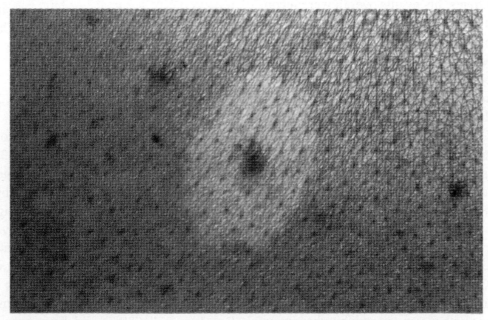

Figure 13–2. A halo nevus demonstrating an area of depigmentation surrounding the pigmented lesion.

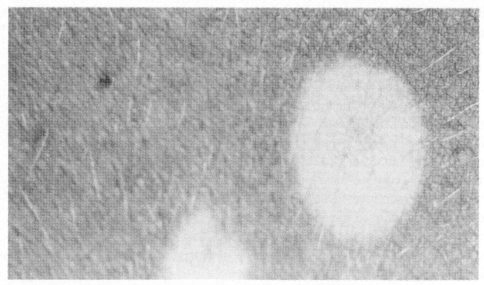

Figure 13–3. A completely regressed halo nevus, with only a residual area of depigmentation.

suggests that CD8+ T cells mediate this effect.[3] If the effect is generalized, widespread leukoderma or vitiligo may be observed (Figure 13–4). When vitiligo occurs, it is typically associated with an improved prognosis, presumably because it indicates that the host immune response is at least partially effective in destroying cells carrying the target epitopes; this is most true of vitiligo associated with therapy. Patients treated with high-dose interleukin-2, for example, may develop vitiligo in the course of their response to therapy.[4]

Regression

Melanoma exhibits evidence of spontaneous involution, or regression, more frequently than other tumor types. This may occur microscopically. Such histologic evidence of regression has long been understood to have prognostic import; although controversial, there is evidence that regression of a primary lesion correlates with a better outcome clinically.[5] Typically, regression is characterized by findings ranging from early melanoma cell degeneration

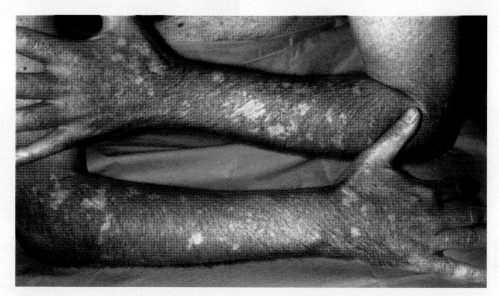

Figure 13–4. Melanoma-associated vitiligo. In this case, the vitiligo arose after dendritic cell vaccination involving the introduction of engineered viruses expressing gp100 and MART-1.

accompanied by lymphocytic infiltration to complete melanoma cell destruction and fibrosis (Figures 13–5 and 13–6).

Regression of clinically evident lesions can also be observed. In the case pictured in Figure 13–7, bacterial infection of the cavity left following resection of a cerebral metastasis took place prior to regression. This may have been an example of the phenomenon studied by Coley and described earlier.[1]

These immunologic observations have long stimulated melanoma researchers to investigate immunologic approaches to the treatment of melanoma. As a result, melanoma has been the model for immunotherapeutic experimentation, and many of the approaches described below will ultimately be tested on other types of cancer as well.

BASIC CONCEPTS OF IMMUNE RESPONSE TO TUMOR

The immune system consists of (1) an innate component that includes effector cells such as macrophages and natural killer (NK) cells and (2) an adaptive component consisting of antigen-specific B and T lymphocytes. Macrophages and NK cells (especially the latter) are thought to play an important role in immune surveillance and tumor immunology in an

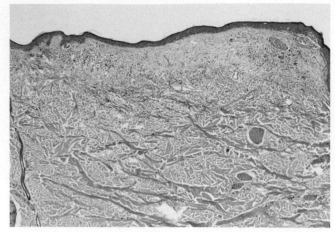

Figure 13–6. Histopathology of regression. The section demonstrates lymphocytic infiltration and melanocytic disruption with fibrosis.

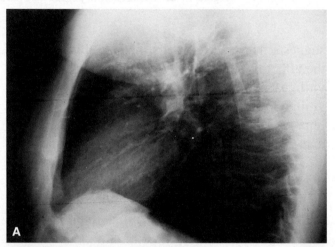

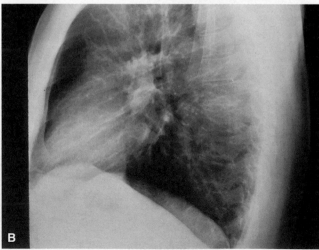

Figure 13–7. Clinical spontaneous regression. *A,* A lateral chest radiograph demonstrates a 2-cm left upper-lobe mass overlying the vertebral column. *B,* A radiograph from approximately 1 year later demonstrates complete spontaneous regression. The patient suffered an intercurrent bacterial brain abscess, and the clinical presentation may be an example of the phenomenon long ago observed by William Coley.

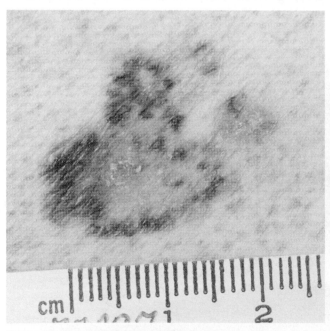

Figure 13–5. A superficial spreading melanoma with an area of depigmentation consistent with regression.

antigen-independent manner. However, most efforts to develop immunologic therapies have employed antigen-specific approaches using B or T cells.

The rationale for attempting to direct B-cell responses at tumors is threefold. First, a wide variety of tumor-associated antigens have been shown to engender an antibody response, and although it is unclear whether these responses are effective in controlling tumors, the observation suggests that the humoral arm of the immune system is capable of recognizing malignancy. Second, patients with antibodies to tumors (either endogenous antibodies or therapeutically engendered antibodies) appear to carry a better prognosis than those without antibody response. And third, several monoclonal antibodies have been tested in hematologic malignancies and solid tumors in the last few years and have been shown to be effective. Thus, the field of antibody-mediated therapy is an emerging one.

Yet, the most developed line of investigation in melanoma has involved the cellular immunologic approach. The clinical observations already mentioned demonstrate a prominent role for TILs, which are predominantly T cells; thus, an understanding of the biology of T lymphocytes is central to reviewing melanoma immunotherapy. T lymphocytes clonally express antigen-specific receptors, namely, T-cell receptors (TCRs) that are generated during lymphocyte differentiation through somatic gene re-arrangement. This somatic re-arrangement of TCR (and immunoglobulin) genes is the molecular basis of the diversity of antigen recognition. Since gene re-arrangement gives rise to cells expressing receptors that recognize autologous self-antigens, it is followed by selection and clonal deletion to remove strongly autoreactive lymphocytes or lymphocytes with high-affinity TCRs in the thymus. However, T cells with low- to intermediate-affinity TCRs (even if they recognize self-antigens) remain in circulation. Thus, all individuals carry T lymphocytes that may recognize self-antigens on normal tissues and (most important) on tumors.

The TCR does not recognize entire native proteins. Instead, it recognizes peptide fragments of antigen presented on the cell surface. In addition, the peptides are not recognized by themselves; they are recognized when they are noncovalently bound by transmembrane glycoproteins encoded by the major histocompatibility complex (MHC) (Figure 13–8). In this way, all T-cell recognition of foreign ("nonself") antigens involves co-recognition of self-MHC molecules, a phenomenon known as MHC restriction. Tumor antigens, which may be self or non-self (mutated or virus modified), can be recognized and targeted by the immune system.

The tumor antigens targeted by T cells are proteins that are processed intracellularly and presented as short peptide fragments, usually 8 to 10 residues, bound in the groove of the tumor MHC class I molecules to be recognized by CD8+ cytotoxic T lymphocytes (CTLs). However, the mere presence of a tumor antigen is not sufficient to trigger an immune response. The second signal, provided either by CD4+ helper T cells or by the interaction between co-stimulatory molecules, is required (Figure 13–9). Once antigen-specific CTLs are activated, they are capable of recognizing and destroying the tumors.

Due to clonal deletion, self-tolerance, and inefficient antigen presentation by tumor cells, most tumors cannot induce effective CTL responses. Strategies for augmenting the antitumor response that have been investigated include stimulating both non-specific and specific antitumor immunity. Modalities for eliciting host immunity to destroy malignant tumors are now entering clinical trials (Table 13–1).

TUMOR CELL–BASED VACCINES

Several strategies have been designed to augment host immune responses to melanoma. One of the first approaches to be widely tested in human subjects was the use of whole melanoma cells, administered autologously or allogeneically. The cells may be administered intact or with some modification or as an extract (Figure 13–10). Data from clinical trials of several types of tumor-based vaccines are available; however, most of these data are from phase I or II studies, and only limited information concerning the therapeutic efficacy of these agents is obtainable.

Autologous Whole-Cell Vaccines

In theory, autologous melanoma cells are potentially optimal tumor vaccines because they carry all the biologically relevant antigens that could be presented to the immune system. Of course, the tumor arose in the host, suggesting that the antigens it carries engender an immune response ineffectively. So the experimental approach has been to attempt to augment the response to the tumor by administration with adjuvants that enhance the response. However, this approach is limited to individuals with sufficient tumor available to prepare a vaccine, and because of self-tolerance, the host may not respond to immunization, despite the use of adjuvants.

Berd and colleagues[6,7] conducted clinical studies in patients with stage IV melanoma, using autolo-

gous tumor. In their studies, autologous whole-cell vaccines were prepared from freshly excised tumor by dissociating the tumor into single-cell suspensions. The cells were cryopreserved in liquid nitrogen and irradiated before vaccination. The autologous whole-cell vaccines were administered by intradermal injections combined with bacille Calmette-Guérin (BCG) as adjuvant in the extremities, with repetition of the cycles every 4 weeks. One nonrandomized trial of this autologous tumor vaccine demonstrated a 12.5 percent response rate.[7] Interestingly, antitumor responses were associated with the development of specific antitumor immunity as

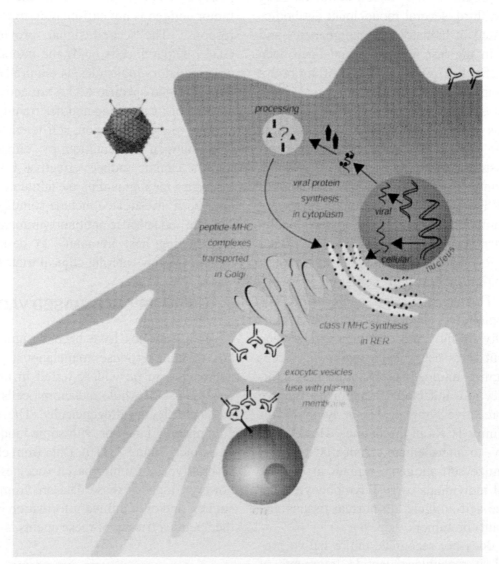

Figure 13–8. Processing of peptides by antigen-presenting cells. Viral or cellular proteins are processed through the proteosomal machinery and transported to the endoplasmic reticulum. There, they are loaded on to major histocompatibility complex (MHC) class I molecules and transported through the Golgi. Peptides complexed with class I molecules and β_2-microglobulin are then transported to the cell surface, where they are recognized by cytolytic T lymphocytes.

assessed by skin test of delayed-type hypersensitivity (DTH), suggesting that an intact host immune response was required for vaccine-induced tumor regression.

Allogeneic Whole-Cell Vaccines

Pioneer work performed by Seigler and colleagues[8-11] has demonstrated that most melanoma cells have "shared" or common antigens that can be recognized by the immune system. Melanoma cells with shared antigens can be lysed by allogeneic CTLs raised in vitro in a human leukocyte antigen (HLA) class I–restricted manner. They can also be used to generate tumor antigen–specific and HLA class I–restricted CTLs from HLA class I–matched peripheral blood mononuclear cells. Furthermore, such CTLs generated against allogeneic tumors are highly toxic to autologous melanomas. The work provides a rationale for immunotherapy for melanoma using allogeneic melanomas. Allogeneic whole-cell vaccines have several advantages, compared with autologous whole-cell vaccines. This approach could be used for any patient and is more convenient since harvesting

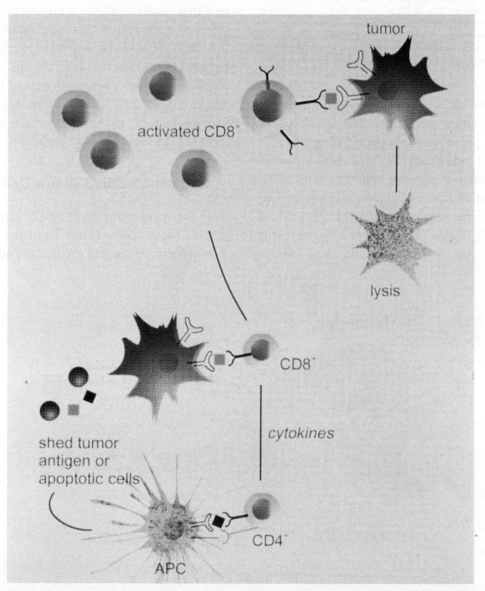

Figure 13–9. A schematic diagram of T-cell recognition and activity against tumors. Antigen-presenting cells (APCs) process antigen shed by tumors or internalized from apoptotic dying cells. These are recognized by CD4 and/or CD8 cells; CD4 helper cells articulate cytokines that stimulate the CD8 CTLs. Activated CTLs then encounter tumor, recognize cognitive antigen, and result in tumor lysis.

Table 13–1. STRATEGIES FOR ANTITUMOR IMMUNOTHERAPY

Nonspecific
    Bacille Calmette-Guérin (BCG)
    Cytokines (IL-2, IFN-α, IFN-γ, GM-CSF, etc)
    Lymphokine-activated killer (LAK) cells
    IL-2 plus LAK cells
Specific
    Tumor-based vaccines
        Autologous or allogeneic whole cells
        Hapten-modified tumor cells
        Gene-modified tumor cells
        Tumor cell lysate
    Purified or recombinant antigens
    Synthetic peptides
    Dendritic cell (DC)–based vaccines
        Antigen-pulsed or tumor lysate–pulsed DCs
        TAA gene–modified DCs
        TAA gene– and cytokine gene–modified DCs
    Adoptive transfer of CTLs or TILs

CTLs = cytotoxic T lymphocytes; GM-CSF = granulocyte-macrophage colony–stimulating factor; IL-2 = interleukin-2; IFN-α = interferon-α; IFN-γ = interferon-γ; TILs = tumor-infiltrating lymphocytes; TAA = tumor-associated antigen.

of autologous tumor is not required. Additionally, the allogeneic vaccines may be more immunogenic because of the presence of allogeneic antigens.

Morton and colleagues[12,13] have used a mixture of three allogeneic melanoma cell lines with a high content of immunogenic melanoma-associated antigens. The vaccine (designated CancerVax) is prepared by equally mixing the three cell lines growing separately in vitro, irradiating them, and freezing them in batches in liquid nitrogen. In several studies, patients received biweekly intradermal injections of CancerVax for 12 weeks, followed by monthly vaccinations for the 1st year and every 2 to 3 months thereafter. In single-institution uncontrolled studies, the median survival period for the immunized group was 23 months versus 7.5 months for historical controls evaluated at the same institution. At 5 years, 25 percent of the CancerVax recipients were alive versus 6 percent of the historical control group. In addition, supporting laboratory data showed that overall survival correlated with the generation of CTLs against autologous tumor cells. These data may suggest that vaccination has a therapeutically beneficial effect. But the results also may be explained by factors that include the selection of better-prognosis patients for vaccination or the correlation of immune responsiveness with a more indolent natural melanoma course. Only randomized trials of the vaccine therapy will address these questions; such trials are presently being conducted.

Hapten-Modified Tumor Cell Vaccines

Both the autologous and the allogeneic administration of tumor cells suffer from the limitation that these vaccine strategies involve the administration of

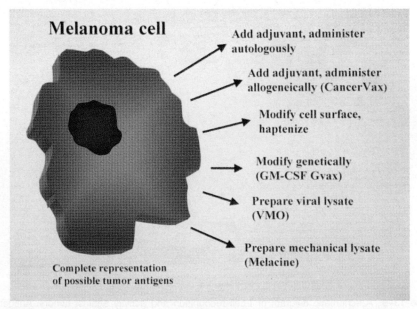

Figure 13–10. Strategies for the use of whole cells in vaccines. Typically, autologous or allogeneic melanoma cells are modified or administered through one of several strategies as illustrated and discussed in the text.

cells that had been ineffective immunogens in the subjects from which they were derived. One attempt to circumvent this limitation has involved the modification of the cell surface antigens to better their immune recognition. It has been reported that presentation of tumor cells conjugated to a strongly immunogenic hapten can induce potent systemic T-cell immunity to parental tumor cells[14] (Figure 13–11). Because of the low immunogenicity of the autologous whole-cell vaccine, Berd and colleagues[15–17] have developed an autologous whole-cell melanoma vaccine modified with such a hapten, dinitrophenyl (DNP), in an effort to increase the vaccine's immunogenicity. Patients immunized with the hapten-modified vaccine have demonstrated inflammatory responses in metastases, including marked infiltration of CD8+ T cells, the presence of messenger ribonucleic acid (mRNA) for interferon-γ (IFN-γ), and the appearance of novel TCR Vβ structures, all suggesting an immune response. Administration of DNP vaccine also results in the regression of measurable metastases. The most common regression has been that of small lung metastases. Administration of DNP vaccine in the postsurgical adjuvant setting for patients with stage III melanoma who had undergone lymphadenectomy resulted in a 5-year relapse-free

survival rate of 45 percent and an overall survival rate of 58 percent.[17] But again, these single-arm studies, lacking a control population, are difficult to interpret; rather than proving a clinical benefit, they suggest a strategy for further randomized studies.

Tumor Lysate Vaccines

Several groups have examined the efficacy of cell lysates of tumor cells as a source of tumor antigen. The purpose of this approach was to maximize antigen availability through cell disruption. Two methods have been used to produce cell lysate vaccines: viral-induced oncolysis and mechanical disruption of cell membranes.

The cell lysate vaccine using virally induced oncolysis was first developed and evaluated by Wallack and colleagues.[18–21] In their studies, four allogeneic melanoma cell lines were infected with a lytic virus, vaccinia. The cells were incubated overnight, and a nucleus-free cell lysate containing membrane fragments of virus-lysed cells was extracted by repeated sonication and centrifugation. The lysates of all four cell lines were pooled to produce a tetravalent vaccinia melanoma oncolysate (VMO) vaccine. A phase III randomized trial of VMO versus vaccinia

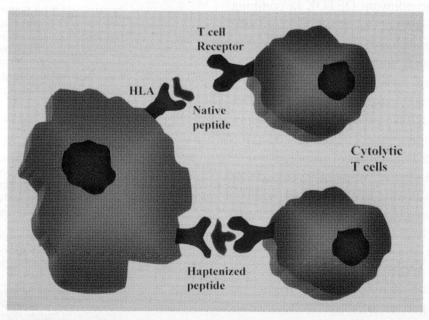

Figure 13–11. Hapten modification of antigens. Native peptides, being self-derived, are poorly recognized by cytolytic T cells. However, chemical modification of antigens (eg, by the introduction of dinitrophenyl [DNP]) results in better recognition and tumor disruption by cytotoxic T lymphocytes.

virus alone was conducted in stage III melanoma patients after surgical resection of involved nodes.[21] In this trial, VMO or vaccinia virus alone was administered intradermally near the sites of nodal basins weekly for 13 weeks and biweekly thereafter for 1 year. No benefit was observed with VMO treatment as assessed by disease-free interval or overall survival upon follow-up at 46.3 months.

A similar strategy[22–24] was also tested in a nonrandomized phase II trial using vaccinia melanoma cell lysate (VMCL). The method used to produce the vaccine is similar to that used by Wallack and colleagues except for the use of only one allogeneic melanoma cell line. A phase II trial of VMCL for stage III melanoma showed a 5-year survival of 60 percent for those treated with VMCL, versus both a historical control group (34% 5-year survival) and a concurrent nonrandomized control group (35% 5-year survival). The final analysis of a 400-patient randomized study of VMCL versus nonimmunotherapy groups is under way.

A tumor cell lysate vaccine using mechanical disruption of cell membranes has also been reported. Using a high-speed tissue homogenizer and freeze-thaw cycles, Mitchell and colleagues created a mixture of mechanical lysates of two melanoma cell lines.[25–28] The lysate was used in combination with an adjuvant DETOX (a combination of detoxified bacterial endotoxin and mycobacterial cell wall skeletons) as a vaccine (Melacine) for injection into patients with metastatic melanoma. Combined results of both phase I and II trials in stage III and IV melanoma patients showed an overall response in 20 of 106 patients; of the 20 patients, 5 had complete responses and 15 experienced partial responses. The median duration of response was 21 months, but overall survival was not increased. The clinical response was strongly correlated with the increase in precursors of CTLs. Failure to generate CTLs was invariably associated with failure of the vaccine to induce tumor shrinkage, and only those patients in whom a cell-mediated response was elicited were capable of rejecting their melanoma. However, only 30 percent of those who generated CTL precursors had an objective long-term remission of more than 1 year in duration. Phase III trials are also under way.

Gene-Modified Tumor Cell Vaccines

One way to enhance the efficacy of a whole-cell vaccine is to conjugate an immunologic molecule to the tumor cell to make it more immunogenic. More recently, however, methods of genetically modifying tumor cells by introducing genes that encode immunomodulatory proteins (eg, cytokines and co-stimulatory molecules) have been explored. These studies have attempted to take advantage of our growing understanding of the cytokines that regulate immune responses. Many murine and human studies have shown that the transduction of melanoma cells with genes encoding cytokines and co-stimulatory molecules leads to increased antitumor immunity against gene-modified tumors as well as parental tumors. Many genes (Table 13–2) have been studied in this manner, including B7, granulocyte-macrophage colony–stimulating factor (GM-CSF),

Table 13–2. CYTOKINES AND THEIR PRINCIPAL FUNCTIONS	
Cytokines	**Principal Functions**
GM-CSF	Activates macrophages; induces granulocytes and monocytes; promotes the differentiation of progenitor cells, monocytes, and Langerhans' cells into dendritic cells
IL-2	Promotes the proliferation and differentiation of immune cells (mainly T cells and NK cells); increases cytokine synthesis by T cells; potentiates Fas-mediated apoptosis of antigen-activated T cells; promotes proliferation and antibody synthesis by B cells
IL-4	Proliferation of T cells; Th2-cell differentiation from naive CD4 helper cells; isotype switching to IgE
IL-6	Synthesis of acute-phase proteins; proliferation of antibody-producing cells
IL-7	Stimulates survival and expansion of immature precursors committed to the B- and T-lymphocyte lineages; growth factor for mature T cells
IFN-γ	Increased microbicidal function of macrophages; increased MHC class I and II expression and antigen processing and presentation to T cells; promotes the differentiation of native CD4 T cells to Th1 effector cells and inhibits the proliferation of Th2 T cells
TNF-α	Stimulates the recruitment of neutrophils and monocytes to sites of infection; activation of neutrophils and monocytes; induces fever, cachexia, and apoptosis of many cell types
Flt-3L	Promotes the proliferation, survival, and differentiation of hematopoietic precursors; expansion of mature dendritic cell subsets

GM-CSF = granulocyte-macrophage colony–stimulating factor; IFN-γ = interferon-γ; IgE = immunoglobulin E; IL = interleukin; MHC = major histocompatibility complex; NK = natural killer; TNF-α = tumor necrosis factor-α.

interleukins-2, -4, -6, and -7 (IL-2, IL-4, IL-6, IL-7), IFN-γ, Flt-3L, and tumor necrosis factor-α (TNF-α). The most potent stimulator of systemic antitumor immunity seems to be GM-CSF.[29,30]

The first such strategy to be clinically tested involved the transduction of melanoma cells with GM-CSF, tested by Dranoff and colleagues.[31] This approach derived from laboratory work that involved exhaustive testing of a variety of cytokine genes as enhancers of immune response. The strategy is illustrated in Figure 13–12. In the mouse model, melanoma cells transduced with the gene for GM-CSF were highly protective against challenge by an otherwise lethal dose of malignant cells.[29] Recently, Soiffer and colleagues[32] reported a phase I clinical trial that investigated this strategy by vaccinating metastatic melanoma patients, using irradiated autologous melanoma cells engineered to secrete human GM-CSF. Immunization sites were intensively infiltrated with T cells, dendritic cells, macrophages, and eosinophils in all 21 evaluable patients. Metastatic lesions resected after vaccination were densely infiltrated with T cells and plasma cells and showed extensive tumor destruction, fibrosis, and edema in 11 of 16 patients examined (Figures 13–13 and 13–14). This trial suggests that autologous melanoma vaccine modified by GM-CSF stimulates potent antimelanoma responses and raises the possibility that this effect is mediated through dendritic cells to GM-CSF.

A similarly tested cytokine is IFN-γ, an immunomodulator with direct and indirect antitumor effects. Interferon-γ, which acts by activating NK cells and CTLs and by up-regulating MHC molecule expression on tumor cells, has been introduced genetically into autologous melanoma cells as a tumor vaccine in clinical trial. Abdel-Wahab and colleagues[33] reported that 8 of 13 patients who completed vaccination demonstrated the development of humoral immunoglobulin G (IgG) response against melanoma. Four patients with IgG response showed tumor response and transient shrinkage of nodular metastasis during the treatment. However, the similar phase I clinical trial conducted by Nemunaitis and colleagues and using autologous melanoma vaccines modified by the INF-γ gene showed no measurable tumor response in the five patients.[34] These variable results underscore the difficulty of testing technologically demanding therapies in a comparative and rigorous fashion.

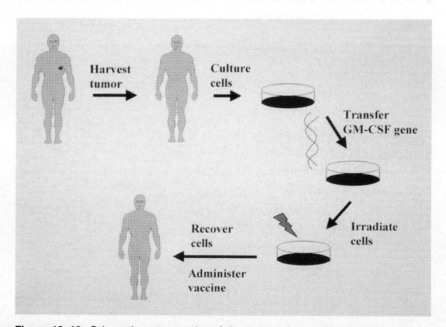

Figure 13–12. Schematic representation of the strategy for vaccination with melanoma cells modified by the granulocyte-macrophage colony–stimulating factor (GM-CSF) gene. A subject with a macroscopic tumor undergoes surgical resection for harvest. Cells are grown in culture. Isolated melanoma cells are then transfected with a retrovirus or adenovirus engineered to encode the GM-CSF gene. After verification of production of the cytokine by the cells, they are irradiated, recovered, and administered back to the patient as a vaccine.

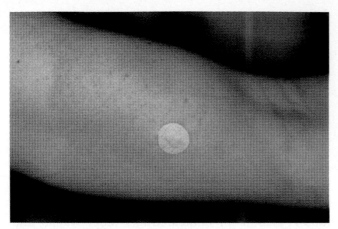

Figure 13–13. Delayed-type hypersensitivity (DTH) reaction at the site of vaccination with autologous melanoma cells modified by the granulocyte-macrophage colony–stimulating factor (GM-CSF) gene. There is an exuberant inflammatory reaction at the site of introduction of the vaccine. (Reproduced with permission from Dranoff G, Soiffer R, Lynch T, et al. A phase I study of vaccination with autologous, irradiated melanoma cells engineered to secrete human granulocyte-macrophage colony stimulating factor. Hum Gene Ther 1997;8:111–23.)

GANGLIOSIDE VACCINES

As an alternative to the use of whole-cell vaccines, attempts have been made to identify those antigens on the melanoma cell surface that are most likely to induce an effective immune response. Thus, vaccine strategies employing individual melanoma cell surface components have also been used. Gangliosides are carbohydrate antigens expressed on several different tumors and are known to be major cell surface constituents of melanoma cells. They are antigens known to be recognized by antibodies but not by T cells. Melanoma tumor cells expressing gangliosides can be lysed by antiganglioside antibodies. In addition, patients mounting an antibody response to ganglioside vaccination appear to have a better prognosis than those not responding.[35] Ganglioside vaccines have been tested in several clinical trials. In a Memorial Sloan-Kettering Cancer Center trial, Livingston and colleagues[35] investigated the use of ganglioside GM_2 mixed with BCG as adjuvant therapy for patients with resected stage III nodal disease. In the study, 122 stage III patients were randomized to vaccination with ganglioside GM_2 plus BCG versus BCG alone. Disease-free survival and overall survival were improved by 18 percent and 11 percent, respectively, but these improvements were not significant. When results were analyzed retrospectively according to the production of anti–ganglioside GM_2 antibody, an advantage was conferred by either endogenous or vaccine-induced anti–ganglioside GM_2 immunity. To increase the immunogenicity of

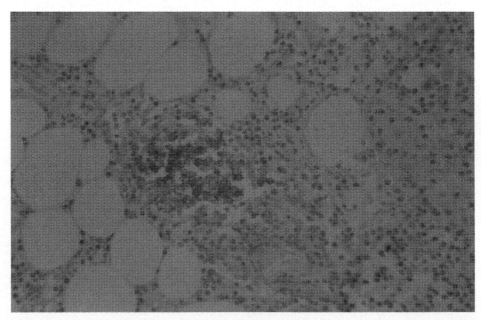

Figure 13–14. Histopathology of a tumor site biopsy specimen after vaccination with autologous melanoma cells modified by granulocyte-macrophage colony–stimulating factor (GM-CSF). This section shows immunoperoxidase for CD1a, a dendritic cell marker, and suggests that GM-CSF stimulates dendritic cell infiltration.

ganglioside GM₂–based vaccine, Chapman and colleagues[36] conjugated ganglioside GM₂ to keyhole limpet hemocyanin (KLH) and used QS21 as adjuvant (GM₂-KLH/QS21). The pilot study demonstrated that the GM₂-KLH/QS21 formulation was more immunogenic than the previous formulation (GM₂/BCG) in inducing immunoglobulin M (IgM) and IgG antibodies against ganglioside GM₂. Based on this preliminary study, a large randomized trial has compared the ganglioside GM₂ vaccine to IFN therapy in the adjuvant treatment of stage III melanoma. Analysis of this trial is ongoing.

TUMOR ANTIGENS

Approaches to Identifying Tumor Antigens

The most promising strategy for specific immunization against melanoma requires the knowledge of the identity of the tumor-associated antigens targeted by the immune response. A number of approaches have been employed to identify these antigens (Figure 13–15). The key to these approaches is the recognition that tumor-infiltrating lymphocytes (TILs) can be used as specific reagents to screen isolated molecules for their antigenic properties. The majority of tumor antigens identified to date that are targets of the immune system are those recognized by tumor-specific CD8+ T cells. The tumor-specific CTLs are usually generated by culturing irradiated melanoma cells with peripheral blood lymphocytes (PBLs) or TILs with IL-2. Those CTLs specifically recognize melanoma cells without significant reaction to normal tissues or other tumors; consequently, they can be used to identify the specific reactive antigens as well. Some of the antigens discovered to date and their characteristics are summarized in Table 13–3.

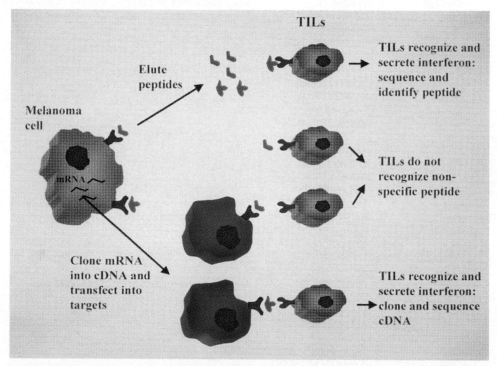

Figure 13–15. Biochemical and genetic strategies for identifying tumor-associated peptides. The melanoma cell, left, displays nonspecific peptides and specific melanoma-associated peptides on the cell surface, the result of translation of messenger ribonucleic acid (mRNA) and antigen processing. The biochemical strategy, top, involves the elution of peptides in solution. The peptides are then screened by tumor-infiltrating lymphocytes (TILs). Cognate TILs recognize the peptides and secrete interferon or lyse target cells pulsed with the peptides. Peptides resulting in activation are then sequenced for identification. In the genetic strategy, below, mRNA is cloned into complementary deoxyribonucleic acid (cDNA) and transfected into target cells. Again, tumor-specific TILs are used to screen targets. Cognate TILs then identify cells containing the cDNA encoding the tumor-specific antigen. The cDNA is isolated and sequenced, yielding the gene encoding the antigen.

Genetic Approach

The genetic approach is the first and most successful approach used to identify a gene encoding a melanoma antigen. The approach uses melanoma-specific CTLs in combination with gene transfection.[37]

Briefly, a eukaryotic expression vector is used to construct a complementary deoxyribonucleic acid (cDNA) library prepared from a melanoma that expresses an appropriate antigen. The library is used to transfect nonmelanoma eukaryotic cells, and transfectants carrying the melanoma antigen are identified by their

Type of MAA	HLA Restriction	Peptide Sequence	Expression	Activation Mechanisms
TSA				
BAGE	–Cw16	AARAVFLAL	Many tumor cells and testis	Ectopic expression of a normal gene
GAGE-1, -2	–Cw6	YRPRPRRY	Many tumor cells and testis	Ectopic expression of a normal gene
MAGE-1	–A1	EADPTGHSY	Many tumor cells and testis	Ectopic expression of a normal gene
	–Cw16	SAYGEPRKL		
MAGE-2	–A2	KWVELVHFL	Many tumor cells and testis	Ectopic expression of a normal gene
	–A2	YLQLVFGIEV		
	–A24	EYLQLVFGI		
MAGE-3	–A1	EVDPIGHLY	Many tumor cells and testis	Ectopic expression of a normal gene
	–A2	FLWGPRALV		
	–A24	TFPDLESEF		
	–B44	MEVDPIGHLY		
	–DR13	AELVHFLLLKYRAR		
	–DR13	LLKYRAREPVTKAE		
MAGE-12	–Cw0702	VRIGHLYIL	Many tumor cells and testis	Ectopic expression of a normal gene
NY-ESO-1	–A2	QLSLLMWWIT	Many tumor cells and testis	Overexpression?
		SLLMWITQC		
		SLLMWWITQCFL		
MSDA				
gp100	–A2	YLEPGPVTA	Melanoma and melanocytes	Overexpression
		LLDGTATLRL		
		KTWGQYWQV		
		ITDQVPFSV		
		VLYRYGSFSV		
		RLPRIFCSC		
	–A3	ALLAVGATK		
	–A3	LIYRRLMK		
	–A3 (A11)	ALNFPGSQK		
	–Cw8	SNDGPTLI		
gp75/TRP-1	–A31	MSLQRQFLR	Melanoma and melanocytes	Overexpression
Melan-A/MART-1	–A2	AAGIGILTV	Melanoma and melanocytes	Overexpression
	–A2	ILTVILGVL		
p15	–A24	AYGLDFYIL	Many normal tissues	Overexpression?
TRP-2	–A31(A33)	LLGPGRPYR	Melanoma and melanocytes	Overexpression
	–Cw8	ANDPIFVVL		
Tyrosinase	–A1	SSDYVIPIGTY	Melanoma and melanocytes	Overexpression
	–A2	MLLAVLYCL		
	–A2	YMDGTMSQV		
	–A24	AFLPWHRLF		
	–B44	SEIWRDIDF		
	–DR4	QNILLSNAPLGPQFP		
	–DR4	SYLQDSDPDSFQD		
SAMA				
β-Catenin	–A24	SYLDSGIHF		Specific amino acid mutation in melanoma
CDK4	–A2	KARDPHSGHFC		Specific amino acid mutation in melanoma
MUM-1	–B44	EEKLIVVLF		Specific amino acid mutation in melanoma

CKD4 = cyclin-dependent kinase 4; HLA = human leukocyte antigen; MAA = melanoma-associated antigen; MSDA = melanoma-specific differentiation antigen; SAMA = specific-amino acid–mutation antigen; TRP = tyrosinase-related protein; TSA = tumor/testis–specific antigen.

ability to stimulate cytokine release from melanoma-specific CTLs or to be killed by melanoma-specific CTLs. Once the gene is identified, the epitope recognized by the CTLs can be established by transfecting gene fragments and using synthetic peptides to sensitize targets for recognition by the CTLs. The advantage of the method is that it results in the identification of not only the peptide antigen but also the gene encoding the protein.

Biochemical Approach

A second approach, involving straightforward biochemistry, was first employed by Cox and colleagues[38] to identify melanoma-antigenic peptides. In this technique, antigenic peptides are isolated from melanoma cell surface HLA class I molecules by acid denaturation and fractionated by reverse-phase high-performance liquid chromatography (RP-HPLC). The fractions are then tested for their ability to sensitize target cells expressing a certain HLA class I molecule for recognition by the appropriate CTL. The candidate antigenic peptides are identified and sequenced by mass spectrometry. These peptides are then synthesized and tested individually to confirm the exact sequences. The major advantage of the approach is that it identifies the naturally processed form of the antigenic peptide and can potentially identify post-translational modification. However, this approach requires relatively complex technology and equipment for mass spectrometric analysis. In addition, it cannot identify the gene encoding the antigen.

Anchor-Motif or Binding-Motif Approach

It has been shown that peptides that bind to class I molecules have a length of 9 to 12 amino residues and characteristically conserved "anchor-motif" amino acids (or "anchor residues"). The anchor motifs serve to facilitate the binding of the peptide to a particular MHC molecule, and motifs for several HLA class I molecules have been identified.[39] With the aid of computer programs, one can use this information to analyze the sequence of potential tumor antigens and predict which peptides from the antigen may bind to a class I molecule and may thus be tumor

antigens. The potential peptides can then be synthesized, and their binding ability can be tested in vitro or predicted with the computer program. The peptides with high binding affinity are then screened for their ability to induce CTL response in vitro or to reconstitute the epitope of melanoma-specific CTLs. The advantage of the approach is that it allows rapid screening of a large number of potential antigens. However, it is limited to known proteins and to those class I molecules whose motif is known. In addition, the CTLs elicited by the peptides identified by this approach must be further tested for their ability to recognize melanomas that express both the appropriate class I antigen and melanoma antigen.

Melanoma Antigens

Through the efforts of several independent research groups, a number of melanoma-associated antigens (MAAs) have been identified. The best-defined MAAs are subdivided into three groups (see Table 13–3): melanoma-specific differentiation antigens (MSDAs), tumor/testis–specific antigens (TSAs), and specific-amino acid–mutation antigens (SAMAs).

Melanoma-Specific Differentiation Antigen

Melanoma-specific differentiation antigens are antigens of melanocytic lineage (eg, gp100/Pmel17, gp75/tyrosinase-related protein 1 [TRP-1], TRP-2, Melan-A/MART-1, p15). These antigens are expressed by tumors and normal cells of melanocytic lineage and by pigmented cells in the retina but not by other tissues or tumors of different histologic origin.

The gene encoding gp100/Pmel17 was originally identified as a melanocyte lineage-specific antigen recognized by the antibody HMB-45.[40] The identification of the protein as an MAA was accomplished when it was demonstrated that the transfection of this gene could reconstitute the epitope recognized by an HLA-A2.1-restricted TIL line.[41–43] Antigenic peptides from this protein were identified independently by several groups. Most of these peptides are restricted by HLA-A2 and can be recognized by TILs and melanoma-specific CTLs[38,41–44] (see Table 13–3). Other HLA loci, A3[45–47] and Cw8,[48] also present gp100 (see Table 13–3). Good potential candidates for immunotherapy are gp100 and its peptides. In support of this, gp100-specific TIL lines have been shown to be effective in adoptive immunotherapy. In addition, immunization of advanced melanoma patients with a gp100 peptide, G209-2M, has also demonstrated an antimelanoma effect.[49]

Using melanoma-specific CTLs derived from PBLs, Melan-A/MART-1 was identified and was named Melan-A.[50] The same gene was identified independently by using HLA-A2-restricted TILs and was named MART-1.[51] Two antigenic peptides were identified by both motif (peptide sequence AAGIGILTV)[51] and biochemical (sequence ILTVILGVL)[52] approaches. However, the two peptides were found to overlap in the amino acid ILTV. Although MART-1 was shown to be recognized by 9 of 10 melanoma-specific TIL lines,[51] it might not be a good candidate for immunotherapy because adoptive transfer of MART-1-specific TILs did not lead to tumor regression.[42]

Tyrosinase is a part of the melanin biosynthesis pathway and catalyses the synthesis of the melanin precursor dihydroxyphenylalanine. The gene encoding tyrosinase was identified by the genetic approach. Presently, five HLA class I–restricted peptides have been identified from tyrosinase (see Table 13–3).[46,53–56]

Interestingly, the HLA-A2-restricted peptide YMDGTMSQV,[53] which was identified by the biochemical approach and is therefore considered a naturally occurring peptide, was first identified as YMNGTMSQV by computer-aided deduction from the tyrosinase gene (binding-motif approach). Both peptides bind equally well to HLA-A2: the naturally occurring peptide sensitizes targets for lysis by CTLs at a 100-fold lower concentration than the deduced version of the peptide. It is hypothesized that naturally processed peptide arises as a result of post-translational modification that converts asparagine (N) to aspartic acid (D) by enzymatic deamidation of N-glycanase. This finding demonstrates that changes in post-translational modification in cancer cells may lead to the generation of new antigens that could induce tumor rejection.

In addition to HLA class I–restricted peptides (see Table 13–3), HLA class II–restricted CD4+ T-cell-specific peptides have also been identified

from tyrosinase.[57] The ability of tyrosinase to provide peptides restricted by both HLA classes I and II may make it an excellent target for immunotherapy because it would presumably be able to stimulate both CD8+ and CD4+ T cells simultaneously.

The tyrosinase-related protein 1 (TRP-1) antigen is identical to a previously reported protein (gp75) that was recognized by IgG from a melanoma patient. The gene encoding TRP-1 antigen was identified using HLA-A31-restricted TILs.[58] However, the antigenic peptide MSLQRQFLR recognized by the TILs was derived from an alternative open reading frame that directs the translation of a 24-amino acid peptide but not from the normal gp75 protein. Thus, translation of alternative open reading frames, a phenomenon reported in some viruses but not previously described in eukaryotic cells, may be a new mechanism for the generation of tumor antigens.

Tyrosinase-related protein 2 (TRP-2) is another member of the tyrosinase family. Like TRP-1, TRP-2 (which has about a 40% amino acid sequence identity with TRP-1) was also identified using HLA-A31-restricted TILs.[59,60] However, the epitope peptide derived from TRP-2 is different from that of TRP-1.

The gene encoding p15 was isolated using HLA-A24-restricted TILs, and a 9mer peptide (AYGLDFYIL) was also identified.[61] Although transcription of p15 mRNA was presented in a wide variety of normal tissues, all the cell lines tested except melanoma were not recognized by the TILs. It appears that the expression of the p15 gene is post-transcriptionally regulated so that melanoma cells (but not other cells) express the protein.

Tumor/Testis–Specific Antigens

The antigens in this group include BAGE, GAGE, MAGE, and NY-ESO-1. They are expressed almost exclusively on various tumors in addition to melanomas but are not expressed in normal tissues except for testis tissue, which does not express MHC molecules.[62]

One of the first human tumor antigens isolated by tumor-specific CTLs was MAGE-1.[63] Recent studies demonstrate that there are at least 12 genes in the MAGE family and that all MAGE genes are located on the long arm of chromosome X.[64] The MAGE-1 gene presents HLA-A1- and HLA-Cw16-restricted epitopes,[65,66] MAGE-2 shows HLA-A2[67] and HLA-A24[68] restriction, and MAGE-3 shows HLA-A1, -A2, -A24, and -B44 restriction.[69–72] Most recently, an HLA-Cw*0702-restricted epitope derived from MAGE-12 was identified from a patient previously immunized with gp100 peptide G209-2M.[73] Of interest, the peptide epitope REPVTKAEML encoded by the homologous region of MAGE-1, -2, -3, and -6 was also identified as a shared HLA-B*3701-restricted antigenic peptide of the four different members of the MAGE family.[74] In addition, HLA-DR13-restricted CD4+ T-cell-specific peptides have been isolated from MAGE-3 using MAGE-3-specific CD4+ T-cell clones.[75] The corresponding antigenic epitopes are shown in Table 13–3.

The other two gene families that encode tumor antigens recognized by melanoma-specific CTLs are BAGE and GAGE. The antigenic peptides identified from BAGE and GAGE are all restricted by HLA-C molecules.[76,77] Until now, no HLA-A-restricted and HLA-B-restricted antigenic peptides from these antigens have been reported.

By screening cDNA expression libraries using antibody from melanoma patients with high-titer antibody against NY-ESO-1, NY-ESO-1 was isolated.[78] It is aberrantly expressed in human cancer. Computer calculation has identified 26 peptides with HLA-A2-binding motifs encoded by NY-ESO-1. Three of those were efficiently recognized by antigen-specific CTLs. Although CTL responses to tumor antigens are of most interest, protective antibody responses to this antigen may occur. Most recently, HLA class II–restricted CD4-positive-specific peptide was also identified from NY-ESO-1 protein.[79]

Specific-Amino Acid–Mutation Antigens

The antigens in this group are encoded by genes that are expressed ubiquitously but that are mutated in tumor cells. These mutations may enable the antigenic peptides to bind to the MHC molecules or generate new epitopes that are recognized as foreign. Some of these mutations are relatively specific, but some, such as mutations in the gene encoding cyclin-dependent kinase 4 (CDK4), have been found in several melanoma lines.[80]

β-Catenin is a cytoplasmic protein that interacts with the cellular adhesion molecule E-cadherin. The antigenic peptide (SYLDSGIHF) identified from β-catenin shows HLA-A24 restriction.[81] However, the cDNA encoding a protein recognized by TILs is different from a previously reported sequence of the gene encoding β-catenin at a single nucleotide, resulting in an amino residue change from serine to phenylalanine.[81] The mutation is at the ninth residue of the peptide, a position that has been shown to be a dominant anchor residue in HLA-A24-binding motif. This mutation is not found in normal cells of the patient and is not found in other tested allogeneic melanoma cells.

The antigenic peptide (EEKLIVVLF) in MUM-1 was identified by HLA-B44-restricted melanoma-specific CTLs.[82] When the sequence of the MUM-1 gene in melanoma cells was compared to that in normal cells, it was found that there was a point mutation in the tumor gene such that a serine (S) residue was replaced with isoleucine (I). Both the mutated and the normal versions of the peptide bind to HLA-B44 equally, but only the mutated one was recognized by CTL.[82]

Another example of mutated peptide was identified in CDK4. The mutation, an arginine (R)-to-cysteine (C) exchange at residue 24, was recognized by CTLs in an HLA-A2-restricted manner.[80] When loaded on T2 cells, both the mutated (KA*R*DPHSGHFC) and normal (KA*C*DPHSGHFC) sequences of the synthetic peptides can be recognized by tumor-specific CTLs. However, wild-type cDNA fragments did not confer CTL recognition after transfection. The result suggested that peptide derived from wild-type DNA is not presented on the cell surface and that the mutation affects peptide processing and/or transportation.

PEPTIDE VACCINES

The molecular identification of MAA and the antigenic epitopes recognized by T cells has opened a new era in the immunotherapy of melanoma. Several small pilot clinical trials have been performed using synthetic antigenic peptides corresponding to defined MAA gp100,[49,83] MAGE-3,[84] and Melan-A/MART-1,[85] injected either alone or combined with an adjuvant such as incomplete Freund adjuvant (IFA) (Table 13–4). Vaccination with synthetic native peptides has been proven to induce systemic immune responses assessed as an increase in specific CTL precursors or enhanced delayed-type hypersensitivity. In addition, these studies also indicate that vaccination with peptide alone or combined with IFA is well tolerated, with only the occasional occurrence of mild fever and inflammation at the site of injection. However, induction of systemic T-cell immunization has not always been associated with clinical response in terms of tumor regression. The reasons for this discrepancy are not clear.

The modified antigenic peptides derived from MAA have also been used in clinical trials for metastatic melanoma patients. This strategy is based on the evidence that the affinity and the stability of the antigenic peptide–HLA class I complex are usually correlated with the immunogenicity of the peptide (Figure 13–16). To date, only one group has reported clinical results with G209-2M peptide derived from gp100.[49] The modified peptide G209-2M has appeared to be more effective than the native peptide in terms of tumor regression. However, tumor regressions were achieved only when exogenous IL-2 was administered during peptide immunization. In addition, therapeutic efficacy did not correlate with the immune response.[49]

Peptide immunization is being actively investigated in other tumor types as well. In the near future, immunotherapy with tumor-derived peptides promises to be a very vigorous area of clinical research.

DEOXYRIBONUCLEIC ACID VACCINES

It has been reported that the delivery of naked DNA encoding a model tumor antigen, OVA, into skin resulted in protective antitumor immunity against an OVA-transfected murine B16 melanoma.[86] Because of the availability of genes encoding MAA and because of the convenience of naked DNA–based vaccines, this approach has attracted great attention as a potent tumor vaccine strategy.[87–91] Using recombinant adenovirus expressing either MART-1 or gp100, Zhai and colleagues[92] demonstrated that immunization of mice with gp100-expressing vector could protect mice from murine melanoma B16 challenge administered intradermally. Based on this finding, Rosenberg and colleagues[93] conducted a phase I clinical trial using the recombinant vector encoding either MART-1 or gp100, alone or combined with the injection of IL-2 (Figure 13–17). In the study, 1 of 16 patients with metastatic melanoma receiving the recombinant adenovirus/MART-1 alone experienced a complete response. However, high levels of neutralizing antibody were found in patients' sera prior to treatment, which might have impaired the efficacy of the vaccines. Recently, Brossart and colleagues[94] have shown that repeated injection of adenovirus-infected dendritic cells (DCs) but not naked virus induced only low titers of neutralizing antibodies. Furthermore, the presence of neutralizing antibodies specific for the virus did not affect the usefulness of infected DCs as the repeated application of virus-infected DCs boosted the CTL response, even in mice previously infected with the recombinant vector. Ongoing clinical trials using DCs infected with recombinant adenovirus encoding MART-1 and gp100 may address the efficacy of virus-infected DCs in human settings.

DENDRITIC CELL–BASED VACCINES

The discovery of the melanoma-specific antigens discussed above has provided an important impetus to the pursuit of strategies for specific antitumor

Table 13–4. MELANOMA-ASSOCIATED ANTIGENIC PEPTIDE–BASED IMMUNOTHERAPY FOR ADVANCED MELANOMA PATIENTS				
Peptide/MAA	HLA Restriction	With IFA	Immune Response	Clinical Response
EVDPIGHLY/MAGE-3	-A1	No	No/minor	Yes
KTWGQYWQV, ITDQVPFSV, YLEPGPVTA/gp100	-A2	Yes	Yes	Yes
AAGIGILTV/MART-1	-A2	Yes	Yes	No
IMQVPFSV/gp100	-A2	Yes	Yes	Yes

HLA = human leukocyte antigen; IFA = incomplete Freund adjuvant; MAA = melanoma-associated antigen.

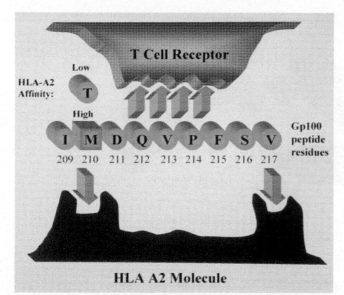

Figure 13–16. Peptide structure and recognition. Illustrated are the gp100-derived peptide G209 and its modification into G209-2M. The nine-amino-acid peptide binds HLA-A2 at positions 210 and 217; interaction occurs through the B and F pockets, respectively, of the HLA-A2 molecule. The central portion of the molecule is recognized by the antigen-specific T-cell receptor. Residues 210 and 217 can be modified. A replacement of the T residue with an M residue at position 210 results in an approximately ninefold increase in the binding affinity of the peptide for HLA-A2. The G209-2M peptide, having been tested in clinical trials, is more immunogenic in stimulating antimelanoma immunity.

immunization. However, the optimal method of delivering antigen to the host has not yet been delineated. An emerging understanding of the molecular and cellular biology of DCs and the development of the techniques for producing large numbers of these cells in vitro have provided a method for potentially delivering antigen via the most potent antigen-presenting cells available.

Antigen Presentation by Dendritic Cells

First described in 1973 by Steinman and Cohn[95] as adherent cells among mouse splenocytes with a distinctive morphology, DCs are now known to be highly specialized and efficient antigen-presenting cells (APCs). Progress in this field has been dependent on the recent development of laboratory techniques for manufacturing large quantities of DCs with reasonably purity. Dendritic cells represent a family of APCs with ubiquitous distributions in trace amounts in tissues and in less than 0.5 percent of blood leukocytes. They probably originate from CD34+ progenitors in the bone marrow, and their

expansion and differentiation are influenced by a variety of cytokines, such as stem cell factor (SCF), IL-3, GM-CSF, and TNF-α.[96]

Dendritic cells reside in tissues of potential antigen entry, where they capture and process antigens efficiently but are poor activators of T cells. When DCs encounter local tissue perturbations such as infections, necrosis, or the entrance of toxic chemicals, they rapidly undergo a maturation process that makes them very potent APCs.[97] The process of maturation is characterized by reduced antigen-capture and processing capacity by up-regulated MHC molecules, adhesion molecules, and co-stimulatory molecules, and by stabilized peptide-MHC complexes on their surface. Dendritic cells then become motile and travel through lymphatic vessels to T-cell areas of lymph nodes, where they form clusters with T cells. The complete maturation of DCs is mediated by the interaction between surface molecules CD40-CD40L and by T-cell-derived cytokines such as IFN-γ. The fully matured DCs are characterized by a loss of phagocytic capacity, further up-regulation of co-stimulatory molecules CD80 and CD86, and increased secretion of cytokines, including TNF-α and IL-12. Dendritic cells are the only natural APCs that have been shown to prime T lymphocytes both in vitro and in vivo. Thereby, DCs serve as sentinels for the immune system, capturing antigen and delivering it in highly immunogenic form for the efficient activation of T cells (Figure 13–18).

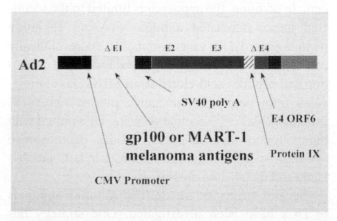

Figure 13–17. Structure of the recombinant adenovirus used for melanoma vaccination. The adenovirus serotype 2 background has been modified with the deletion of the E1 and E4 regions. A region encoding gp100 or MART-1 has been inserted in its place. This virus has been used in clinical trials both at the National Institutes of Health (NIH) and at Harvard to stimulate antimelanoma immunity.

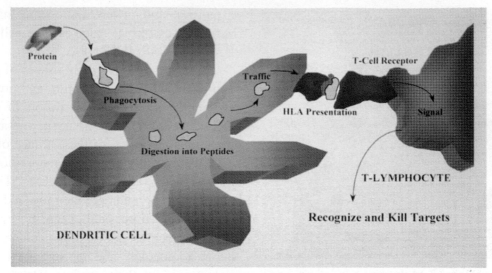

Figure 13–18. The function of dendritic cells in antigen presentation. The dendritic cell is an efficient antigen-presenting cell (APC). It phagocytoses protein, processes the protein into peptides, and presents peptide on the surface in the context of the human leukocyte antigen (HLA) molecule. The HLA-bound peptide is then recognized by the T-cell receptor, stimulating T-cell killing.

Approaches to Using Dendritic Cells for Cancer Therapy

Figures 13–19 and 13–20 outline present strategies to design DC-based cancer vaccines. Dendritic cells pulsed with MHC class I–restricted peptides derived from model tumor antigens have been studied extensively in animals and have demonstrated potent antitumor responses in both protective and therapeutic models.[98–101] However, the peptides derived from model tumor antigens are usually highly immunogenic and thus quite unlike those expressed in most human cancers. In addition, the approach is limited to the identified tumor-associated antigens (TAAs). To study peptide-pulsed DC vaccination in a more clinically relevant setting, several groups used lysate and unfractionated peptides acid-eluted from MHC class I molecules from poorly immunogenic murine tumors as immunogens.[102,103] Vaccination using DCs pulsed with tumor lysates and stripped peptides demonstrated markedly specific antitumor responses in both prophylactic and therapeutic models.

Several strategies for delivering tumor antigens to DCs have been investigated. One strategy has been to introduce the genes encoding TAA directly into DCs. This approach allows DCs to process and present tumor-antigenic peptides on both class I and class II molecules. Vaccination with DCs transfected with cDNA and RNA encoding tumor antigens induced potent antitumor immunity.[91,104–106] In addition, DC vaccines modified with gene-encoding TAA not only elicited multiple epitope-specific CD8 T-cell responses but also antigen-specific CD4 responses.[91] Recombinant viruses have proven to be a highly efficient means of introducing TAA genes into DCs. Adenovirus, poxvirus, and retroviral vectors encoding tumor antigens have been used to infect DCs and induce protective and therapeutic tumor immunity. Alternative strategies that have also been used include direct fusion of DCs with tumor, allowing provision of the whole array of tumor antigens in the context of MHC and co-stimulatory molecules of DCs.[107] Recently, Celluzzi and Falo[108] demonstrated that simple coculturing of DCs with tumor for several hours ex vivo yields an effective immunogen in prophylactic mouse tumor models.

The identification of MAAs and their corresponding antigenic epitopes recognized by melanoma-specific CTLs has resulted in clinical trials using the peptides either alone or with adjuvants. Although vaccination with the peptides readily induced immune response as already discussed, no significant tumor regression was observed.[49,109] However, preclinical data suggest that antigen presentation by DCs might substantially augment the immunogenicity of MAA peptides. Hu and colleagues[110] and Mukherji and colleagues[111] showed that immunization with DCs pulsed with MAGE-1 peptide could elicit autologous melanoma-reactive CTLs in patients with advanced melanoma. However, no significant clinical responses were observed in spite of the presence of CTLs in tumor sites.

One promising clinical trial was performed by Nestle and colleagues, who reported a 31 percent response rate in terms of tumor regression in melanoma patients receiving peptide-pulsed or melanoma lysate–pulsed DCs.[112] In their study, monocyte-derived DCs were pulsed with a cocktail of MAA peptides (gp100, MART-1, MAGE-1, MAGE-3 or tyrosinase) chosen to match the individual patient's HLA class I molecules. Dendritic cells pulsed with autologous melanoma lysate were

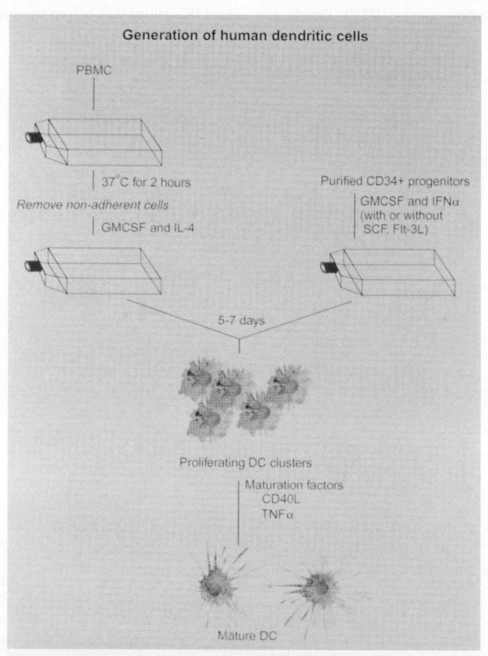

Figure 13–19. Laboratory production of dendritic cells. Peripheral blood mononuclear cells (PBMCs) are grown in the laboratory for 2 hours, after which dendritic precursors adhere to laboratory ware. Alternatively, CD34+ progenitors can be grown. Cells are then grown for up to a week in granulocyte-microphage colony–stimulating factor (GM-CSF) and interleukin-4 (IL-4) and harvested for use as dendritic cells.

used for patients whose HLA haplotype was inappropriate for the known peptides. In addition, the DC vaccines were also pulsed with KLH to prime CD4+ T cells that could provide helper signals for activation and expansion of antigen-specific CD8+ killer cells. The resultant DC vaccines were injected directly into uninvolved lymph nodes under ultrasonographic guidance. Nearly 70 percent of patients (11 of 16) revealed immune response as assessed by delayed-type hypersensitivity (DTH). Peptide-spe-

cific CTLs were also generated from the skin biopsy specimens of some patients. Tumor regression was observed in 5 of 16 patients (31%), 2 of them with complete responses lasting over 15 months. Response sites were noted not only in the skin but also in visceral sites such as the lung and pancreas, suggesting that systemic vaccination results from inventions bodes well for the future of this therapy.

A second trial from the University of Pittsburgh used DCs pulsed with polyepitope peptides. Among

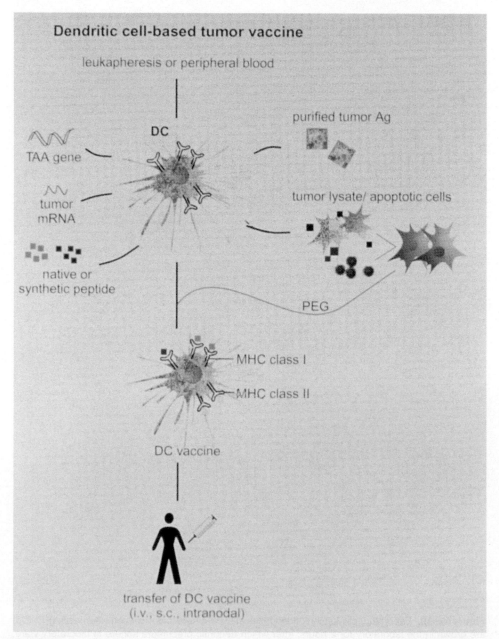

Figure 13–20. Strategy for using dendritic cells as a tumor vaccine. Patients undergo withdrawal of peripheral blood or leukapheresis. Dendritic cells are grown in the laboratory and are exposed to antigen by one of several methods. Cells are then harvested and injected as a dendritic cell vaccine.

the 20 patients with advanced melanoma who received DCs, 1 patient showed a complete response, 2 patients showed partial response, and 2 patients showed stable disease.

In our own hands, DC vaccination appears promising. Figure 13–21 illustrates one outcome of vaccination using DCs transfected with adenovirus engineered to express MART-1 and gp100: vitiligo. This finding suggests that such immunization strategies successfully induce antimelanocyte immunity.

Several other groups in the United States and other countries have been performing active clinical trials using DC-based vaccine for melanoma immunotherapy. Although these ongoing clinical trials will continue to address the safety of DC-based vaccination, they should also provide further information about the efficacy of DC vaccination, optimal approaches to delivering melanoma antigens to DCs, and the dose-response relationship of the vaccines.

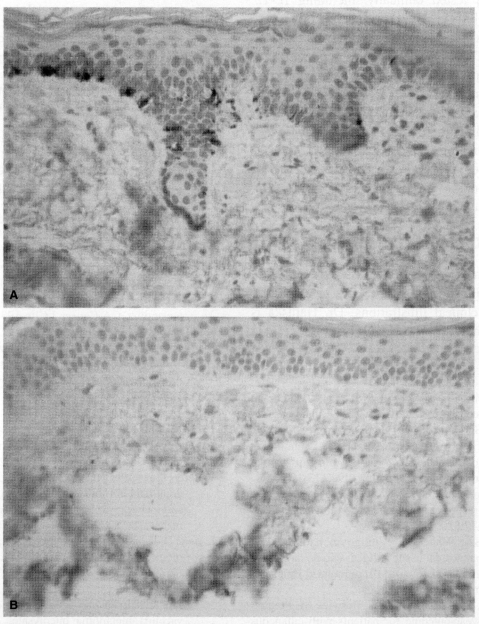

Figure 13–21. Histopathology of dendritic cell vaccine–induced vitiligo. *A,* An area of normal skin from a subject stained with MART-1. The MART-1-positive cells, dark brown, are normal melanocytes. *B,* An area of vitiligo, also stained with MART-1. The melanocytes, normally present at the epidermal-dermal junction as seen in panel *A,* are absent.

FUTURE DIRECTIONS

Immunotherapy is a promising modality for the specific treatment of melanoma and for wider application to other malignancies; however, the field is in its infancy. The clinical phenomena that provide the observational underpinning for this field are clearcut and striking, but the field has yet to develop clearly successful therapies. As a result, immunotherapy promises to be a very active area of investigation in the near future. New cytokines are being developed and tested clinically, including IL-12, CD40L, and Flt-3L. New cellular therapies are emerging, including refinements in DC therapy, the production of T cells specifically designed with anti-tumor specificity, and engineered cells. Antigen discovery projects will clearly feed into this effort, and with the maturation of the Human Genome Project, the understanding of tumor antigens is expanding. In the future, immunotherapy will remain a vigorous intellectual discipline, and experimental therapy for melanoma promises to continue to be at the forefront of this wave of research.

ACKNOWLEDGMENTS

Thanks to Simonne Longerich for assistance in preparing the illustrations and to Dr. Arthur Sober for providing clinical illustrations. Dr. Haluska is supported by the Cancer Research Institute.

REFERENCES

1. Conforti AM, Ollila DW, Kelley MC, et al. Update on active specific immunotherapy with melanoma vaccines. J Surg Oncol 1997;66:55–64.
2. Becker JC, Guldberg P, Zeuthen J, et al. Accumulation of identical T cells in melanoma and vitiligo-like leukoderma. J Invest Dermatol 1999;113:1033–8.
3. Zeff RA, Freitag A, Grin CM, Grant-Kels JM. The immune response in halo nevi. J Am Acad Dermatol 1997;37:620–4.
4. Rosenberg SA, White DE. Vitiligo in patients with melanoma: normal tissue antigens can be targets for cancer immunotherapy. J Immunother Emphasis Tumor Immunol 1996;19:81–4.
5. Barnhill RL, Fine JA, Roush GC, Berwick M. Predicting five-year outcome for patients with cutaneous melanoma in a population-based study [published erratum appears in Cancer 1997 Jan 15;79(2):423]. Cancer 1996;78:427–32.
6. Berd D, Mastrangelo MJ. Active immunotherapy of human melanoma exploiting the immunopotentiating effects of cyclophosphamide. Cancer Invest 1988;6:337–49.
7. Berd D, Maguire HC Jr, McCue P, Mastrangelo MJ. Treatment of metastatic melanoma with an autologous tumor-cell vaccine: clinical and immunologic results in 64 patients. J Clin Oncol 1990;8:1858–67.
8. Crowley NJ, Darrow TL, Seigler HF. Generation of autologous tumor-specific cytotoxic T-cells using HLA-A region matched allogeneic melanoma. Curr Surg 1989;46:393–6.
9. Crowley NJ, Slingluff CL Jr, Darrow TL, Seigler HF. Generation of human autologous melanoma-specific cytotoxic T-cells using HLA-A2-matched allogeneic melanomas. Cancer Res 1990;50:492–8.
10. Crowley NJ, Darrow TL, Quinn-Allen MA, Seigler HF. MHC-restricted recognition of autologous melanoma by tumor-specific cytotoxic T cells. Evidence for restriction by a dominant HLA-A allele. J Immunol 1991;146:1692–9.
11. Darrow TL, Slingluff CL Jr, Seigler HF. The role of HLA class I antigens in recognition of melanoma cells by tumor-specific cytotoxic T lymphocytes. Evidence for shared tumor antigens. J Immunol 1989;142:3329–35.
12. Morton DL, Foshag LJ, Hoon DS, et al. Prolongation of survival in metastatic melanoma after active specific immunotherapy with a new polyvalent melanoma vaccine [published erratum appears in Ann Surg 1993 Mar;217(3):309]. Ann Surg 1992;216:463–82.
13. Morton DL, Barth A. Vaccine therapy for malignant melanoma. CA Cancer J Clin 1996;46:225–44.
14. Fujiwara H, Aoki H, Yoshioka T, et al. Establishment of a tumor-specific immunotherapy model utilizing TNP-reactive helper T cell activity and its application to the autochthonous tumor system. J Immunol 1984;133:509–14.
15. Berd D, Murphy G, Maguire HC Jr, Mastrangelo MJ. Immunization with haptenized, autologous tumor cells induces inflammation of human melanoma metastases. Cancer Res 1991;51:2731–4.
16. Berd D, Maguire HC Jr, Schuchter LM, et al. Autologous hapten-modified melanoma vaccine as post-surgical adjuvant treatment after resection of nodal metastases. J Clin Oncol 1997;15:2359–70.
17. Berd D, Kairys J, Dunton C, et al. Autologous, hapten-modified vaccine as a treatment for human cancers. Semin Oncol 1998;25:646–53.
18. Wallack MK, Bash JA, Leftheriotis E, et al. Positive relationship of clinical and serologic responses to vaccinia melanoma oncolysate. Arch Surg 1987;122:1460–3.
19. Wallack MK, Sivanandham M, Balch CM, et al. A phase III randomized, double-blind multiinstitu-

tional trial of vaccinia melanoma oncolysate-active specific immunotherapy for patients with stage II melanoma. Cancer 1995;75:34–42.

20. Wallack MK, Sivanandham M, Ditaranto K, et al. Increased survival of patients treated with a vaccinia melanoma oncolysate vaccine: second interim analysis of data from a phase III, multi-institutional trial. Ann Surg 1997;226:198–206.

21. Wallack MK, Sivanandham M, Balch CM, et al. Surgical adjuvant active specific immunotherapy for patients with stage III melanoma: the final analysis of data from a phase III, randomized, double-blind, multicenter vaccinia melanoma oncolysate trial. J Am Coll Surg 1998;187:69–77.

22. Hersey P. Evaluation of vaccinia viral lysates as therapeutic vaccines in the treatment of melanoma. Ann N Y Acad Sci 1993;690:167–77.

23. Hersey P. Melanoma vaccines. Current status and future prospects. Drugs 1994;47:373–82.

24. Hersey P. Active immunotherapy with viral lysates of micrometastases following surgical removal of high risk melanoma. World J Surg 1992;16:251–60.

25. Mitchell MS, Harel W, Kempf RA, et al. Active-specific immunotherapy for melanoma. J Clin Oncol 1990; 8:856–69.

26. Mitchell MS, Harel W, Kan-Mitchell J, et al. Active specific immunotherapy of melanoma with allogeneic cell lysates. Rationale, results, and possible mechanisms of action. Ann N Y Acad Sci 1993;690:153–66.

27. Mitchell MS. Active specific immunotherapy of melanoma. Br Med Bull 1995;51:631–46.

28. Mitchell MS. Perspective on allogeneic melanoma lysates in active specific immunotherapy. Semin Oncol 1998;25:623–35.

29. Dranoff G, Jaffee E, Lazenby A, et al. Vaccination with irradiated tumor cells engineered to secrete murine granulocyte-macrophage colony-stimulating factor stimulates potent, specific, and long-lasting antitumor immunity. Proc Natl Acad Sci U S A 1993; 90:3539–43.

30. Mach N, Gillessen S, Wilson SB, et al. Differences in dendritic cells stimulated in vivo by tumors engineered to secrete granulocyte-macrophage colony-stimulating factor or Flt3-ligand. Cancer Res 2000;60:3239–46.

31. Dranoff G, Soiffer R, Lynch T, et al. A phase I study of vaccination with autologous, irradiated melanoma cells engineered to secrete human granulocyte-macrophage colony stimulating factor. Hum Gene Ther 1997;8:111–23.

32. Soiffer R, Lynch T, Mihm M, et al. Vaccination with irradiated autologous melanoma cells engineered to secrete human granulocyte-macrophage colony-stimulating factor generates potent antitumor immunity in patients with metastatic melanoma. Proc Natl Acad Sci U S A 1998;95:13141–6.

33. Abdel-Wahab Z, Weltz C, Hester D, et al. A phase I clinical trial of immunotherapy with interferon-gamma gene-modified autologous melanoma cells: monitoring the humoral immune response [published erratum appears in Cancer 1999 Oct 1; 86(7):1380]. Cancer 1997;80:401–12.

34. Nemunaitis J, Bohart C, Fong T, et al. Phase I trial of retroviral vector-mediated interferon (IFN)-gamma gene transfer into autologous tumor cells in patients with metastatic melanoma. Cancer Gene Ther 1998;5:292–300.

35. Livingston PO, Wong GY, Adluri S, et al. Improved survival in stage III melanoma patients with GM2 antibodies: a randomized trial of adjuvant vaccination with GM2 ganglioside. J Clin Oncol 1994;12: 1036–44.

36. Chapman PB, Morrissey DM, Panageas KS, et al. Induction of antibodies against GM2 ganglioside by immunizing melanoma patients using GM2-keyhole limpet hemocyanin + QS21 vaccine: a dose-response study. Clin Cancer Res 2000;6:874–9.

37. Brichard V, Van Pel A, Wolfel T, et al. The tyrosinase gene codes for an antigen recognized by autologous cytolytic T lymphocytes on HLA-A2 melanomas. J Exp Med 1993;178:489–95.

38. Cox AL, Skipper J, Chen Y, et al. Identification of a peptide recognized by five melanoma-specific human cytotoxic T cell lines. Science 1994;264: 716–9.

39. Engelhard VH. Structure of peptides associated with class I and class II MHC molecules. Annu Rev Immunol 1994;12:181–207.

40. Adema GJ, de Boer AJ, van't Hullenaar R, et al. Melanocyte lineage-specific antigens recognized by monoclonal antibodies NKI-beteb, HMB-50, and HMB-45 are encoded by a single cDNA. Am J Pathol 1993;143:1579–85.

41. Kawakami Y, Eliyahu S, Sakaguchi K, et al. Identification of the immunodominant peptides of the MART-1 human melanoma antigen recognized by the majority of HLA-A2-restricted tumor infiltrating lymphocytes. J Exp Med 1994;180:347–52.

42. Kawakami Y, Eliyahu S, Jennings C, et al. Recognition of multiple epitopes in the human melanoma antigen gp100 by tumor-infiltrating T lymphocytes associated with in vivo tumor regression. J Immunol 1995;154:3961–8.

43. Bakker AB, Schreurs MW, de Boer AJ, et al. Melanocyte lineage-specific antigen gp100 is recognized by melanoma-derived tumor-infiltrating lymphocytes. J Exp Med 1994;179:1005–9.

44. Tsai V, Southwood S, Sidney J, et al. Identification of subdominant CTL epitopes of the GP100 melanoma-associated tumor antigen by primary in vitro immunization with peptide-pulsed dendritic cells. J Immunol 1997;158:1796–802.

45. Skipper JC, Kittlesen DJ, Hendrickson RC, et al. Shared epitopes for HLA-A3-restricted melanoma-reactive human CTL include a naturally processed epitope from Pmel-17/gp100. J Immunol 1996;157:5027–33.

46. Kawakami Y, Robbins PF, Wang X, et al. Identification of new melanoma epitopes on melanosomal proteins recognized by tumor infiltrating T lymphocytes restricted by HLA-A1, -A2, and -A3 alleles. J Immunol 1998;161:6985–92.

47. Kawashima I, Tsai V, Southwood S, et al. Identification of gp100-derived, melanoma-specific cytotoxic T-lymphocyte epitopes restricted by HLA-A3 supertype molecules by primary in vitro immunization with peptide-pulsed dendritic cells. Int J Cancer 1998;78:518–24.

48. Castelli C, Tarsini P, Mazzocchi A, et al. Novel HLA-Cw8-restricted T cell epitopes derived from tyrosinase-related protein-2 and gp100 melanoma antigens. J Immunol 1999;162:1739–48.

49. Rosenberg SA, Yang JC, Schwartzentruber DJ, et al. Immunologic and therapeutic evaluation of a synthetic peptide vaccine for the treatment of patients with metastatic melanoma. Nat Med 1998;4:321–7.

50. Coulie PG, Brichard V, Van Pel A, et al. A new gene coding for a differentiation antigen recognized by autologous cytolytic T lymphocytes on HLA-A2 melanomas. J Exp Med 1994;180:35–42.

51. Kawakami Y, Eliyahu S, Delgado CH, et al. Cloning of the gene coding for a shared human melanoma antigen recognized by autologous T cells infiltrating into tumor. Proc Natl Acad Sci U S A 1994;91:3515–9.

52. Castelli C, Storkus WJ, Maeurer MJ, et al. Mass spectrometric identification of a naturally processed melanoma peptide recognized by CD8+ cytotoxic T lymphocytes. J Exp Med 1995;181:363–8.

53. Skipper JC, Hendrickson RC, Gulden PH, et al. An HLA-A2-restricted tyrosinase antigen on melanoma cells results from posttranslational modification and suggests a novel pathway for processing of membrane proteins. J Exp Med 1996;183:527–34.

54. Wolfel T, Van Pel A, Brichard V, et al. Two tyrosinase nonapeptides recognized on HLA-A2 melanomas by autologous cytolytic T lymphocytes. Eur J Immunol 1994;24:759–64.

55. Kang X, Kawakami Y, el-Gamil M, et al. Identification of a tyrosinase epitope recognized by HLA-A24-restricted, tumor-infiltrating lymphocytes. J Immunol 1995;155:1343–8.

56. Brichard VG, Herman J, Van Pel A, et al. A tyrosinase nonapeptide presented by HLA-B44 is recognized on a human melanoma by autologous cytolytic T lymphocytes. Eur J Immunol 1996;26:224–30.

57. Topalian SL, Gonzales MI, Parkhurst M, et al. Melanoma-specific CD4+ T cells recognize nonmutated HLA-DR-restricted tyrosinase epitopes. J Exp Med 1996;183:1965–71.

58. Wang RF, Parkhurst MR, Kawakami Y, et al. Utilization of an alternative open reading frame of a normal gene in generating a novel human cancer antigen. J Exp Med 1996;183:1131–40.

59. Wang RF, Johnston SL, Southwood S, et al. Recognition of an antigenic peptide derived from tyrosinase-related protein-2 by CTL in the context of HLA-A31 and -A33. J Immunol 1998;160:890–7.

60. Wang RF, Appella E, Kawakami Y, et al. Identification of TRP-2 as a human tumor antigen recognized by cytotoxic T lymphocytes. J Exp Med 1996;184:2207–16.

61. Robbins PF, el-Gamil M, Li YF, et al. Cloning of a new gene encoding an antigen recognized by melanoma-specific HLA-A24-restricted tumor-infiltrating lymphocytes. J Immunol 1995;154:5944–50.

62. Fork HE, Wagner RF Jr, Wagner KD. The Texas peer education sun awareness project for children: primary prevention of malignant melanoma and nonmelanocytic skin cancers. Cutis 1992;50:363–4.

63. van der Bruggen P, Traversari C, Chomez P, et al. A gene encoding an antigen recognized by cytolytic T lymphocytes on a human melanoma. Science 1991;254:1643–7.

64. De Plaen E, Arden K, Traversari C, et al. Structure, chromosomal localization, and expression of 12 genes of the MAGE family. Immunogenetics 1994;40:360–9.

65. Traversari C, van der Bruggen P, Luescher IF, et al. A nonapeptide encoded by human gene MAGE-1 is recognized on HLA-A1 by cytolytic T lymphocytes directed against tumor antigen MZ2-E. J Exp Med 1992;176:1453–7.

66. van der Bruggen P, Szikora JP, Boel P, et al. Autologous cytolytic T lymphocytes recognize a MAGE-1 nonapeptide on melanomas expressing HLA-Cw*1601. Eur J Immunol 1994;24:2134–40.

67. Visseren MJ, van der Burg SH, van der Voort EI, et al. Identification of HLA-A*0201-restricted CTL epitopes encoded by the tumor-specific MAGE-2 gene product. Int J Cancer 1997;73:125–30.

68. Tahara K, Takesako K, Sette A, et al. Identification of a MAGE-2-encoded human leukocyte antigen-A24-binding synthetic peptide that induces specific antitumor cytotoxic T lymphocytes. Clin Cancer Res 1999;5:2236–41.

69. Gaugler B, Van den Eynde B, van der Bruggen P, et al. Human gene MAGE-3 codes for an antigen recognized on a melanoma by autologous cytolytic T lymphocytes. J Exp Med 1994;179:921–30.

70. van der Bruggen P, Bastin J, Gajewski T, et al. A peptide encoded by human gene MAGE-3 and presented by HLA-A2 induces cytolytic T lymphocytes that recognize tumor cells expressing MAGE-3. Eur J Immunol 1994;24:3038–43.

71. Oiso M, Eura M, Katsura F, et al. A newly identified MAGE-3-derived epitope recognized by HLA-A24-restricted cytotoxic T lymphocytes. Int J Cancer 1999;81:387–94.

72. Fleischhauer K, Fruci D, Van Endert P, et al. Characterization of antigenic peptides presented by HLA-B44 molecules on tumor cells expressing the gene MAGE-3. Int J Cancer 1996;68:622–8.

73. Panelli MC, Bettinotti MP, Lally K, et al. A tumor-infiltrating lymphocyte from a melanoma metastasis with decreased expression of melanoma differentiation antigens recognizes MAGE-12. J Immunol 2000;164:4382–92.

74. Tanzarella S, Russo V, Lionello I, et al. Identification of a promiscuous T-cell epitope encoded by multiple members of the MAGE family. Cancer Res 1999; 59:2668–74.

75. Chaux P, Vantomme V, Stroobant V, et al. Identification of MAGE-3 epitopes presented by HLA-DR molecules to CD4(+) T lymphocytes. J Exp Med 1999; 189:767–78.

76. Boel P, Wildmann C, Sensi ML, et al. BAGE: a new gene encoding an antigen recognized on human melanomas by cytolytic T lymphocytes. Immunity 1995;2:167–75.

77. Van den Eynde B, Peeters O, De Backer O, et al. A new family of genes coding for an antigen recognized by autologous cytolytic T lymphocytes on a human melanoma. J Exp Med 1995;182:689–98.

78. Jager E, Chen YT, Drijfhout JW, et al. Simultaneous humoral and cellular immune response against cancer-testis antigen NY-ESO-1: definition of human histocompatibility leukocyte antigen (HLA)-A2-binding peptide epitopes. J Exp Med 1998;187: 265–70.

79. Jager E, Jager D, Karbach J, et al. Identification of NY-ESO-1 epitopes presented by human histocompatibility antigen (HLA)-DRB4*0101-0103 and recognized by CD4(+) T lymphocytes of patients with NY-ESO-1-expressing melanoma. J Exp Med 2000; 191:625–30.

80. Wolfel T, Hauer M, Schneider J, et al. A p16INK4a-insensitive CDK4 mutant targeted by cytolytic T lymphocytes in a human melanoma. Science 1995; 269:1281–4.

81. Robbins PF, el-Gamil M, Li YF, et al. A mutated beta-catenin gene encodes a melanoma-specific antigen recognized by tumor infiltrating lymphocytes. J Exp Med 1996;183:1185–92.

82. Coulie PG, Lehmann F, Lethe B, et al. A mutated intron sequence codes for an antigenic peptide recognized by cytolytic T lymphocytes on a human melanoma. Proc Natl Acad Sci U S A 1995;92:7976–80.

83. Salgaller ML, Marincola FM, Cormier JN, Rosenberg SA. Immunization against epitopes in the human melanoma antigen gp100 following patient immunization with synthetic peptides. Cancer Res 1996;56:4749–57.

84. Marchand M, van Baren N, Weynants P, et al. Tumor regressions observed in patients with metastatic melanoma treated with an antigenic peptide encoded by gene MAGE-3 and presented by HLA-A1. Int J Cancer 1999;80:219–30.

85. Cormier JN, Salgaller ML, Prevette T, et al. Enhancement of cellular immunity in melanoma patients immunized with a peptide from MART-1/Melan A. Cancer J Sci Am 1997;3:37–44.

86. Condon C, Watkins SC, Celluzzi CM, et al. DNA-based immunization by in vivo transfection of dendritic cells. Nat Med 1996;2:1122–8.

87. Corr M, Lee DJ, Carson DA, Tighe H. Gene vaccination with naked plasmid DNA: mechanism of CTL priming. J Exp Med 1996;184:1555–60.

88. Corr M, Tighe H, Lee D, et al. Costimulation provided by DNA immunization enhances antitumor immunity. J Immunol 1997;159:4999–5004.

89. Conry RM, LoBuglio AF, Loechel F, et al. A carcinoembryonic antigen polynucleotide vaccine has in vivo antitumor activity. Gene Ther 1995;2:59–65.

90. Schreurs MW, de Boer AJ, Figdor CG, Adema GJ. Genetic vaccination against the melanocyte lineage-specific antigen gp100 induces cytotoxic T lymphocyte-mediated tumor protection. Cancer Res 1998; 58:2509–14.

91. Yang S, Vervaert CE, Burch J Jr, et al. Murine dendritic cells transfected with human GP100 elicit both antigen-specific CD8(+) and CD4(+) T-cell responses and are more effective than DNA vaccines at generating anti-tumor immunity. Int J Cancer 1999;83: 532–40.

92. Zhai Y, Yang JC, Kawakami Y, et al. Antigen-specific tumor vaccines. Development and characterization of recombinant adenoviruses encoding MART-1 or gp100 for cancer therapy. J Immunol 1996;156: 700–10.

93. Rosenberg SA, Zhai Y, Yang JC, et al. Immunizing patients with metastatic melanoma using recombinant adenoviruses encoding MART-1 or gp100 melanoma antigens. J Natl Cancer Inst 1998;90: 1894–900.

94. Brossart P, Goldrath AW, Butz EA, et al. Virus-mediated delivery of antigenic epitopes into dendritic cells as a means to induce CTL. J Immunol 1997;158: 3270–6.

95. Steinman RM, Cohn ZA. Identification of a novel cell type in peripheral lymphoid organs of mice. I. Morphology, quantitation, tissue distribution. J Exp Med 1973;137:1142–62.

96. Shortman K, Caux C. Dendritic cell development: multiple pathways to nature's adjuvants. Stem Cells 1997;15:409–19.

97. Banchereau J, Steinman RM. Dendritic cells and the control of immunity. Nature 1998;392:245–52.

98. Porgador A, Gilboa E. Bone marrow-generated dendritic cells pulsed with a class I-restricted peptide are potent inducers of cytotoxic T lymphocytes. J Exp Med 1995;182:255–60.

99. Porgador A, Snyder D, Gilboa E. Induction of antitumor immunity using bone marrow-generated dendritic cells. J Immunol 1996;156:2918–26.

100. Mayordomo JI, Zorina T, Storkus WJ, et al. Bone marrow-derived dendritic cells pulsed with synthetic tumour peptides elicit protective and therapeutic antitumour immunity. Nat Med 1995;1:1297–302.

101. Celluzzi CM, Mayordomo JI, Storkus WJ, et al. Peptide-pulsed dendritic cells induce antigen-specific CTL-mediated protective tumor immunity. J Exp Med 1996;183:283–7.

102. Yang S, Darrow TL, Vervaert CE, Seigler HF. Immunotherapeutic potential of tumor antigen-pulsed and unpulsed dendritic cells generated from murine bone marrow. Cell Immunol 1997;179:84–95.

103. Zitvogel L, Mayordomo JI, Tjandrawan T, et al. Therapy of murine tumors with tumor peptide-pulsed dendritic cells: dependence on T cells, B7 costimulation, and T helper cell 1-associated cytokines. J Exp Med 1996;183:87–97.

104. Song W, Kong HL, Carpenter H, et al. Dendritic cells genetically modified with an adenovirus vector encoding the cDNA for a model antigen induce protective and therapeutic antitumor immunity. J Exp Med 1997;186:1247–56.

105. Specht JM, Wang G, Do MT, et al. Dendritic cells retrovirally transduced with a model antigen gene are therapeutically effective against established pulmonary metastases. J Exp Med 1997;186:1213–21.

106. Boczkowski D, Nair SK, Snyder D, Gilboa E. Dendritic cells pulsed with RNA are potent antigen-presenting cells in vitro and in vivo. J Exp Med 1996;184:465–72.

107. Gong J, Chen D, Kashiwaba M, Kufe D. Induction of antitumor activity by immunization with fusions of dendritic and carcinoma cells. Nat Med 1997;3:558–61.

108. Celluzzi CM, Falo LD Jr. Physical interaction between dendritic cells and tumor cells results in an immunogen that induces protective and therapeutic tumor rejection. J Immunol 1998;160:3081–5.

109. Marchand M, Weynants P, Rankin E, et al. Tumor regression responses in melanoma patients treated with a peptide encoded by gene MAGE-3 [letter]. Int J Cancer 1995;63:883–5.

110. Hu X, Chakraborty NG, Sporn JR, et al. Enhancement of cytolytic T lymphocyte precursor frequency in melanoma patients following immunization with the MAGE-1 peptide loaded antigen presenting cell-based vaccine. Cancer Res 1996;56:2479–83.

111. Mukherji B, Chakraborty NG, Yamasaki S, et al. Induction of antigen-specific cytolytic T cells in situ in human melanoma by immunization with synthetic peptide-pulsed autologous antigen presenting cells. Proc Natl Acad Sci U S A 1995;92:8078–82.

112. Nestle FO, Alijagic S, Gilliet M, et al. Vaccination of melanoma patients with peptide- or tumor lysate-pulsed dendritic cells. Nat Med 1998;4:328–32.

14

Melanoma: Chemotherapy, Cytokine Therapies, and Biochemotherapy

JARED A. GOLLOB, MD

MICHAEL B. ATKINS, MD

Melanoma will be diagnosed in an estimated 47,700 Americans in 2000, and 7,700 will die of metastatic disease.[1] Although excision of limited metastatic disease can occasionally provide durable benefit, the majority of patients with distant metastases require a systemic treatment approach. Commonly used treatment modalities for metastatic melanoma have included cytotoxic chemotherapy and immunotherapy, alone or in combination. This chapter will review the clinical experience with cytotoxic chemotherapy, administered either as single agents or in combination chemotherapy regimens, and cytokine-based immunotherapy, focusing on interleukin-2 (IL-2), interferon-α (IFN-α), and newer agents such as interleukin-12 (IL-12). In addition, this chapter will review the experience with biochemotherapy regimens that involve the addition of IL-2 and/or IFN-α to cytotoxic chemotherapy.

CYTOTOXIC CHEMOTHERAPY

Dacarbazine and Temozolomide

The chemotherapeutic agents with reproducible activity against melanoma include dacarbazine (DTIC), the platinum analogues, nitrosourea agents, and tubular toxins such as vinca alkaloids and taxanes.[2] The activities of these various agents are summarized in Table 14–1.

Dacarbazine is the most active single agent, with response rates ranging from 15 to 20 percent. How-

ever, the majority of responses are only partial, and the median response duration is only 4 to 6 months.[3] Long-term follow-up of patients treated with DTIC alone shows that less than 2 percent of patients can be anticipated to survive for 6 years.[4] While DTIC remains the only Food and Drug Administration (FDA)–approved cytotoxic drug for the treatment of metastatic melanoma, there are no phase III trial data available to support a survival benefit for DTIC relative to a "no treatment" control.

Dacarbazine is well tolerated, and its major side effects are limited to nausea and vomiting. Bone marrow suppression is modest, and both alopecia and fatigue are minimal, allowing most patients to maintain their normal level of activity while undergoing therapy. Commonly used schedules of DTIC include

Table 14–1. CHEMOTHERAPY DRUGS ACTIVE IN METASTIC MELANOMA			
Agent	N	Response Rate (%)	95% CI (%)
Decarbazine (DTIC)	1,936	20	18–22
Temozolomide	56	21	11–32
Cisplatin	188	23	17–29
Carboplatin	43	16	5–27
Carmustine (BCNU)	122	18	11–25
Lomustine (CCNU)	270	13	9–17
Fotemustine	153	24	17–31
Vinblastine	62	13	5–21
Vindesine	273	14	10–18
Paclitaxel (Taxol)	65	18	9–28
Docetaxel (Taxotere)	26	15	2–29

CI = confidence interval; N = population size.

200 mg/m^2/d intravenously (IV) for 5 days or 850 to 1,000 mg/m^2 IV over 1 hour, with cycles of DTIC administered every 3 to 4 weeks. Neither the response rate nor the duration of response appears to be affected by the schedule of administration. The use of powerful new antiemetic agents has significantly reduced the emetogenic effects of DTIC, allowing the more convenient 1-day schedule of therapy to be administered in an outpatient setting.

Temozolomide (TMZ), an analogue of DTIC, has recently been tested in patients with melanoma. At physiologic pH, temozolomide chemically degrades to MTIC (the active metabolite of DTIC) via a process that does not require metabolic activation.[5] In contrast to DTIC, TMZ is well absorbed orally and is capable of penetrating into the central nervous system (CNS). The ability of TMZ to enter the CNS is probably responsible for its activity in primary brain tumors, a finding that led to its recent approval by the FDA for the treatment of patients with anaplastic astrocytoma.

In a phase II study in patients with metastatic melanoma (conducted by the Cancer Research Campaign),[6] TMZ was well tolerated, and it produced objective responses in 21 percent of patients, including complete responses in 5 percent. One of 4 patients with cerebral metastases had regression of their CNS disease. In a European phase III trial involving 305 patients with metastatic melanoma, TMZ was compared to DTIC. Patients with CNS metastases were excluded from this trial. Patients received either TMZ 200 mg/m^2/d orally for 5 days every 4 weeks or DTIC 250 mg/m^2/d intravenously for 5 days every 3 weeks. Responses were observed in 13.5 percent of patients receiving TMZ and in 12.1 percent of patients treated with DTIC.[7] Median survival was 7.7 months for TMZ and 6.4 months for DTIC ($p = .20$). Temozolomide was well tolerated, and quality of life assessments favored the TMZ arm over DTIC.

Other Agents

Cisplatin and carboplatin have shown modest activity in patients with metastatic melanoma. Single-agent cisplatin has been tested at doses up to 200 mg/m^2 and has produced response rates ranging from 0 to 53 percent (mean, 15 to 20%).[2] Evidence that the activity of cisplatin may be dose dependent has come from a review of single-arm studies. Cisplatin administered at doses up to 150 mg/m^2 in combination with amifostine (WR2721), a thiol derivative with protective effects on bone marrow and kidney, produced tumor responses in 53 percent of patients.[8] However, responses were all partial, and the median response duration was only 4 months. A randomized phase II trial conducted by the Eastern Cooperative Oncology Group (ECOG) compared cisplatin at 150 mg/m^2 plus WR2721 to cisplatin alone at 120 mg/m^2. While both regimens showed activity, unacceptable renal and gastrointestinal toxicity, as well as ototoxicity, was observed on both arms of the study.[2] Carboplatin has been less extensively tested in melanoma,[9] and its value relative to cisplatin, DTIC, TMZ, or other single agents remains to be determined.

The nitrosoureas, including carmustine (BCNU), lomustine (CCNU), and semustine (methyl CCNU), have produced overall response rates of 13 to 18 percent.[2,3] Alopecia is more pronounced and hematologic toxicity (especially thrombocytopenia) more prolonged with these agents compared with either DTIC or cisplatin. While the nitrosoureas are able to cross the blood-brain barrier, the effectiveness of these agents in the treatment or prevention of CNS metastases has yet to be demonstrated. Fotemustine is a chlorethyl nitrosourea that crosses the blood-brain barrier more rapidly and that has been extensively studied in Europe. Although it has induced responses in melanoma patients with CNS metastases[10] as well as in uveal melanoma patients with liver metastases,[11] multicenter trials conducted by the European Organization for Research and Treatment of Cancer (EORTC) have failed to show activity superior to that of other nitrosoureas.[10,12] Fotemustine remains unavailable in the United States even though it is considered first-line therapy for metastatic melanoma in some European countries.

Microtubule toxins (such as vinblastine or vindesine)[13] and agents that interfere with microtubule disassembly (such as the taxanes)[14,15] have also shown modest activity in patients with metastatic melanoma. This activity has led to the use of vinblastine in some combination chemotherapy and biochemotherapy regimens and to the use of paclitaxel as second- or third-line chemotherapy.

Combination Chemotherapy

Combination chemotherapy regimens have produced response rates of 30 to 50 percent in single-institution phase II trials involving patients with metastatic melanoma. Two of the most active regimens reported are the three-drug combination of cisplatin/vinblastine/DTIC (CVD) developed by Legha and colleagues[16] and the four-drug combination of cisplatin/DTIC/BCNU/tamoxifen (CDBT) developed by Del Prete and colleagues.[17]

The CVD regimen was initially reported to have a response rate of 40 percent, with 4 percent complete responses (CRs) and a median response duration of 9 months. In a randomized multi-institutional trial comparing CVD to DTIC alone, the initial analysis suggested that CVD was superior with regard to response rate, duration of response, and survival.[18] However, a recent update of this trial shows that the overall response rates were only 19 percent for CVD and 14 percent for DTIC (Table 14–2), with no differences in either response duration or survival (A. Buzaid, MD, personal communication).

In 1992, the results of a prospective randomized trial of DTIC plus tamoxifen versus DTIC alone[19] suggested that the combination might be more effective (see Table 14–2). A 28 percent response rate and a 41-week median survival was reported for patients treated with DTIC plus tamoxifen whereas the response rate with DTIC alone was only 12 percent,

with a 23-week median survival. The benefit of tamoxifen was attributed to the potentiation of the action of the cytotoxic chemotherapy rather than to tamoxifen's antiestrogenic effects. However, in a recent large-scale four-arm phase III ECOG trial[20] examining the effect of adding either tamoxifen and/or IFN-α to DTIC (Figure 14–1), patients treated with the combination of DTIC plus tamoxifen fared no better than those receiving DTIC alone (response rates of 18 and 15 percent, respectively).

Cisplatin/DTIC/BCNU/tamoxifen (CDBT, also known as the Dartmouth regimen) was originally reported to have produced responses in 46 percent of 141 patients (16 complete responses [CRs] and 49 partial responses [PRs]), with a median response duration of more than 7 months.[21] In phase II studies without tamoxifen, response rates as low as 10 percent were observed.[22] However, a randomized phase III trial by the National Cancer Institute (NCI) of Canada comparing CDBT to cisplatin/DTIC/BCNU (CDB) showed a response rate of 30 percent for the CBDT arm but no benefit to the addition of tamoxifen[23] (see Table 14–2). Another trial, performed by the North Central Cancer Treatment Group, produced similar results.[24] Finally, a randomized phase III trial performed by a consortium including ECOG and Memorial Sloan-Kettering Cancer Center showed no benefit for CDBT compared to DTIC alone[25] (see Table 14–2). In this trial of 240 patients, the response to DTIC was 10.2 percent versus 18.5

Table 14–2. RECENT PHASE III CHEMOTHERAPY TRIALS				
Protocol, Principal Investigator (Reference)	Study Design	N	Major RR (%)	Comments
MD Anderson, Buzaid (19)	CVD vs DTIC	150	19 14	No difference in response duration or survival
Italian Oncology Group, Cocconi (20)	DTIC vs DTIC + tam	52 60	12 28	Improved RR and survival in women only for DTIC + tamoxifen
ECOG* 3690, Falkson (21)	DTIC vs DTIC + IFN vs DTIC + tam vs DTIC + IFN + tam	69 68 66 68	15 21 18 19	No benefit to addition of IFN and/or tamoxifen to DTIC
Canadian Oncology Group, Rusthoven (24)	CDB vs CDBT	100 104	21 30	No benefit to addition of tamoxifen to CDB
ECOG* 91-140, Chapman (26)	DTIC vs CDBT	118 108	10 18.5	No significant difference in RR; survival equivalent; toxicity greater with CDBT

*Eastern Cooperative Oncology Group.
CDB = cisplatin/dacarbazine/carmustine; CDBT = cisplatin/dacarbazine/carmustine/tamoxifen; CVD = cisplatin/vinblastine/dacarbazine; DTIC = dacarbazine; IFN = interferon; N = number of patients; RR = response rate; tam = tamoxifen.

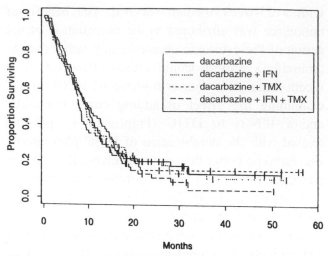

Figure 14–1. The addition of interferon-α (IFN-α) and/or tamoxifen (TMX) to dacarbazine does not improve survival compared to treatment with dacarbazine alone in patients with metastatic melanoma. Shown are the Kaplan-Meier survival plots for melanoma patients randomly assigned to one of four dacarbazine-based treatment arms on the Eastern Cooperative Oncology Group (ECOG) E3690 protocol.

percent for CDBT, and the median survival time from randomization was 7 months, with no significant difference between the two regimens (Figure 14–2). However, myelotoxicity, nausea/vomiting, and fatigue were more frequent with CDBT. Findings from these phase III trials (comparing CVD, DTIC plus tamoxifen, or CDBT to DTIC alone) present no evidence to support these regimens over sin-

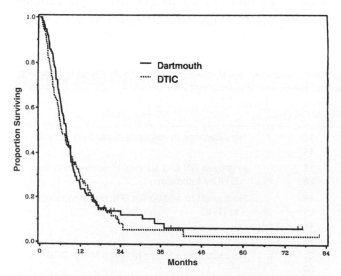

Figure 14-2. Impact on overall survival of the Dartmouth regimen versus dacarbazine (DTIC) in patients with metastatic melanoma. The Kaplan-Meier survival plots show no difference ($p = .51$) in overall survival for patients randomized to treatment with DTIC (median survival, 6.4 months) versus those treated with the Dartmouth regimen (median survival, 7.7 months).

gle-agent DTIC in the treatment of patients with metastatic melanoma. The randomized trials have demonstrated that combination chemotherapy yields slightly higher response rates than single agents but at the cost of increased toxicity and without additional clinical benefit.

CYTOKINE-BASED IMMUNOTHERAPY

Clinical and laboratory observations suggesting that host immunologic responses may influence the course of melanoma stimulated the investigation of immunotherapeutic approaches to the treatment of metastatic disease. While a number of cytokines have been tested in patients with metastatic melanoma, the two that have been the most extensively studied and which have reproducible antitumor activity are IFN-α and IL-2. Another potent immunostimulatory cytokine, IL-12, has also undergone testing in melanoma patients over the past 5 years and may have a role in the treatment of this disease in combination with either IFN-α or IL-2.

Interferon-α

Interferon-α was the first recombinant cytokine to be investigated clinically for metastatic melanoma. The antitumor effects of IFN-α have been attributed both to its ability to stimulate lymphocyte tumoricidal activity and to its direct antiproliferative effect on melanoma cells.[26] It has also recently been shown to have antiangiogenic properties that may contribute to its ability to mediate tumor regression.[27] Phase I and II trials initiated with IFN-α alone in the 1980s yielded an aggregate response rate of 16 percent in published studies.[28] Approximately one-third of the responses to IFN-α were complete. In contrast to responses to cytotoxic chemotherapy, responses to IFN-α could be delayed and were observed as late as 6 months after the start of therapy. Although some of the responses were durable, the median duration of response was only 4 months.

Effective doses of IFN-α have ranged from 10 MU/m²/d to 50 MU/m² three times per week. Uninterrupted treatment has been more effective than cyclic interrupted schedules, regardless of the route of administration. Tumor responses to IFN-α have largely been confined to patients with small-volume cutaneous or soft-tissue disease,[29] thus limiting the usefulness of single-agent IFN-α in the general metastatic melanoma population.

Interleukin-2

Interleukin-2 was first identified in 1976 as a T-cell growth factor whereas the isolation of copy deoxyribonucleic acid (cDNA) was described in 1983. Recombinant IL-2 was shown to have potent immunomodulatory and antitumor activity in a number of murine tumor models.[30] Animal models indicated that the response to IL-2 was dose dependent; this eventually led to the development of high-dose IL-2 regimens for clinical investigation. The antitumor effect of IL-2 appears to be a function of this cytokine's ability to stimulate natural killer (NK)–cell and T-cell cytolytic activity and interferon-γ (IFN-γ) production,[31] as well as its ability to potentiate nitric oxide and tumor necrosis factor-α (TNF-α) production by macrophages and dendritic cells.

Early trials used high-dose intravenous bolus recombinant IL-2 either alone or in combination with lymphokine-activated killer (LAK) cells. The high-dose regimen consisted of 600,000 to 720,000 IU/kg/dose administered IV every 8 hours on days 1 to 5 and again on days 15 to 19, with a maximum of 28 doses per course (Figure 14–3). This regimen resulted in an overall response rate of 15 to 20 percent, with CRs in 4 to 6 percent of patients.[32–35] In a retrospective analysis of 270 patients treated in all

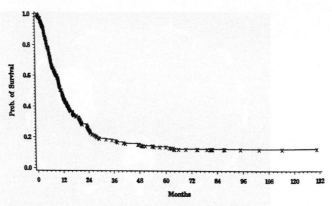

Figure 14–4. Survival curve for 270 patients with metastatic melanoma treated with high-dose interleukin-2 (IL-2). Shown is the Kaplan-Meier plot of survival for 270 patients treated in eight clinical trials of high-dose IL-2 conducted between 1985 and 1993. Median survival was 11.4 months.

trials involving high-dose intravenous-bolus IL-2 conducted between 1985 and 1993,[36] the response rate was 16 percent, the median response duration was 8.9 months (range 4 to more than 106 months), and the median survival was 11.4 months (Figure 14–4). Seventeen patients experienced a complete response; 10 of the complete responders remained progression-free at 5 years (Figure 14–5). Responses were less frequent in patients with a poor performance status or in those who had received prior systemic therapy. However, in contrast to the responses to IFN-α, responses to IL-2 were seen with equal frequency in patients with visceral metastases and/or large tumor burdens (Figure 14–6). At a minimum follow-up of 4 years, 47 percent of all responders

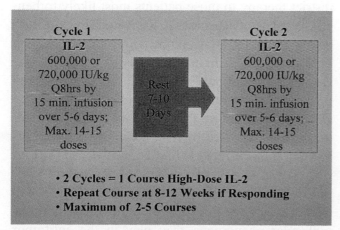

Figure 14–3. Dosing schema for the intravenous bolus (IVB) high-dose interleukin-2 (IL-2) regimen.

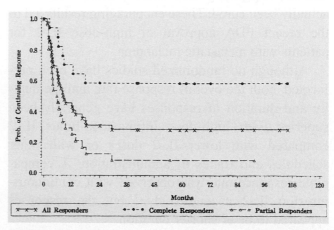

Figure 14–5. Response duration curves for 270 patients with metastatic melanoma treated with high-dose interleukin-2 (IL-2). Durable responses were seen in 59 percent of patients who had a complete response to high-dose IL-2.

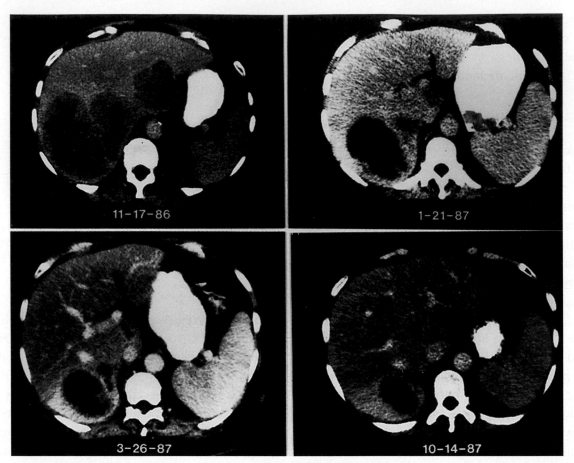

Figure 14–6.   Response of visceral melanoma metastases to high-dose interleukin-2 (IL-2). Computed tomography scans performed over a 1-year period in a patient with melanoma show regression of bulky hepatic metastases after high-dose IL-2 therapy.

remained alive; 12 (28%) of the responding patients were progression free. In addition, no patient responding for longer than 30 months had progressed, suggesting that some patients may have actually been cured. These encouraging results led to the recent FDA approval of high-dose IL-2 for patients with metastatic melanoma.

Although no randomized studies have been performed, both the overall response rate and the quality and duration of responses have generally been superior with high-dose intravenous-bolus IL-2 compared with lower IL-2 doses or with other schedules and routes of administration. A comparable response rate was observed with continuous-infusion IL-2 in one study,[37] but the responses appeared to be of shorter duration.

Response to IL-2 has correlated with the total amount of IL-2 received,[38] as well as with the Cw7 human leukocyte antigen (HLA) phenotype, the development of vitiligo (Figures 14–7 and 14–8) or autoimmune thyroid dysfunction, and low pretreatment serum levels of C-reactive protein and interleuken-6 (IL-6).[39] However, efforts to confirm these response correlates or to use such parameters to restrict therapy to those patients most likely to benefit have been unsuccessful. Resistance to IL-2 therapy is attributed to a number of factors, including tumor-induced immune suppression mediated via Fas/FasL interactions[40] and T-cell receptor dysfunction caused by diminished zeta-chain expression.[41] One study has shown that T-cell receptor abnormalities can be reversed by IL-2 therapy[42] and that this reversal may correlate with tumor response to IL-2. Correlative laboratory studies performed in conjunction with current and future clinical trials will be necessary to elucidate the roles these various molecular phenomena may play in the antitumor effects of IL-2.

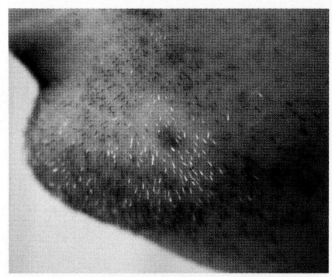

Figure 14–7. Interleukin-2 (IL-2)-induced vitiligo in a patient treated with high-dose IL-2 for metastatic melanoma. A halo of depigmentation is seen around a subcutaneous melanoma metastasis in a patient responding to high-dose IL-2 therapy.

Although high-dose bolus IL-2 is capable of inducing durable complete responses in patients with metastatic melanoma, its widespread use has been limited by the extensive multiorgan toxicity of this regimen. Side effects with high-dose IL-2 include hypotension, cardiac arrhythmias, pulmonary edema, fever, capillary leak syndrome, and (rarely) death.[43] Bacterial infection, particularly catheter-related sepsis, contributed significantly to the toxicity of IL-2 administration in early high-dose IL-2 trials and was responsible for all 6 deaths in those studies.[36] Antibiotic prophylaxis has greatly reduced the incidence of catheter-related sepsis and has thereby improved the safety of IL-2 therapy. As high-dose IL-2 can cause potentially life-threatening toxicity, its use is necessarily limited to patients with excellent organ function who are treated by experienced clinicians in specialized programs capable of providing intensive care unit–level monitoring and intervention.

Animal models and studies of the in vivo effects of IL-2 in humans have provided evidence that the toxic effects of IL-2 (especially hypotension and capillary leak syndrome) are partly due to endothelial cell activation and injury mediated by IL-2-induced cytokines and nitric oxide[44–47] as well as by activated lymphocytes and platelets[48–51] (Figure 14–9). Interleukin-2–induced proinflammatory cytokines (including IL-1, TNF-α, and IL-6) and

nitric oxide, products of macrophage activation, do not appear to be critical to the antitumor effect of IL-2—an effect that may be more dependent on tumor lysis mediated directly by activated T cells and NK cells. This has suggested that it may be possible to enhance the therapeutic index of high-dose IL-2 by dissociating its toxic effects from its antitumor effects. One of the first toxicity reduction strategies to be considered was the use of corticosteroids[52] (see Figure 14–9). For example, in both humans and animals, dexamethasone prevents the induction of TNF-α by IL-2. This, in turn, is associated with a diminution of toxicities related to IL-2, including fever and hypotension. However, corticosteroids such as dexamethasone also interfere with the antitumor activity of IL-2[53] and thus limit the utility of this approach. Techniques such as the coadministration of high-dose IL-2 with soluble receptors to TNF (sTNFR:IgG)[54] or IL-1 (sIL-1R)[55] or with methylxanthine-derived inhibitors of TNF or IL-1 signal transduction (pentoxifylline or CT1501R) have shown promise in animal models and were able to inhibit some of the biologic effects of high-dose IL-2 in patients without interfering with its antitumor effects (see Figure 14–9). Unfortunately, none of these agents were able to significantly block IL-2 toxicity as measured either by the ability to administer more IL-2 or by the induction of less toxicity with the same amount of IL-2.

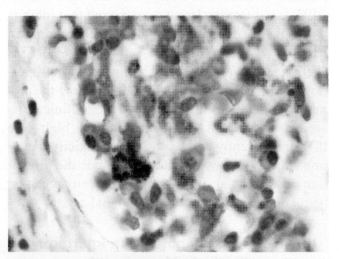

Figure 14–8. Pathology of responding subcutaneous melanoma metastasis following high-dose interleukin-2 (IL-2) therapy. A biopsy specimen of a subcutaneous metastasis with associated vitiligo following IL-2 therapy shows an infiltrate composed of lymphocytes, plasma cells, and melanin-laden macrophages, with no viable tumor cells.

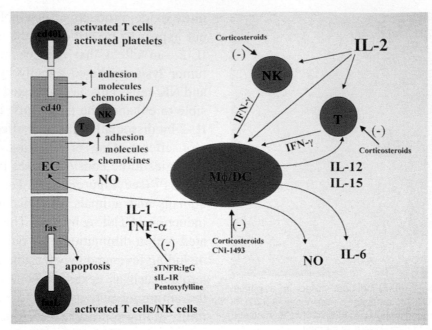

Figure 14–9.   Model of the mechanisms underlying immune activation and toxicity mediated by high-dose interleukin-2 (IL-2). The diagram shows how the liberation of proinflammatory cytokines and nitric oxide (NO) from activated lymphocytes, macrophages (Mϕ), and dendritic cells (DC) is central to the vascular toxicity of high-dose IL-2, including hypotension and capillary leak syndrome. Also shown is how vascular toxicity induced by IL-2 involves endothelial cell (EC) activation and injury through interactions with activated lymphocytes and platelets and stimulation by proinflammatory cytokines. The targets of prior and current strategies to reduce the toxicity of high-dose IL-2 are also shown. (INF-γ = interferon-γ; NK = natural killer cell; T = T cell; TNF-α = tumor necrosis factor-α.)

The successful dissociation of IL-2 toxicity from its antitumor effects may require the use of multiple cytokine antagonists or novel inhibitors of IL-2-derived proinflammatory cytokines with broader effects. One such potential agent, CNI-1493, is a guanylhydrazone compound that inhibits macrophage production of TNF-α, IL-1, and nitric oxide in response to IL-2[56] (see Figure 14–9). This agent protects rats from IL-2 toxicity without perturbing the antitumor effects, thus allowing the animals to tolerate 10 times more IL-2.[57] Clinical trials with this agent in conjunction with high-dose IL-2 are currently under way. Future toxicity reduction strategies may also need to include the disruption of potential interactions between activated lymphocytes/platelets and endothelial cells.

Interleukin-2 Combined with Interferon-α or Activated Lymphocytes

Preclinical data showing that IFN-α could up-regulate major histocompatability complex (MHC) and tumor-associated antigen expression in tumor cells suggested that IFN-α might increase the vulnerability of tumor cells to attack by T cells activated by IL-2. Despite these promising preclinical investigations and some encouraging early clinical results, the combination of IL-2 and IFN-α has not been superior to high-dose IL-2 alone.[58] One potential exception is the regimen involving "decrescendo" continuously infused high-dose IL-2 in combination with IFN-α. This regimen had a response rate comparable to that of high-dose bolus IL-2, but with far less toxicity.[59] Responses were seen in 31 percent of patients, including 22 percent of patients who had progressed following DTIC therapy. A median survival of 17 months was reported. Given the reported tolerability of this regimen, these encouraging results warrant independent confirmation.

Early animal models indicated that the activity of IL-2 was optimal when high doses were combined with peripheral blood lymphocytes (LAK cells) activated by IL-2. However, randomized trials comparing IL-2 plus LAK cells with high-dose IL-2 alone failed to show sufficient benefit from the addition of LAK cells to justify LAK-cell use.[60,61] Clinical trials of IL-2 in combination with autologous tumor-infiltrating lymphocytes (TILs) showed responses in 29 (34%) of 86 patients.[62] Responses were seen in some patients who had received prior IL-2, perhaps indicating enhanced potency for the IL-2 plus TILs combination. Unfortunately, only 5 responses were complete, and all partial responses except 1 were less than 10 months in duration. In addition, as a total of 121 patients were enrolled in order to treat the 86, the true response rate for IL-2 plus TILs was actually closer to 24 percent. It is unlikely, therefore, that IL-2 plus TILs is sufficiently superior to IL-2 alone to warrant the time, commitment, and expense necessary to employ this treatment modality.

Interleukin-12

Interleukin-12 (IL-12) is a powerful stimulator of cellular immune responses directed against infectious pathogens and tumor cells.[63] In animal models, IL-12 has potent antitumor activity against melanoma, renal cell cancer, sarcoma, and bladder cancer.

Interleukin-12 activates lymphocytes, antigen-presenting cells (APCs), B cells, and neutrophils although its antitumor activity has been linked to CD8-positive T-cell[64] and NK T-cell activation[65] and to the production of IFN-γ.[66] The antitumor activity of IL-12 appears to be due to the direct killing of tumor cells by activated effector cells as well as to antiangiogenic effects of IL-12 mediated in part by IFN-γ (Figure 14–10). In phase I and phase II clinical trials of recombinant human IL-12 performed over the past 5 years, antitumor responses in patients with metastatic melanoma or renal cell cancer have been observed.[67] However, compared with high-dose IL-2, response rates have been low, ranging from 0 to 7 percent. Studies in humans and animals treated with IL-12 have shown that the low response rate to IL-12 in cancer patients is due in part to a partly schedule-dependent rapid down-modulation of immune activation by IL-12[68,69] (Figure 14–11). Strategies, including the addition of IL-2 or IFN-α to IL-12, for potentiating the in vivo antitumor activity of IL-12 and for overcoming the early dampening of IL-12-induced immune activation are currently being tested in clinical trials in patients with metastatic melanoma or renal cell cancer.

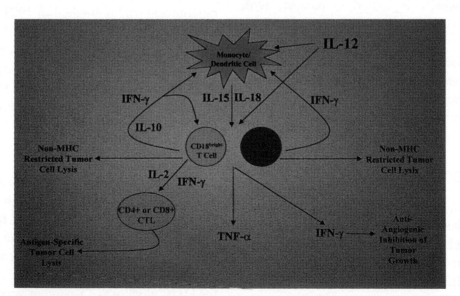

Figure 14–10. Model of the mechanisms through which interleukin-12 (IL-12) mediates immune activation and tumor regression. The diagram shows the central role that antigen-presenting cells (including monocytes and dendritic cells) and certain IL-12–responsive subsets of T cells and natural killer (NK) cells play in immune activation mediated by the combination of IL-12 plus co-stimulatory cytokines such as interleukins-15 and -18 (IL-15 and IL-18). Also shown is the central role of IL-12–induced interferon-γ (IFN-γ) in tumor regression mediated through the direct killing of tumor cells by activated lymphocytes as well as through antiangiogenic mechanisms. (MHC = major histocompatability complex; TNF-α = tumor necrosis factor-α.)

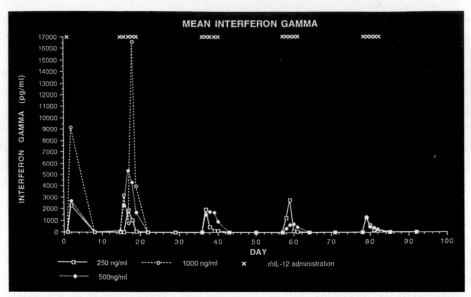

MEAN INTERFERON GAMMA

Figure 14–11. The magnitude of immune activation induced by interleukin-12 (IL-12) diminishes with successive cycles of IL-12. Among cohorts of patients treated at different dose levels on the first phase I trial of intravenous (IV) IL-12, interferon-γ (IFN-γ) production was maximal during the first cycle of therapy and diminished thereafter with successive cycles of IL-12. (X = test dose; XXXXX = 5-day treatment cycle with IL-12.) (Reproduced with permission from Atkins MB, Robertson MJ, Gordon M, et al. Phase I evaluation of intravenous recombinant human interleukin-12 in patients with advanced malignancies. Clin Cancer Res 1997;3(3):409–17.)

Other Cytokines

Interferon-γ, TNF-α, interleukin-4 (IL-4), and IL-6 have been extensively evaluated in patients with metastatic melanoma and have been found to be largely inactive.[39] Tumor necrosis factor-α may be useful when added to melphalan and hyperthermia in isolated limb perfusion therapy for locoregionally recurrent extremity melanomas.[70] Tumor necrosis factor is currently being examined in a randomized phase III trial in this setting.

BIOCHEMOTHERAPY

Because both chemotherapy and cytokine-based immunotherapy have proven (albeit limited) activity in metastatic melanoma, many investigators have examined whether the combination of these two treatment modalities can improve the response rate and have a greater impact on survival.

Combinations of Dacarbazine with Interferon-α or Interleukin-2

In mice, cytotoxic chemotherapy can enhance the immunomodulatory effects of cytokines such as IFN-α and IL-2. Consequently, DTIC has been administered in combination with either IFN-α or IL-2 to patients with metastatic melanoma. A small randomized trial published in 1991 compared DTIC to DTIC plus high-dose IFN-α.[71] The IFN-α was administered initially as a high-dose intravenous induction over 3 weeks, then subcutaneously thrice weekly throughout the cycles of DTIC administration. In this study, the combination of DTIC plus IFN-α produced 12 complete and 4 partial responses in 30 patients, compared with only 2 complete and 4 partial responses in 30 patients treated with DTIC alone. Median response durations and survival were also significantly prolonged with the DTIC-plus-IFN-α regimen. However, a recent four-arm phase III ECOG trial[20] investigating these same regimens failed to confirm these initial encouraging observations (see Table 14–2). In this trial, the response rate for DTIC alone was 15 percent versus 21 percent for DTIC plus IFN-α. Overall, there was no response, time to treatment failure, or survival advantage attributable to the addition of IFN-α to DTIC (see Figure 14–1). Based on this trial and data from other randomized studies, there is no convincing evidence to support the addition of IFN-α to DTIC. In clinical trials examining the addition of IL-2 to DTIC, the toxicity has been considerable, and response rates have remained in the range of only 13 to 30 percent.[72,73]

Interleukin-2 and Cisplatin-Based Biochemotherapy

While the combination of DTIC with IFN-α or IL-2 has not been superior to chemotherapy or immunotherapy alone, more encouraging results have been observed with regimens that combine cisplatin-based chemotherapy with either high-dose IL-2 alone or lower doses of IL-2 combined with IFN-α.[74–79] Composite results from a variety of inpatient regimens show a response rate of approximately 50 percent, with 10 to 20 percent CRs and median survival of 11 to 12 months. Partial responses were usually of short duration (median, 4 to 6 months) and were not associated with prolonged survival. In some studies, up to 60 percent of complete remissions appeared to be durable[79] (Figure 14–12). Overall, about 10 percent of all patients treated with cisplatin-based biochemotherapy regimens remained disease free for greater than 2 years; relapses after 2 years were uncommon.[79] In contrast to responses to chemotherapy alone, responses to cisplatin-based therapy were seen in all sites with equal frequency (Figure 14–13), and no clear dose-response effect for IL-2 was evident. Although some investigators reported partial regression of small CNS metastases in some patients,[74] most trials

excluded patients with CNS disease, and in fact, the CNS was a common site of initial relapse after treatment with biochemotherapy.[77]

Responses to cisplatin-based biochemotherapy were seen in patients previously treated with chemotherapy[78] and appeared to be associated with the development of vitiligo.[74] The cisplatin appeared to be required for synergy with IL-2 and/or IFN-α,[78] and activity appeared to be greatest when the chemotherapy was administered first.[75] Early trials showed that cytotoxic chemotherapy did not interfere with ongoing responses to immunotherapy,[76] thus enabling closer integration of these two treatment modalities.

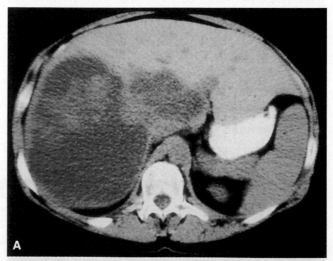
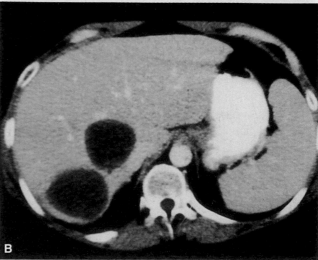

Figure 14–13. Regression of hepatic melanoma metastases in a patient treated with biochemotherapy. Shown are computed tomography (CT) scans of the liver performed *A*, before, and *B*, after concurrent biochemotherapy consisting of cisplatin, dacarbazine, vinblastine, interleukin-2 (IL-2), and interferon-α (IFN-α).

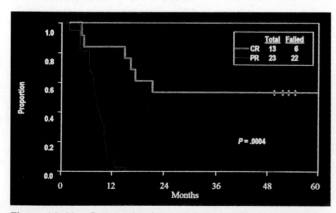

Figure 14–12. Progression-free survival according to response in melanoma patients treated with biochemotherapy. Shown are progression-free survival curves for patients achieving either a partial response (PR) or a complete response (CR) following treatment with a sequential biochemotherapy regimen containing cisplatin, dacarbazine, vinblastine, interleukin-2 (IL-2), and interferon-α.

The apparent higher response rate and the 10 percent durable CR rate suggest that these combination regimens may be superior to either chemotherapy or immunotherapy alone and that synergistic interactions between IL-2 and the cisplatin-based chemotherapy might be contributing to these improved results. Two compilations of data from large numbers of patients suggest that biochemotherapy produces response rates superior to those of either chemotherapy or immunotherapy alone. Keilholz and colleagues collected data on 631 patients treated with IL-2, either alone or in combination with IFN-α and/or cytotoxic drugs.[80] In this analysis, patients receiving IL-2, IFN-α, and chemotherapy had a response rate of 44.8 percent, compared with response rates of 20.8 and 14.9 percent for IL-2 plus IFN-α and for IL-2 alone, respectively. Median survival, however, did not differ between these three groups. Allen and colleagues performed a meta-analysis of 168 published trials involving 7,711 patients with metastatic melanoma treated with chemotherapy, immunotherapy based on IL-2, or biochemotherapy.[81] Here, the combination of

IL-2, IFN-α, and chemotherapy again had a significantly greater response rate. Unfortunately, the early biochemotherapy regimens described above involved intensive inpatient treatment as well as substantial toxicity, expense, and patient time commitment, making more widespread use or phase III investigation impractical.

Attempts have been made to enhance the tolerability and practicality of inpatient biochemotherapy. Regimens producing toxicity acceptable for more widespread inpatient (or even outpatient) use while retaining comparable antitumor activity to prior biochemotherapy regimens have recently been developed. The most promising of these approaches are detailed in Table 14–3. Legha and colleagues developed a regimen in which CVD chemotherapy was administered concurrently with IL-2 and IFN-α.[82] Therapy was administered in an inpatient setting over 5 days every 3 weeks for a maximum of 6 cycles. Tumor responses were seen in 34 of 53 patients (response rate [RR] of 64%, with 11 CRs and 23 PRs), with a median response duration of 6.5 months. Five patients (9%) remained in continuous CR for 50

Table 14–3. SECOND–GENERATION PHASE II BIOCHEMOTHERAPY TRIALS

Author (Reference)	Study Design	N	No. of Responses CR	No. of Responses PR	Overall RR (%)	Comments
Inpatient Regimens						
Legha (83)	Concurrent CVD/IL-2/IFN	53	11	23	64	Median response duration, 6.5 mo; 9% continuous CR 50 to > 61 mo
McDermott (84)	Modified CVD/IL-2/IFN	40	8	11	48	Responses in IFN-treated patients; CNS relapses frequent in responders
O'Day (85)	CVD/tamoxifen with concurrent decrescendo IL-2/IFN	45	10	15	57	No CRs in patients that had received prior chemotherapy
Outpatient Regimens						
Flaherty (86)	Cisplatin/D/IL-2 (IVB)	32	5	8	41	
Flaherty (87)	CD/IL-2(SC)/IFN vs	38	1	6	19	Randomized phase II CWG trial; IV IL-2 better than SC
	CD/IL-2(IV)IFN	44	5	11	37	
Thompson (88)	CDBT/IL-2 (SC)/IFN	53	10	12	42	Median survival, 11 mo
Atzpodien (89)	CDBT/IL-2 (SC)/IFN	27	3	12	55	
	Carboplatin D/IL-2 (SC)/IFN	40	3	11	35	

CNS = central nervous system; CR = complete response; CVD = cisplatin/vinblastine/dacarbazine; CWG = Cytokine Working Group; CD = cisplatin/dacarbazine; D = dacarbazine; CDBT = cisplatin/dacarbazine/carmustine/tamoxifen; IFN = interferon α; IL-2 = interleukin-2; IV = intravenous; IVB = intravenous bolus; N = number of patients; PR = partial response; RR = response rate; SC = subcutaneous.

to more than 61 months. The main side effects included myelosuppression with a 54 percent incidence of febrile neutropenia, nausea/vomiting/anorexia, fluid retention, and hypotension. The antitumor activity appeared equivalent to that of the other biochemotherapy regimens described above whereas the toxicity was more manageable. McDermott and colleagues recently completed a phase II pilot trial of a version of the Legha regimen that was modified to further reduce toxicity and enhance convenience.[83] Modifications included the implementation of antibiotic prophylaxis, the use of granulocyte colony–stimulating factor (G-CSF) to prevent febrile neutropenia, more aggressive antiemetics, the elimination of long-term central venous access, and restriction to a maximum of 4 cycles of therapy. Toxicity was considerably more manageable, and tumor responses were seen in 19 (48%) of 40 evaluable patients (8 CRs, 11 PRs). Responses were observed in all disease sites, including liver and bone (see Figure 14–4), and in 11 (48%) of 23 patients who had previously been treated with IFN-α. Unfortunately, 11 of the responders, including 4 patients who had achieved a CR, subsequently relapsed in the CNS. O'Day and colleagues[84] modified the Legha regimen by adding tamoxifen and administering the IL-2 in a "decrescendo" fashion similar to that described by Keilholz and colleagues. To prevent febrile neutropenia and infection, G-CSF was also added. Tumor responses were seen in 57 percent, and 23 percent achieved a CR. No CRs were seen in the patients who had received prior chemotherapy. Treatment was well tolerated, and the majority of patients were discharged from the hospital on day 5. Re-admission for toxicity was required in only 6 percent of cycles.

Flaherty and colleagues developed an outpatient biochemotherapy regimen, in which patients received cisplatin and DTIC on day 1 and boluses of intravenous IL-2 (24 MIU/m^2) on days 4 to 8 of a 21-day cycle[85] (see Table 14–3). The response rate was 41 percent. A similar regimen that included IFN-α was tested by the Cytokine Working Group.[86] In a randomized phase II trial, patients were assigned to receive IL-2 by either subcutaneous or intravenous injection. Tumor responses were seen in 37 percent of patients (12% CR and 25% PR) on the intravenous arm and in 19 percent of patients (3% CR and 16% PR) on the subcutaneous arm. Toxicity was comparable, except for a higher incidence of neutropenia on the intravenous arm. Thompson and colleagues evaluated an outpatient regimen consisting of cisplatin, DTIC, and BCNU on day 1 plus daily tamoxifen (CDBT) and subcutaneous IL-2 and IFN-α on days 3 to 9.[87] Grade 3 nausea occurred in 32 percent of patients, and hospitalization for intravenous hydration was necessary in 11 percent of treatment cycles. A response rate of 42 percent (10 CRs and 12 PRs) was observed in 53 patients, with a median overall survival of 11 months. Atzpodien and colleagues[88] reported on outpatient regimens using either carboplatin plus DTIC or CBDT for several cycles followed by subcutaneous IL-2 and IFN-α. These regimens produced responses in 35 and 55 percent of patients, respectively, with minimal reported toxicity. Whether these regimens are truly suitable for routine outpatient use and how they compare with either chemotherapy alone or the more thoroughly tested inpatient biochemotherapy regimens remains to be determined.

Randomized Trials of Interleukin-2-Based Biochemotherapy

Several randomized phase III trials comparing biochemotherapy to either IL-2/IFN-α or chemotherapy have been performed. Initial results have been disappointing (Table 14–4). In both the multicenter EORTC trial[89] comparing biochemotherapy to IL-2/IFN-α and the NCI Surgery Branch trial[90] comparing biochemotherapy to chemotherapy, response rates were higher for the biochemotherapy arm. However, this improved antitumor activity did not translate into any improvement in overall survival or any increase in the percentage of patients obtaining a durable complete response.

Although requiring confirmation, the lack of survival benefit in these two studies calls into question the value of biochemotherapy relative to chemotherapy or immunotherapy alone. Additional phase III trials comparing biochemotherapy to chemotherapy or immunotherapy are necessary to determine the value of this approach. Legha and his colleagues at the M.D. Anderson Cancer Center have recently completed accrual to a study compar-

Table 14–4. RANDOMIZED PHASE III BIOCHEMOTHERAPY TRIALS

Protocol, Principal Investigator (Reference)	Study Design	N	No. of Responses CR	No. of Responses PR	Overall RR (%)	Comments
EORTC,* Keilholz (90)	Decrescendo IL-2/IFN vs descrescendo IL-2/IFN + cisplatin	138	— —	— —	18 33	RR and progression-free survival better with addition of cisplatin; no difference in overall survival
NCI† Surgery Branch, Rosenberg (91)	Cisplatin/DTIC/tam vs cisplatin/DTIC/tam + IL-2/IFN	52 50	4 3	10 19	27 44	Short duration of PRs in both arms; no significant difference in RR or survival
MD Anderson Cancer Center, Legha	CVD vs CVD/IL-2/IFN					Completed accrual
EORTC,* Keilholz	Cisplatin/DTIC/IFN vs cisplatin/DTIC/IFN/IL-2					Completed accrual
ECOG‡-SWOG§ 3695, Atkins/Flaherty	CVD vs modified CVD/IL-2/IFN					Under way

*European Organization for Research and Treatment of Cancer.
†National Cancer Institute.
‡Eastern Cooperative Oncology Group.
§Southwest Oncology Group.
CR = complete response; CVD = cisplatin/vinblastine/dacarbazine; DTIC = dacarbazine; IFN = interferon α; IL-2 = interleukin-2; PR = partial response; RR = response rate; tam = tamoxifen.

ing their CVD/IL-2/IFN-α regimen to CVD alone. The EORTC is conducting a study comparing cisplatin/DTIC/IFN-α to the same regimen plus "decrescendo" IL-2. In addition, a phase III intergroup trial comparing the biochemotherapy regimen of McDermott and colleagues to CVD was initiated in early 1998. Results from all of these phase III trials should be available within the next 2 years and should firmly define the role of biochemotherapy in the treatment of this disease.

Future Applications of Biochemotherapy for Metastatic Melanoma

Efforts to reduce the incidence of CNS relapse associated with biochemotherapy have focused on the drug temozolomide because of its superior ability to penetrate into the CNS. Studies involving biochemotherapy regimens in which temozolomide is substituted for DTIC are currently under way at several institutions (Figure 14–14). Others have focused on moving biochemotherapy into the neoadjuvant or adjuvant setting. In addition to a lower tumor burden, these earlier disease settings also offer the potential advantage of a lower likelihood of CNS involvement. The Southwest Oncology Group (SWOG) and ECOG will soon be opening a phase

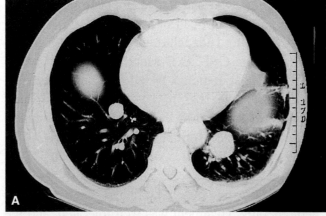

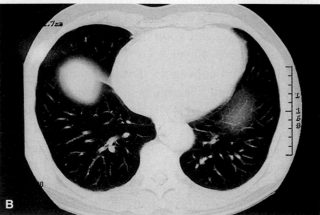

Figure 14–14. Regression of pulmonary melanoma metastases in a patient treated with temozolomide-based biochemotherapy. Shown are computed tomography (CT) scans of the lungs performed *A*, before, and *B*, after biochemotherapy consisting of temozolomide, cisplatin, dacarbazine, interleukin-2 (IL-2), and interferon-α (IFN-α).

III trial comparing the biochemotherapy regimen of McDermott and colleagues to high-dose IFN-α as adjuvant therapy for stage 3 patients with disease involving multiple regional lymph nodes.

REFERENCES

1. Landis SH, Murray T, Bolden S, Wingo PA. Cancer statistics, 1999. CA Cancer J Clin 1999;49:8–31.
2. Atkins MB. The role of cytotoxic chemotherapeutic agents either alone or in combination with biological response modifiers. In: Kirkwood JK, editor. Molecular diagnosis, prevention and therapy of melanoma. Hamilton (ON): BC Decker Inc; 1997. p. 219–51.
3. Houghton AN, Legha S, Bajorin DF. Chemotherapy for metastatic melanoma. In: Balch CM, Houghton AN, Milton, et al, editors. Cutaneous melanoma. Philadelphia: J.B. Lippincott Company; 1992. p. 498–508.
4. Hill GJ, Krementz ET, Hill HZ. Dimethyl triazeno imidazole carboxamide and combination therapy for melanoma. IV. Late results after complete response to chemotherapy (Central Oncology Group protocols 7130, 7131, and 7131A). Cancer 1984;53: 1299–305.
5. Stevens MFG, Hickman JA, Langdon SP, et al. Antitumor activity and pharmacokinetics in mice of 8-carbamoyl-2-methylimidazo {5, 1-d} 1, 2, 3, 5-tetrazin-4(3H)-one (CCRG 81045; M&B 39831), a novel drug with potential as an alternative to dacarbazine. Cancer Res 1987;47:5846–52.
6. Bleehen NM, Newlands SM, Thatcher LN, et al. Cancer Research Campaign phase II trial of temozolomide in metastatic melanoma. J Clin Oncol 1995;13: 910–3.
7. Middleton M, Gore W, Tilgen G, et al. A randomized phase III study of temozolomide (TMZ) versus dacarbazine (DTIC) in the treatment of patients with advanced metastatic melanoma. Proc Am Soc Clin Oncol 1999;18:536a.
8. Glover D, Glick JH, Weiler C, et al. WR2721 and high-dose cisplatin: an active combination in the treatment of metastatic melanoma. J Clin Oncol 1987;5: 574–8.
9. Evans LM, Casper ES, Rosenbluth R. Participating community oncology program investigators: phase II trial of carboplatin in advanced malignant melanoma. Cancer Treat Rep 1987;71:171–2.
10. Khayat D, Avril M, Auclerc G, et al. Clinical value of the nitrosourea fotemustine in disseminated malignant melanoma: overview of 1,022 patients including 144 patients with cerebral metastases. Proc Am Soc Clin Oncol 1993;12:393a.
11. Leyvras S, Spataro B, Bauer J, et al. Hepatic arterial chemotherapy for liver metastases from ocular melanoma. Proc Am Soc Clin Oncol 1996;15:435a.
12. Jacquillat C, Khayat D, Banset P, et al. Final report of the French multicenter phase II study of the nitrosourea fotemustine in 153 evaluable patients with disseminated malignant melanoma including patients with cerebral metastases. Cancer 1990;56:1873–8.
13. Quagliana JM, Stephens M, Baker LH, et al. Vindesine in patients with metastatic malignant melanoma. A Southwest Oncology Group study. J Clin Oncol 1984;4:316–9.
14. Einzig AI, Hochster H, Wiernik PH, et al. A phase II study of taxol in patients with malignant melanoma. Invest New Drugs 1991;9:59–64.
15. Bedikian A, Legha S, Jenkins J, et al. Phase II trial of docetaxel in patients with advanced melanoma previously untreated with chemotherapy. Proc Am Soc Clin Oncol 1995;14:412a.
16. Legha SS, Ring S, Papadopoulos N, et al. A prospective evaluation of a triple-drug regimen containing cisplatin, vinblastine and DTIC (CVD) for metastatic melanoma. Cancer 1989;64:2024–9.
17. Del Prete SA, Maurer LH, O'Donnell J. Combination chemotherapy with cisplatin, carmustine, dacarbazine and tamoxifen in metastatic melanoma. Cancer Treat Rep 1984;69:1403–5.
18. Buzaid AC, Legha S, Winn R, et al. Cisplatin (C), vinblastine (V), and dacarbazine (D) (CVD) versus dacarbazine alone in metastatic melanoma: preliminary results of a phase II cancer community oncology program (CCOP) trial. Proc Am Soc Clin Oncol 1993;12:389a.
19. Cocconi G, Bella M, Calabresi F, et al. Treatment of metastatic malignant melanoma with dacarbazine plus tamoxifen. N Engl J Med 1992;327:516–23.
20. Falkson CI, Ibrahim J, Kirkwood J, et al. Phase III trial of dacarbazine versus dacarbazine with interferon α2b versus dacarbazine with tamoxifen (TMX) versus dacarbazine with interferon α2b and tamoxifen in patients with metastatic malignant melanoma: an Eastern Cooperative Oncology Group study (E3690). J Clin Oncol 1998;16:1743–51.
21. Mastrangelo MJ, Berd D, Bellet RE. Aggressive chemotherapy for melanoma. PPO Updates 1991;5: 1–5.
22. McClay EF, Mastrangelo MJ, Berd D, et al. Effective combination chemo/hormonal therapy for malignant melanoma: experience with three clinical trials. Int J Cancer 1992;50:553–6.
23. Rusthoven JJ, Quirt IC, Iscoe NA, et al. Randomized, double-blind placebo-controlled trial comparing the response rates of carmustine, dacarbazine, and cisplatin with and without tamoxifen in patients with metastatic melanoma. National Cancer Institute of Canada Clinical Trials Group. J Clin Oncol 1996; 14:2083–90.

24. Creagan ET, Suman VJ, Dalton RJ, et al. Phase III clinical trial of the combination of cisplatin, dacarbazine, and carmustine with or without tamoxifen in patients with advanced malignant melanoma. J Clin Oncol 1999;17:1884–90.

25. Chapman PB, Einhorn LH, Meyers ML, et al. Phase III multicenter randomized trial of the Dartmouth regimen versus dacarbazine in patients with metastatic melanoma. J Clin Oncol 1999;17:2745–51.

26. Sreevalsan T. Biologic therapy with interferon-α and β: preclinical studies. In: DeVita VT, Hellman S, Rosenberg SA, editors. Biologic therapy of cancer. 2nd ed. Philadelphia: J.B. Lippincott Company; 1995. p. 347–64.

27. Slaton JW, Perrotte P, Inoue K, et al. Interferon-alpha-mediated down-regulation of angiogenesis-related genes and therapy of bladder cancer are dependent on optimization of biological dose and schedule. Clin Cancer Res 1999;5:2726–34.

28. Agarwala SS, Kirkwood JM. Interferon in melanoma. Curr Opin Oncol 1996;8:167–74.

29. Creagan ET, Ahmann DL, Frytak S, et al. Phase II trials of recombinant leukocyte A interferon in disseminated malignant melanoma: results in 96 patients. Cancer Treat Rep 1986;70:619–24.

30. Rosenberg SA, Mule JJ, Speiss PJ, et al. Regression of established pulmonary metastases and subcutaneous tumor mediated by systemic administration of high-dose recombinant interleukin 2. J Exp Med 1985;161:1169–88.

31. Lotze MT. Biologic therapy with interleukin-2: preclinical studies. In: DeVita VT, Hellman S, Rosenberg SA, editors. Biologic therapy of cancer. 2nd ed. Philadelphia: J.B. Lippincott Company; 1995. p. 207–33.

32. Dutcher JP, Creekmore S, Weiss GR, et al. A phase II study of interleukin-2 and lymphokine-activated killer cells in patients with metastatic malignant melanoma. J Clin Oncol 1989;7:477–85.

33. Parkinson DR, Abrams JS, Wiernik PH, et al. Interleukin-2 therapy in patients with metastatic malignant melanoma. A phase II study. J Clin Oncol 1990;8:1650–6.

34. Rosenberg SA, Yang JC, Toapplian SL, et al. Treatment of 283 consecutive patients with metastatic melanoma or renal cell cancer using high-dose bolus interleukin-2. JAMA 1994;271:907–13.

35. Rosenberg SA, Yang JS, White DE, et al. Durability of complete responses in patients with metastatic cancer treated with high-dose interleukin-2: identification of the antigens mediating response. Ann Surg 1998;228:307–19.

36. Atkins MB, Lotze M, Dutcher JP, et al. High-dose recombinant interleukin-2 therapy for patients with metastatic melanoma: analysis of 270 patients treated from 1985–1993. J Clin Oncol 1999;17:2105–16.

37. Legha SS, Gianan MA, Plager C, et al. Evaluation of interleukin-2 administered by continuous infusion in patients with metastatic melanoma. Cancer 1996;77:89–96.

38. Royal RE, Steinberg SM, Krouse RS, et al. Correlates of response to IL-2 therapy in patients treated for metastatic renal cell cancer and melanoma. Cancer J Sci Am 1996;2:91.

39. Atkins MB. Immunotherapy and experimental approaches for metastatic melanoma. Hematol Oncol Clin North Am 1998;12:877–902.

40. Hahne M, Rimoldi D, Schroter M, et al. Melanoma cell expression of Fas (Apo 1/CD95) ligand: implications for tumor immune escape. Science 1996;274: 1363–6.

41. Zea AH, Curti BD, Longo DL, et al. Alterations in T cell receptor and signal transduction molecules in melanoma patients. Clin Cancer Res 1995;1: 1327–35.

42. Rabinowich H, Banks M, Reichert TE, et al. Expression and activity of signaling molecules in T lymphocytes obtained from patients with metastatic melanoma before and after interleukin 2 therapy. Clin Cancer Res 1996;2:1263–74.

43. Gollob JA, Atkins MB. The treatment of metastatic renal cell cancer with high-dose interleukin 2. In: Vogelzang NJ, Scardino PT, Shipley WU, Coffey DS, editors. Comprehensive textbook of genitourinary oncology. 2nd ed. Baltimore: Lippincott Williams and Wilkins; 1999. p. 207–18.

44. Pugin J, Ulevitch RJ, Tobias PS. Tumor necrosis factor-alpha and interleukin-1 beta mediate human endothelial cell activation in blood at low endotoxin concentrations. J Inflamm 1995;45:49–55.

45. Ruegg C, Yilmaz A, Bieler G, et al. Evidence for the involvement of endothelial cell integrin alphaV-beta3 in the disruption of the tumor vasculature induced by TNF and IFN-gamma. Nat Med 1998;4:408–14.

46. Pober JS. Activation and injury of endothelial cells by cytokines. Pathol Biol (Paris) 1998;46:159–63.

47. Kilbourn RG, Owen-Schaub LB, Cromeens LB, et al. N^G methyl arginine, an inhibitor of nitric oxide formation, reverses IL-2-mediated hypotension in dogs. J Appl Physiol 1994;76:1130–7.

48. Yellin MJ, Brett J, Baum D, et al. Functional interactions of T cells with endothelial cells: the role of CD40L-CD40-mediated signals. J Exp Med 1995; 182:1857–64.

49. Henn V, Slupsky JR, Grafe M, et al. CD40 ligand on activated platelets triggers an inflammatory reaction of endothelial cells. Nature 1998;391:591–4.

50. Karmann K, Min W, Fanslow WC, et al. Activation and homologous desensitization of human endothelial cells by CD40 ligand, tumor necrosis factor, and interleukin 1. J Exp Med 1996;184:173–82.

51. Rafi AQ, Zeytun A, Bradley MJ, et al. Evidence for the involvement of Fas ligand and perforin in the induction of vascular leak syndrome. J Immunol 1998; 161:3077–86.

52. Mier JW, Vachino G, Klempner MS, et al. Inhibition of interleukin-2-induced tumor necrosis factor release by dexamethasone: prevention of an acquired neutrophil chemotaxis defect and differential suppression of interleukin-2-associated side effects. Blood 1990;76:1933–40.

53. Papa MZ, Vetto JT, Ettinghausen SE, et al. Effect of corticosteroids on the antitumor activity of lymphokine-activated killer cells and interleukin 2 in mice. Cancer Res 1986;46:5618–23.

54. DuBois JS, Trehu EG, Mier JW, et al. Randomized placebo-controlled trial of high-dose interleukin-2 in combination with a soluble p75 tumor necrosis factor receptor immunoglobulin G chimera in patients with advanced melanoma and renal cell cancer. J Clin Oncol 1997;15:1052–62.

55. McDermott DF, Trehu EG, Mier JW, et al. A two-part phase I trial of high-dose interleukin 2 in combination with soluble (Chinese hamster ovary) interleukin 1 receptor. Clin Cancer Res 1998;4:1203–13.

56. Bianchi M, Bloom O, Raabe T, et al. Suppression of proinflammatory cytokines in monocytes by a tetravalent guanylhydrazone. J Exp Med 1996; 183:927–36.

57. Kemeny MM, Botchkina GI, Ochani M, et al. The tetravalent guanylhydrazone CNI-1493 blocks the toxic effects of interleukin-2 without diminishing antitumor efficacy. Proc Natl Acad Sci U S A 1998;95:4561–6.

58. Sparano JA, Fisher RI, Sunderland M, et al. Randomized phase III trial of treatment with high-dose interleukin-2 either alone or in combination with interferon alfa-2a in patients with advanced melanoma. J Clin Oncol 1993;11:1969–77.

59. Keilholz U, Scheibenbogen C, Brossart P, et al. Interleukin-2-based immunotherapy and chemoimmunotherapy in metastatic melanoma. Recent Results Cancer Res 1995;139:383–90.

60. Rosenberg SA, Lotze MT, Muul LM, et al. A progress report on the treatment of 157 patients with advanced cancer using lymphokine-activated killer cells and interleukin-2 or high-dose interleukin-2 alone. N Engl J Med 1987;316:889–97.

61. McCabe MS, Stablein D, Hawkins MJ, et al. The modified group C experience-phase III randomized trials of IL-2 vs. IL-2/LAK in advanced renal cell carcinoma and advanced melanoma. Proc Am Soc Clin Oncol 1991;10:213a.

62. Rosenberg SA, Yannelli JR, Yang JC, et al. Treatment of patients with metastatic melanoma with autologous tumor-infiltrating lymphocytes and interleukin 2. J Natl Cancer Inst 1994;86:1159–66.

63. Trinchieri G. Interleukin-12: a proinflammatory cytokine with immunoregulatory functions that bridges innate resistance and antigen-specific adaptive immunity. Annu Rev Immunol 1995;13:251–76.

64. Brunda MJ, Luistro L, Warrier RR, et al. Antitumor and antimetastatic activity of interleukin 12 against murine tumors. J Exp Med 1993;178:1223–30.

65. Cui J, Shin T, Kawano T, et al. Requirement for Vα14 NKT cells in IL-12-mediated rejection of tumors. Science 1997;278:1623–6.

66. Nastala CL, Edington ED, McKinney TG, et al. Recombinant IL-12 administration induces tumor regression in association with IFN-γ production. J Immunol 1994;153:1697–706.

67. Gollob JA, Atkins MB. Clinical trials of interleukin-12 in oncology. Curr Opin Oncol Endoc Metabol Invest Drugs 1999;1:260–71.

68. Atkins M, Robertson M, Gordon M, et al. Phase I evaluation of intravenous recombinant human interleukin 12 in patients with advanced malignancies. Clin Cancer Res 1997;3:409–17.

69. Coughlin CM, Wysocka M, Trinchieri G, et al. The effect of interleukin 12 desensitization on the antitumor efficacy of recombinant interleukin 12. Cancer Res 1997;57:2460–7.

70. Lienard D, Ewalenko P, Delmotte JJ, et al. High-dose recombinant tumor necrosis factor alpha in combination with interferon gamma and melphalan in isolation perfusion of the limbs for melanoma and sarcoma. J Clin Oncol 1992;10:52–60.

71. Falkson CI, Falkson G, Falkson HC. Improved results with the addition of interferon α2b to dacarbazine in the treatment of patients with metastatic malignant melanoma. J Clin Oncol 1991;9:1403–8.

72. Stoter G, Aamdal S, Rodenhuis S, et al. Sequential administration of recombinant human interleukin-2 and dacarbazine in metastatic melanoma: a multicenter phase II study. J Clin Oncol 1991;9:1687–91.

73. Dummer R, Gore ME, Hancock BW, et al. A multicenter phase II clinical trial using dacarbazine and continuous infusion interleukin-2 for metastatic melanoma. Clinical data and immunomonitoring. Cancer 1995;75:1038–44.

74. Richards JM, Gale D, Mehta N, et al. Combination of chemotherapy with interleukin-2 and interferon alpha for the treatment of metastatic melanoma. J Clin Oncol 1999;17:651–7.

75. Legha SS, Buzaid AC. Role of recombinant interleukin-2 in combination with interferon alpha and chemotherapy in the treatment of advanced melanoma. Semin Oncol 1993;2 Suppl 9:27–32.

76. Demchak PA, Mier JW, Robert NJ, et al. Interleukin-2 and high-dose cisplatin in patients with metastatic melanoma: a pilot study. J Clin Oncol 1991;9:1821–30.

77. Atkins MB, O'Boyle KR, Sosman JA, et al. Multi-institutional phase II trial of intensive combination chemoimmunotherapy for metastatic melanoma. J Clin Oncol 1994;12:1553–60.

78. Antoine EC, Benhammouda A, Bernard A, et al. Salpetiere Hospital experience with biochemotherapy in metastatic melanoma. Cancer J Sci Am 1997; 3:S16–21.

79. Legha SS, Sigrid R, Eton O, et al. Development and results of biochemotherapy in metastatic melanoma: the University of Texas M.D. Anderson Cancer Center Experience. Cancer J Sci Am 1997;3:S9–15.

80. Keilholz U, Conradt C, Legha SS, et al. Results of interleukin-2-based treatment in advanced melanoma: a case record-based analysis of 631 patients. J Clin Oncol 1998;16:2921–9.

81. Allen IE, Kupelnick B, Kumashiro M, et al. Efficacy of interleukin-2 in the treatment of metastatic melanoma: systematic review and meta-analysis. Cancer Ther 1998;1:168–72.

82. Legha SS, Ring S, Eton O, et al. Development of a biochemotherapy regimen with concurrent administration of cisplatin, vinblastine, dacarbazine, interferon alpha and interleukin-2 for patients with metastatic melanoma. J Clin Oncol 1998;16:1752–9.

83. McDermott DF, Mier JW, Lawrence DP, et al. A phase II pilot trial of concurrent biochemotherapy with cisplatin, vinblastine, dacarbazine (CVD), interleukin-2 (IL-2) and interferon alpha-2B (IFN) in patients with metastatic melanoma. Proc Am Soc Clin Oncol 1998;17:507a.

84. O'Day SJ, Gamman G, Boasberg PD, et al. Advantages of concurrent biochemotherapy modified by decrescendo interleukin-2, granulocyte colony-stimulating factor, and tamoxifen for patients with metastatic melanoma. J Clin Oncol 1999;17:2752–91.

85. Flaherty LE, Robinson W, Redman BG, et al. A phase II study of dacarbazine and cisplatin in combination with outpatient administered interleukin-2 in metastatic malignant melanoma. Cancer 1993;71: 3520–5.

86. Flaherty LE, Atkins M, Sosman J, et al. Randomized phase II trial of chemotherapy and outpatient biotherapy with interleukin-2 and interferon alpha (IFN) in metastatic melanoma. Proc Am Soc Clin Oncol 1999;18:536a.

87. Thompson J, Gold P, Fefer A. Outpatient chemo-immunotherapy for patients with metastatic melanoma. Cancer J Sci Am 1997;3:S29–36.

88. Atzpodien J, Lopez E, Hanninen A, et al. Chemoimmunotherapy of advanced malignant melanoma: sequential administration of subcutaneous interleukin-2 and interferon-alpha after intravenous dacarbazine and carboplatin or intravenous dacarbazine, cisplatin, carmustine and tamoxifen. Eur J Cancer 1995;31A:876–81.

89. Keilholz U, Goey SH, Punt CJ, et al. Interferon alfa-2a and interleukin-2 with or without cisplatin in metastatic melanoma: a randomized trial of the European Organization for Research and Treatment of Cancer Melanoma Cooperative Group. J Clin Oncol 1997;15:2579–88.

90. Rosenberg SA, Yang JC, Schwartzentruber DJ, et al. Prospective randomized trial of the treatment of patients with metastatic melanoma using chemotherapy with cisplatin, dacarbazine, and tamoxifen alone or in combination with interleukin-2 and interferon alfa-2b. J Clin Oncol 1999;17:968–75.

15

Treatment of Nonmelanoma Skin Cancer

ABEL TORRES, MD, JD
JOSE R. PEÑA, MD
ARTURO SAAVEDRA, MD

This chapter reviews the treatment of nonmelanoma skin cancers (NMSCs)—primarily, basal cell carcinoma (BCC) and squamous cell carcinoma (SCC). The treatment of some rarer forms of skin cancer will also be covered. (A discussion of radiation therapy for NMSC is presented elsewhere in this atlas.)

TREATMENT MODALITIES FOR BASAL AND SQUAMOUS CELL CARCINOMAS

The ease of the skin for access makes it possible to treat BCC and SCC with a variety of ablative or surgical techniques. Several well-established techniques include (1) electrodessication and curettage, (2) cryosurgery, (3) radiation therapy, (4) excision, and (5) Mohs' micrographic surgery (MMS). Some newer therapies include laser surgery, photodynamic therapy, and immunomodulatory ablation.

Electrodessication and Curettage

Electrodessication and curettage (ED&C) is a technique that removes the cancer by curetting (scraping) it off of the skin surface. Tumor tissue is usually more friable than normal tissue; it forms poor epithelial attachments and is consequently more easily curetted than normal tissue. Curettage is accomplished through the use of a curette, which is a long, thin instrument with a loop of sharp metal at one end, similar to a vegetable peeler (Figure 15–1). The curette is used to scrape off the visible tumor. Curet-

tage is followed by application of an electrical current to the wound (electrodessication). An electrical device called a hyfrecator or Bovie (Figure 15–2), which produces the electric current, is used for hemostasis and to destroy residual tumor cells and subclinical tumor extensions. This process of curettage followed by electrodessication is usually repeated from one to three times, with the goal of complete ablation of the cancer. Cure rates for the treatment of BCC and SCC with ED&C vary, depending on the experience of the operator, the location, and the histologic nature of the lesion. These cure rates are presented later in this chapter in a comparative analysis with the other ablative and surgical modalities. Electrodessication and curettage

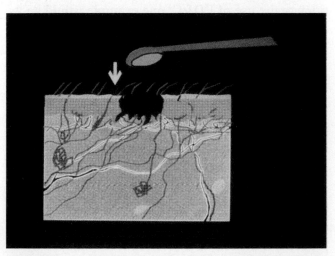

Figure 15–1. Curettage accomplished through the use of a curette —a long, thin instrument with a loop of sharp metal at one end.

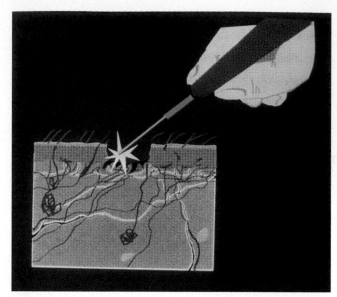

Figure 15–2. Application of an electrical current to the wound to destroy residual tumor (electrodessication).

offers a rapid way to eradicate primary superficial BCCs and SCCs on skin that lends itself to curettage, such as the thick skin of the back. The resultant wounds heal by secondary intention (granulation), and ED&C sometimes may result in a better cosmetic outcome than results from excision. However, healing can sometimes be prolonged, and scars can be hypopigmented, depressed, or hypertrophic. In the hands of operators who are well versed in its proper indications and use, ED&C can be a useful tool and can be especially helpful in those patients with multiple lesions. There are few contraindications to the use of ED&C; one example would be its use in patients with implanted electrical devices such as pacemakers or defibrillators. Advocates of ED&C point out that most of these devices are well insulated or that ED&C can still be safely used in these patients with proper placement of grounding plates, the use of bipolar electrodes, and careful monitoring of these devices. Detractors of the technique point to the inability to adequately determine margin control as the major limitation of its usefulness. (For an excellent discussion of the technique of cutaneous electrosurgery and for instruction on the procedure, the reader is referred to *Cutaneous Electrosurgery* by Jack Sebben, published in 1989 by Year Book Medical Publishers.)

Cryosurgery

Cryosurgery uses liquid nitrogen (–195.8°C) to freeze tumor-involved tissue and ablate cancer cells. Adequate control of the depth and intensity of the freezing allows the superficial destruction of a lesion such as an actinic keratosis or the extensive necrosis of deeper cancerous cells. The equipment necessary is simple and may consist of a cryogenic spray device (Figure 15–3) or cotton-tipped applicators with a cryogen canister (a specially vented thermos). Usually, treatment of cancerous lesions is best accomplished through more than one freeze-thaw cycle (Figure 15–4). This approach seems to afford the greatest chance for the destruction of cancerous tissue. The mechanism of action is thought to be cellular destruction by crystal formation, with cell membrane leakage on the first freeze-thaw cycle and cell destruction on subsequent freeze-thaw cycles. Ideally, thermocouples should be used to measure the temperatures and the depth of the freeze in the dermis or subcutis. However, this is not always practical, and experienced operators are often comfortable estimating the breadth and depth of freeze on the basis of varying formulas and/or experience. Treatment of BCC usually requires at least two freeze-thaw cycles, with a freeze colder than –40° to –50°F and at least 60 seconds of thaw time advocated for adequate ablation.[1] Cryosurgery has been effectively used for BCCs and selected low-risk SCCs.[2] In both BCC and SCC, the types of lesions amenable to cryosurgery are small to medium, superficial, well-delineated, and well-differentiated

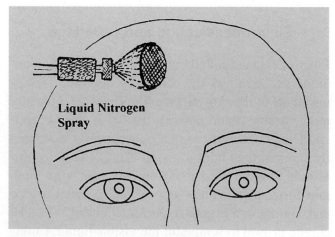

Liquid Nitrogen Spray

Figure 15–3. Cryogenic spray device.

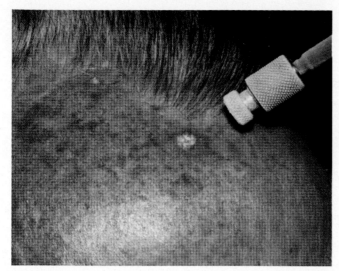

Figure 15–4. Freeze and thawing of multiple skin lesions.

skin cancers.[3] Cryosurgery is useful for patients with implanted electrical devices (pacemakers, defibrillators, etc.) or in patients for whom surgery may pose a higher risk. (The cure rates for cryosurgery are presented later in this chapter in a comparative analysis with other ablative and surgical modalities.) Among the few contraindications to the use of cryosurgery are disorders associated with cold intolerance, as is found in cold urticaria and cryoglobulinemia.

The tissue response after cryosurgery consists of immediate and delayed edema, blister formation, and necrosis with subsequent sloughing and eschar formation (Figure 15–5). As with ED&C, the resultant wounds heal by secondary intention, and this procedure sometimes results in a better cosmetic outcome than results from excision. However, healing can sometimes be prolonged, and scars can be hypopigmented, depressed, or hypertrophic, similar to those seen after ED&C. In addition, tissue retraction of tissue-free margins can sometimes be seen and can result in deformity of an alar rim or ear. Cryosurgery can be a very useful tool in the hands of operators who are well versed with its proper indications and use. It can be especially helpful in patients with multiple lesions or patients who are not good candidates for other therapies. Detractors of the technique point to the inability to adequately determine margin control as the major limitation of its usefulness. (For an excellent discussion of the technique of cutaneous cryosurgery and for instruc-

tion on the procedure, the reader is referred to *Cryosurgical Treatment of Skin Cancer,* by E.G. Kuflik and A.A. Gage, published in 1990 by Igaku-Shoin Medical Publishers, and/or "Cryosurgery," by G.F. Graham, in *Atlas of Cutaneous Surgery*, edited by J.K. Robinson, K.A. Arndt, P.E. LeBoit, and B.V. Wintroub and published in 1996 by W.B. Saunders.)

Laser Ablation

Superficially invasive or in situ skin cancers such as SCC and superficial BCC have been successfully treated by using carbon dioxide (CO_2) laser ablation.[4] The destructive method used is similar to that of ED&C, but advocates contend that superpulsed and ultrapulsed CO_2 lasers can limit the depth of penetration as compared to ED&C, resulting in a more superficial destruction and thus a more elegant and faster wound healing response. However, this same advantage may be a disadvantage, in that deeper extension down follicular structures could be missed by a very precise superficial ablative modality such as the CO_2 laser. Yet, in some areas with sparse or absent follicular structures (such as the genitals), the CO_2 laser can be successfully used with less risk of problematic scarring.[4,5] Laser ablation has also been used as a substitute for electrical current in ED&C, to avoid the unpredictable nature of tissue penetration by an electrical current; possible interference with electrical implanted devices by the ED&C current would also be avoided. The advantages of the laser ablation approach are

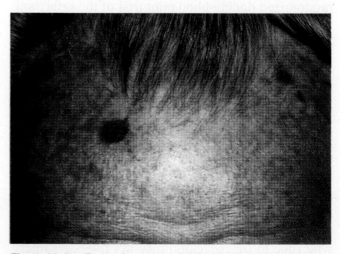

Figure 15–5. Eschar formation, after liquid nitrogen therapy.

unclear at this time, but it shows promise as a treatment modality, and more experience with its use should be welcome.

Photodynamic Therapy

Photodynamic therapy (PDT) involves systemically or topically administering an agent, such as 5-aminolevulinic acid, that is selectively absorbed by cancerous cells, rendering them photosensitive. Exposure to a high-intensity light results in a chemical reaction in these cells, leading to cell death.[6] In early studies, PDT successfully treated some superficial BCCs and SCCs.[7,8] Success with this modality in treating skin cancers is still to be fully achieved, but the procedure shows sufficient promise. The Federal Drug Administration (FDA) recently approved 5-aminolevulinic acid for PDT.

Immunomodulatory Ablation

Imiquimod (Aldara, 3M Pharmaceuticals) is a newer chemical compound that has emerged as a promising new treatment of BCC and possibly of SCC.[9] The topical use of this drug had been developed to treat anogenital condylomata acuminata and other human papillomavirus infections.[10] Imiquimod is not an antiviral or antineoplastic drug; rather, it is an immunomodulating drug that stimulates production of interferon-α (IFN-α) subtypes 1, 2, 5, 6, and 8 and tumor necrosis factor-α (TNF-α).[11] Because intralesional IFN has been used somewhat effectively in BCC, Beutner and colleagues[12] conducted a randomized double-blind pilot trial of the safety and efficacy of imiquimod 5% cream in the treatment of BCC. The BCCs responded in the patients who were dosed twice daily, once daily, and three times weekly; efficacy seemed to drop off with less frequent use. Adverse events were predominantly local reactions that correlated to frequency of use and stopped with withdrawal of treatment. Only nonaggressive BCCs, superficial and nodular, were involved in this study. Although this was a small pilot study (n = 35), the results are very promising for the nonsurgical treatment of such a common malignancy. This holds especially true for patients who (due to other factors) may not tolerate surgery

or for tumor sites that are not amenable to excision. More studies are needed before the value of using imiquimod to treat BCC can be established.

Surgical Excision

Surgical excision is the treatment modality that is generally considered to be the standard of care in the treatment of NMSC. It involves the physical removal of the cancer through the use of a cutting device (usually a cold steel scalpel), with a small margin of surrounding clinically normal skin. The excised specimen is sent to pathology for examination and margin assessment (see discussion of the limitations of pathology, below). The resultant surgical wound defect can usually be closed primarily through approximation of the tissue margins (Figure 15–6), or through a skin flap or skin graft, or occasionally through secondary intention. The type of repair depends mostly on the size and location of the surgical wound defect.

Excision of NMSC without a prior biopsy is advocated by some physicians and health maintenance organizations as a means of cutting down on health care costs, in that the excision could serve as both a diagnostic and therapeutic biopsy. However, this approach ignores the fact that all NMSCs are not alike and require different approaches to treatment. For instance, due to subclinical extension of the tumor, dermatofibrosarcoma protuberans (DFSP) requires a different treatment approach with respect to margins than would a nodular BCC. Sim-

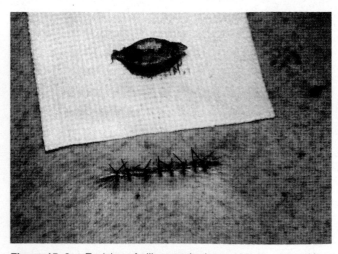

Figure 15–6.   Excision of ellipse and primary closure of the skin.

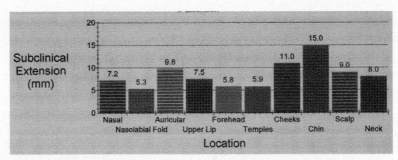

Figure 15–7. Subclinical extension of morpheaform basal cell carcinoma. (Adapted from Salasche SJ, Amonette RA. Morpheaform basal cell epitheliomas. A study of subclinical extensions in a series of 51 cases. J Dermatol Surg Oncol 1981;7:387–93.)

ilarly, not all BCCs and SCCs are clinically or histologically alike, and both cancers show variability of subclinical extension. This variability of subclinical tumor extension was highlighted in a study performed by Salasche and Amonette in 1981 at the University of Tennessee.[13] In their study of 51 patients with morpheaform BCC, Salasche and Amonette found the average lateral subclinical extension to be 7.2 mm (Figure 15–7). Similarly, in their review of the treatment of SCC of the skin and lip (1940 to 1992), Rowe, Carroll, and Day (all of the University of Texas Health Science Center at San Antonio) showed that SCCs differ in their aggressiveness and require varying margins of excision, based on such factors as histologic evidence of perineural involvement, histologic differentiation, and size of lesion[14] (Figure 15–8). Thus, treatment for a particular skin cancer should be individualized to the patient and to the type of lesion. A biopsy of the lesion for histologic confirmation and classification prior to treatment seems a prudent and logical

initial step, from which a reasonable treatment approach can be formulated.

If a biopsy is a prudent initial surgical step, then what is the appropriate method for sampling tissue? A 1999 study by Russell, Carrington, and Smoller, at the University of Arkansas for Medical Sciences,[15] compared the histologic findings of the shave (tangential) biopsy versus the punch (cylindrical) biopsy technique for subtype diagnosis of BCC (86 cases: 57 punch biopsies and 29 shave biopsies). They found that shave biopsies and punch biopsies resulted in essentially equivalent diagnostic accuracy rates of 75.9 and 80.7 percent, respectively (Figure 15–9). For the 20 percent of cases for which the first biopsy was inadequate, or where one needs to clearly differentiate between morpheaform and nodular BCC or other NMSC, a second deeper excisional biopsy can be performed. However, the reliability of a second biopsy has been questioned, as shown by a study performed by one of the authors (Torres and colleagues at Loma Linda University and the Uni-

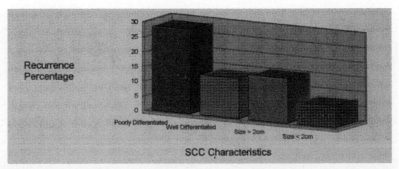

Figure 15–8. Comparison of recurrence rate for SCC. (Adapted from Rowe DE, Carroll J, Day CL. Prognostic factors for local recurrence, metastasis, and survival rates in squamous cell carcinoma of the skin, ear, and lip. J Am Acad Dermatol 1992;26:976–90.)

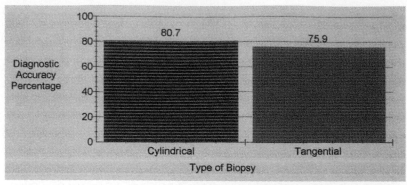

Figure 15–9. Biopsy method: cylindrical (punch) versus tangenital (shave). (Adapted from Russell BE, Carrington PR, Smoller BR. Basal cell carcinoma: a comparison of shave biopsy techniques in subtype diagnosis. J Am Acad Dermatol 1999;41:69–71.)

versity of San Francisco) in 1992. The study, which involved 291 patients (167 men and 133 women; ages 23 to 95 years; 91.8% with BCC and 8.2% with SCC, on all areas of the head and neck), looked at whether a second biopsy after an initial diagnostic shave or punch biopsy can be reliable for determining residual tumor.[16] It was found that 63 percent or more of subsequent biopsies for skin cancer may yield false-negative results and can be interpreted to cast doubt on the usefulness of a second biopsy versus just proceeding with surgery (Figure 15–10). Yet, this study dealt with lesions that were so small that they were no longer clinically evident at the time of presentation for treatment, and it did not deal with lesions such as SCCs, which may have deeper components unaffected by the initial shave biopsy. In fact, the study underscored the fact that deeper tumor components could still be found at a subsequent excisional surgery or biopsy. However, the study did

emphasize that once a BCC has been histologically diagnosed, it is not generally useful to repeat a biopsy but is rather more prudent to excise the lesion. To further underscore this point, a study by Holmkvist, Rogers, and Dahl in 1999 at Boston University looked at the incidence of residual BCCs in patients who appeared to be clinically tumor free after biopsy (41 BCC patients: 27 women and 14 men; ages 31 to 77 years; lesions on head and neck areas). Holmkvist and colleagues found that tumor was still present in 66 percent of the cases and concluded that even though the tumor may appear to be clinically removed, the patients are at risk for recurrence if they receive no further treatment (Figure 15–11).[17]

Surgical excision is touted as the "gold standard" for treatment once the diagnosis is established through a biopsy. In part, this is because of the ability of surgical excision to provide tissue for margin assessment as a means of judging the adequacy of

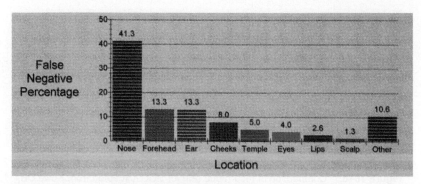

Figure 15–10. Reliability of second biopsies for residual tumor. (Adapted from Torres A, Seeburger J, Robinson D, Glogau R. The reliability of a second biopsy for determining residual tumor. J Am Acad Dermatol 1992;27:70–3.)

cancer removal. Margins can be assessed either through the use of permanent paraffin-embedded sections or through the preparation of frozen-section tissue. Permanent sections offer the advantage of usually being easier to prepare and are more consistent in quality. They have the disadvantage of taking longer to prepare, usually necessitating the closure of the defect without knowing the adequacy of the margin removed at the time of surgery. Frozen sections, on the other hand, enable the operator to assess the adequacy of margin removal at the time of surgery, but the quality of the slides, accuracy of interpretation, and speed of preparation will vary with laboratory experience. In both permanent- and frozen-section tissue processing, the traditional approach has been to have a pathologist or dermatopathologist interpret the slides. This is advocated (1) because of the experience of these professionals in interpreting slides, (2) to separate the process of surgery, and (3) to free the surgeon from determining the adequacy of tumor removal. This is an important point because, as some surgeons have commented, "Difficulties in closing the defect may tempt the surgeon to make too narrow an excision, in which case the tumor will recur."[18] There are certainly advantages to having the pathologist involved in this process, but it also adds an extra cost to the procedure. The cost of frozen sections is usually greater than that of permanent sections alone, since permanent sections will also be performed traditionally to confirm the frozen-section interpretation. Furthermore, there are usually added costs to the patient when frozen sections are performed, resulting from the traditional use of an operating room or outpatient surgical facility instead of the operator's clinic or office. This results in room use fees, nursing time fees, and (often) anesthesiologist fees, in addition to fees for the pathologist while the operator waits for the frozen-section results. In a study by Cataldo, Stoddard, and Reed in 1989, a review of 450 BCC cases (347 primary, 103 recurrent, with 180 cases undergoing frozen-section evaluation at the time of surgery; 2-mm margins) treated by a single plastic surgeon from 1973 to 1989 was undertaken to look at this issue.[19] The frozen sections at that institution cost $120 for the first slide and $70 for each subsequent slide. A negative result entailed five slides at a cost of $400, with the added cost of 20 additional minutes of operative and anesthesia time, amounting to approximately $5 to $15 per minute at the hospital, depending on whether surgery was performed at the day stay center or in the operative suite. The study's authors estimated that margin verification by frozen sections would result in $500 to $700 in added costs.[19] More than 10 years have elapsed since then, and those costs could be lower today (although in keeping with the inflation of health care costs over the past 10 years, it is more likely that the actual costs are higher). In addition, there is the capability today of performing immunoperoxidase stains and fast permanent microwave sections that can both add to the accuracy and costs of microscopic slide interpretations. The development of MMS has been an effort to address the concerns surrounding the need to obtain adequate and accurate tissue margins while keeping costs in check. Before MMS is discussed, however, an issue that must be addressed is whether margins matter.

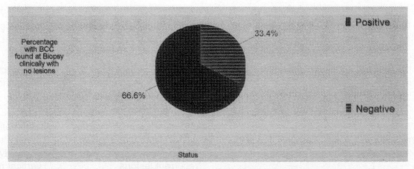

Figure 15–11.   Residual BCC after biopsy versus no residual BCC found. (Adapted from Holmkvist KA, Rogers GS, Dahl PR. Incidence of residual basal cell carcinoma in patients who appear tumor free after biopsy. J Am Acad Dermatol 1999;41:600–5.)

The Meaning of Surgical Margins: Do Margins Matter?

Unlike margin recommendations for melanoma, recommendations for surgical margins in the excision of NMSC vary widely and depend mostly on the tumor's histologic type, on whether the lesion is a primary or recurrent one, and on clinical characteristics such as location and size. Although exten-

sive, most of the literature is retrospective, and only a few prospective clinical studies have been conducted to adequately assess whether subclinical extension is predictive of recurrence, metastasis, or other comorbidities. Furthermore, the need to control for multiple variables (such as age, sex, and differences in populations; clinical exclusion criteria; study designs; follow-up periods; and ways of presenting data) makes a general comparison of stud-

Study	Characteristics	Margins	Results	Comments
Table 15–1. SELECTED LITERATURE FOR MARGINS IN THE TREATMENT OF BASAL CELL CARCINOMA				
Bart et al	N = 468; recurrent = 27	3–5 mm	5-year cumulative recurrence = 6.8%	Retrospective analysis; no routine histologic examination for adequacy of margins
Burg et al	N = 72	Used Mohs' to remove lesion; compared size of the defect to recommended margins	Average subclinical extension = 7.6 ± 4.5 mm	Subclinical extension varied according to tumor characteristics
Griffith et al	N = 634 recurrent = 13%	Varied from 2–3 mm to 1 cm, depending on physician	1.4% recurrence for tumors followed for 3–14 years	Recommends 2–3 mm for small lesions, at least 5 mm for high-risk lesion
Epstein	N = 131	1.5–2 mm minimum	Accurate visual diagnosis within 1 mm 94% of the time	Examined extension of margins by step sectioning
Macomber et al	N = 673; follow-up available in 159 cases	Recommends 5 mm	98.1% cure rate at 5 years	No clear correlation between margin size and outcome
Beirne et al	N = 169 (mixed basal and squamous cell lesions)	Recommends 5–10 mm	No recurrences after 2–6 years of follow-up	No correlation between margins and outcome
Blomqvist et al	N = 406 patients	At least 3 mm	2% recurrence after 6 months	No prospective data
Shanoff et al	N = 1,168 lesions	No mention	5.5% recurrence after "wide excision"	Correlates pathologic reports to recurrence
Ghauri et al	N = 108 lesions	At least 2 mm	7.7% recurrence	Clear margins in 87.5% of cases
Cataldo et al	N = 950 lesions	At least 2 mm	13% positive margins for primary tumors, 40% for recurrent tumors	Few data on margins; mostly focuses on indications for frozen section in treatment
Wolf et al	N = 117 lesions	Used Mohs' until margins were tumor free	Minimum margin of 4 mm required to eradicate 95% of tumors	One of two studies with prospective evaluation of variable margins and lateral subclinical extension (vertical margins not evaluated); no long-term follow-up
Salasche et al	N = 51 lesions	Used Mohs' to determine subclinical extension	Average subclinical extension = 7.2 ± 3.8 mm	Stratifies according to histology, location, duration
Dixon et al	N = 631 cases; recurrent = 30	None available	Distance to closest resection margin = 0.313 mm for primary tumors, 0.843 mm for recurrences	Retrospective study on pathology slides; no prospective data
Breuninger et al	N = 1,757 primary lesions	2–6 mm (average = 3.8 mm)	Subclinical extension varies according to diameter and histology, for primary versus recurrent lesions (prospective data)	Mathematical functions were derived to calculate probability of positive lateral and vertical margins for variable clinical margins used

Mohs' = Mohs' micrographic surgery; N = population studied.

Table 15–2. SELECTED LITERATURE FOR MARGINS IN THE TREATMENT OF SQUAMOUS CELL CARCINOMA

Study	Characteristics	Margins	Results	Comments
Brodland et al	N = 141 primary lesions	Used Mohs' until clear margins were achieved	High-risk tumors require at least 6-mm margins; 4 mm is adequate for all others	Prospective evaluation of variable margins and tumor-free sections; good stratification of high-risk factors
Bumstead et al	N = 71 auricular lesions	Used Mohs' and compared necessary margins to recommended excision margins	21% of tumors would have been inadequately excised if conventional treatments were used	Recommends Mohs' for these lesions to limit excess removal of healthy skin and prevent "inadequate excision"
Hoffman et al	N = 7 penile lesions	Retrospectively identified margins used	3 patients were treated with margins < 10 mm, with no recurrences after 22.7 months	Challenged use of 15–25-mm margins, or total penectomy as guideline for excision
Ghauri et al	N = 110 lesions	At least 2 mm	10.3% recurrence	Clear margins in 92.6% of cases
Friedman et al	N = 63 in trunk or extremities only	Retrospectively examined tumor thickness, invasion, and histologic grade; no mention of margins	Recurrent tumors were at least 4 mm thick; fatal tumors were at least 10 mm thick	Examined depth of invasion, histologic grade, and tumor thickness as prognostic factors
Dinehart et al	N = 27 metastatic tumors	Retrospective evaluation of pre- and postoperative size and depth of defect	Postoperative size and depth of defect were statistically higher for metastatic than non-metastatic lesions	Stratified data according to location and other variables such as histologic grade
Beirne et al	N = 169 (mixed basal and squamous cell lesions)	Recommends 5–10 mm	No recurrences after 2–6 years of follow-up	No correlation between margins and clinical outcome
Moller et al	N = 186 SCCs, 25 "probable" SCCs	Not available or evaluated	Metastasis is dependent foremost on the anatomic site	Duration and size of lesion also predictive of metastasis

Mohs' = Mohs' micrographic surgery; N = population studied; SCC = squamous cell carcinoma.

ies and a statistical analysis of pooled data difficult to accomplish. More important, most studies have examined lateral extension of tissue as a measure guiding surgical therapy; but with the exception of those that involve SSC, only a few studies have attempted to examine vertical extension as a predictor of how wide surgical margins should be in the treatment of NMSC. The final answers await properly designed and conducted prospective studies. Nevertheless, data from our review of the literature (Tables 15–1 and 15–2) support our knowledge of cancer in general, in that the chance of recurrence is greater when margins are positive for tumor involvement. One study that has been extensively cited over the years as supporting the position that margins are not that important in the treatment of BCC is the one by Pascal, Hobby, Lattes, and Crikelair[20] (Figure 15–12). This study looked at the recurrence of primary BCC over the 10-year period of 1945 to 1955, relative to incomplete versus complete excision of the tumor as established by permanent-section evaluation after excision. Of the 361 patients, 143 patients were seen regularly for the 10-year period and were included; the remaining 218 were excluded. The lesions were evaluated by the pathologist as being either adequately or inadequately excised or suboptimal in excision if tumor extended to within one high-power field (400×) of an edge. Of 42 tumors that were inadequately excised, only 14 (33%) were reported to recur; of 17 tumors suboptimally excised, only 12 percent recurred[20] (see Figure 15–12). This study has resulted in many surgeons concluding that margins in and of themselves are not the only factor in deciding tumor recurrence since only "one-third" of inadequately excised tumors recurred. One hypothesis put forward is that in the case of BCC, once you remove the bulk of the tumor, the body's immune surveillance system can then overcome the tumor because of the decreased tumor burden. Thus, some

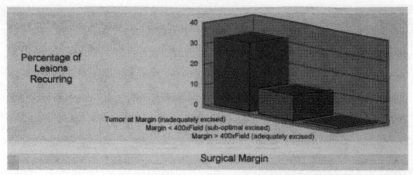

Figure 15–12. Recurrence of incompletely excised versus completely excised BCC. Adapted from Pascal RR, Hobby LW, Lattes R, Crikelair GF. Prognosis of "incompletely excised" versus "completely excised" basal cell carcinoma. Plastic and Reconstructive Surgery 1968;41:328–32.

individuals advocate unaggressive removal of BCC tumor, with the limited goal of reducing tumor burden and in the belief that the body will destroy the tumor in two-thirds of cases. Unfortunately, this logic does not take into account other studies that contradict the results of Pascal and colleagues and especially ignores the fact that their study dealt with a small number of primary BCCs—not recurrent lesions—and failed to address multiple variables.

An important study that contradicted the study by Pascal and colleagues was that of Shanoff and colleagues from the Division of Plastic Surgery at the Baylor University College of Medicine conducted in 1967, a year before the Pascal study.[21] This study looked at a total of 1,168 BCCs in 625 patients treated over the 15-year period from 1948 to 1963. (There were 218 multiple lesions, 1% of the patients were female, and 450 BCCs undergoing surgery were included in the study.) Among other factors it evaluated was the recurrence of BCCs if the margins were involved (narrow vs wide margins).[21] Like Pascal and colleagues,[20] they found even less recurrence with positive margins, in that only 19 percent of patients with positive margins had recurrences (Figure 15–13). More significant (and appearing to contradict the results of Pascal and colleagues) was that 67 percent of patients with a tumor-free but narrow margin had recurrence of the BCC (see Figure 15–13). This casts doubt on the theory that tumor will be destroyed by inflammation and that margins are not important. But how is it that a patient with a tumor-free margin can have a recurrence but a patient with a tumor-involved margin does not always have a recurrence? Perhaps the answer lies more in the process used to assess the adequacy of tumor removal rather than in any factor related to the tumor or the body's immune response.

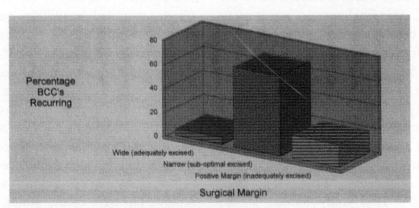

Figure 15–13. BCC recurrence and tissue margins. (Adapted from Shanoff LB, Spira M, Hardy B. Basal cell carcinoma: a statistical approach to rational management. Plast Reconstr Surg 1967;39:619–24.)

Tissue Processing for Microscopic Evaluation

Figures 15–14 and 15–15 depict and explain current methods commonly used to process tissue specimens for microscopic evaluation of margins. As can be seen, the commonly used techniques of tissue "bread-loafing" and cross-margin sectioning can result in the pathologist interpreting the tumor as having been completely removed when the margins are in fact involved with tumor. This can explain why a narrow margin will allow recurrence: tumor can still be present even though interpreted otherwise.

An explanation for a decreased tumor recurrence when margins are interpreted as involved can be attributed partly to the fact that the margin being evaluated is not the patient's true margin but rather the margin of the tissue removed. This may or may not be indicative of true continuation of tumor at the margin of the wound itself. Furthermore, in a study carried out by Abide, Nahai, and Bennett in 1984 at Emory University, an attempt was made to correlate the consistency of margin interpretation by 11 pathologists with the understanding of their criteria by the 25 plastic surgeons with whom they worked.[22] What Abide and colleagues found was surprising (Figure 15–16): there was a wide variation in the interpretation of the margins. What constituted tumor involvement versus being close to the margins varied: what one pathologist described as close was considered positive by another or narrow by yet another (see Figure 15–16). To further compound the problem, Abide and colleagues found that the plastic surgeons often were not even aware of what criteria were being used by the pathologists.[22] Thus, phraseology used in interpreting tumor margins presently is varied and confusing and may account

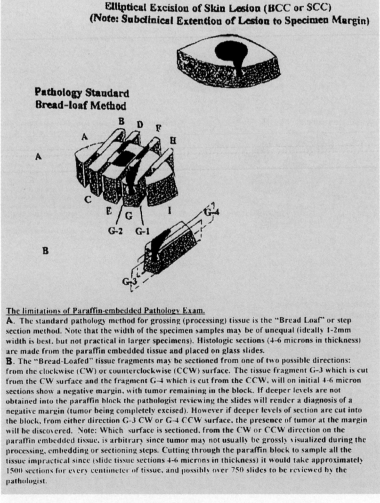

Elliptical Excision of Skin Lesion (BCC or SCC)
(Note: Subclinical Extention of Lesion to Specimen Margin)

Pathology Standard
Bread-loaf Method

The limitations of Paraffin-embedded Pathology Exam.
A. The standard pathology method for grossing (processing) tissue is the "Bread Loaf" or step section method. Note that the width of the specimen samples may be of unequal (ideally 1-2mm width is best, but not practical in larger specimens). Histologic sections (4-6 microns in thickness) are made from the paraffin embedded tissue and placed on glass slides.
B. The "Bread-Loafed" tissue fragments may be sectioned from one of two possible directions: from the clockwise (CW) or counterclockwise (CCW) surface. The tissue fragment G-3 which is cut from the CW surface and the fragment G-4 which is cut from the CCW, will on initial 4-6 micron sections show a negative margin, with tumor remaining in the block. If deeper levels are not obtained into the paraffin block the pathologist reviewing the slides will render a diagnosis of a negative margin (tumor being completely excised). However if deeper levels of section are cut into the block, from either direction G-3 CW or G-4 CCW surface, the presence of tumor at the margin will be discovered. Note: Which surface is sectioned, from the CW or CCW direction on the paraffin embedded tissue, is arbitrary since tumor may not usually be grossly visualized during the processing, embedding or sectioning steps. Cutting through the paraffin block to sample all the tissue impractical since (slide tissue sections 4-6 microns in thickness) it would take approximately 1500 sections for every centimeter of tissue, and possibly over 750 slides to be reviewed by the pathologist.

Figure 15–14. Pitfalls of bread-loaf method of tissue processing.

for some of the confusion surrounding the significance of tissue margins. What one pathologist calls an involved margin would not show tumor recurrence if interpreted as close by another pathologist. If tissue margins are important and yet there is confusion in the communication between pathologists and surgeons, then one solution is to rely on visual determinations of margins or, better yet, some objective data that establish minimum margins for most tumors. The validity of this approach is the subject of the following discussion.

Evaluation of Subclinical Extension

Surgeons often express confidence in their abilities to recognize ("eyeball") visible margins, and perhaps this is justified. Yet, as a group they have long recognized that skin cancer commonly exhibits subclinical extensions beyond the visible margins.[18] As

a result, multiple studies have been performed to assess what normal tissue margin beyond the visible tumor margin is necessary when excising skin cancer. Many of these studies are described above in Tables 15–1 and 15–2. Typical of several of these studies is the retrospective chart review by Blomqvist, Eriksson, and Lauritzen in their 1982 study at the University of Gothenburg. They reviewed the hospital records of 406 patients (204 men and 202 women) with BCCs, 79 percent of which were on the head and neck. They recommended that a 3-mm margin should be used for excising all BCCs.[18] They emphasized the importance of obtaining clear margins so that, besides achieving complete removal of the tumor, a primary closure (such as a skin flap) would not have to be sacrificed if the initial resection were inadequate. Although commendable for emphasizing the importance and need for margins beyond visible tumor, the study reinforced prior

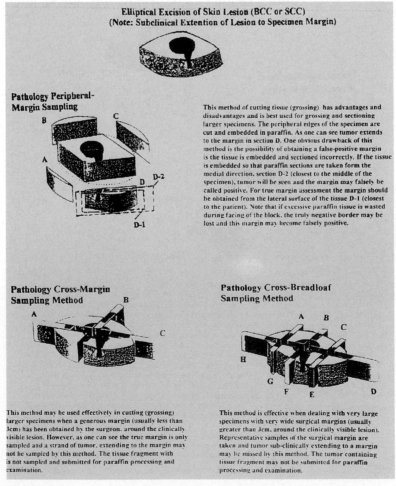

Figure 15–15.   Different methods of tissue processing and their pitfalls.

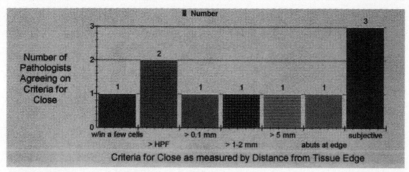

Figure 15–16. Pathologists' interpretation of surgical margins. (Adapted from Abide JM, Nahai F, Bennett RG. The meaning of surgical margins. Plast Reconstr Surg 1984;73:492–7.)

studies that proposed a "one-size-fits-all" solution to a problem that is not so easily solved. A prospective study by Wolf and Zitelli, from the Department of Dermatology at the University of Pittsburgh School of Medicine in 1986, evaluated the subclinical extensions of 117 BCCs treated with MMS.[23] Wolf and Zitelli marked the skin in 2-mm increments from the visible tumor margin preoperatively and then excised the tumor with the frozen-section control of MMS. They found that a minimum of 4 mm of margin was necessary to eradicate tumor in 95 percent of BCCs, but their finding of the variable subclinical extensions for BCCs was more important (Figure 15–17).

Not only did this study show a need sometimes for a margin that was greater than the 3-mm margin advocated by Blomqvist and colleagues,[18] but it also highlighted the point that to remove a 4-mm margin for all primary BCCs would result in a needless sacrifice of normal tissue in the majority of patients who required a margin of less than 3 mm. Similarly,

a prospective study by Brodland and Zitelli at the Department of Dermatology of the Mayo Clinic in 1992 involved 111 patients treated for primary invasive SCC and looked at the subclinical extension of SCCs.[24] Brodland and Zitelli used the same approach outlined above for the BCC study and found that clinically definable SCCs needed a margin of 4 mm for removal of more than 95 percent of tumors and that high-risk tumors needed a margin of 6 mm for removal of more than 95 percent of tumors. As in the BCC study, however, the majority of SCCs required a margin of only 2 mm for complete tumor removal, and a 4- or 6-mm margin would have sacrificed excess normal tissue (Figure 15–18).

The results of these studies are in keeping with the study by Cataldo, Stoddard, and Reed in 1989,[19] which reviewed 450 BCC cases treated by a single plastic surgeon from 1973 to 1989 and which looked at the usefulness and cost-effectiveness of excisional surgery with frozen-section control in the treatment of BCCs (2-mm margins; 347 primary, 103 recur-

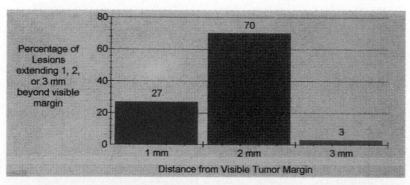

Figure 15–17. Measurements of minimal tumor (BCC) extension (subclinical extension). (Adapted from Wolf DJ, Zitelli JA. Surgical margins for basal cell carcinoma. Arch Dermatol 1987;123:340–4.)

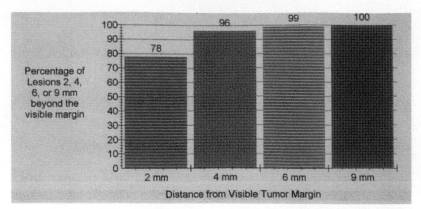

Figure 15–18. Tumor clearance versus margins in SCC. (Adapted from Broadland DG, Zitelli JA. Surgical margins for excision of primary cutaneous squamous cell carcinoma. J Am Acad Dermatol 1992;27:241–8.)

rent, with 180 undergoing frozen-section evaluation at the time of surgery).[19] As previously noted (see p. 6), verification by frozen sections would result in $500 to $700 in added costs for the surgery. However, Cataldo and colleagues[19] pointed out that the added cost would be justified for the 24 percent of patients with recurrent tumors who would have to undergo re-excision, since re-excision would result in greater cost than would be incurred if frozen sections had initially been used in the excision of recurrent tumors (Figure 15–19).

Cataldo and colleagues found that for those with primary lesions (nonrecurrent tumors), only 10 percent had positive margins on frozen sections and that the cost of frozen sections would not justify their use initially. However, they added that for those primary tumors with indistinct margins resembling recurrent tumors, frozen sections might still be justified. Thus, it appears that in establishing tumor-free margins for

BCC and SCC, it is prudent to consider a method that ensures adequacy of tissue margins, such as excision with frozen-section control or MMS, rather than relying on visual margins or fixed 3-mm margins.

Mohs' Micrographic Surgery

Mohs' chemosurgery was developed by Frederic Mohs in 1941, after he observed that the application of a 20 percent zinc chloride paste (hence the "chemo" in chemosurgery) to tumor-bearing tissue resulted in excellent preservation of histologic detail. He then applied the use of this paste to surgical excisions combined with the use of horizontal (as opposed to conventional vertical—bread-loafing and cross-sectioning) tumor processing. In addition, he added tissue scoring (marking the normal wound edges with small scalpel cuts) together with tissue color coding (marking the excised tissue with col-

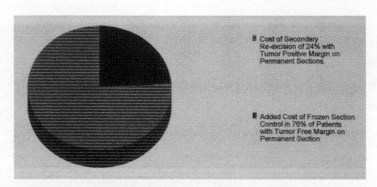

Figure 15–19. Comparison of cost of secondary procedure versus frozen section for recurrent tumors. (Adapted from Cataldo PA, Stoddard PB, Reed WF. Use of frozen section analysis in the treatment of basal cell carcinoma. Am J Surg 1990;159:561–3.)

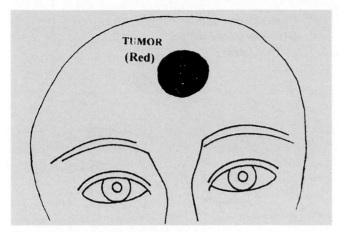

Figure 15–20. Tumor on forehead.

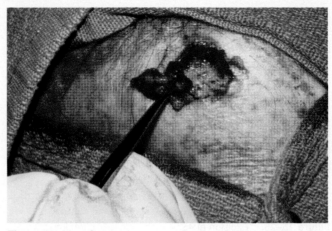

Figure 15–22. Curettage.

ored dyes to correlate with the scalpel cuts) as opposed to the traditional practice of placing a suture at one end of a specimen. Last, he eliminated the confusion in communication between the pathologist and surgeon by training in the histologic evaluation of skin cancer and serving as both surgeon and microscopic slide interpreter when performing an excision of a skin cancer with MMS. In the 1970s, Dr. Ted Tromovich, at the University of California in San Francisco (UCSF), established that frozen-section capabilities had progressed to the point that the same technique could be carried out without the discomfort and delays caused by the use of zinc chloride paste. This resulted in the technique we now know as MMS.

A study by Dr. Timothy Johnson at UCSF highlighted how curettage prior to an excision helps delineate the extent of BCC tumor involvement. This has resulted in the evolution of MMS in such a way that curettage of the BCC or SCC is usually the first step performed, followed by excision of the lesion at 45°, including 1 mm or more of surrounding normal tissue (Figures 15–20 to 15–26). The skin is then scored (Figures 15–27 and 15–28), the excised tissue

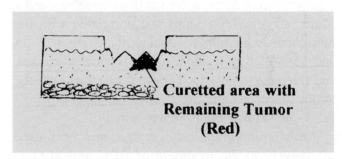

Figure 15–23. Wound, post curettage.

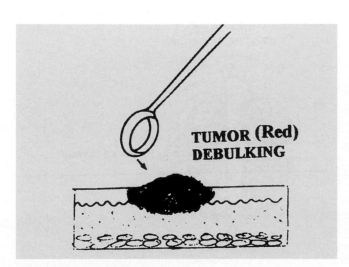

Figure 15–21. Curettage.

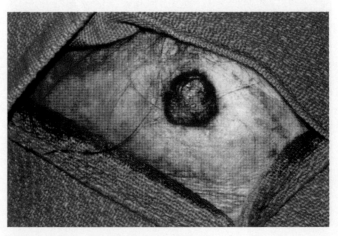

Figure 15–24. Wound, post curettage.

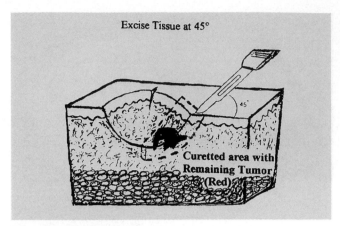

Figure 15–25.   Excision at 45°.

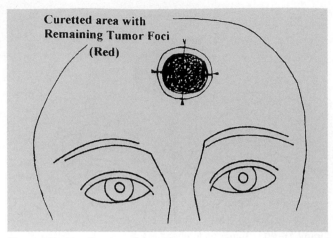

Figure 15–27.   Scoring of the skin.

is color coded with inks, and a corresponding anatomic map is prepared (Figures 15–29 to 15–31). The tissue is then inverted on a flat surface. The initial 45° incision angle allows the epidermal edge to be placed at the same plane as the bottom (center) of the specimen to permit processing by horizontal sections (Figures 15–32 to 15–34). The sections are then evaluated microscopically by the Mohs' surgeon (the Mohs' surgeon receives training in the evaluation of histopathology during a dermatology residency and a Mohs' surgery fellowship) and correlated with the initial map to pinpoint residual tumor (Figures 15–35 and 15–36). Any residual tumor is then re-excised, and the process described above is repeated until the tumor has been completely removed (Figures 15–37 to 15–39). The defect is then repaired.

Mohs' micrographic surgery has now been used extensively in the treatment of BCC and SCC as

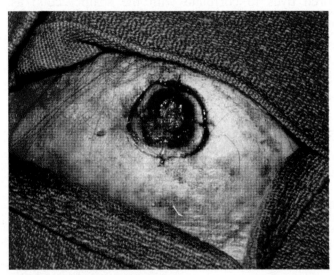

Figure 15–28.   Scoring of the skin.

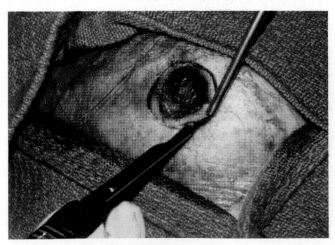

Figure 15–26.   Excision at 45°.

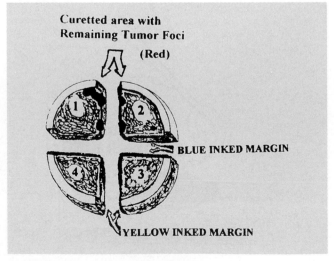

Figure 15–29.   Color coding of tissue.

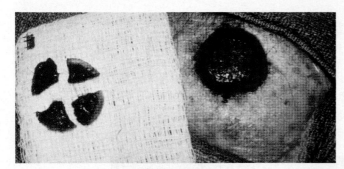

Figure 15–30. Color coding of tissue.

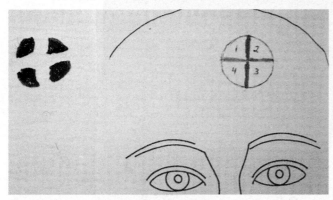

Figure 15–31. Anatomic map and coding.

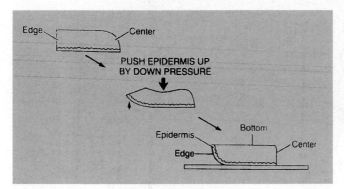

Figure 15–32. Horizontal section processing.

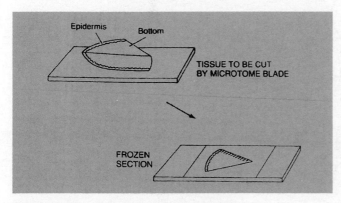

Figure 15–33. Horizontal section processing.

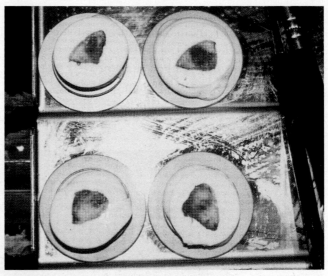

Figure 15–34. Cutting horizontal sections.

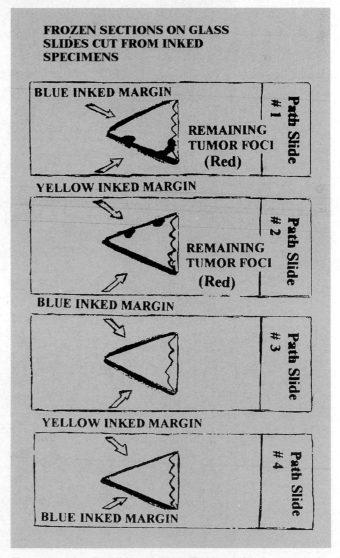

Figure 15–35. Residual tumor identified in sections.

well as DFSP, atypical fibroxanthoma (AFX), and (less commonly) malignant fibrous histiocytoma (MFH) and other NMSCs. This microscopically controlled surgical method has proved better at long-term tumor removal than the usual visual-inspection method of margin assessment. A comparative analysis of the various ablative and surgical modalities in the next section discusses how MMS can improve on the benefits offered by conventional excision of skin cancer, with or without frozen-section control or other ablative and surgical modalities.

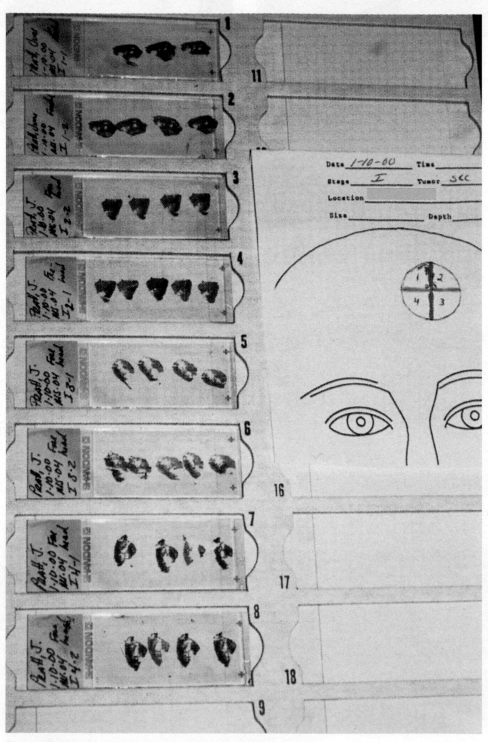

Figure 15–36.   Residual tumor correlated with anatomic mapping.

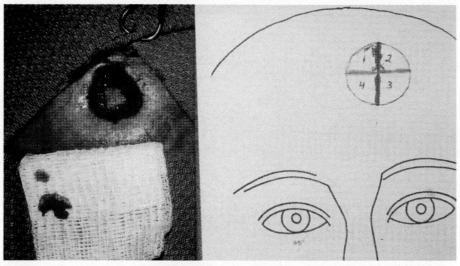

Figure 15–37. Second-stage Mohs' excision, using anatomic map (one skin margin and deep).

TREATMENT EFFECTIVENESS OF ABLATIVE AND SURGICAL MODALITIES: A COMPARATIVE ANALYSIS

It must be emphasized that there is currently no randomized study of primary or recurrent BCCs or SCCs treated by the different treatment modalities. This is important because even when using strict criteria in selecting studies for review, it is difficult (if not impossible) to compare results between studies. The studies report recurrence rates in various manners, such as (a) < 5, 5, and > 5 years after treatment and (b) inclusion of all treated tumors, even those lost to follow-up. Although extensive, most of the literature is retrospective, and only a few prospective clinical studies have been conducted to adequately assess whether subclinical extension is predictive of recurrence, metastasis, or other comorbidities. Furthermore, the need to control for multiple variables such as age and sex, differences in populations, clinical exclusion criteria, study designs, and ways of presenting data makes a general comparison of data and a statistical analysis of pooled data difficult to accomplish. As a result, some have advocated that techniques such as MMS should not be used until proven in a randomized controlled double-blind trial. Unfortunately, the same would probably have to be said about all of the treatment modalities for

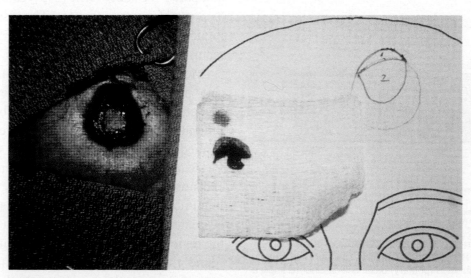

Figure 15–38. Color coding and creation of a new anatomic map.

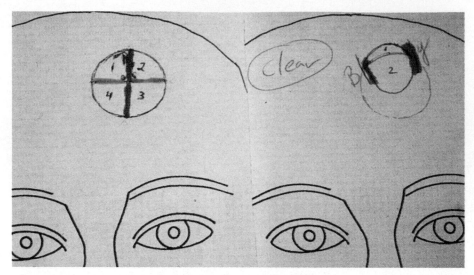

Figure 15–39. Final versus initial map showing clearance of tumor.

NMSC, and this approach would make no sense in view of the data supporting the various treatment modalities. Likewise, a randomized controlled double-blind trial to evaluate the treatment effectiveness of the various treatment modalities would be impeded by the ethical dilemma of patient autonomy and allowing the patient to choose a treatment on the basis of current information and standards. Nevertheless, such a trial would be welcome although it will be difficult, time consuming, and in need of ethical limits. Until then, surgeons have to rely on data from the reviews available regarding the effectiveness of various treatment modalities for NMSC.

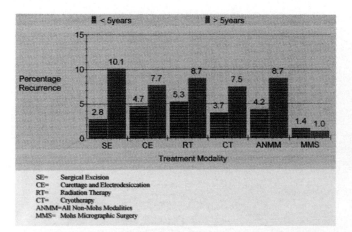

Figure 15–40. Short- and long-term recurrence of primary BCC. (Adapted from Rowe DE, Carroll RJ, Day CL. Long-term recurrence rates in previously untreated (primary) basal cell carcinoma: implications for patient follow-up. J Dermatol Surg Oncol 1989;15:315–28.)

Treatment of Primary (Untreated) Basal Cell Carcinoma

An attempt to address the issue of treatment of primary BCC is provided by the study performed by Rowe, Carroll, and Day, which looked at the long-term recurrence rates in previously untreated (primary) BCC.[25] In this study, Rowe and colleagues reviewed the literature on BCCs treated between 1947 and 1991. Hundreds of articles involving well over 18,883 cases of BCCs were systematically reviewed to determine the effectiveness of surgical excision, radiotherapy, cryotherapy, ED&C, and MMS in the treatment of BCCs. The results were compared for short-term (< 5 years) and long-term (> 5 years) recurrence rates. The results are noted in Figure 15–40 and indicate that MMS has the lowest recurrence rate.

More recently, Thissen, Neumann, and Schouten[26] also performed a systematic review of treatment modalities for primary BCCs (Table 15–3). They limited their study to prospective analyses performed after 1970 that tracked 50 or more lesions for 5 or more years after treatment with surgical excision, radiotherapy, cryotherapy, ED&C, MMS, immunotherapy, and PDT. Of 298 studies that they evaluated, only 18 met their criteria for inclusion in the review, for a total of 9,930 primary BCCs. They found a recurrence rate of less than 10 percent at 5 years for surgical excision, radiotherapy, cryother-

		Primary BCC			Recurrent BCC			
Modality and Study	Comments	No. of Patients	> 5-yr Follow-up	Unavailable for Follow-up	Absolute No. of Patients	Raw Rate[†]	Strict Rate[‡]	Cumulative 5-yr Rate[§]
Radiotherapy								
Silverman et al 1992	1955–1982	862	470	392	—	—	—	7.4
ED&C								
Kopf et al 1977	1958–1962	597	—	—	108	18.1	—	18.8
Kopf et al 1977	1970	91	—	—	7	7.7	—	9.6
Kopf et al 1977	1962–1973	210	—	—	8	3.8	—	5.7
Launis 1993		356	—	—	22	6.2	—	—
McDaniel 1983	Curettage only	644	328	318	28	4.3	8.5	—
Silverman et al 1991	1955–1982	2,314	1,110	1,204	—	—	—	13.2
Cryosurgery								
Nordin et al 1997	Nose > 10 mm	61	50	11	1	1.6	2.0	—
Lindgren and Larko 1997	Eyelid	214	140	64	0	0.0	0.0	0.0
Anders et al 1995	Eyelid	254	202	52	7	2.8	3.5	3.5
Fraunfelder et al 1984	Eyelid ≤ 10 mm	181[‖]	115	66	6	3.3	5.2	4.7
	Eyelid >10 mm	88[‖]	49[#]	39	10	11.4	20.4	16.5
Recurrence rate (mean)						3.0 (24/798)	4.3 (24/556)	—
Surgical excision								
Baur et al 1977	High number unavailable	443	74	369	6	1.4	8.1	8.0
Germann et al 1992		272	—	—	8	2.9	—	3.2
Silverman et al 1992	1955–1982	588	289	299	—	—	—	4.8
Recurrence rate (mean)								5.8**
MMS								
Julian and Bowers 1997	1981–1995	145	117	28	1	0.7	0.8	—
Mohs et al 1988	Ear	1,032[‖]	748	284	13	1.3	1.7	—
Mohs 1986	Eyelid	1,483[‖]	1,124	359	7	0.5	0.6	—
Recurrence rate (mean)						0.8 (21/2, 660)	1.1 (21/1, 989)	—

Table 15–3. REVIEW OF TREATMENT MODALITIES FOR BASAL CELL CARCINOMA 1970 TO 1997*

BCC = basal cell carcinoma; ED&C = electrodessication and curettage; MMS = Mohs' micrographic surgery.
*Dashes indicate that data are unavailable.
[†]Raw recurrence rate: absolute number of patients with recurrence divided by number of patients with primary BCCs at the start of study.
[‡]Strict recurrence rate: absolute number of patients with recurrence divided by number of patients with primary BCC observed for at least 5 years.
[§]Life-table cumulative 5-year recurrence rate: values are recorded from the cited study.
[‖]The number of patients with primary BCC at the start of study is not mentioned (total number of patients with BCC minus the number with treated recurrent BCC observed for > 5 years).
**Small group (number < 50).
[#]Calculated.
Adapted from Thissen MR, Neumann MH, Schouten LJ. A systematic review of treatment modalities for primary basal cell carcinomas. Arch Dermatol 1999;135:1177–83.

apy, ED&C, and MMS (see Table 15–3). They concluded that the results for immunotherapy and PDT are less impressive and that these techniques should be considered investigative. It should be noted that an analysis of the studies reviewed by Thissen and colleagues[26] revealed that greater than 94 percent of the cases Thissen and colleagues used to compare recurrence rates for MMS were based on tumors of the eyelids and ears treated with MMS, as opposed to the articles reviewing surgical excisions that did not involve these areas. This calls Thissen and colleagues' conclusions comparing MMS to surgical excision into question since lesions in the eye and ear areas are well known to have higher rates of recurrence.

Treatment of Primary (Untreated) Squamous Cell Carcinoma

Rowe, Carroll, and Day[14] reviewed all studies in the literature between 1940 and 1992 looking at the prognostic factors for local recurrence, metas-

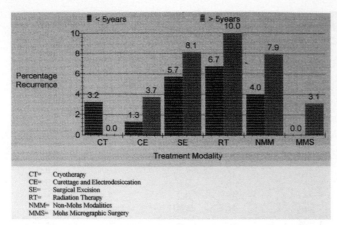

Figure 15–41. Short- and long-term recurrence of primary SCC. (Adapted from Rowe DE, Carroll RJ, Day CL. Prognostic factors for local recurrence, metastasis, and survival rates in squamous cell carcinoma of the skin, ear, and lip. J Am Acad Dermatol 1992;26: 976–90.)

tasis, and survival rates for SCC of the skin, ear, and lip. Hundreds of articles, involving well over 7,447 cases of SCCs, were systematically reviewed for the effectiveness of surgical excision, radiotherapy, cryotherapy, ED&C, and MMS in the treatment of primary SCCs.[14] The results were compared for short-term (< 5 years) and long-term (> 5 years) recurrence rates (Figure 15–41). In addition, the results were compared for the influence of tumor variables on local recurrence and metastasis (Figure 15–42). A comparison of MMS versus non-MMS modalities for some of these variables was also performed (Figure 15–43). The results show that MMS seems to provide the lowest short- and long-term recurrence rates for treating primary SCC.

Treatment of Recurrent (Previously Treated) Basal Cell Carcinoma

Rowe, Carroll, and Day reviewed all studies conducted from 1945 to 1989 looking at short-term versus long-term recurrence rates for the treatment of recurrent BCCs. Fifty articles, involving well over 4,387 cases of recurrent BCCs, were systematically reviewed for the effectiveness of surgical excision, radiotherapy, cryotherapy, ED&C, and MMS in the treatment of BCC.[27] After the exclusion of 12 studies, the results of 38 independent observations were compared for short-term (< 5 years) and long-term (> 5 years) recurrence rates (Figure 15–44). Rowe and colleagues concluded that (a) MMS is the treatment of choice for recurrent BCC, (b) radiation therapy offers a better cure than other non-MMS treatment modalities when the lesion is small, and (c) ED&C should not be used to treat recurrent BCCs.

Treatment of Recurrent (Previously Treated) Squamous Cell Carcinoma

An even smaller number of studies can be found for a comparative analysis of treatment modalities for SCC than for BCC. Another study by Rowe, Carroll, and Day reviewed all studies in the literature between 1940 and 1992 looking at the prognostic factors for local recurrence, metastasis, and survival rates in squamous cell carcinoma of the skin, ear, and lip. Published studies involving well over 736 cases of recurrent SCCs were systematically reviewed for the effectiveness of surgical excision,

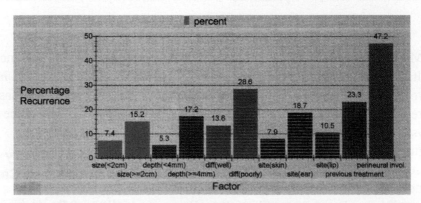

Figure 15–42. Influence of tumor variables on SCC recurrence. (Adapted from Rowe DE, Carroll RJ, Day CL. Prognostic factors for local recurrence, metastasis, and survival rates in squamous cell carcinoma of the skin, ear, and lip. J Am Acad Dermatol 1992;26:976–90.)

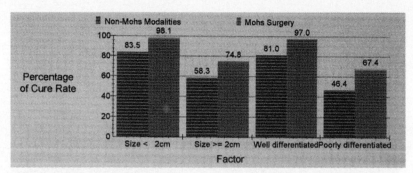

Figure 15–43. Cure rates by Mohs' versus non-Mohs' surgery according to SCC variables. (Adapted from Rowe DE, Carroll RJ, Day CL. Prognostic factors for local recurrence, metastasis, and survival rates in squamous cell carcinoma of the skin, ear, and lip. J Am Acad Dermatol 1992;26:976–90.)

radiotherapy, cryotherapy, ED&C, and MMS in the treatment of SCCs.[14] The results were compared for short-term (< 5 years) and long-term (> 5 years) recurrence rates. The results (Figure 15–45) again point to the low recurrence rate with MMS.

If recurrence rate were the only criterion to be used in deciding upon the best treatment for primary and recurrent BCCs and SCCs, it seems clear that Mohs' surgery would be the superior modality when one looks at the review of all studies to date. In the case of primary (untreated) BCCs, Thissen and colleagues cast doubt on whether MMS is any more effective than the other treatment modalities, but as noted above, their use of MMS studies revolving around the treatment of lesions at a higher risk of recurrence raises questions about their conclusions. Furthermore, treatment should not be based on

recurrent rates alone but also on the effect on metastasis and mortality, which MMS seems to address at least as well as (if not measurably better than) the other treatment modalities. The decreased morbidity due to the tissue-sparing advantage of MMS is another important feature of this treatment. Nevertheless, the choice of treatment for BCC and SCC as well as other NMSCs should be individualized for each patient, taking into account recurrence, risk of metastasis, tumor location, size, histologic characteristics, cosmesis, tissue sparing, and cost. Note that in the studies by Rowe and colleagues looking at follow-up of BCC and SCC, the majority of recurrences are seen within 5 years but that not all recurrences are seen until more than 10 years.[14,26,27] Thus, patients treated for NMSC would be well served by a follow-up of more than 5 years (Figure 15–46).

Treatment of Dermatofibrosarcoma Protuberans

The main goal in the treatment of DFSP is to excise sufficient tissue to prevent local recurrence although occasional metastasis has been reported with this tumor.[28] Recurrence rates after surgical excision have been reported in the range of 11 to 73 percent.[29] In one study of 17 cases by Pack and Tabah, a 24 percent recurrence rate was reported.[30] In a study of 98 cases, Taylor and Helwig reported a 49 percent recurrence rate, and in a study of 119 cases by Hajdu, a 53 percent recurrence rate was noted.[31,32] These and other studies have led to the recommendation that DFSP be excised with wide (> 3 cm) margins. Yet even these aggressive approaches have

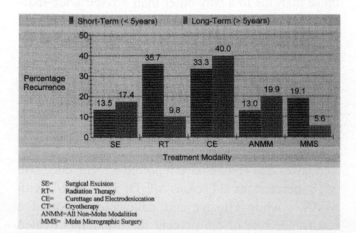

Figure 15–44. Recurrence of previously treated basal cell carcinoma. (Adapted from Rowe DE, Carroll RJ, Day CL. Mohs' surgery is the treatment of choice for recurrent (previously treated) basal cell carcinoma. J Dermatol Surg Oncol 1989;15:424–31.)

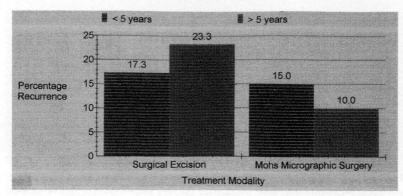

Figure 15–45. Recurrence of previously treated SCC (short-term versus long-term). (Adapted from Rowe DE, Carroll RJ, Day CL. Prognostic factors for local recurrence, metastasis, and survival rates in squamous cell carcinoma of the skin, ear, and lip. J Am Acad Dermatol 1992;26:976–90.)

had inconsistent results. In one study of 7 patients by Bendix-Hansen and colleagues, no recurrences were reported during a follow-up period of 4 to 13 years.[33] Yet in a study of 10 cases by Roses and colleagues, a 20 percent recurrence rate was reported,[34] and in another (of 27 cases, by McPeak and colleagues), a recurrence rate of 11 percent was reported in a follow-up period of 3 to 15 years.[35] This study is consistent with a study performed by Gloster, Harris, and Roenigk at the Mayo Clinic in 1996, who performed wide excisions on 39 patients and reported a recurrence rate of 10 percent. Their review of the world literature of 15 articles encompassing 489 patients revealed an average recurrence rate of 18 percent.[36]

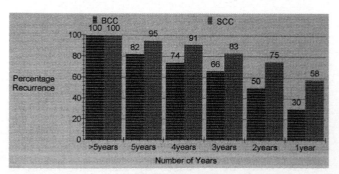

Figure 15–46. Time to appearance of recurrences for BCC versus SCC. (Adapted from Rowe DE, Carroll RJ, Day CL. Prognostic factors for local recurrence, metastasis, and survival rates in squamous cell carcinoma of the skin, ear, and lip. J Am Acad Dermatol 1992;26:976–90. Rowe DE, Carroll RJ, Day CL. Long-term recurrence rates in previously untreated (primary) basal cell carcinoma: implications for patient follow-up. J Dermatol Surg Oncol 1989;15:315–28. Rowe DE, Carroll RJ, Day CL. Mohs' surgery is the treatment of choice for recurrent (previously treated) basal cell carcinoma. J Dermatol Surg Oncol 1989;15:424–31.)

In 1995, Parker and Zitelli, at the University of Pittsburgh, performed a study on 20 patients who were undergoing treatment with Mohs' surgery for DFSP from 1985 to 1993.[29] They marked the clinically involved margin and then removed additional margins of 0.4 to 1.0 cm of normal-appearing tissue as indicated by microscopic evaluations of the removed tissue for residual tumor. They found that it took at least a 2.5-cm margin to excise all of the DFSPs but that margins were variable and that DFSPs could be removed in their entirety, with smaller margins for some tumors. Dawes and Hanke complicated the matter even further by reporting that 2 of 26 patients (7.6%) required surgical margins of greater than 3 cm for complete removal of DFSPs (Figure 15–47).[37] Thus, DFSPs usually require extensive surgical margins, but there is a need to establish these margins in a way other than a fixed wide-margin approach since many DFSPs can be removed with smaller margins and because large margins offer no guarantee that the tumor will be removed.

There has been an increasing use of MMS for the treatment of DFSP since this would eliminate the use of arbitrary fixed wide margins and allow the tracing out of the numerous and diffuse extensions seen with DFSP (Figure 15–48).

Dawes and Hanke have reported a recurrence rate of 8 percent in 24 cases of DFSP treated with MMS,[37] while Gloster and colleagues reported a recurrence rate of 6.6 percent in 15 patients treated with MMS.[36] On the other hand, Huether and colleagues reported a recurrence rate of 3.0 percent in 38 patients,[38] and Haycox and colleagues reported a

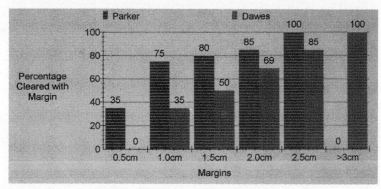

Figure 15–47. Surgical margins and tumor clearance for DFSP. (Adapted from Parker TL, Zitelli JA. Surgical margins for excision of dermatofibrosarcoma protuberans. J Am Acad Dermatol 1995;32:233–6. Dawes KW, Hanke WC. Dermatofibrosarcoma protuberans treated with Mohs micrographic surgery/cure rates and surgical margins. Dermatol Surg 1996;22:530–4.)

recurrence rate of 2.4 percent for 169 cases of DFSP treated with MMS.[39] The latter study compares favorably with a world literature review of 11 articles by Gloster and colleagues that arrived at a combined recurrence rate of 1.6 percent.[36] It appears that when the use of MMS versus the use of wide excision for treating DFSP are compared, MMS seems to offer the advantages of lower recurrence rates as well as frozen-section control so that smaller tumors can be removed with smaller margins yet avoids the possibility that tumors requiring margins larger than 3 cm will be undertreated. The tissue-sparing effect of MMS for DFSP is supported by the study of Dawes and Hanke, who further compared the amount of tissue that would be removed with a fixed 3-cm margin with that actually removed with MMS for 24 cases and found that a mean of 43 cm of normal tissue would have been spared if all the lesions they studied had been treated with the MMS technique (Figure 15–49).[37] The tissue-sparing effect of MMS in a recent case of DFSP that was treated by the authors is illustrated in Figures 15–50 and 15–51.

Yet the promise of better results with MMS has to be tempered with the fact that although the majority of DFSPs are reported to recur within 3 years,[37–39] there are reports of DFSP recurring as late as 19 to 23 years.[28,29,37] In fact, Dawes and Hanke reported that their two recurrences occurred 6 and 12 years after MMS. Thus, one must be careful interpreting the studies since most studies have not followed patients in the long term. Nevertheless, the data are even more sketchy for excisions, and the

recurrence rate for excisions is very likely to be higher than that for MMS on long-term follow-up.

Treatment of Atypical Fibroxanthoma

Data regarding the surgical outcomes in the treatment of atypical fibroxanthoma (AFX) and malignant fibrous histiocytoma (MFH) are even more limited than those available on the treatment of DFSP. Like DFSP, AFX is uncommon, but it can invade locally, recurs after excision 2 to 20 percent of the time, and metastasizes only rarely and usually after a recurrence.[40] Traditionally, treatment for these lesions is by conservative surgical removal, and if margin control is not achieved during surgery, a 1-cm margin with extension into the subcutaneous

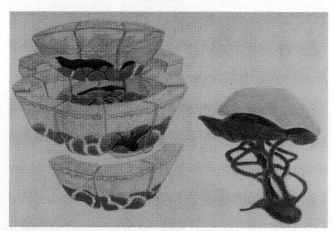

Figure 15–48. Diagrammatic representation of extensions of a DFSP. (Reprinted with permission from Haycox CL, Odland PB, Olbricht SM, et al. Dermatofibrosarcoma protuberans (DFSP) growth characteristics based on tumor modeling and a review of cases treated with Mohs micrographic surgery. Ann Plast Surg 1997;38:246–51.)

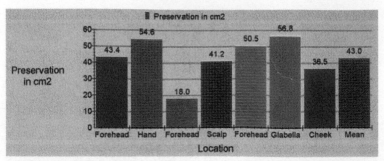

Figure 15–49.   Tissue preservation with MMS versus 3-cm margins for seven DFSP lesions. (Adapted from Dawes KW, Hanke WC. Dermatofibrosarcoma protuberans treated with Mohs' micrographic surgery/cure rates and surgical margins. Dermatol Surg 1996;22:530–4.)

tissue is recommended.[41] Nevertheless, "dimensions that constitute adequate margins have not been precisely defined."[40] Recently, AFX has been regarded as a superficial variant of MFH, and because of its low-grade (but real) malignant potential, the goal is complete resection.[42]

To compare wide excision and MMS in the treatment of AFX, Davis and colleagues retrospectively evaluated 44 cases. Of this group, 19 lesions were treated with MMS, without evidence of recurrence during a mean follow-up period of 29.6 months. The remainder of the patients were treated with wide local excision, with margins ranging from 0.3 to 2.6 cm (mean of 0.7 cm), and showed a recurrence

rate of 12 percent after a follow-up period of 73.6 months.[40] Mohs' micrographic surgery was reported to be more effective at treating these lesions, despite the larger sizes treated by this modality (average of 1.5 cm; range, 0.5 to 3.9 cm) in comparison to those treated with wide local excision (average of 1.1 cm; range, 0.4 to 2.0 cm). It is important to note, however, that follow-up periods were shorter and therefore biased in favor of MMS. Nevertheless, MMS was recommended as the treatment of choice for these lesions because of its ability to ensure local tumor clearance and conserve "normal tissue in functionally and cosmetically important areas without additional surgical risk to the patient."[40] Huether

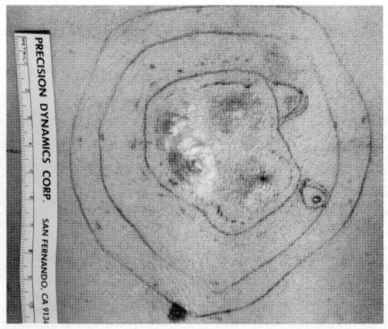

Figure 15–50.   DFSP, with depiction of possible surgical margins for excision using standard surgery.

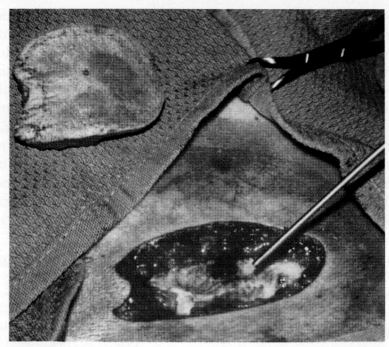

Figure 15–51. DFSP after excision with Mohs' surgery, showing the difference between actual margins with Mohs' surgery (defect) versus expected margin with standard excision (broken line).

and colleagues have also confirmed this recommendation.[38] In their review of the literature, they identified several reports outlining the successful treatment of these lesions with MMS although none included more than six patients. Their series, compiled from 29 patients over 18 years, reported a local recurrence rate of 6.9 percent after treatment with MMS, over a mean follow-up of 3.3 years.[38] No comparisons to other treatment modalities were made in this report although the rate of recurrence after MMS compares favorably to the general recurrence rate of upwards of 10 percent; in the case of wide excision, most recurrences were within a year after treatment.[41]

Treatment of Malignant Fibrous Histiocytoma

Unlike DFSP and AFX, MFH can be highly aggressive, and about 10 percent of cases may present after a metastasis.[43] Several histologic types of MFH have been described, and although some consider AFX to be a superficial version of MFH,[42] the latter tumor can also invade deeply or arise in muscle or other deeper subcutaneous tissue. These deeper tumors have a worse prognosis, and treatment involves aggressive

and wide deep excision.[43] Unfortunately, despite 3- to 5-cm margins around these lesions, MFH has been reported to recur in 30 to 40 percent of cases.[43,44]

Unlike other spindle cell tumors that have been treated successfully with Mohs' chemosurgery, treatment of MFH by this modality has not yielded

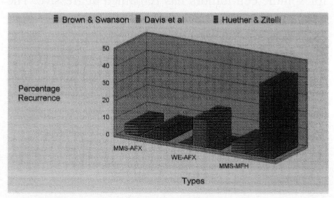

Figure 15–52. Treatment for AFX and MFH. (AFX = atypical fibroxanthoma; MFH = malignant fibrous histiocytoma; MMS = Mohs' micrographic surgery; WE = wide excision.)(Adapted from Brown MD, Swanson NA. Treatment of malignant fibrous histiocytoma and atypical fibrous xanthomas with micrographic surgery. J Dermatol Surg Oncol 1989;15:1287–92. Davis JL, Randle HW, Zalla MJ, et al. A comparison of Mohs micrographic surgery and wide excision for the treatment of atypical fibroxanthoma. Dermatol Surg 1997;23:105–10. Huether MJ, Zitelli JA, Brodland DG. Mohs micrographic surgery for the treatment of spindle cell tumors of the skin (unpublished data).

consistent results. Brown and Swanson reported a 6 percent recurrence rate in the treatment of both MFH and AFX, without detailing the histology of these recurrent tumors.[44] Nonetheless, even if all recurrences in this series were due to MFH, a 6 percent recurrence rate compares favorably to rates currently reported after wide excision.[44] Although recurrence rates with excision vary in the literature, some have reported a 44 percent recurrence rate after wide excision,[38] a 71 percent rate after "complete" excision, and up to 50 to 90 percent recurrence if positive resection margins are reported after surgical removal of the tumor.[45]

In a retrospective analysis of 7 cases treated by Mohs' chemosurgery, Huether and colleagues reported 3 recurrences and a recurrence rate of 43 percent. However, of these tumors, 2 were recurrent at the time of referral for Mohs' surgery, and the average follow-up period in this study was 3.8 years.[38] It is noteworthy that most MFHs recur within the first 2 years following diagnosis.[43] Thus, recurrence rates after treatment with Mohs' surgery vary widely, and specific indications for the treatment of these lesions by either Mohs' surgery or wide excision are more difficult to delineate than in the case of other spindle cell tumors (see Figure 15–52).

Due to the relatively low incidence of these spindle cell tumors and the general lack of data from which to make more conclusive recommendations, treatment for spindle cell tumors has remained aggressive. The treating clinician is encouraged to individualize treatment decisions according to the clinical characteristics of the tumor, taking into account the potential of the tumor for deep invasion and the desire to salvage as much normal skin as possible, especially in anatomically high-risk locations. Mohs' surgery should be considered under these circumstances.

CONCLUSION

At present, the treatment of NMSC should be aimed at complete removal of the lesion. Although treatment recommendations vary according to tumor histology, size, and other features, prospective data are still necessary. Most reports regarding surgical margins cannot be readily pooled or compared, due to differences in study designs, population studied, status of the tumors, and other confounders. Nevertheless, the stratification of lesions according to risk factors and studies performed extending longer than 5 years have elucidated the need to individualize therapy according to tumor characteristics, as outlined in this chapter. As future prospective studies are performed and variables are standardized, the treatment of these lesions will follow more specific recommendations, and lower recurrence rates can be anticipated. At this time, the MMS technique is becoming established as the best method of margin control and may lead to the lowest long-term recurrence rate after tumor removal.

REFERENCES

1. Kuflik EG, Gage AA. Cryosurgical treatment for skin cancer. New York: Igaku-Shoin; 1990. p. 35–51.
2. Kuflik EG. Cryosurgery updated. J Am Acad Dermatol 1994;31:925–44.
3. Graham GF. Cryosurgery. In: Robinson JK, Arndt KA, LeBoit PE, Wintroub BU, editors. Atlas of cutaneous surgery. Philadelphia: W.B. Saunders; 1996.
4. Greenbaum SS, Glogau RG. CO_2 laser treatment of erythroplasia of queyrat. J Dermatol Surg Oncol 1979;5:803–6.
5. Adams EL, Price NM. Treatment of basal cell carcinomas with a carbon-dioxide laser. J Dermatol Surg Oncol 1979;5:803–6.
6. Henderson BW, Doherty TJ. How does photodynamic therapy work? Photochem Photobiol 1992;55:145–57.
7. Keller GS, Razam NJ, Doiron DR. Photodynamic therapy for nonmelanoma skin cancer. Facial Plast Surg 1989;6:180–4.
8. Wilson BD, Mang TS, Stoll H, et al. Photodynamic therapy for the treatment of basal cell carcinoma. Arch Dermatol 1992;128:1597–601.
9. Kashani-Sabet M. Toward the biologic treatment of nonmelanoma skin cancer. J Am Acad Dermatol 1999;41:1018–9.
10. Beutner KR, Spruance SL, Hougham AJ, et al. Treatment of genital warts with an immune-response modifier (imiquimod). J Am Acad Dermatol 1998;38:230–9.
11. Lipper GM, Arndt KA, Dover JS. Recent therapeutic advances in dermatology. JAMA 2000;238:175–7.
12. Beutner KR, Geisse JK, Helman D, et al. Therapeutic response of basal cell carcinoma to the immune response modifier imiquimod 5% cream. J Am Acad Dermatol 1999;41:1002–7.
13. Salasche SJ, Amonette RA. Morpheaform basal-cell epitheliomas. A study of subclinical extensions in a

series of 51 cases. J Dermatol Surg Oncol 1981; 7:387–93.

14. Rowe DE, Carroll RJ, Day CL. Prognostic factors for local recurrence, metastasis, and survival rates in squamous cell carcinoma of the skin, ear and lip. J Am Acad Dermatol 1992;26:976–90.

15. Russell BE, Carrington PR, Smoller BR. Basal cell carcinoma: a comparison of shave biopsy techniques in subtype diagnosis. J Am Acad Dermatol 1999;41:69–71.

16. Torres A, Seeburger J, Robinson D, Glogau R. The reliability of a second biopsy for determining residual tumor. J Am Acad Dermatol 1992;27:70–3.

17. Holmkvist KA, Rogers GS, Dahl PR. Incidence of residual basal cell carcinoma in patients who appear tumor free after biopsy. J Am Acad Dermatol 1999; 41:600–5.

18. Blomqvist G, Eriksson E, Lauritzen C. Surgical results in 477 basal cell carcinomas. Scand J Plast Reconstr Surg 1982;16:283–5.

19. Cataldo PA, Stoddard PB, Reed WF. Use of frozen section analysis in the treatment of basal cell carcinoma. Am J Surg 1990;159:561–3.

20. Pascal RR, Hobby LW, Lattes R, Crikelair GF. Prognosis of "incompletely excised" versus "completely excised" basal cell carcinoma. Plast Reconstr Surg 1968;41:328–32.

21. Shanoff LB, Spira M, Hardy B. Basal cell carcinoma: a statistical approach to rational management. Plast Reconstr Surg 1967;39:619–24.

22. Abide JM, Nahai F, Bennet RG. The meaning of surgical margins. Plast Reconstr Surg 1984;73:492–7.

23. Wolf DJ, Zitelli JA. Surgical margins for basal cell carcinoma. Arch Dermatol 1987;123:340–4.

24. Brodland DG, Zitelli JA. Surgical margins for excision of primary cutaneous squamous cell carcinoma. J Am Acad Dermatol 1992;27:241–8.

25. Rowe DE, Carroll RJ, Day CL. Long-term recurrence rates in previously untreated (primary) basal cell carcinoma: implications for patient follow-up. J Dermatol Surg Oncol 1989;15:315–28.

26. Thissen MR, Neumann MH, Schouten LJ. A systematic review of treatment modalities for primary basal cell carcinomas. Arch Dermatol 1999;135: 1177–83.

27. Rowe DE, Carroll RJ, Day CL. Mohs surgery is the treatment of choice for recurrent (previously treated) basal cell carcinoma. J Dermatol Surg Oncol 1989; 15:424–31.

28. Gloster HM. Dermatofibrosarcoma protuberans. J Am Acad Dermatol 1996;35:355–74.

29. Parker TL, Zitelli JA. Surgical margins for excision of dermatofibrosarcoma protuberans. J Am Acad Dermatol 1995;32:233–6.

30. Pack GT, Tabah EJ. DFSP: a report of 39 cases. Arch Surg 1951;62:391–411.

31. Taylor HB, Helwig EB. Dermatofibrosarcoma protuberans: a study of 115 cases. Cancer 1962;15:717–25.

32. Hadju SI. Pathology of soft tissue tumors. Philadelphia: Lea & Febiger; 1979.

33. Bendix-Hansen K, Myhre-Jensen O, Kaae S. Dermatofibrosarcoma protuberans. A clinicopathological study of nineteen cases and review of world literature. Scand J Plast Reconstr Surg 1983;17:247–52.

34. Roses DF, Valensi Q, LaTrenta G, Harris MN. Surgical treatment of dermatofibrosarcoma protuberans. Surg Gynecol Obstet 1986;162:449–52.

35. McPeak CJ, Cruz T, Nicastri AD. Dermatofibrosarcoma protuberans: an analysis of 86 cases—five with metastasis. Ann Surg 1967;166:803–16.

36. Gloster HM, Harris KR, Roenigk RK. A comparison between Mohs micrographic surgery and wide surgical excision for the treatment of dermatofibrosarcoma protuberans. J Am Acad Dermatol 1996;35:82–7.

37. Dawes KW, Hanke CW. Dermatofibrosarcoma protuberans treated with Mohs micrographic surgery: cure rates and surgical margins. Dermatol Surg 1996;22:530–4.

38. Huether MJ, Zitelli JA, Brodland DG. Mohs micrographic surgery for the treatment of spindle cell tumors of the skin [unpublished].

39. Haycox CL, Odland PB, Olbricht SM, et al. Dermatofibrosarcoma protuberans (DFSP) growth characteristics based on tumor modeling and a review of cases treated with Mohs micrographic surgery. Ann Plast Surg 1997;38:246–51.

40. Davis JL, Randle HW, Zalla MJ, et al. A comparison of Mohs micrographic surgery and wide exision for the treatment of atypical fibroxanthoma. Dermatol Surg 1997;23:105–10.

41. Hess KA, Hanke ZW, Estes NC, Shideler SJ. Chemosurgical reports: myxoid dermatofibrosarcoma protuberans. J Dermatol Surg Oncol 1985;11:268–71.

42. Mikhail GR. Mohs micrographic surgery. Philadelphia: W.B. Saunders Co.; 1991.

43. Maloney ME, Torres A, Hoffman TJ, Helm KF. Surgical dermatopathology. Malden: Blackwell Science; 1999.

44. Brown MD, Swanson NA. Treatment of malignant fibrous histiocytoma and atypical fibrous xanthomas with micrographic surgery. J Dermatol Surg Oncol 1989;15:1287–92.

45. Weiss SW, Enzinger FM. Malignant fibrous histiocytoma. An analysis of 200 cases. Cancer 1978;41: 2250–66.

16

Radiation Therapy

C. C. WANG, MD, FACR

The skin has three layers—an outermost epidermis, a middle dermis, and an inner subcutis—and is associated with a variety of structures and cell types, all of which can give rise to malignant tumors. This chapter discusses radiation therapy techniques useful in treating the variety of malignancies arising in the skin.

Malignant tumors arising from the skin include basal cell carcinoma (BCC), squamous cell carcinoma (SCC), lymphoma, malignant melanoma, malignant fibrohistiocytoma, angiosarcoma, and skin appendage carcinoma. The adnexal tumors consist of sebaceous gland carcinoma and meibomian, eccrine, and apocrine gland carcinomas. The common BCCs (so-called rodent ulcers) appear typically as pearly firm elevations with occasional central ulceration surrounded by minute capillaries and are commonly found on the skin of the eyelids, head, and neck (eg, the eyelid, nose, and nasolabial sulcus). Squamous cell carcinoma is less common and manifests various forms, including superficial multicentric, nodular or noduloulcerative, pigmented, morphealike or sclerosing, and the adenoid cystic variety. It is unreliable to differentiate between BCC and SCC on clinical grounds; it is therefore important that a tissue biopsy specimen be obtained before any form of treatment is given.

Other uncommon tumors of the skin include mycosis fungoides, lymphomas, and leukemic infiltrates. These tumors involve multiple sites as a generalized process, and their local problems may require local radiation therapy.

Since most of the skin cancers involving the trunk and the unexposed portions of the body are dealt with by surgery, this chapter primarily reviews radiation therapy for BCC and SCC of the skin arising in the head and neck region and for some other cancers of radiotherapeutic interest.

SELECTION OF THERAPY AND INDICATIONS

There are many ways to treat skin cancers. These include surgical excision, curettage, radiation therapy,[1–3] cryosurgery,[4] Mohs' micrographic surgery,[5] and topical 5-fluorouracil (5-FU) cream.[6] Although Mohs' procedure can be used for treatment of BCC of the skin, it is better reserved for the management of advanced lesions and/or recurrent tumors after curative procedures. For early and moderately advanced lesions, surgery and irradiation remain the mainstays of curative procedures.

Surgery is the treatment of choice for the following skin cancers:

1. Small lesions that can be treated by excision expediently, without sequential dysfunction or esthetic impairment
2. Small lesions of the neck and scalp
3. Lesions of the dorsum of the hand or arising from scars, thermal burns, or chronic radiation dermatitis
4. Lesions arising in atrophic and aged skin, lupus vulgaris, and infected tumors in the pinna of the ear with chondritis
5. Large destructive lesions where extensive loss of soft tissue is evident and where plastic repair is necessary if cure is by radiation therapy
6. Extensive tumor infiltrating the underlying bone
7. Skin appendage carcinomas and invasive melanomas

Radiation therapy is the treatment of choice for the following skin cancers:

1. Carcinomas arising in the midline of the face, eyelids, nose and lip, and the so-called facial triangle (Figure 16–1)
2. Large deeply infiltrative lesions of the skin of the face (without bone involvement)
3. Basal cell carcinoma and SCC arising in the skin of the auricle
4. Lesions involving the commissure of the mouth
5. Lesions arising in the pre- and postauricular areas and the nasolabial sulcus

Squamous cell carcinomas of the skin may involve the regional lymph nodes. The incidence of metastases, however, is low (about 5 to 10%);[7] elective nodal treatment either by neck dissection or by radiation therapy for clinically uninvolved neck nodes is not indicated. For the clinically positive

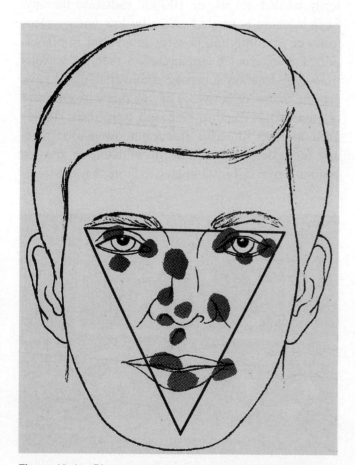

Figure 16–1. Diagram showing the so-called facial triangle and illustrating the various sites of cancer of the skin most suitable for radiation therapy.

nodal metastasis, radical nodal dissection (with or without adjuvant radiation therapy) is warranted.

EVALUATION OF SKIN CANCERS

The size, thickness, and margins of the lesion must be carefully assessed before a radiotherapeutic procedure is considered. The margins are best evaluated with bright light and the aid of magnifying glasses. The lesion should be palpated gently. The surrounding hair follicles, skin texture, and color should be carefully compared with the normal skin and with the lesion. The use of a Wood's lamp (ultraviolet light) may aid differentiation between the tumor and the adjacent normal skin. Unfortunately, carcinoma and keratosis cannot be differentiated with the aid of a Wood's lamp alone.

When the lesion is situated on the skin of the cheek and lip, bidigital palpation by gloved fingers may help determine the depth of infiltration of the lesion. When the lesion is fixed to the adjacent bone, appropriate radiographic studies, including computed tomography (CT) scans, should be performed to evaluate the possibility of bone involvement.

RADIOTHERAPEUTIC MODALITIES AND ACCESSORIES

Most of the superficial cancers of the skin currently are treated by low-energy electrons, commonly 6- to 9-MeV electrons. Low-megavoltage photons (4 to 6 MeV) are used for treatment of large and thick invasive tumors and regional lymph node metastases. Basal cell carcinoma of the eyelid is best treated by low-energy x-rays such as those used by the Phillips 50-kV contact unit (Figure 16–2).

In addition to external beam therapy, brachytherapy can be used. The afterloading interstitial implant procedure is preferred, using angiocath applicators and iridium-192 sources. For the past 4 years, a high-dose-rate (HDR) iridium-192 source has been available at the Massachusetts General Hospital (MGH), and large fractions (ie, 3 to 4 Gy bid) are given as a boost, fractionated for 2 to 3 days. Important, the optimal treatment of skin cancers requires the availability of various treatment modalities to achieve the best local control and cosmesis.

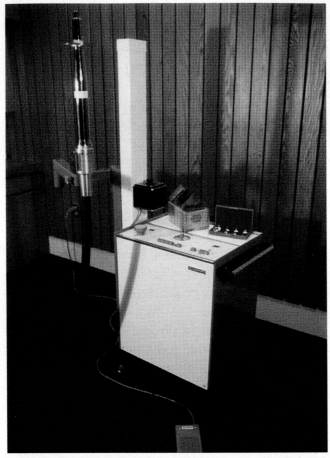

Figure 16–2. The Phillips 50-kV contact machine, used for the treatment of small carcinomas of the eyelid.

As a general rule, the lesions on a curved surface are preferably treated by electrons and those on a flat surface by photons (x-rays) alone or combined with brachytherapy or with electrons.

For radiation therapy of skin cancers, lead shields are used for proper exposure of the lesion and for protection of the adjacent normal tissues. Individually made lead cutouts (especially for the eye) and nose and gum shields are used for the treatment of appropriate tumors (Figures 16–3 and 16–4). For electron beam therapy, 6- to 9-MeV beams are frequently used. The low-energy electrons have skin-sparing characteristics, and a thin layer of bolus must be added on the surface of the tumor to achieve maximum density (Dmax) on the skin, as shown in Figure 16–5. Individual cerrobends cut out with the appropriate aperture are made to shape the lesion and are placed under the window of the linear accelerator. These simple gadgets are extremely important for the treatment of skin cancers.

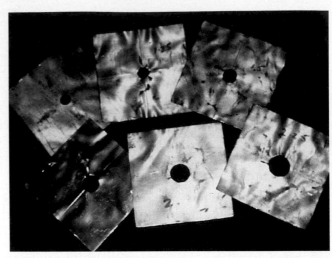

Figure 16–3. Special lead sheets and cutouts tailor-fit to the shape and size of lesions (for use with the 50-kV contact machine).

RADIATION THERAPY DOSAGES AND FRACTION SIZE

Any lesion thicker than 1.0 cm cannot be satisfactorily treated by 50- or 100-kV radiation therapy. Such a lesion is treated either by low-energy electrons or in combination with interstitial implantation. For external beam radiation therapy, various time-dose-fraction schemes[8] are available and have proven to be effective. The cosmetic results are related to the fraction size and total dose. Tables 16–1 to 16–3 illustrate fractionated radiation therapy for lesions 1.5 to 2.0 cm in diameter and for lesions 5 to 6 cm in diameter.[1,9] Note that the treat-

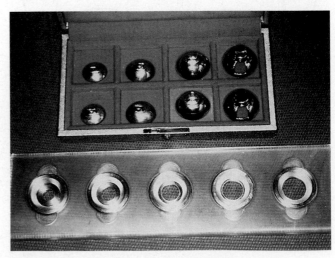

Figure 16–4. Top tray holds lead eye shields for radiation therapy of the eyelid. Bottom tray holds lead "nipple" cutouts suitable for treatment of cancer of the inner canthus of the eye.

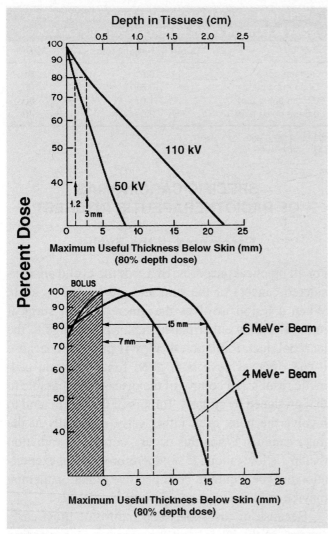

Figure 16–5. Comparison of percent-depth-dose data of radiations versus maximal therapeutic thickness of the lesions suitable for radiation therapy.

ment schemes are extremely variable, depending on aspects such as the availability of treatment machine time, the patient population (ie, young or old, male or female), and the likelihood of the patient's long-term survival. The program of radiation therapy for skin cancer that has been used at the MGH for the past 35 years and that has proven to be highly effective, giving acceptable cosmetic results, is as follows:

1. For small lesions 0.5 cm to 1.0 cm in diameter, a single treatment of 24 Gy is curative. It is rarely used, but it may be given to debilitated and aged patients who have difficulties attending daily radiation therapy sessions on an outpatient basis.

Table 16–1. FRACTIONATION RADIATION THERAPY FOR SKIN CANCER*

Study Author (Center)	Dose Fractionation†	Reference
Fitzpatrick (PMH)	35 Gy/5 Gy/F/ 5 days	9
Moss (OU)	45 Gy/ 3–4 Gy/F/ 3–4 weeks	1
Wang (MGH)	45 Gy/9 Gy/F/ 1 week, or	—
	45 Gy /5 Gy/F/ 2 weeks, or	—
	52 Gy/4 Gy/F/ 2.5 weeks	—

*1.5 to 2.0 cm in diameter.
†No differences in dosage for squamous cell and basal cell carcinomas.
F = fraction; MGH = Massachusetts General Hospital; OU = Oregon University; PMH = Princess Margaret Hospital.

2. For lesions 1.5 to 2.5 cm in size, 45 Gy in 5 fractions or 45 Gy in 9 fractions is commonly used, depending on the patient's skin and age and on the availability of daily sessions.

3. For a somewhat larger lesion, or highly desirable cosmesis, a prolonged course of treatment is prescribed (eg, 52 Gy divided into 13 daily fractions).

4. Large tumors are treated with 60 Gy in 25 fractions.

5. For large lesions suitable for combined external beam radiation and interstitial implants, a total dose between 65 and 70 Gy is generally planned (eg, 30 Gy in 10 daily fractions by x-rays or electrons plus 30 to 35 Gy by implant).

6. For permanent local control of most small- to medium-sized carcinomas of the skin, experience has shown that the isobioeffect of a time-dose-fraction (TDF) relationship value of 120 to 130 (as shown in Figure 16–6) is required. For larger and thicker lesions, a higher dose is required.

Table 16–2. FRACTIONATION RADIATION THERAPY FOR SKIN CANCER*

Center	Dose Fractionation (TDF†)
PMH	7 Gy × 5 (113)
U Oregon	3 Gy × 15 (92)
U Florida	3 Gy × 15 (92) or 4 Gy × 10 (96)
U Arizona	7 Gy × 5 (113) or 5 Gy × 8 (108)
U Alabama	9 Gy × 5 (167)
Christie	10 Gy × 3 (123) or 20 Gy × 1
MGH	9 Gy × 5 (167) or 5 Gy × 9 (123), or
	4 Gy × 13 (125), or
	20–23 Gy × 1 (rarely used)

MGH = Massachusetts General Hospital; PMH = Princess Margaret Hospital.
*1.5 to 2.0 cm in diameter.
†TDF = time-dose-fraction formulation (biologic equivalent isoeffects). These numbers are used to compare various treatment schemes.

Table 16–3. FRACTIONATION RADIATION THERAPY FOR SKIN CANCER*	
Center	Dose Fractionation
PMH	3 Gy × 20 or 4 Gy × 10
	3 Gy × 15 plus implant
U Oregon	3 Gy × 20
U Florida	1.8 Gy × 35
U Arizona	3 Gy × 20
U Alabama	3 Gy × 10 plus implant 35 Gy
Christie	35 Gy plus implant
	Implant to 60 Gy alone
MGH	4 Gy × 13 or 3 Gy × 20
	3 Gy × 10 plus implant

*5.0 to 6.0 cm in diameter.
MGH = Massachusettts General Hospital; PMH = Princess Margaret Hospital.

Tables 16–4 and 16–5 present data related to 6- and 9-MeV electron dose distribution at depth for the daily clinical management of skin carcinoma.

RADIOTHERAPEUTIC RESULTS

Carcinoma of the skin is highly curable by radiation therapy, with local control rates of 90 percent or higher. When BCC involves bone, the local control rate is poor; however, the patient may live with the disease for many years, and a relentless surgical approach could therefore be rewarding. Metastatic SCC of the skin to the regional nodes has a poor prognosis, with a 3-year no-evidence-of-disease (NED) rate of approximately 30 percent.

Table 16–6 shows the results of the treatment of skin cancer as reported in the literature.[10–12]

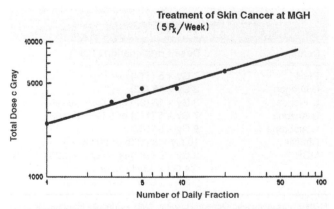

Figure 16–6. Isobioeffect line for treatment of small- to medium-sized cancers of the skin at the Massachusetts General Hospital, (MGH). Time-dose-fraction (TDF) values range from 125 to 135.

Table 16–4. DAILY MANAGEMENT OF SKIN CANCER BY 6-MeV ELECTRON BEAM RADIATION WITH 0.5 CM BOLUS*		
	Depth in Patient (cm)	% DD
Surface dose	0.0	84
Dose maximum	0.5	100
0.5 cm bolus plus	1.0	80
0.5 cm bolus plus	2.0	40

*Varian 2100 C data.
DD = depth dose.

SPECIFIC CARCINOMAS OF RADIOTHERAPEUTIC INTEREST

Carcinoma of the Eyelid

For all practical purposes, BCCs of the eyelid are considered cancers of the skin and are treated as such. When a lesion involves the inner canthus, surgical removal means either plastic repair or damage to the lacrimal duct. Radiation therapy is preferred because it can often achieve both good functional and cosmetic results and control of the disease comparable to that produced by surgery. Tumors of the canthi tend to involve the bony orbit rather early, especially at the inner canthus. When this occurs, control by radiation therapy is low (about 25%); therefore, orbital exenteration may be required. Postoperative radiation therapy may be considered as an adjuvant procedure.

Because of the superficial nature of most early cancers of the eyelid and the necessity for avoiding irradiation of the underlying radiosensitive structures of the eye, radiation therapy must be highly individualized. Radiation of low penetration is highly desirable, such as 4- to 6-MV electrons or 50-kV x-rays with a Phillips contact machine (the only kilovoltage machine used for clinical radiation therapy at the MGH at the present time).

The doses used for the treatment of carcinoma of the eyelid are similar to those used in radiation ther-

Table 16–5. DAILY MANAGEMENT OF SKIN CANCER BY 9-MeV ELECTRON BEAM RADIATION WITH 1.0 CM BOLUS*		
	Depth in patient (cm)	% DD
Surface dose	0.0	90
Dose maximum	0.6	100
1.0 cm bolus plus	1.0	82
1.0 cm bolus plus	2.0	55

*Varian 2100 C data.
DD = depth dose.

Table 16–6. LOCAL CONTROL AFTER TREATMENT OF SKIN CANCER AS REPORTED IN LITERATURE			
	Result	Comment	Reference
Study			
del Regato	594/654 pts	93.0% by RT	10
Lauritzen	2802/2900 pts	96.5% by S or RT	11
Freeman	2235/2288 pts	98.0% by S or RT	12
Cancer type			
Sweat gland (well differentiated)	70.0% 5-yr survival	—	10
Merkel cell carcinoma	50.0%	—	10

RT = radiation therapy; S = surgery; pts = patients.

apy for carcinoma of the skin: for small lesions, 45 Gy in 5 daily fractions; for moderately advanced lesions, 45 Gy in 2 weeks; and for large lesions, 4 Gy per fraction for 13 days.

Squamous cell carcinoma of the eyelid is an uncommon disease, and its management is identical to that of BCC in terms of extent of coverage and radiation dose and fractionation. Metastases from carcinoma of the eyelid occur in about 10 percent of cases and carry a grave prognosis. The parotid lymph nodes are the most common site of involvement. The management of such metastases requires a combination of surgical resection and radiation therapy. Sebaceous gland carcinoma of the eyelid is rare, with a high incidence of regional lymph node and distant metastases (approximately 25%).[13] For good local control and satisfactory cosmesis of small lesions, radiation therapy is the treatment of choice.[13] The large infiltrative tumors associated with orbital invasion are better managed by surgical resection with adjuvant postoperative radiation therapy. Owing to its high propensity for lymph node metastases, elective ipsilateral parotid and neck irradiation with 45 to 50 Gy in 4 weeks appears worthwhile.

The results of radiation therapy for carcinoma of the eyelid are shown in Table 16–7.[9,14,15]

Carcinoma of the Skin Overlying the Nasal Cartilage and the Nasolabial Sulcus

Carcinomas arising from the bridge and tip of the nose and nasal alae present a difficult problem for radiation dosimetry.[2,3] The so-called saddle lesion, covering both nasal alae, is best treated by low-energy electrons and/or an interstitial implant. The nasal cartilage has a high tolerance to radiation, and radiochondritis following a therapeutic dose of radiother-

apy has not been encountered in the author's practice.

Carcinoma arising from the nasolabial sulcus tends to burrow beneath the skin and into the premaxillary fossa and adipose tissue so that the true tumor extension often escapes accurate detection. The treatment of choice for these lesions is a combination of external beam therapy and interstitial implant.

Carcinoma of the Skin of the Auricle of the Ear

When a lesion on the skin of the auricle of the ear is infected and deeply ulcerative, exposing the cartilage, surgical excision is preferred. For early superficial lesions arising from the pinna or concha of the ear, radiation therapy alone may be used with good local control and cosmetic results (Table 16–8).[10,16] Because of the irregular curvature of the surface of the auricle of the ear, radiation therapy for this kind of lesion often results in "hot" spots and "cold" spots in the irradiated field, which may result in radiochondritis or local recurrence. The treatment of choice for these lesions is low-energy electrons, with which the incidence of radiochondritis is much lessened.

Carcinoma of the Skin Overlying the Pre- or Postauricular Sites

Carcinomas arising from pre- or postauricular sites should not be treated by external beam radiation alone

Table 16–7. LOCAL CONTROL OF CARCINOMA OF THE EYELID: REPORTED RESULTS		
Study	Results	Reference
del Regato	108/117 (92%)	14
Wildermuth and Evans	67/71 (93%)	15
Fitzpatrick	1106/1166 (95%)	9
Wang	290/300 (97%)	—

Table 16–8. LOCAL CONTROL OF CARCINOMA OF THE SKIN OVER THE NOSE AND EAR: REPORTED RESULTS		
Study	**Results**	**Reference**
del Regato	53/56 (95%)	10
Fitzpatrick		16
Nose	285/320 (89%)	
Ear	672/743 (90%)	

because the inclusion of the temporomandibular joint (TMJ) or temporal bone in the area irradiated may result in complications such as TMJ ankylosis or temporal bone necrosis. These lesions can be managed satisfactorily by a combination of low-energy electron beam radiation and interstitial implant.

MISCELLANEOUS SKIN TUMORS OF RADIOTHERAPEUTIC INTEREST

Carcinomas of Skin Appendages

Carcinomas of sebaceous glands, eccrine sweat glands, and apocrine glands may occur in the head and neck region.[17,18] Sebaceous gland carcinoma occurs most frequently on the eyelid, as a malignant lesion of the meibomian gland. Widespread aggressive metastatic disease is often seen with the eyelid lesions. Carcinomas of eccrine sweat glands and apocrine glands are locally invasive and tend not to metastasize. Treatment of these malignant appendage tumors is mostly by radical resection. The role of radiation therapy is not well recognized. This author's experience, however, indicates that these lesions respond to high-dose (ie, 70 to 75 Gy) irradiation well and with good local control. If the lesions remain localized yet unresectable, a trial course of radiation therapy is worthwhile.[13]

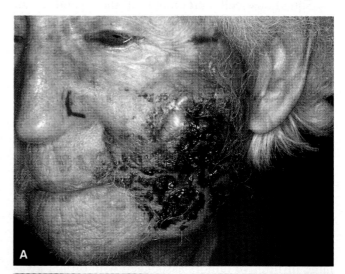

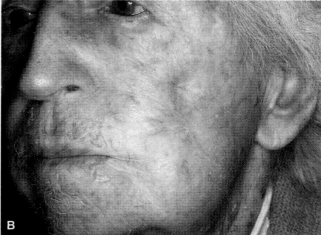

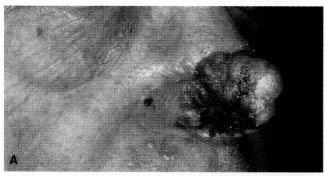

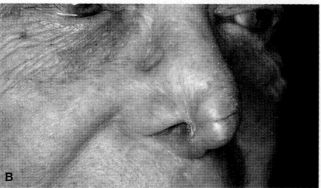

Figure 16–7. *A,* Pretreatment photograph of an 83-year-old male with a recurrent basal cell carcinoma on the right nasal ala, previously treated by excision and skin graft. The recurrent lesion was treated with 12-MV electrons for 30 Gy in 10 daily fractions, followed by an interstitial implant of 30 Gy in 60 hours. *B,* Post–radiation therapy photograph 2¹/₂ years after implant. The patient showed no evidence of disease.

Figure 16–8. *A,* Pretreatment photograph of an 87-year-old female with an enlarging lesion in the left cheek; biopsy revealed well-differentiated squamous cell carcinoma, with no regional adenopathy. Radiation therapy was given, using a combination of 12- and 15-MV electrons for 30 Gy and lateral wedge pair cobalt-60 x-rays for 40 Gy in 45 days. The total time-dose-fraction (TDF) value was 136. *B,* Post–radiation therapy photograph 1 year after treatment.

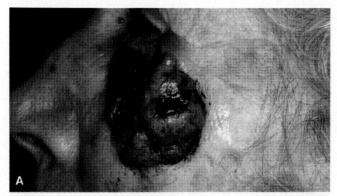

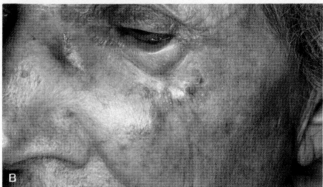

Figure 16–9. *A*, Photograph, taken before radiation therapy, of an 83-year-old female with large mobile and exophytic basal cell carcinoma of the left malar region involving the lower eyelid. Radiation therapy consisted of 45 Gy, using 9-MeV electrons with a 0.5-cm bolus in 9 daily fractions. Three weeks later, an additional 10 Gy was given in a single treatment, using a 6-MeV electron beam. The patient's eye was protected, and the time-dose-fraction (TDF) value was 145.8. *B*, Post–radiation therapy photograph 1¹/₂ years later.

Merkel Cell Tumor

Merkel cell tumors[19–22] are small-cell neuroendocrine undifferentiated neoplasms of the skin that occur on sun-exposed areas, particularly on the face and arms in elderly men and women. Merkel cell tumors not infrequently run a fulminating clinical course with regional and distant metastases. These tumors are quite radiosensitive and respond to a modest dose of radiation therapy. Generally, a dose of 45 to 50 Gy in 3 to 4 weeks is sufficient for local control. Because of this tumor's propensity for distant metastases, the eventual outcome of patients is extremely poor. Chemotherapy has been used, but its efficacy remains primarily palliative.[20]

Keratoacanthoma

Keratoacanthoma is a benign lesion and is histologically similar to well-differentiated carcinoma. It can rapidly grow to 1 to 2 cm.[23,24] This lesion is often umbilicated and covered with a central keratin plug. The diagnosis can often be made on clinical grounds. Biologically, although keratoacanthomas may undergo spontaneous resolution (leaving a depressed scar), those occurring on the eyelid, nose, and lip may cause significant loss of soft tissue, with resultant facial and functional deformity, and therefore require radiation therapy for local control.

A dose of 25 Gy in 1 week, or its equivalent, is sufficient for most lesions. If the tumor fails to show

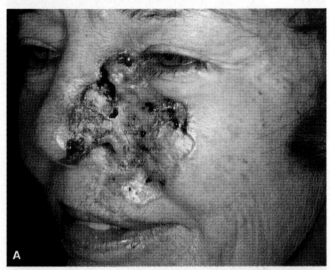

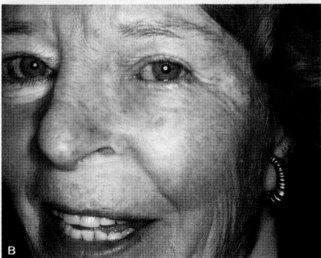

Figure 16–10. *A*, Pretreatment photograph of a 63-year-old female who had a scaly eczematoid squamous cell carcinoma on the left side of her face and nose for 5 years. The lesion was freely mobile from the underlying structures and was 7 × 7 cm in size. There was no parotid or cervical adenopathy. The lesion was treated with 64 Gy in 25 fractions over 35 elapsed days, with good response. *B*, Postradiation photograph showing excellent response with good cosmesis. Five years after radiation therapy, the patient showed no evidence of disease.

good regression in 2 weeks with such doses, an additional higher-radiation dose (60 to 65 Gy) should be given as if the tumor were a squamous cell carcinoma.

Lentigo Maligna

Circumscribed precancerous melanosis, or melanotic freckle of Hutchinson, is a noninvasive melanotic lesion occurring primarily on the faces of elderly persons. It is usually a flat tan lesion with irregular borders and areas of lighter pigmentation. The treatment of choice is surgical excision. In areas of cosmetic and functional importance such as the eyelid, the pinna of the ear, and the bridge and ala of the nose, radiation therapy is used in lieu of surgery and can achieve satisfactory local control.[25] Doses similar to those for the treatment of carcinoma of the skin are recommended (ie, 45 Gy in 9 daily fractions or its equivalent).

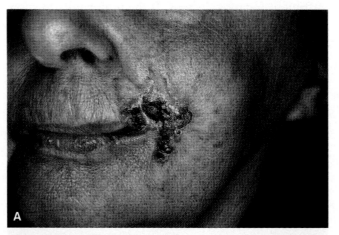

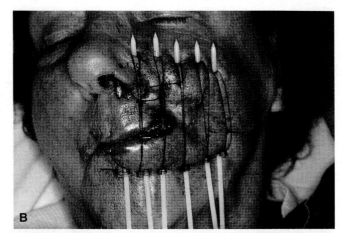

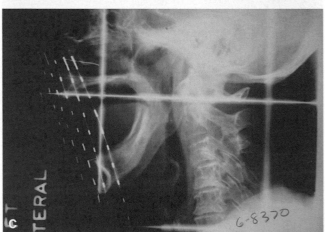

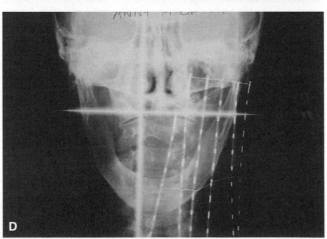

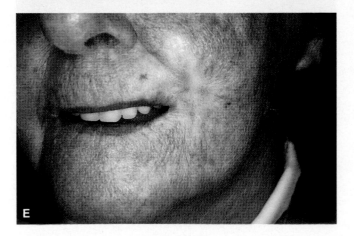

Figure 16–11. *A,* A 73-year-old female with an infiltrative pigmented lesion on the left side of the anterior face and lip commissure. A biopsy specimen of the lesion indicated basal cell carcinoma. The lesion was treated with 6-MeV electrons in 3 Gy per fraction per day for 10 days. Two weeks later, the lesion was treated by 30 Gy in 3 days with a single-plane interstitial implant; teeth and gums were shielded. The patient was last seen 4 years after radiation. There was no evidence of recurrence, and the skin and subcutaneous tissues were in good condition. *A,* Pretreatment photograph. *B,* Photograph showing interstitial angiocaths in place. *C* and *D,* Radiographs showing implant applicators in place. *E,* Post-treatment photograph showing good cosmetic results.

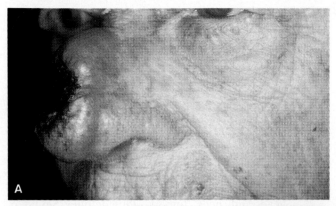

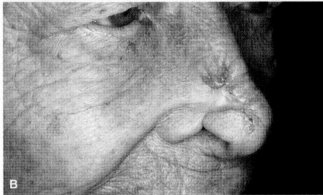

Figure 16–12. A 93-year-old female noted a rapidly enlarging mass on the nose for 3 months; a biopsy showed squamous cell carcinoma. The clinical course was that of keratoacanthoma. The lesion was treated with 32 Gy in 10 days with 4 Gy per fraction of 12-MV electrons. The tumor completely vanished, leaving a relatively normal-looking nose. *A,* Photograph of patient before radiation therapy. *B,* Photograph of patient after radiation therapy.

Kaposi's Sarcoma

Kaposi's sarcoma[26,27] is a multicentric incurable lesion. The tumors are extremely radiosensitive, and a single dose of 10 or 15 Gy in 3 fractions should produce lasting regression in small symptomatic lesions. Kaposi's sarcoma associated with acquired immunodeficiency syndrome (AIDS) can also be irradiated, with good local control. A dose of 25 to 30 Gy in 1 week (or its biologic equivalent) should suffice. Unfortunately, the survival of AIDS patients is short in terms of months.

SUMMARY

Cancers of the skin of the head and neck are very common. Basal cell and squamous cell carcinomas are the common histologic types and are curable in about 90 to 95 percent of patients in the early stage.

The selection of various treatment methods is highly important in their management and depends, for example, on the availability and skill of the specialists, the location and size of the lesion, the cosmetic and functional results anticipated after treatment, and the cost, effects, and inconvenience for the patient. Many small accessible BCCs of the face can be expediently treated by excisional biopsy, electrodesiccation, and curettage. Large and superficial lesions arising in difficult sites where surgery may result in significant cosmetic mutilation are best dealt with by radiation therapy. Surgical excision may be used for large deeply infiltrative lesions with bone involvement in accessible locations.

The use of radiation therapy for Merkel cell tumor, keratoacanthoma, lentigo maligna, and Kaposi's sarcoma has been gradually recognized and may be rewarding in selected cases.

Radiation therapy for carcinoma of the skin requires careful planning; techniques with various energies of photons and electrons, intermixed with

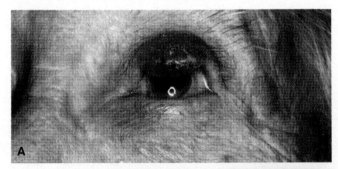

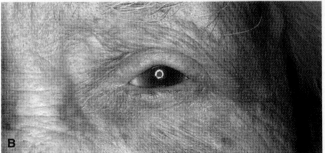

Figure 16–13. *A,* Pretreatment photograph of a 98-year-old woman who had a small lump in the left upper eyelid for 6 months. An incisional biopsy revealed a Merkel cell tumor. The patient also had a 2.0-cm metastatic left preauricular lymph node. The eyelid lesion was treated with 51 Gy in 16 days (eye protected), and the left parotid node was treated with a separate field to 60 Gy in 29 days, using a combination of electrons and cobalt-60 (^{60}Co) radiation bid with 2 Gy per fraction. *B,* Post-treatment photograph. Both lesions disappeared completely after the treatment. The patient developed fulminating cervical and supraclavicular metastatic lesions and received chemotherapy for palliation.

brachytherapy; and greater professional skills, ingenuity, and individuality. Proper selection of radiations and fraction size, with careful protection of adjacent and underlying structures, can result in extremely high cure rates and excellent cosmesis without complications. This requires personal interest and enthusiasm on the part of the radiation oncologist.

REFERENCES

1. Moss WT, Bran WN, Battifora H. Metastasis of squamous cell carcinoma of the skin by region and frequency of surgical control of metastasis. In: Moss WR, Brand WN, Battifora AH, editors. Radiation oncology. 5th ed. St Louis: C.V. Mosby Co.; 1979.

2. del Regato JA, Vuksanovic M. Radiotherapy of carcinomas of the skin overlying the cartilages of the nose and ear. Radiology 1962;79:203–8.

3. Parker RG, Wildermuth O. Radiation therapy of lesions overlying cartilage. Cancer 1962;15:57–65.

4. Zacarian S, editor. Cryosurgical advances in dermatology and tumors of head and neck. Dermatology. Springfield (IL): Charles C. Thomas; 1977.

5. Mohs EE. Chemosurgery: microscopically controlled surgery for skin cancer. Springfield (IL): Charles C. Thomas; 1978. p. 263–7.

6. Klein E, Helen F, Milgram H, et al. Tumors of the skin, effects of local use of cytostatic agents. Skin 1962; 1:89.

7. Preston DS, Stern RS. Nonmelanoma cancers of the skin. N Engl J Med 1992;327:1649–62.

8. Strandquist M. Time-dose relationship. Acta Radiol 1944;Suppl 55:1.

9. Fitzpatrick PJ, Jamieson DM, Thompson GA, et al. Tumors of the eyelids and their treatment by radiotherapy. Radiology 1972;104:661–5.

10. del Regato JA. Ackerman and del Regato's Cancer—diagnosis, treatment and prognosis. 6th ed. St. Louis: Mosby; 1985. p. 203–6.

11. Lauritzen RE, Johnson RE, Spratt JS Jr. Pattern of recurrences in basal cell carcinoma. Surgery 1965; 57:813–6.

12. Freeman RG, Duncan WC. Recurrent skin cancer. Arch Dermatol 1973;107:395–9.

13. Pardo F, Wang CC, Albert D, et al. Sebaceous carcinoma of the ocular adnexae: a role of radiotherapy. Int J Radiat Oncol Biol Phys 1989;18:643–7.

14. del Regato JA. Roentgen therapy of carcinoma of the eyelids. Radiology 1949;52:564–73.

15. Wildermuth O, Evans JC. The special problem of cancer of the eyelid. Cancer 1956;9:837–41.

16. Fitzpatrick PJ. Radiation therapy of tumors of the skin of the head and neck. In: Thawley, Panje, Batsakis, Lindberg, editors. Comprehensive management of head and neck tumors. Philadelphia: Saunders Company; 1987. p. 1208–20.

17. Miller WL. Sweat gland carcinoma. Am J Clin Pathol 1967;47:767.

18. Wertkin MG, Bauer JJ. Sweat gland carcinoma. Arch Surg 1976;111:884–5.

19. Sibley RK, Dehner LP, Rosai J. Primary neuroendocrine (Merkel cell?) carcinoma of the skin. Am J Surg Pathol 1985;9(2):–95–108.

20. George TK, Santagnese A, Bennett JM. Chemotherapy for metastatic Merkel cell carcinoma. Cancer 1985; 56:1034–8.

21. Goepfert H, Remmier D, Silva E, Wheeler B. Merkel cell carcinoma (endocrine carcinoma of the skin) of the head and neck. Arch Otolaryngol 1984;110: 707–12.

22. Warner TF, Uno H, Hafez GR, et al. Merkel cells and Merkel cell tumors: ultrastructure, immunocytochemistry and review of the literature. Cancer 1983;52:238–45.

23. Finley AG. Keratoacanthoma. Aust J Dermatol 1954; 2:144.

24. Shimm D, Duttenhaver J, Doucette J, et al. Radiation therapy of keratoacanthomas. Int J Radiat Oncol Biol Phys 1983;9:759–61.

25. Harwood AR. Conventional radiotherapy in the treatment of lentigo maligna and lentigo melanoma. J Am Acad Dermatol 1982;6:310–2.

26. O'Brien PH, Brasfield RD. Kaposi's sarcoma. Cancer 1966;19:1497–9.

27. Holecek MJ, Harwood AR. Radiotherapy of Kaposi's sarcoma. Cancer 1978;41:1733.

17

Treatment of Primary Cutaneous Lymphomas

HOSSAMELDIN NAEEM, MD
SOLA X. CHENG
THOMAS S. KUPPER, MD

CUTANEOUS T-CELL LYMPHOMA

The treatment of primary cutaneous lymphoma depends on the extent of disease (stage) at diagnosis. Patients with disease that is clinically limited to the skin (eg, mycosis fungoides, stages I and IIA) can often achieve durable remissions with one of the available skin-directed therapies. In contrast, first-line therapy for patients with extracutaneous disease involves at least one systemic therapy, sometimes with the addition of another adjuvant therapy from either the skin-directed or the systemic therapeutic category. In addition, modalities from both therapeutic categories may be employed as maintenance therapies.

While it is likely that most of the malignant cells in early-stage disease reside predominantly in the skin, the malignant cells in cutaneous T-cell lymphoma (CTCL), unlike carcinoma or sarcoma cells, arise from lymphocytes that normally traffic through blood, tissue, and lymph nodes. It is not surprising, then, that patients with skin-limited stage IA disease in fact have polymerase chain reaction (PCR)–demonstrated clonal populations in the peripheral blood.[1] The paradox is that most patients can achieve durable remission of their disease by a therapy directed solely at the skin. One possible explanation is that early in disease, the malignant T cells behave much like normal cutaneous T cells, which display strong "homing" tendencies to the tissue where they first encountered antigen. They thus spend the majority of their time in, and may be

dependent upon, the skin. With the accumulation of progressive mutations later in disease, the malignant T cells' dependence on skin diminishes, resulting in clinically apparent extracutaneous disease. With this working model, a reasonable approach to choosing therapy is to treat the compartment where identifiable malignant cells exist by standard clinical criteria (such as palpable or radiographic adenopathy, circulating abnormal cells on peripheral blood smear, or an elevated CD4-CD8 ratio). Finally, the indolent but potentially progressive nature of CTCL makes treatment of this disease a process that involves constant re-evaluation. Because recurrent disease is almost always accompanied by skin findings, it can be readily detected with regular follow-up.

Skin-Directed Therapies

Topical Corticosteroids

Corticosteroids have proven to be the cornerstone of topical treatment for a wide array of skin disorders. They have been shown to have multiple immunomodulatory and anti-inflammatory effects via such mechanisms as the down-regulation of cytokine production through the inhibition of NF-KB, a transcription factor that promotes the expression of many inflammatory mediators.[2] Corticosteroids inhibit cell-cell interactions involved in the amplification of the immune response, interfere with lymphocyte adhesion to endothelial cells and with their subsequent extravasation into tissues, and induce apoptosis of lymphocytes by both biochemical and oncogene pathways.[3] These anti-inflammatory and immunomodulatory effects have made topical corticosteroids useful in both acute and chronic inflammatory disorders while their proapoptotic effects have established systemic corticosteroids as part of standard treatment of acute lymphoblastic leukemia, Hodgkin's and non-Hodgkin's lymphomas, and other neoplasms. These mechanisms also make corticosteroids a logical and attractive agent in the treatment of CTCL.

Topical corticosteroids are a mainstay of induction and maintenance of remission in patients with early-stage disease. In a prospective study of 79 patients with patch- and plaque-stage disease, daily use of topical corticosteroids for 3 to 6 months resulted in complete remission in 63 percent of patients and partial remission in 31 percent, for a total response rate of 94 percent. Post-treatment biopsies performed in 7 patients revealed histologic clearing, which correlated with the clinical improvement observed.[4] Although the long-term use of potent topical corticosteroids can lead to atrophy of the skin, formation of striae, and (in rare cases) adrenal suppression, alternating the use of superpotent (class I) and midpotent (class III) agents or using corticosteroids as adjuvants to other therapies rather than as the primary therapy can be used to address patch- and plaque-stage disease, without significant side effects.

Topical Chemotherapy

The two alkylating agents mechlorethamine hydrochloride (nitrogen mustard [NM]) and bischloro nitrosourea (carmustine [BCNU]) are cytotoxic chemotherapeutic agents used as topical therapy for CTCL. Nitrogen mustard exerts most of its effects during the G1 and S phases of the cell cycle. It is thought to prevent the separation of strands necessary for normal cell division by cross-linking deoxyribonucleic acid (DNA) and may also act by alkylating and thus blocking transcription factor–binding sites on DNA. Its selective action in lymphoid tissue prompted its use as a systemic agent in CTCL as early as 1947.

Over time, NM has proven to be effective in the treatment of stage I CTCL.[5] In 1977, Vonderheid and colleagues reported induction of remission in 68 percent of patients treated with daily topical NM over several months, and a subsequent (albeit smaller) study reported 87 percent complete remission with daily therapy.[6,7] Although these results are impressive, NM can be complicated to use in practice as it is a carcinogen and a potential environmental contaminant. Nitrogen mustard is dispensed as a powder, which is dissolved in tap water by the patient and applied carefully to affected areas with gloves and gauze or a paintbrush. An ointment form is available and may be easier to use. To decrease local irritation, risk of secondary cutaneous malignancies, and other potential complications, patients should apply the solution carefully, washing off all spills, and should avoid sunlight as ultraviolet B (UVB) radiation will increase the risk of carcinogenesis. Irritant dermatitis with erythema, edema, and (occasionally) vesicle formation is a common adverse effect, occurring in 50 to 60 percent of patients, and can be addressed by diluting the medication. Reversible hyperpigmentation, especially of formerly diseased skin, is also common. Delayed-type hypersensitivity, which occurs in up to 35 percent of patients, is actually thought to contribute to its therapeutic effect. Induction of tolerance to NM through intravenous administration has actually been associated with a subsequent loss of treatment efficacy. Immediate-type hypersensitivity, however, carries a risk of anaphylaxis and should therefore prompt discontinuation of the drug.

Carmustine (BCNU) also acts as an alkylating agent. However, its use is not clearly associated with an increased incidence of cutaneous malignancies.[5] Like NM, BCNU is available in powder and ointment forms, but it is used more often than NM for total-body treatment. The majority of patients experience macular erythema, resembling a sunburn reaction, 2 to 8 weeks after initiation of treatment with BCNU. In severe reactions, skin tenderness and cutaneous telangiectasias may follow and remain for months after the erythema has cleared. Reversible leukopenia occurs in about 4 percent of patients. Monitoring the leukocyte count is especially important in patients applying BCNU to their total body surface and who are using either the ointment form of the drug or the more highly concentrated solution. (For further details on the use of these two agents, the reader is referred to Ramsay, Meller, and Zackheim's excellent review in *Hematology/Oncology Clinics of North America.*[5])

Phototherapy

Perhaps the most widely used skin-directed therapies for early-stage CTCL are psoralen plus ultraviolet A (PUVA) photochemotherapy and UVB photototherapy. Radiation (the term is derived from the name of the Egyptian sun god Ra) within the UVB (290 to 320 nm) and ultraviolet A (UVA) (320 to 400 nm) spectra has both beneficial and harmful effects on skin. Psoralen plus ultraviolet A has demonstrated efficacy in a variety of T-cell-mediated diseases such as psoriasis, vitiligo, and graft-versus-host disease. The observation that CTCL often affects covered areas of the body while sparing sun-exposed skin may have led to the application of PUVA to the treatment of CTCL, first reported by Gilchrest and colleagues in 1976. The effects of ultraviolet radiation on immune functions in skin fall into three categories: (1) effect on soluble mediators, (2) effect on surface membrane protein expression, and (3) induction of apoptosis. In general, UVB is active on epidermal keratinocytes and Langerhans' cells while UVA penetrates deeper into the dermis and can reach dermal fibroblasts, dendritic cells, endothelial cells, and infiltrating inflammatory cells. Ultraviolet radiation has been shown to decrease interleukin-7 (IL-7) expression and to increase the expression of interleukin-10 (IL-10). Ultraviolet B and PUVA down-regulate the expression of surface molecules such as major histocompatibility complex II (MHC-II) and intercellular adhesion molecule 1 (ICAM-1) by generating singlet oxygen, DNA adducts, and pyrimidine dimers, further dampening antigen-presenting functions and other cell-cell interactions. They also induce apoptosis through both protein synthesis–dependent (late) and protein synthesis–independent (early) pathways.[8,9]

Psoralens are phototoxic furocoumarin compounds that, when activated by UVA light, bind covalently to pyrimidine bases in DNA. They are inactivated in the liver, with a plasma half-life of 1 hour, and are cleared by the kidney 24 hours after administration. One-and-a-half to 2 hours prior to each UVA treatment, the patient takes an oral dose of 8-methoxypsoralen (0.65 mg/kg). Escalating doses of UVA are administered three times weekly until a maintenance dose that induces complete remission is achieved. The frequency (but not the UVA dose) is then decreased gradually, and the patient may be maintained on once-monthly therapy for more than a year after remission. A 1995 review by Herrmann and colleagues reported complete response in 90 percent of patients with stage IA disease, 76 percent with stage IB disease, 78 and 59 percent with stages IIA and IIB disease, 61 percent with stage III disease, and 40 percent with stage IV disease.[10] Both clearing of the skin and a durable remission were found to be much more likely with earlier stages of disease.[10] The most frequently reported acute adverse effects are an erythematous macular reaction (similar to sunburn), pruritus, and nausea. Symptom control with emollients and other agents is usually satisfactory, and most patients eventually tolerate the therapy well. To prevent PUVA-induced cataracts, patients must wear wraparound dark glasses during the day of their treatment. When used in the long term, PUVA can lead to solar elastosis, solar lentigines, and other manifestations of photo-aging. In addition, patients with underlying photosensitive conditions such as lupus erythematosus, porphyria, and xeroderma pigmentosa, as well as patients with severe hepatic and renal impairment, should not receive PUVA therapy.[11]

Ultraviolet B therapy does not involve ingestion of a drug, but its goals are very similar to those of PUVA therapy. Rates of remission are slightly more modest than those achieved with PUVA therapy, and 74 percent of patients with predominantly stage IA disease achieve complete remission. Recently, the use of narrowband (311 nm) UVB has been found to have increased efficacy and decreased toxicity when compared with conventional UVB.[12] Unlike PUVA therapy patients, patients on UVB therapy cannot be maintained on once-monthly or even less frequent treatments for 1 or more years following induction of remission. With both UVB and PUVA therapies, re-treatment with light is often a viable option if relapse occurs.

The formation of DNA adducts with activated psoralen and thymine dimers with UVB forms a theoretic basis for mutagenesis and increased skin cancer risk in patients undergoing light therapy. This increased risk is supported by a 16-center study by Stern and Laird, which followed up 1,380 patients who had undergone long-term PUVA therapy for psoriasis. A small but not statistically significant increase in melanoma risk and a small but significant increase in risk of basal cell carcinomas were seen. A marked and significant increased risk of squamous cell carcinomas was also reported; roughly one-quarter of patients who received high doses developed these cancers. Furthermore, the study found a correlation between cumulative dose received and the degree of increased risk of squamous cell carcinomas.[13] Although the CTCL patient population may have inherent differences in ultraviolet-induced skin cancer risk, it is reasonable to infer that they would also be susceptible to PUVA-related cutaneous malignancy. Increased incidence of these skin cancers has also been reported specifically in CTCL patients who have undergone PUVA therapy.[10] Therefore, before initiation of light therapy, careful consideration of other treatment options is advised for patients with a history of melanoma or nonmelanoma skin cancer or with a history of arsenic exposure.

Electron Beam Therapy

Radiation has a long history in the treatment of CTCL. Earlier x-ray therapy was limited by the problem of effectively treating a wide field such as the human skin surface while delivering a total dose of radiation that was safe. In 1940, Trump and colleagues replaced photon-based radiation with radiation from accelerated electrons. Total-skin electron beam (TSEB) therapy has since undergone many modifications and advances to achieve the goal of delivering a sufficient dose to the target tissue volume while minimizing the radiation of normal tissue.

The basic mechanism of radiation therapy is direct toxicity to tumor cells within the target volume. Since most patients with CTCL have disease involving the dermis, that target volume consists of tissue approximately 5 mm deep to the skin surface. Electron energy decays in tissue much faster than

photon energy, and by delivering beams at various angles of appropriate energy levels, it is now possible to effectively irradiate the target volume while sparing deeper tissues such as bone marrow. A large treatment room, flattening filters, and scattering foils are additional tools used to deliver the most uniform dose possible to the complex surface of the human body. Most centers use a dual fixed-angle six-field method or a rotation method, with the patient standing approximately 7 m from the electron source and assuming different positions during treatment. Naturally shielded areas such as the scalp, perineum, inframammary folds, and plantar surfaces receive additional therapy while areas such as the hands, which receive higher doses due to their geometry, may be shielded during treatment. Typically, a total radiation dose of 36 Gy is administered over a 10-week period. For foci of deeper disease, such as involved lymph nodes or thick plaques or tumors, beam energy levels can be adjusted to deliver higher doses to those areas only (spot therapy).[14,15]

Total-skin electron beam therapy has proven to be extremely effective in the treatment of CTCL. Because it has the ability to penetrate deeper tissue through the use of higher-energy electron beams, it is the treatment of choice for tumor-stage disease. In their study summarizing 35 years of experience with almost 1,000 patients at Stanford University and the Hamilton Clinic, Hamilton, Ontario, Canada, Jones and colleagues reported complete-remission rates of 84 to 96 percent in patients with stage IA disease. Of these patients, 40 to 60 percent remained disease free 5 years after completion of therapy. An inverse relationship between stage of disease and remission rates was found, with remission rates of 56 to 81 percent in stage IB disease and 64 to 74 percent in stage IIA disease; 5-year disease-free rates were 10 to 25 percent in these two groups of patients. A study of 45 stage III and stage IV patients at Yale University and at the Hamilton Clinic found that with higher doses of radiation, 100 percent of stage III patients and 74 percent of stage IV patients had complete clinical remission of disease and that 69 and 36 percent, respectively, were free of recurrence at 5 years. The addition of PUVA therapy after completion of TSEB therapy was shown to further extend remission in stage I patients, with no relapses in the stage IA

TSEB-plus-PUVA group and a crude 5-year relapse rate of 36 percent in the TSEB-only group.[16]

Acute toxic effects of TSEB therapy most commonly include erythema and pruritus (especially at sites of disease), soreness, edema, xerosis, and desquamation. As a result of radiation to the adnexa, almost all patients experience total-body alopecia, nail plate loss, and anhidrosis, all of which typically resolve within 6 months after completion of therapy. In men, sperm production may temporarily decrease. Chronic toxicity consists of xerosis and cutaneous telangiectasia. There is little evidence that TSEB therapy alone increases the incidence of skin cancers. Patients who have undergone radiation therapy or who have pacemakers are candidates for TSEB therapy but may require a lower dose or additional shielding.[13]

Systemic Therapies

Retinoid Therapy

The retinoids are a group of vitamin A analogues that bind (like the natural hormone) to retinoid receptors in the nucleus to modify gene expression. There are six retinoid receptor subtypes, which fall into two categories: retinoid-A receptors (RARs) and retinoid-X receptors (RXRs). These receptors target genes that influence different cellular processes; bound RARs promote cellular differentiation and proliferation while RXRs steer cells towards apoptosis and inhibit the growth of many types of cell lines in vitro.[17] The cytosolic retinoic acid–binding proteins (CRABPs) I and II are another pathway by which retinoids exert their effects. Recently, the RXR-selective compound bexarotene has been used in phase I and II trials against cancers such as squamous cell carcinomas of the head and neck and has been approved by the Food and Drug Administration (FDA) as a therapy for advanced CTCL. Classic nonselective retinoids have a long history of use in the treatment of CTCL but are perhaps better known for their role in the treatment of disorders of proliferation and keratinization, such as psoriasis and Darier's disease, and in the treatment of severe acne vulgaris.[18]

Oral retinoids have been used successfully in treating CTCL; isotretinoin and etretinate monother-

apy (1 mg/kg) have yielded response rates of about 60 percent. Etretinate may be more effective than isotretinoin and has also been shown to enhance response when used with PUVA therapy (Re-PUVA) in patients whose disease was initially resistant to PUVA.[19] Retinoids combined with interferon-α (IFN-α) therapy (3 MU three times weekly) and retinoids combined with extracorporeal photopheresis have also been used, with higher reported rates of remission than those seen with retinoids alone.[19–23] Most of the clinical experience with bexarotene has been with the oral form although a topical gel is also available. In patients with early-stage patch or plaque disease, response rates of up to 80 percent were observed with oral therapy (300 mg/kg/day) at the M.D. Anderson Cancer Center.[24] Although responses as early as 4 to 8 weeks have been reported, the authors' experience has found that the time lag from the initiation of treatment to the beginning of clinical response can be as long as 12 to 14 weeks.

Retinoids are known to have the side effects of xerosis, mucocutaneous toxicity (cheilitis, conjunctivitis), headache (including a low incidence of pseudotumor cerebri), arthralgias and myalgias, and leukopenia, as well as metabolic changes such as hyperlipidemia, reversible and asymptomatic elevations in hepatic enzymes, and hypercalcemia.[25] The RXR-selective retinoid bexarotene carries fewer side effects and does not cause mucocutaneous toxicity, which is thought to be mediated via RARs. Hyperlipidemia is common and often marked and can usually be controlled with 3-hydroxy-3-methylglutaryl–coenzyme A (HMG-CoA) reductase inhibitors (statins) as well as micronized fenofibrate (Tricor). Central hypothyroidism via a thyroid hormone–independent suppression of thyroglobulin production is another reversible and treatable side effect of bexarotene.[26] Leukopenia, particularly neutropenia, can also be seen and is usually transient. It is therefore important to establish baseline values for fasting blood lipids, liver function tests (aspartate transaminase [AST], alanine transaminase [ALT], and total bilirubin), complete blood count with differential, and thyroid-stimulating hormone (TSH) and T4 before instituting retinoid therapy, particularly bexarotene therapy. Lipid elevation in response to bexarotene therapy is usually seen 2 to 4 weeks after initiating therapy, and lipid-lowering therapy should be instituted. Thereafter, lipid levels should be monitored every 4 to 8 weeks, with a total plasma triglyceride level of 400 as an upper limit for the continuation of bexarotene; other laboratory values should be monitored as needed.[17,27]

Extracorporeal Photopheresis

Extracorporeal photopheresis (ECP) is a method developed by Edelson in 1981 specifically to treat CTCL. In ECP, patients take an oral dose of 8-methoxypsoralen (8-MOP). Their blood is then exposed, outside of the body, to UVA light, thereby activating the psoralen within white blood cells; the blood is subsequently returned to the patient. About 10 percent of the total lymphocytes are treated in one session, and because activated psoralens form adducts with pyrimidine bases (see PUVA section in "Phototherapy," above), anucleate blood components such as red blood cells and platelets are not affected. In addition, ECP is not broadly immunosuppressive and does not prevent primary responses to vaccines and other antigens.[28] The technique was FDA-approved for use in advanced CTCL in 1988 and is more likely to be effective in patients with peripheral blood involvement. As a lymphocyte-targeted therapy, ECP has also been effectively used in the treatment of systemic sclerosis, graft-versus-host disease, and rheumatoid arthritis and for the prevention of postoperative rejection of cardiac transplants.[29]

The mechanism whereby ECP destroys malignant T cells is not completely understood. Clearly, the DNA photoadducts formed with psoralens lead to DNA damage, with inhibition of DNA synthesis; however, mechanisms other than cross-link formation are also involved in DNA damage.[30] The intervening steps between DNA damage and cell death are also being elucidated; these may include depletion of cell stores of adenosine triphosphate (ATP) and nicotinamide adenine dinucleotide (NAD) caused by poly-adenosine diphosphate (ADP) ribosylation at sites of DNA strand breaks.[31] Even more intriguing is the observation that repeated treatment of a small fraction of lymphocytes can lead to durable remissions. It is postulated that the re-infusion of psoralen-altered lymphocytes incites a heightened immune response and that ECP-induced mutations enhance the antigenicity of the tumor cells with an "autovaccination effect."[32] Regardless, 90 percent of treated T cells are found to be nonviable 96 hours after treatment. Extracorporeal photopheresis has also been demonstrated to (1) increase and even reverse the aberrant ratio of CD8+ to CD4+ that is often observed, enhancing cytotoxic responses against tumor cells; (2) induce expression of IFN-α and tumor necrosis factor-α (TNF-α); and (3) restore the Th1-Th2 imbalance seen in patients with advanced CTCL.[33,34]

As in PUVA therapy, patients undergoing ECP take a dose of psoralen 2 hours prior to initiation of UVA exposure, to maximize plasma concentrations during irradiation. After whole blood is removed from the patient and centrifuged, the plasma and leukocyte-rich fraction are passed through a clear plastic cassette, where they are exposed to UVA light for 3 hours, and are then re-infused into the patient. In a recent modification, 8-MOP is added directly into the leukocyte-rich fraction, thus eliminating the nausea and other side effects that often accompany psoralen ingestion, while ensuring optimum psoralen levels in the irradiated blood. Treatment typically occurs on 2 consecutive days every 3 to 4 weeks, and response is often heralded by an initial increase in erythema and pruritus followed by a cephalad-to-caudad clearing. Most patients who will respond do so in the first 6 to 8 months of treatment. Erythrodermic patients with a total leukocyte count of < 15,000 and a percentage of at least 15% of CD8+ cells in the blood are considered the best responders. Other features are history of primary erythroderma, short duration of disease, immunocompetence, and absence of lymph node or visceral disease. Continuation of treatment is periodically re-evaluated, and leukocytopenia is the only clear contraindication to therapy, aside from technical difficulties with venous access. In Edelson's 1987 study of 37 erythrodermic patients, a 73 percent response rate was reported, with a 64 percent decrease in the skin score designating severity of disease. Mean time to development of a response was between 4 and 5 months.[35] In 1999, Jiang and colleagues observed 41 patients with stages III and IV disease who had failed multiple previous modalities and found a 20 percent complete-response rate after 10 to 13 months of treatment; 60 percent of the patients were partial responders, and 20 percent were nonresponders.[37] Other studies have reported similar findings, with complete-response rates of 15 to 25 percent.[38] The impact of ECP on overall survival has not been well studied, and large-scale multicenter randomized trials comparing ECP with chemotherapy and other therapies for advanced disease are called for.[39]

Side effects associated with ECP are few and minimal and consist primarily of transient nausea from psoralen ingestion. Hypotension during treatment and catheter-related infection are rare (< 5% of patients), and although herpes zoster, herpes simplex virus (HSV), disseminated fungal, and other infections have been reported during therapy, these infections are seen in the setting of advanced CTCL, regardless of treatment modality.[35] As mentioned above, ECP is not an immunosuppressive therapy; in fact, it may even enhance specific segments of the immune response.

Cytokine Therapy

Immunologic abnormalities seen in advanced CTCL include a diminution in cell-mediated immunity, with a decreased capacity to produce cytokines such as IFN-γ and IL-2, produced by Th1 CD4 cells, and markedly low levels of IL-12. Interleukin-2 and IL-12 both augment the activity of natural killer (NK) cells and cytotoxic T cells, and IL-12 promotes the differentiation of CD4 cells to the Th1 subtype. In addition, the malignant T cells in CTCL produce elevated levels of the cell-mediated immunosuppressive cytokines IL-10 and IL-4, further worsening the Th1-Th2 imbalance and weakening the host's natural cytotoxic antitumor response. These observations have led to the administration of exogenous cytokines in an attempt to reverse these immune abnormalities and enhance the host's immune-mediated destruction of malignant T cells.[40]

Interferons (IFNs) are divided into the type 1 IFNs, which include IFN-α and IFN-β and which share a cell surface receptor, and the type 2 IFN (IFN-γ), which binds a receptor distinct from the type 1 IFNs. The alpha interferons in clinical use are recombinant molecules and include IFN-α2a (Roferon-A) and IFN-α2b (Intron A). There is no apparent difference in clinical performance between the two molecules. Once bound to their surface receptor, IFNs induce changes in the expression of 50 to 100 genes, including the cell surface antigens MHC-I and MHC-II.[41] The downstream effects cascade through multiple levels of mediators to produce an immune response. In CTCL, specifically, IFN-α strongly inhibits the ability of malignant T cells to proliferate in response to growth-stimulatory factors and also inhibits their production of IL-4 and IL-5.[42]

Most clinical experience has been with IFN-α. It was first found to have activity against CTCL when it was used in high doses (50 million units/m²) at the National Cancer Institute. Since then, several trials using low-dose (usually 3 million units/m²) and intermediate-dose (18 to 36 million units/m²) IFN-α given three times weekly have resulted in encouraging results, with higher tolerability than is seen with the high dose. In a literature review, Bunn and colleagues reported that intermediate-dose therapy in two series of 15 and 20 patients yielded response rates of 75 to 85 percent.[43] Overall, there was an objective response in 60 percent of 110 patients, with complete remissions seen more often in earlier stages of disease. However, there is some evidence that the immunophenotype of the malignant T cells is more important than the disease stage in predicting response to therapy, and CD5- and CD7-negative clones may be more resistant to therapy.[44] In addition to monotherapy, IFN-α has been used in combination with various other treatment modalities (see "Combination Therapies," below). Experience with IFN-β is very limited. Its unique tissue affinity lends it to intralesional use because plasma levels are undetectable after intralesional injection.[41] In a single trial of 16 patients with advanced disease, IFN-γ showed a response rate of 31 percent.[45] More clinical experience is needed before the utility of IFN-γ can be assessed.

Interferon-α is usually given subcutaneously or intramuscularly three times per week. About 90 percent of patients experience flulike side effects of fever and chills, headache, and myalgias, and many will have nausea and vomiting and loose stools. To minimize the occurrence of these side effects, treatment can be initiated at 1.0 to 1.5 MU/m² and escalated to 3 to 5 MU/m². Acetaminophen premedication and dosing at bedtime are other ways to reduce these side effects, which tend to diminish over the duration of treatment. Reversible dose-related leukopenia is seen in 40 percent of patients, changes of mental status (including depression and confusion) are seen in 33 percent, and the most significant dose-dependent toxicities are fatigue and anorexia. Asymptomatic hepatic enzyme elevation and telogen effluvium are also seen. Response can occur after 2 to 5 months of therapy; maximal response may require longer therapy, and the dose may be increased as tolerated if no response is seen. Neutralizing antibody develops in many if not most of treated patients, but it is not clear that its presence alters treatment efficacy.[45,46]

Interleukin-2 and IL-12 are other cytokines that have been used in the treatment of CTCL. There is limited experience with either as monotherapy. One small study of IL-2 monotherapy reported complete and durable remission in 3 and partial remission in 2 of 7 patients with advanced disease.[47] However, IL-2 may stimulate the growth of tumor cells, and this must be weighed against the magnitude of the resulting antitumor response. Interleukin-12 reverses the immunologic defects of malignant T cells in vitro.[48] There have been few reports of the use of IL-12 in clinical trials.

Ontak

Ontak (DAB_{389}-IL-2) is a recombinant fusion protein produced by the expression of a recombinant gene in *Escherichia coli*. It is composed of the enzymatic (fragment A) and translocation (fragment B) portions of diphtheria toxin fused to the human IL-2 gene. It specifically binds the human IL-2 receptor (IL-2R). After being endocytosed into an acidic vesicle, Ontak releases fragment A into the cytosol, where it catalyzes ADP ribosylation of elongation factor 2, inhibiting protein synthesis and causing cell death.[49,50] The IL-2 receptor exists in low-, intermediate-, and high-affinity forms. The high-affinity form, a three-chain receptor that includes CD25, is found on activated proliferating T cells and recently activated B cells, and Ontak is selectively cytotoxic for cells with CD25 expression.[51] Ontak has been used with varying success in lymphocyte-mediated diseases such as psoriasis and Hodgkin's and non-Hodgkin's lymphomas.[52] An earlier version of the protein was constructed and purified by Williams and colleagues in 1987; in 1990, molecular modifications resulted in the present Ontak protein, which has greater affinity for CD25 than its predecessor and more favorable pharmacokinetics and toxicity profiles.[53] Anti-interleukin-2 and anti–diphtheria toxin antibodies and soluble IL-2 receptors have been detected in the blood of many patients, both prior to and during treatment with Ontak, but there is no clear relationship between their presence or titers and clinical response to Ontak.[52] Reported expression of CD25 in CTCL varies widely and has been estimated at 62 percent in the largest study. However, its presence or absence in skin biopsy specimens does not correlate definitively with clinical response. Some patients with relapse of disease that was CD25 negative on biopsy have responded to subsequent courses of Ontak therapy, and other patients with evidence of adequate CD25 expression on biopsy have done less well.[24,52]

Ontak first showed activity against CTCL during phase I trials in 1998. Thirty-seven percent of 35 CTCL patients responded to doses ranging from 6 to 31 μg/kg/d, with complete remission achieved in 14 percent. In a later study of 35 CTCL patients, 27 percent responded in a median period of 2 months, with durable remissions of 12 to 16 months.[53] In a double-blind two-arm study comparing doses of 9 and 18 μg/kg/d in 71 patients with multiple-treatment-resistant CTCL, 30 percent of patients achieved partial or complete responses, with a median of 7 months of therapy.[54] Ontak is administered intravenously over 15 to 80 minutes for 5 consecutive days at 21-day intervals, for a minimum of six cycles. The most commonly encountered associated adverse effects are fever and chills (74% of patients), nausea and vomiting, light-headedness, and hypotension (50% of patients). A mild capillary leak syndrome characterized by hypoalbuminemia, hypotension, and edema has also been seen. Anaphylaxis, a rare but potentially life-threatening reaction to Ontak, may be mitigated by pretreatment with dexamethasone and antihistamines (Decadron). Laboratory test abnormalities include elevation of hepatic transaminases and transient changes in lymphocyte counts, but no evidence of immune dysfunction has been reported. Patients usually start at a dose of 9 μg/kg/day and may progress to the highest approved dose, 18 μg/kg/d. Higher doses are limited by symptoms of severe lethargy and fatigue. At present, candidates for therapy include patients with stages IB to III disease who have not responded or relapsed after four or more treatment modalities and patients with stage IV disease who have failed at least one modality and who have greater than 20 percent of skin biopsy specimen tumor cells staining positive for CD25.[50] More data regarding the efficacy of Ontak in patients with less than 20 percent CD25 positivity on biopsy and in patients with various antibody profiles are needed before these guidelines can be better defined.

Single-Agent and Multiagent Chemotherapy

Many single-agent and multiagent chemotherapies have been used, predominantly in CTCL patients who have had disease resistance to other therapies and for those who have nodal or visceral disease on presentation. As many as 60 to 80 percent of patients show at least partial response; however, disease remission induced by chemotherapy is usually short-lived, and palliation remains the primary goal.[38,55]

Methotrexate, cisplatin, etoposide, bleomycin, cladribine, fludarabine, vinblastine, systemic corticosteroids, and other agents that have demonstrated effectiveness in lymphoid malignancies have been used in the treatment of CTCL, with comparable total-response rates in the range of 60 to 70 percent.[55,56] Of these, methotrexate (MTX) has demonstrated a relatively high rate of complete response; in low doses (25 to 50 mg/wk), it is considered a first-line therapy for patients with erythrodermic CTCL. Methotrexate is an antimetabolite used as a single agent in rheumatologic and autoimmune disease and in many multiagent chemotherapies for malignancy. Haynes and Van Scott first described its efficacy in the treatment of CTCL in 1970.[57] Total response rates are typically around 60 percent, and one study of 17 stage III CTCL patients reported a 41 percent complete-response rate with low-dose MTX and a 5-year survival of 70 percent.[58] Methotrexate is given as a weekly oral dose. It is metabolized by the hepatic P450 microsomal system and thus has many potential drug interactions. Major toxicities include

reversible leukopenia and myelosuppression, elevated hepatic enzymes and hepatic fibrosis, and pulmonary fibrosis. Frequent monitoring of complete blood count (cbc) and liver function enzymes is required, and liver biopsy may also be indicated.[56,59] Other side effects include mucositis, nausea, vomiting, diarrhea, and cutaneous erosions.

Pentostatin, a nucleoside analogue that inhibits adenosine deaminase, has also been used, alone and with IFN-α in the treatment of CTCL. In 1991, Cummings and colleagues reported that 4 of 8 CTCL patients in a phase II trial of pentostatin achieved a partial but fairly durable response (16 months).[60] More recent literature regarding pentostatin monotherapy showed an overall response rate of between 40 and 71 percent and complete-response rates of between 7 and 25 percent.[61–63] Combination therapy with high-dose intermittent IFN did not show a higher response rate than pentostatin used alone.[61] The major toxicities observed were granulocytopenia, a prolonged depression in CD4 counts, nausea and vomiting, renal insufficiency, elevated hepatic enzymes, and non-neutropenic fever.

The antimetabolite fludarabine has also shown some promise although overall and complete-response rates were not as good as those with some other agents and although significant bone marrow suppression was seen.[64,65] Data on other single-agent chemotherapies are limited, with small numbers of patients in each stage of disease; an analysis (by Bunn and colleagues in 1994) of 528 patients in multiple studies revealed an overall response rate of 62 percent and a complete-response rate of 32 percent, with a median duration of 3 to 22 months. However, although more data are available regarding the use of MTX than of other agents, no particular agent has been shown to have superior efficacy.[38]

Various combinations of chlorambucil, cyclophosphamide, vincristine, etoposide, doxorubicin, bleomycin, methotrexate, and prednisone have been employed in the treatment of advanced CTCL.[56] The inclusion of Adriamycin in a regimen has been associated with slightly higher rates but shorter duration of complete response.[55] Well-recognized combinations include cyclophosphamide, Adriamycin, vincristine, and prednisone (CHOP); idarubicin, etoposide, cyclophosphamide, vincristine, prednisone, and bleomycin (VICOP-B); and etoposide, vincristine, doxorubicin, cyclophosphamide, and prednisone (EPOCH). An analysis by Bunn and colleagues of 331 patients predominantly with advanced CTCL in several trials revealed an overall response rate of 81 percent and a complete-response rate of 38 percent.[38] These rates were only marginally higher than those seen with single-agent chemotherapy, and none of the patients with advanced disease were cured. In a randomized study at the National Cancer Institute, no survival advantage was seen for patients on multiagent chemotherapy as opposed to patients treated with topical NM. Furthermore, the toxicities associated with multiagent chemotherapy (particularly bone marrow suppression) were a source of significant morbidity and mortality in the multiagent chemotherapy arm. In summary, multiagent chemotherapy helps control advanced disease that has resisted skin-directed and other systemic therapies. The duration of response can be expected to range from 5 months to a few years. As no clear survival advantage has been demonstrated, the benefits in terms of quality of life and symptom control offered by multiagent chemotherapy must be weighed in each individual case against the significant toxicities and risks that such therapy carries.

Combination Therapies

Many combinations of IFN, retinoid, TSEB, and ECP therapies have been tried, and several reports have been subsequently generated. Although studies of combination therapies are not rare, very few individual combinations have been studied in large numbers of patients. Of these combinations, IFN-α therapy combined with PUVA has been shown in two small studies to yield significantly greater complete-response and overall response rates than either therapy alone. Another benefit of this combination is that it spares patients a significant amount of PUVA exposure and the concomitant dose-related increase in skin cancer risk. Interferon plus PUVA was also shown in one randomized prospective multicenter study of 98 patients to be superior to the combination of IFN and retinoids despite the observation that retinoids enhance the antiviral activity of IFN in vitro.[66,67] In this study, the IFN/PUVA group achieved a 70 per-

cent complete-response rate in a shorter period of time than did the IFN/retinoid group, which achieved a 38 percent complete-response rate.

Other promising combinations include the maintenance of TSEB-induced remission with PUVA, the combination of ECP with IFN, and the combination of electron beam therapy (EBT) and ECP. The prolongation of TSEB-induced remission by PUVA has been documented by Quiros and colleagues in a study of 114 patients with stage I disease.[68] The combination of ECP and IFN has been supported by two case reports and one small study of 31 patients with advanced disease.[69–71] A single study of 44 patients reported an 81 percent 3-year disease-free survival with a combination of ECP and TSEB therapy, compared with a 3-year disease-free survival of 49 percent with TSEB therapy alone.[72] While these combinations offer some patients an increased rate of complete response to treatment and a longer period of remission, experience with them is too limited to uniformly recommend them for a particular category of patients.

PRIMARY CUTANEOUS B-CELL LYMPHOMA

White primary cutaneous B-cell lymphomas (PCB-CLs) constitute approximately 20 to 25 percent of all cutaneous lymphomas[73,74] in European centers. Zachheim and colleagues[73] found a significantly lower frequency of 4.5 percent in US institutions. By definition, they are limited to the skin at the time of diagnosis and 6 months after. They are classified into (1) primary cutaneous follicular center cell lymphoma (PCFCCL) and marginal-zone B-cell lymphoma (MZL) (synonymous terms are mucosa-associated lymphoid tissue [MALT]–like lymphoma or primary cutaneous immunocytoma), both of which have an excellent prognosis and a 5-year survival rate of greater than 95 percent; (2) primary cutaneous large B-cell lymphoma (PCLBCL) of the leg, (3) intravascular large B-cell lymphoma, and (4) plasmacytoma. The latter three subtypes carry a more guarded prognosis, with frequent extracutaneous spread. Electron beam therapy, with either local or extended-field radiation or with orthovoltage radiation, can be used in the treatment of PCBCL; the choice of treatment depends primarily on the type of PCBCL, the number and distribution of lesions, and the age and general medical condition of the patient.[75] In the rare event of extracutaneous spread, multiagent chemotherapy is indicated. The specific regimen is guided by histologic subtype and does not differ from the general oncologic approach to lymphomas.

Radiation Therapy

Localized and extended-field electron beam radiation is an extremely effective treatment for most localized forms of primary cutaneous disease. Widespread skin involvement necessitates treatment with extended-field or orthovoltage radiation whereas localized-beam therapy is effective treatment for limited lesions. In one study that compared 55 patients with various types of PCBCLs, all 40 patients treated with radiation therapy had complete remission of their disease, with a 5-year survival rate of 89 percent. Patients with PCLBCL of the leg were disproportionately represented among the 8 patients in this group who had relapse of their disease.[76] Similar findings are reported in slightly smaller studies.[77,78] For multifocal skin disease, multiagent chemotherapy was found to offer neither higher response rates nor longer survival rates in two small series although the length of remission was slightly longer for patients with more aggressive disease who were treated with chemotherapy.[76,78]

Chemotherapy

Multiagent chemotherapy with regimens such as CHOP is employed earlier and more frequently for the more aggressive subtypes of PCBCL. In these subtypes, radiation may still be a useful first-line therapy, but recurrent disease is more often extracutaneous and is thus better addressed by chemotherapy. For advanced stages of PCBCL, chemotherapy is the treatment of choice, and radiation therapy may be useful for palliation of symptoms.

Other Therapies

The use of antibiotics in the treatment of PCBCL is based on the observation that some indolent PCBCLs

are linked to infection by *Borrelia burgdorferi*, analogous to the association of MALT-like lymphomas with *Helicobacter pylori* infection.[79-82] In patients with serologic or molecular evidence of *B. burgdorferi* infection, treatment with antibiotics may result in complete remission and should be attempted first. Subcutaneous injections of IFN-α2a have been found to induce remission of generalized lesions in a few patients. Recently, Heinzerling and colleagues reported that the injection of the anti-CD20 monoclonal antibody rituximab resulted in the dramatic resolution of lesions in two patients with recurrent disease.[83]

In conclusion, the cornerstones of the treatment of PCBCL are electron beam radiation therapy and multiagent chemotherapy, with the former playing a more palliative role in advanced disease. Antibiotics and immunomodulatory treatments, including anti-CD20 monoclonal antibody, can be helpful in select cases, and further investigation is required before they can be incorporated into standard therapy.

REFERENCES

1. Veelken J, Wood GS, Sklar J. Molecular staging of cutaneous T-cell lymphoma: evidence for systemic involvement in early disease. J Invest Dermatol 1995;104:889–94.
2. Barnes PJ, Karin M. Nuclear factor-kappa b: a pivotal transcription factor in chronic inflammatory diseases. N Engl J Med 1997 Apr 10;336:1066–71.
3. Pitzalis C, Pipitone N, Bajocchi G, et al. Corticosteroids inhibit lymphocyte binding to endothelium and intercellular adhesion. J Immunol 1997;158:5007–16.
4. Zackheim HS, Kashani-Sabet M, Amin S. Topical corticosteroids for mycosis fungoides. Arch Dermatol 1998;124:949–54.
5. Ramsay DL, Meller JA, Zackheim HS. Topical treatment of early cutaneous T-cell lymphoma. Hematol Oncol Clin North Am 1995;9:1031–56.
6. Vonderheid EC, Van Scott EJ, Johnson WC, et al. Topical chemotherapy and immunotherapy of mycosis fungoides: intermediate-term results. Arch Dermatol 1977;113:454–62.
7. Hamminga L, Herman J, Noordijk EM, et al. Cutaneous T-cell lymphoma: clinico-pathological relationships, therapy and survival in ninety-two patients. Br J Dermatol 1982;107:145–56.
8. Krutmann J, Morita A. Mechanisms of ultraviolet B and UVA phototherapy. J Investig Dermatol Symp Proc 1999;4:70–2.

9. Beissert S, Schwarz T. Mechanisms involved in ultraviolet light-induced immunosuppression. J Investig Dermatol Symp Proc 1999;4:61–4.

10. Herrmann JJ, Roenigk HH, Honigsmann H. Ultraviolet radiation for treatment of cutaneous T-cell lymphoma. Hematol Oncol Clin North Am 1995;9:1077–88.

11. Morison WL, Baughman RD, Day RD, et al. Consensus workshop on the toxic effects of long-term PUVA therapy. Arch Dermatol 1998;134:595–8.

12. Clark D, Dawe RS, Evans AT, et al. Narrowband TL-01 phototherapy for patch-stage mycosis fungoides. Arch Dermatol 2000;136:748–52.

13. Stern RS, Laird N. The carcinogenic risk of treatments for severe psoriasis. Cancer 1994;73:2759.

14. Jones GW, Hoppe RT, Glatstein E. Electron beam treatment for cutaneous T-cell lymphoma. Hematol Oncol Clin North Am 1995;9:1057–76.

15. Voss N, Kim-Sing C. Radiotherapy in the treatment of dermatologic malignancies. Dermatol Clin 1998; 16:313–20.

16. Jones G, Rosenthal D, Wilson LD. Total skin electron radiation for patients with erythrodermic cutaneous T-cell lymphoma (mycosis fungoides and the Sézary syndrome). Cancer 1999;85:1985–95.

17. Rizvi NA, Marshall JL, Dahut W, et al. A phase I study of LGD1069 in adults with advanced cancer. Clin Cancer Res 1999;5:1658–64.

18. Orfanos CE, Zouboulis CC, Almond-Roesler B, Geilen CC. Current use and future potential role of retinoids in dermatology. Drugs 1997;53:358–88.

19. Lim HW, Harris HR. Etretinate as an effective adjunctive therapy for recalcitrant palmar/plantar hyperkeratosis in patients with erythrodermic cutaneous T-cell lymphoma undergoing photopheresis. Dermatol Surg 1995;21:597–9.

20. Duvic M, Lemak NA, Redman JR, et al. Combined modality therapy for cutaneous T-cell lymphoma. J Am Acad Dermatol 1996;34:1022–9.

21. Dreno B, Claudy A, Meynadier J, et al. The treatment of 45 patients with cutaneous T-cell lymphoma with low doses of interferon-2a and etretinate. Br J Dermatol 1991;125:456–9.

22. Zachariae H, Thestrup-Pedersen K. Interferon-α and etretinate combination treatment of cutaneous T-cell lymphoma. J Invest Dermatol 1990;95:206S–8S.

23. Knobler RM, Trautinger F, Tadaszkiewica T, et al. Treatment of cutaneous T-cell lymphoma with a combination of low-dose interferon alfa-2b and retinoids. J Am Acad Dermatol 1991;24:247–52.

24. Duvic M, Cather JC. Emerging new therapies for cutaneous T-cell lymphoma. Dermatol Clin 2000;18(1): 147–56.

25. Shalita AR. Mucocutaneous and systemic toxicity of retinoids: monitoring and management. Dermatologica 1987;175 Suppl 1:151–7.

26. Sherman SI, Gopal J, Haugen BR, et al. Central hypothyroidism associated with retinoid X receptor-selective ligands. N Engl J Med 1999;340:1075–9.

27. Miller VA, Benedetti FM, Rigas JR, et al. Initial clinical trial of a selective retinoid X receptor ligand, LGD1069. J Clin Oncol 1997;15:790–5.

28. Suchin KA, Cassin M, Washko R, et al. Extracorporeal photochemotherapy does not suppress T- or B-cell responses to novel or recall antigens. J Am Acad Dermatol 1999;41:980–6.

29. Rook AH, Suchin KR, Kao DMF, et al. Photopheresis: clinical applications and mechanism of action. J Investig Dermatol Symp Proc 1999;4:85–90.

30. Lim HW, Edelson RL. Photopheresis for the treatment of cutaneous T-cell lymphoma. Hematol Oncol Clin North Am 1995;9:1117–26.

31. Marks DI, Rockman SP, Oziemski MA, Fox RM. Mechanisms of lymphotoxicity induced by extracorporeal photochemotherapy for cutaneous T-cell lymphoma. J Clin Invest 1990;86:2080–5.

32. Taylor A, Gasparro FP. Extracorporeal photochemotherapy for cutaneous T-cell lymphoma and other diseases. Semin Hematol 1992;29(2):132–41.

33. Vowels BR, Cassin M, Boufal MH, et al. Extracorporeal photochemotherapy induces the production of tumor necrosis factor-alpha by monocytes: implications for the treatment of cutaneous T-cell lymphoma and systemic sclerosis. J Invest Dermatol 1992;98:686–92.

34. Miracco C, Rubegni P, De Aloe G, et al. Extracorporeal photochemotherapy induces apoptosis of infiltrating lymphoid cells in patients with mycosis fungoides in early stages: a quantitative histological study. Br J Dermatol 1997;137:549–57.

35. Edelson R, Berger C, Gasparro F, et al. Treatment of cutaneous T-cell lymphoma by extracorporeal photochemotherapy: preliminary results. N Engl J Med 1987;316:297–303.

36. Demierre MG, Foss FM, Koh HK. Proceedings of the international consensus conference on cutaneous T-cell lymphoma treatment recommendations. J Am Acad Dermatol 1997;36:460–6.

37. Jiang SB, Dietz SB, Kim M, Lim HW. Extracorporeal photochemotherapy for cutaneous T-cell lymphoma: a 9.7-year experience. Photodermatol Photoimmunol Photomed 1999;15(5):161–5.

38. Bunn PA, Hoffman SJ, Norris D, et al. Systemic therapy of cutaneous T-cell lymphomas (mycosis fungoides and the Sézary syndrome). Ann Intern Med 1994;121:592–602.

39. Stevens SR, Bowen GM, King LE, et al. Effectiveness of photopheresis in Sezary syndrome. Arch Dermatol 1999;135:995–7.

40. Rook AH, Yoo EK, Grossman DJ, et al. Use of biological response modifiers in the treatment of cutaneous T-cell lymphoma. Curr Opin Oncol 1998;10:170–4.

41. Stadler R, Ruszczak A. Interferons: new additions and indications for use. Dermatol Clin 1993;11(1):187–99.

42. Rook AH, Gottlieb SL, Wolfe JT, et al. Pathogenesis of cutaneous T-cell lymphoma: implications for the use of recombinant cytokines and photopheresis. Clin Exp Immunol 1997;107 Suppl 1:16–20.

43. Bunn PA, Norris DA. Therapeutic role of interferons and monoclonal antibodies in cutaneous T-cell lymphomas. J Invest Dermatol 1990;95 (6 Suppl):209S–12S.

44. Springer EA, Kuzel TM, Variakojis D, et al. Correlation of clinical responses with immunologic and morphologic characteristics in patients with cutaneous T-cell lymphoma treated with interferon alfa-2a. J Am Acad Dermatol 1993;29:42–6.

45. Ross C, Tingsgaard P, Jorgensen H, Vejlsgaard GL. Interferon treatment of cutaneous T-cell lymphoma. Eur J Haematol 1993;51:63–72.

46. Olsen EA, Bunn PA. Interferon in the treatment of cutaneous T-cell lymphoma. Hematol Oncol Clin North Am 1995;9:1089–106.

47. Marolleau JP, Baccard M, Flageul B, et al. High-dose recombinant interleukin-2 in advanced cutaneous T-cell lymphoma. Arch Dermatol 1995;131:574–9.

48. Rook AH, Kubin M, Fox FE, et al. The potential therapeutic role of interleukin-12 in cutaneous T-cell lymphoma. Ann N Y Acad Sci 1996 Oct 31;795:310–8.

49. LeMaistre CF, Saleh MN, Kuzel TM, et al. Phase I trial of a ligand fusion-protein (DAB389IL-2) in lymphomas expressing the receptor for interleukin-2. Blood 1998;91:399–405.

50. Foss FM, Saleh MN, Krueger JG, et al. Diphtheria toxin fusion proteins. Curr Top Microbiol Immunol 1998;234:63–81.

51. Nichols J, Foss F, Kuzel TM, et al. Interleukin-2 fusion protein: an investigational therapy for interleukin-2 receptor expressing malignancies. Eur J Cancer 1997;33 (Suppl 1):S34–6.

52. Foss FM, Borkowski TA, Gilliom M, et al. Chimeric fusion protein toxin DAB486-IL-2 in advanced mycosis fungoides and the Sézary syndrome: correlation of activity and interleukin-2 receptor expression in a phase II study. Blood 1994;84:1765–74.

53. Saleh MN, LeMaistre CF, Kuzel TM, et al. Antitumor activity of DAB389IL-2 fusion toxin in mycosis fungoides. J Am Acad Dermatol 1998;39:63–73.

54. Olsen EA, Duvic M, Martin A, et al. Pivotal phase III trial of two dose levels of DAB-IL2 (Ontak) for the treatment of cutaneous T-cell lymphoma. J Invest Dermatol 1998;110:678 (Abstract).

55. Rosen ST, Foss FM. Chemotherapy for mycosis fungoides and the Sézary syndrome. Hematol Oncol Clin North Am 1995;9:1109–16.

56. Zackheim HS. Cutaneous T-cell lymphoma: update of treatment. Dermatology 1999;199:102–5.

57. Haynes HA, Van Scott EJ. Therapy of mycosis fungoides lymphoma. Proc Natl Cancer Conf 1970;6:553–7.

58. Zackheim H, Epstein EH. Low-dose methotrexate for the Sézary syndrome. J Am Acad Dermatol 1989; 21:757–62.

59. Zackheim HS, Kashani-Sabet M, Hwang ST. Low-dose methotrexate to treat erythrodermic cutaneous T-cell lymphoma: results in twenty-nine patients. J Am Acad Dermatol 1996;34:626–31.

60. Cummings FJ, Kim K, Neiman RS, et al. Phase III trial of pentostatin in refractory lymphomas and cutaneous T-cell disease. J Clin Oncol 1991;9:565–71.

61. Foss FM. Activity of pentostatin (Nipent) in cutaneous T-cell lymphoma: single-agent and combination studies. Semin Oncol 2000;27 (2 Suppl 5):58–63.

62. Kurzrock R, Pilat S, Duvic M. Pentostatin therapy of T-cell lymphomas with cutaneous manifestations. J Clin Oncol 1999;17:3117–21.

63. Ho AD, Suciu S, Stryckmans P, et al. Pentostatin in T-cell malignancies. Leukemia Cooperative Group and the European Organization for Research and Treatment of Cancer. Semin Oncol 2000;27(2 Suppl 5):52–7.

64. Nikko AP, Pandya AG. Successful treatment of Sézary syndrome with lymphomatous transformation to large cell lymphoma with fludarabine phosphate. Arch Dermatol 1996;132:978–9.

65. Foss FM, Kuzel TM. Experimental therapies in the treatment of cutaneous T-cell lymphoma. Hematol Oncol Clin North Am 1995;9:1125–37.

66. Stadler R, Otte HG, Luger T, et al. Prospective randomized multicenter clinical trial on the use of interferon-2a plus acitretin versus interferon-2a plus PUVA in patients with cutaneous T-cell lymphoma stages I and II. Blood 1998;92:3578–81.

67. Fox FE, Kubin M, Cassin M, et al. Retinoids synergize with interleukin-2 to augment IFN-gamma and interleukin-12 production by human peripheral blood mononuclear cells. J Interferon Cytokine Res 1999 Apr;19:407–15.

68. Quiros PA, Jones GW, Kacinski BM, et al. Total skin electron beam therapy followed by adjuvant psoralen/ultraviolet-A light in the management of patients with T1 and T2 cutaneous T-cell lymphoma (mycosis fungoides). Int J Radiat Oncol Biol Phys 1997;38:1027–35.

69. Rook AH, Prystowsky MB, Cassin M, et al. Combined therapy for Sézary syndrome with extracorporeal photochemotherapy and low-dose interferon alfa therapy: clinical, molecular, and immunologic observations. Arch Dermatol 1991;127:1535–40.

70. Haley HR, Davis DA, Sams WM. Durable loss of a malignant T-cell clone in a stage IV cutaneous T-cell lymphoma patient treated with high-dose interferon and photopheresis. J Am Acad Dermatol 1999;41:880–3.

71. Gottlieb SL, Wolfe JT, Fox FE, et al. Treatment of cutaneous T-cell lymphoma with extracorporeal photo-

pheresis monotherapy and in combination with recombinant interferon alfa: a 10-year experience at a single institution. J Am Acad Dermatol 1996; 35:946–57.

72. Wilson LD, Jones GW, Kim D, et al. Experience with total skin electron beam therapy in combination with extracorporeal photopheresis in the management of patients with erythrodermic (T4) mycosis fungoides. J Am Acad Dermatol 2000;43:54–60.

73. Burg G, Dummer R, Kerl H. Classification of cutaneous lymphomas. Dermatol Clin 1994 Apr;12(2):213–7.

74. Willemze R, Kerl H, Sterry W, et al. EORTC classification for primary cutaneous lymphomas: a proposal from the Cutaneous Lymphoma Study Group of the European Organization for Research and Treatment of Cancer. Blood 1997 Jul 1;90:354–71.

75. Zackheim HS, Vonderheid EC, Ramsay DL, et al. Relative frequency of various forms of primary cutaneous lymphomas. J Am Acad Dermatol 2000 Nov; 43(5):793–6.

76. Rijlaarsdam JU, Toonstra J, Meijer OW, et al. Treatment of primary cutaneous B-cell lymphomas of follicle center cell origin: a clinical follow-up study of 55 patients treated with radiotherapy or polychemotherapy. J Clin Oncol 1996 Feb;14:549–55.

77. Kirova YM, Piedbois Y, Le Bourgeois JP. Radiotherapy in the management of cutaneous B-cell lymphoma. Our experience in 25 cases. Radiother Oncol 1999 Jul;52(1):15–8.

78. Bekkenk MW, Vermeer MH, Geerts ML, et al. Treatment of multifocal primary cutaneous B-cell lymphoma: a clinical follow-up study of 29 patients. J Clin Oncol 1999 Aug;17:2471–8.

79. Isaacson PG, Spencer J. Is gastric lymphoma an infectious disease? Hum Pathol 1993 Jun;24:569–70.

80. Garbe C, Stein H, Dienemann D, Orfanos CE. *Borrelia burgdorferi*-associated cutaneous B cell lymphoma: clinical and immunohistologic characterization of four cases. J Am Acad Dermatol 1991Apr;24(4): 584–90.

81. Isaacson PG. Gastric lymphoma and *Helicobacter pylori*. N Engl J Med 1994 May 5;330:1310–1.

82. Wotherspoon AC, Ortiz-Hidalgo C, Falzon MR, Isaacson PG. *Helicobacter pylori*–associated gastritis and primary B-cell gastric lymphoma. Lancet 1991 Nov 9;338(8776):1175–6.

83. Heinzerling L, Dummer R, Kempf W, et al. Intralesional therapy with anti-CD20 monoclonal antibody rituximab in primary cutaneous B-cell lymphoma. Arch Dermatol 2000;136:374–8.

18

Prevention of Skin Cancer

ROBIN MARKS, MBBS, MPH, FRACP, FACD
DAVID HILL, PhD

One of the unique features of skin cancers is that the vast majority of them are easily seen in the early stages because they are on the surface of the body. For this reason, these tumors should theoretically be amenable to a public health approach to detecting them at a stage at which they might be easily cured. As well, our knowledge of causation means that it should also be possible to prevent the development of skin cancers that might otherwise occur.

PREVENTION THROUGH REDUCED EXPOSURE TO CAUSES (PRIMARY PREVENTION)

Applying Knowledge of Causation

The capacity to prevent the occurrence of a condition is determined by an understanding of its cause(s) and the ability to modify exposure to the cause(s). The causes of skin cancer are covered in Chapters 1 to 3, where it is shown that both constitutional (genetic) and environmental factors have been identified. Predominant among the causal factors are skin type (color, reaction to sunlight, tendency to develop freckles and melanocytic nevi) and exposure to solar radiation (ultraviolet radiation [UVR] predominantly in the ultraviolet B [UVB] range). Hence, the primary strategy to reduce skin cancer at a population level is to minimize exposure to the sun when UVR is most intense, particularly among those fair-skinned people who are most susceptible.

In practice, in Western industrialized countries, most people's opportunities for intense solar UVR exposure are limited to recreation in summer. This means that without taking precautions, many people will suffer repeated sunburn. Hence, the simple public health message to moderate sun exposure, particularly in summer, and sufficiently to reduce sunburn, is the one message that will do the greatest good for the greatest number of people if heeded.

Ultraviolet Radiation Varies by Time of Day and Time of Year

Ultraviolet radiation reaches the earth's surface from dawn to dusk, reaching its peak level at solar noon (1:00 pm during daylight saving time). The earth's atmosphere provides a natural barrier that filters solar UVR so that the farther UVR has to travel through the atmosphere, the less of it reaches the earth's surface. A straight line drawn from the sun to the earth's surface passes through the least thickness of atmosphere in the equatorial regions (at the equinox) whereas UVR passes through a much greater thickness of atmosphere to reach the poles. This is why UVR is most intense at the equator and diminishes as latitude increases. For the same reason, UVR levels are greater at high altitudes.

Ultraviolet radiation levels also change by time of day as the earth rotates through its axis. At solar noon, solar radiation travels the least distance to pass through the atmosphere. At either side of solar noon, there is greater rotation of the earth relative to the sun and consequently more atmosphere through which solar UVR passes before reaching the earth's surface.

The seasonal changes in the axis about which the earth rotates also affect the distance through the atmosphere that UVR must pass to reach the earth's surface. As well, the *differential* in ground level ambient UVR between latitudes is less in summer than in winter (Figure 18–1). This explains why midsummer sunburn is possible even in high latitudes.

Given the demonstrated filtering effect of the "clear" atmosphere, it is only to be expected that cloud cover (and even air pollution) over cities could reduce the UVR reaching the earth's surface. However, cloud is water vapor, which filters out proportionally more infrared radiation (heat) than UVR. This can be very deceptive because clouds reduce the temperature more than they reduce UVR, thus giving those who believe that temperature reflects the UVR risk a false sense of security. Clouds also scatter UVR; on cloudy days, there may thus be more reflected UVR from the sky than there might be from direct sunlight on a cloud-free day.

Finally, depletion of stratospheric ozone (theoretically, at least) increases UVR exposure at ground level. Fortunately, the implementation of international treaties (commencing in 1988 and progressively upgraded since then) has successfully reversed the manufacture, use, and release of ozone-depleting chemicals in the last decade, thus reversing the long-term increase in ozone depletion.

Barriers to Solar Ultraviolet Radiation

Very few materials transmit UVR without some reduction as a result of filtration or reflection by the material. Even clear 3-mm window glass blocks at least 90 percent of the UVB passing through it. Almost any opaque substance can be used as a barrier to prevent or reduce the amount of UVR reaching the skin. Some materials are better than others, but in general, the more opaque the material (ie, the less visible light it transmits), the better a UVR filter it will be.

Clothing

The most obvious and efficient barrier for personal use is clothing, and clothed areas of skin are effectively protected in most instances. Exceptions may occur when loosely woven fabrics that transmit UVR are worn. Under test conditions, some loosely woven fabrics have been found to transmit up to 20 percent of erythemal UVR.[1] But the majority of summer fabrics that are tested are very effective barriers.[1] An important finding is that fabrics transmit more UVR when wet than when dry, particularly loosely woven fabrics. Thus, the quality of clothing worn during water activities is important for most people. Most of the time, the amount of UVR that reaches skin through clothing is probably negligible. The main points to be understood about clothing for sun protection are when and under what conditions it is important to wear it.

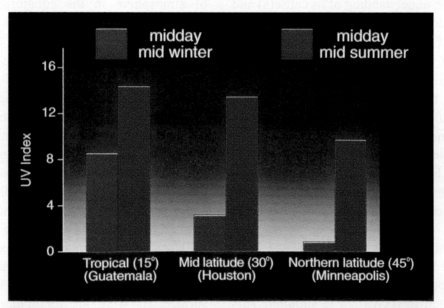

Figure 18–1. Variation in midsummer and midwinter midday ultraviolet (UV) radiation levels depends on latitude.

A hat can protect the scalp; it can also protect the face and the neck, as long as the face and neck remain shaded by the hat. Figure 18–2 provides an indication of the level of protection given to the face by hats with varying brim sizes. A factor to consider in assessing the effectiveness of hats is the amount of reflected UVR reaching the face.

Shade provided by opaque manufactured materials, such as roofs and walls of buildings, and "natural" shade, such as the foliage of trees, block or reduce solar UVR. However, it is possible for UVR to be reflected off concrete, turbulent water, snow, and buildings and thus to reach the skin indirectly. While it is easy to understand why and how shade reduces UVR exposure, it is not so obvious how much the combination of shade and appropriate activity scheduling would reduce UVR exposure. A person who plays a 4-hour game of golf between 10:00 am and 2:00 pm (solar time) on a clear midsummer day will receive at least five times the UVR exposure that will be received by a person who plays the first nine holes between 8:00 am and 10:00 am and completes the round between 2:00 pm and 4:00 pm.

Chemical Sunscreens

When clothing, natural shade, and scheduling are not appropriate or possible, chemical sunscreens can provide considerable protection. These products are divided into absorbents and reflectants. The reflectants tend to reduce radiation across the whole of the solar spectrum whereas the absorbents work predominantly in the UVR range (Table 18–1).

The relative efficacy of the chemical absorbents is measured in the laboratory, and a sun protection factor (SPF) grading is given. This figure is derived from the proportional increase in the amount of erythemal UVR required to produce minimal erythema in human volunteers when a sunscreen is applied as compared to the amount of UVR required when their skin is unprotected. For example, a product that requires four times the amount of UVR needed to produce minimal erythema in unprotected skin is labeled SPF 4. Looked at in another way, an SPF-4 sunscreen filters out 75 percent of incident UVR (Figure 18–3).

It can be seen from Figure 18–3 that there is relatively little increase in filtration of UVR for very large increases in SPF after an SPF of around 10 (90% filtration) is reached. Most health organizations recommend an SPF of at least 15 to allow for inadequate application, which substantially reduces the efficacy of the product. In fact, the most frequent reason for sunscreen failure (ie, a person getting burnt while using one) is lack of adequate application, rather than inadequate SPF activity.

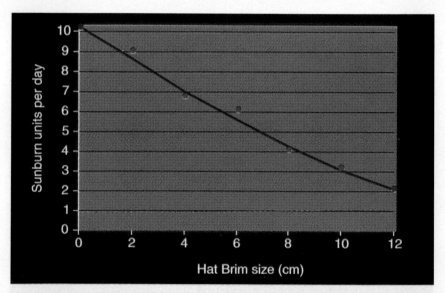

Figure 18–2. Reduction in erythemal ultraviolet B (UVB) (sunburn units) to the head and neck with increasing brim size on hats. (Data from Dr. W. Ryman, Skin and Cancer Foundation, Sydney, Australia)

Table 18–1. COMMONLY USED SUNSCREEN CHEMICALS

Physical blockers(reflectants)
  Zinc oxide
  Talc
  Titanium dioxide
  Red petrolatum

Chemical absorbers
  UVB absorbers
    Salicylates
      Octyl salicylate
      Homosalate
    Cinnamates
      Octyl and isoamyl methoxycinnamate
    Camphor derivatives
      4-Methylbenzylidene
      Camphor
    Aminobenzoates
      Aminobenzoic acid (PABA)
      Padimate O (octyl dimethyl PABA)
      Methyl anthranilate
  UVA absorbers
    Benzophenones*
      Benzophenone-6
      Oxybenzone
    Dibenzoylmethanes
      Dibenzoylmethane
      Avobenzone (butylmethoxydibenzoylmethane)

*Benzophenones absorb in the UVB, UVA, and UVC ranges.
UVA = ultraviolet A; UVB = ultraviolet B; UVC = ultraviolet C.

One of the traps in promoting sunscreens is the tendency to relate their efficacy to "sunburn times." For example, some people have suggested that the use of a product with an SPF of X will allow people to remain X times longer in the sun before sunburn occurs. Unfortunately, the dose of radiation received outdoors is not a constant as it is in the laboratory under product-testing conditions. Time of day, time of year, cloud cover, latitude, altitude, atmospheric particulate matter, UVR reflection, natural skin color, and epidermal thickness all make a difference to the UVR dose received and thus to the likelihood of sunburn occurring at any particular time. (It would require chaos theory for an individual to work out their own "sunburn time" at a given moment!) Thus, it is misleading (and possibly risky) to recommend the use of SPF numbers as a way to calculate how much time one could spend outdoors without burning.

Irritant contact dermatitis from sunscreens is common, particularly around the eyes and on the often hairy forearms of men. However, true allergic contact dermatitis to a sunscreen's active chemicals is rare; when it does occur, it is most commonly due to either the preservatives or the perfumes in the products.

Studies of Sun-Related Behavior

Given that solar UVR exposure is so clearly determined by individual actions, the study of "sun-related" behavior assists in developing public health promotion strategies to reduce skin cancer. Sun-related behavior has been defined as "any behavior that increases or decreases the exposure of skin or eyes to solar UVR."[2] It can include the use of cloth-

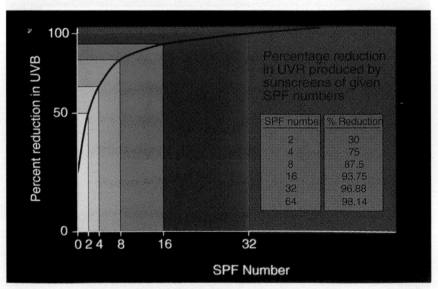

Figure 18–3. Reduction in ultraviolet radiation (UVR) with increasing sun protection factor (SPF) number, showing an exponential relationship.

ing and hats, the use of sunscreens, shade-seeking activity, scheduling, and even the choice of latitude and altitude for locating home, work, or recreation.

Most studies of sun-related behavior have relied upon self-reporting methods, but objective measures have also been used.[3] Patches that are sensitive to UVR can be worn on the skin throughout the day to quantify exposure. The objectivity of such measures is somewhat offset by the possibility that recruiting research subjects to wear such patches sensitizes the subjects and thereby influences the way they behave (the "Hawthorne effect"). This would be a problem if one were attempting to study naturally occurring sun-related behavior.

Studies of sun-related behavior fall into two broad categories: those designed to understand its correlates and determinants through cross-sectional surveys and occasional longitudinal studies and those that attempt to intervene to induce change in sun-related behavior. Knowledge of correlates or risk factors assists in directing interventions to those most in need (eg, certain age groups) and in changing determinants that are modifiable in principle (eg, misbeliefs about sun protection).

To test interventions, appropriate outcome measures (dependent variables) need to be specified. Ultimately, of course, changes in skin cancer incidence or mortality are what is of interest, but more short-term measures are needed to guide ongoing prevention research. Self-reported recent sunburn has been used as an intermediate marker of skin cancer risk.[2] Sunburn is a measure of biologically active sunlight reaching the skin. It correlates highly with ambient UVR levels and is person specific in that it depends on the skin phenotype, the degree of melanization (natural and acquired), the degree of epidermal thickening, and the amount of applied protection.

Using sunburn as the outcome variable in a multivariate analysis of data collected from sample surveys throughout an Australian summer, researchers evolved a picture of the determinants of sunburn.[2] Table 18–2 shows the multiple causes of harmful levels of sun exposure. Ambient solar UVR plays an important role (linear relationship), but the relationship between temperature and sunburn was curvilinear, suggesting that people were cued to take precautions when the temperature outdoors was very high. The period of highest sunburn occurrence was midsummer, followed by early summer—a warning that people may get inadvertently sunburned early in the summer season. Sunburn was most common at younger ages. In this study, there was little gender difference. Skin type was a major determinant—despite evidence from elsewhere that people with highly sensitive skin are the greatest users of protective clothing, hats, and sunscreens. Important, the study showed that the body exposure index (a composite measure of coverage and time spent outside) co-determines the risk of sunburn. That is, at a population level, behavioral differences *do* affect risk.

Table 18–2. PREDICTORS OF WEEKEND SUNBURN IN SUMMER: VICTORIA, AUSTRALIA, 1989			
Variable	Odds Ratio	Variable	Odds Ratio
UVR	(2.10)*	Age (yr)	
3 pm temperature (°C)		14–19	1.00
18°	1.00	20–29	0.65
19–22°	2.24*	30–39	0.56*
23–27°	2.21*	40–54	0.52*
28°+	1.35	55+	0.33*
Season		Skin type	
Early summer	1.00	Highly sensitive	1.00
Midsummer	1.53	Moderately sensitive	0.79
Late summer	0.67	Not sensitive	0.28*
Sex			
Male	1.00	Body exposure index	(1.12)*
Female	0.90		

*p < .05 for difference between 1.
( ) treated in analysis as a continuous variable.
UVR = ultraviolet radiation.

Can Sun-Related Behaviors Be Changed?

A number of intervention studies have shown that it is possible to change sun-related behavior through health education and broader health promotion strategies. More interventions aimed at changing the behavior of children and their caregivers seem to have been evaluated than those aimed at adults.[4] The examples below illustrate the range of target populations, settings, and techniques that have been investigated.

Caregivers to Infants

Rodrigue[5] recruited mothers of infants and children aged 6 months to 10 years into a program to increase skin cancer knowledge and promote healthier "sun-safe" attitudes, beliefs, and behavior toward sun exposure. Mothers who received a comprehensive educational intervention showed significant improvements over a 12-week period.

Schoolchildren

Over a period of 3 years, a school-based intervention was tested among students in grades 8 to 10 in a study in Queensland, Australia.[6] Among these students, the greatest improvement was found in knowledge; effects on sun-protection behavior were minimal and not sustained, suggesting the need to complement school health education with community activities and structural changes to the physical and social environments that affect sun protection.

Swimming-Pool Patrons

Lombard and colleagues trained lifeguards at community swimming pools to model and advocate sun-protection behaviors while on duty.[7] Observation at the end of the intervention period showed significant effects on patron behavior.

Vacationers

In Australian and UK settings, Segan and Dey and their respective colleagues[8,9] attempted to educate holiday travelers heading for sunny destinations about sun-protection practices and followed up subjects upon their return from vacation. Minimal effects were found at best, suggesting that more intensive interventions at such holiday destinations would be needed to supplement predeparture "inoculative" approaches.

Outdoor Workers

Borland and colleagues[10] allocated outdoor telecommunications workers to receive sun-protection messages (or not) at their base depots and unobtrusively observed the shirt- and hat-wearing behavior of workers at outdoor workplaces in summer. Workers based at depots where the educational messages had been in place were observed to be better protected than those based at control depots.

Inhabitants of Seaside Communities

Miller and colleagues[11] implemented a community program in a US eastern seaboard population, in which the emphasis was mainly on solar protection for children. They found that a combination of community activism, publicity campaigns, and behavioral interventions was associated with improved sun-protection knowledge, attitudes, and practices in parents, caregivers, and children.

Whole Populations

Hill and colleagues[12] showed that over the first 2 years of SunSmart community health promotion campaigns, compared to baseline, the population of Victoria, Australia held increasingly favorable beliefs and attitudes toward sun protection, showed high levels of sun-protection behavior and, important, had a significantly reduced incidence of summer weekend sunburn, after controlling for ambient UVR levels and other potential confounding factors on the days when behavioral measures were taken.

Have Prevention Programs Reduced Skin Cancer Rates?

No data from controlled trials are available to demonstrate that programs to change behavior reduce skin cancer at a population level. However, trials of sunscreen use have shown that sunscreens reduce the incidence of actinic keratosis and squamous cell carcinoma (SCC).[13,14] As well, Australian trends in the incidence rates of melanoma and non-melanoma skin cancer suggest that Australian prevention programs are having an effect.[15,16] Reductions in age-specific incidence rates are occurring in the younger age groups, where the effects of reductions in population exposure to an environmental carcinogen (such as UVR) would first be observed.

PREVENTION THROUGH EARLY DETECTION (SECONDARY PREVENTION)

Screening for Skin Cancer: General Principles

The public health approach to early detection (secondary prevention) involves the ability to detect abnormalities that might suggest the need for further investigation and possibly treatment, all of which implies screening. Screening relies on the following general principles, many of which apply to skin cancers.

The Incidence Should Be High

As reported earlier in this book, the criterion of high incidence certainly applies to melanoma, SCC, and basal cell carcinoma (BCC) in the United States and many other countries where there is a fair-skinned population that is exposed to a hot sunny climate.

The Disease Causes Considerable Morbidity and Mortality

Once again, a previous chapter on the epidemiology of skin cancer confirms that this is indeed the case with skin cancer.

Early Treatment of the Disease Can Reduce the Associated Morbidity and/or Mortality

Morbidity related to tumor invasion can occur in areas such as the nose, the eyelid, the lips, and the ear, where both the tumor and the therapeutic approach to removal can be associated with not only extensive tissue loss but also possibly compromised

function. Thus, early treatment should prevent unnecessary morbidity.

The case survival rate from SCC is high because the vast majority of tumors are detected at a very early stage. The mortality rate has been falling in recent decades.[17] This has been attributed to the increased accessibility and use of medical services and the consequent treatment of these tumors at an earlier stage.

For melanoma, long-term follow-up studies have clearly established that survival can be influenced by treatment when the tumor is thin.[18] Thus, melanoma fits well with the concept that early treatment can reduce both morbidity and mortality. In fact, some people have questioned whether some of the very favorable outcomes from early treatment of melanoma may be because the tumors being treated, although they are invasive tumors, have no metastatic potential at the time they are removed.[19] This leads to the next principle of screening.

The Natural History of the Tumors Should Be Known

In general, BCCs are slowly growing tumors that enlarge over a period of years. On the other hand, SCCs generally tend to enlarge over a period of months once they become clinically apparent. The natural history of melanoma appears to be variable although there are very few data of good quality available as bases for assessment. The growth pattern of melanoma may vary; tumors that grow relatively slowly over months to a year or more in a thin stage (the lateral-growth phase) may enter a more rapidly growing deeply invasive phase (the vertical-growth phase). This tends to be the case with the superficial spreading melanomas. On the other hand, primary nodular melanomas may enter the vertical-growth phase and become deeply invasive within months.

Other public health pointers in natural history include characteristic signs of each of these tumors, which may indicate to those affected the need to consult a physician. For both BCC and SCC, the classic description is that of a red scaling lesion that is not healing and that is increasing in size. In the case of a very slow growing BCC that is predominantly infiltrating, there may not be easily describable characteristics. In the early stages, an SCC may resemble an actinic keratosis. This creates problems of specificity in the clinical descriptions that might be promoted to the public.

Actinic keratosis occurs far more commonly than true invasive SCC, in a ratio of between 500:1 and 1,000:1. On the other hand, actinic keratosis has been shown to be a risk factor for all skin cancers and may be of value as part of a screening program in identifying those people who are at high risk for true invasive skin cancer and who need to be carefully examined.[20]

For both superficial spreading and lentigo maligna melanoma, the acronym "ABCDE" has been promoted to indicate the clinical signs of early tumors. A stands for asymmetry, B for border irregularity, C for color variegation, and DE for diameter enlarging (Table 18–3). A seven-point checklist refining the clinical characteristics to major and minor signs has been produced for medical practitioners. Of these characteristics, border irregularity was shown to be the most powerful predictor of melanoma although it had a positive predictive value of only 13 percent.[21]

The ABCDE formula applies to the clinical signs of a pigmented lesion that might be of concern. One of the most powerful predictors of malignancy for melanoma, as it is for all skin cancers, is a recent change in the appearance of the suspected lesion. However, this is difficult to quantify.

Because of the rapidly invasive nature of nodular melanomas, they contribute proportionally more to mortality data than do the superficial spreading or lentigo maligna melanomas. The latter two melanoma types are, of course, more suitable tumors for screening than the former.

There is an Acceptable, Safe, Noninvasive Screening Test that is not Expensive

For skin cancer, the screening test is physical inspection, either by eye or assisted by a dermatoscope (in the case of pigmented lesions). There has also been recent interest in computerized digital imaging as a way of recording and assessing pigmented lesions. The use of standardized photographs for comparison studies has been promoted for following up people with a large number of pigmented lesions.

Table 18–3. CLINICAL SIGNS OF EARLY MELANOMA	
Acronym Component	Meaning
A	Asymmetrical lesion
B	Border irregularity
C	Color variegation within the lesion
DE	Diameter enlarging

Visual inspection in screening involves inspection by the individuals themselves (ie, skin self-examination) or inspection by a professional. The professional may be a medical practitioner, either a generalist or a specialist trained in skin cancer. Other professional observers have included nurse practitioners, pharmacists, and others who might have an opportunity to inspect the skin in detail, such as physiotherapists and other manipulative therapists, occupational therapists, and even people such as hairdressers. Under these conditions, the screening is the mere detection of some abnormality that requires attention from a medical practitioner rather than the making of a specific diagnosis.

Professional screening includes surveillance of groups that are at very high risk of skin cancer; opportunistic screening of people who consult the medical professional for another reason; population-based screening; and the availability of highly specific skin cancer or pigmented-lesion clinics that people at risk can either attend of their own volition or be referred to by a medical practitioner.

Self-Examination

A variety of techniques for self-examination of skin have been recommended, such as the American Cancer Society's technique illustrated in Figure 18–4. There have been no studies that demonstrate the effi-

Table 18–4. SCREENING APPROACHES FOR EARLY DETECTION OF SKIN CANCER	
Self-screening	Regular self-examination of skin
Opportunistic screening (case finding)	Sporadic examination of patients (particularly elderly) who present for another medical reason
Surveillance	Regular examination of individuals with previously demonstrated very high risk of skin cancer
Mass screening	Regular population-based screening of normal asymptomatic individuals

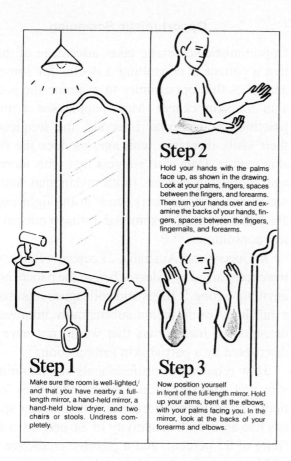

Step 1

Make sure the room is well-lighted, and that you have nearby a full-length mirror, a hand-held mirror, a hand-held blow dryer, and two chairs or stools. Undress completely.

Step 2

Hold your hands with the palms face up, as shown in the drawing. Look at your palms, fingers, spaces between the fingers, and forearms. Then turn your hands over and examine the backs of your hands, fingers, spaces between the fingers, fingernails, and forearms.

Step 3

Now position yourself in front of the full-length mirror. Hold up your arms, bent at the elbows, with your palms facing you. In the mirror, look at the backs of your forearms and elbows.

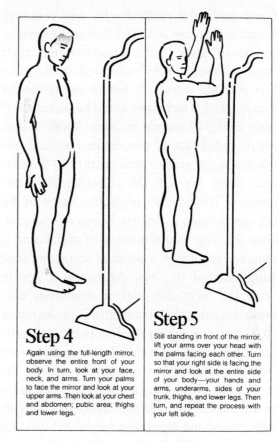

Step 4

Again using the full-length mirror, observe the entire front of your body. In turn, look at your face, neck, and arms. Turn your palms to face the mirror and look at your upper arms. Then look at your chest and abdomen; pubic area; thighs and lower legs.

Step 5

Still standing in front of the mirror, lift your arms over your head with the palms facing each other. Turn so that your right side is facing the mirror and look at the entire side of your body—your hands and arms, underarms, sides of your trunk, thighs, and lower legs. Then turn, and repeat the process with your left side.

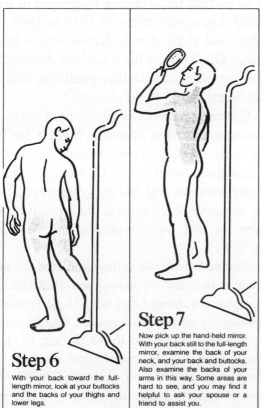

Step 6

With your back toward the full-length mirror, look at your buttocks and the backs of your thighs and lower legs.

Step 7

Now pick up the hand-held mirror. With your back still to the full-length mirror, examine the back of your neck, and your back and buttocks. Also examine the backs of your arms in this way. Some areas are hard to see, and you may find it helpful to ask your spouse or a friend to assist you.

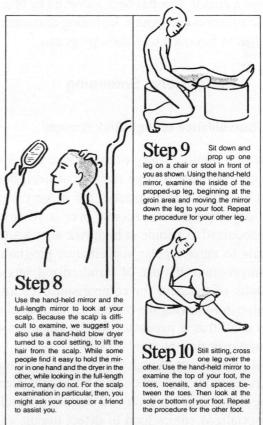

Step 8

Use the hand-held mirror and the full-length mirror to look at your scalp. Because the scalp is difficult to examine, we suggest you also use a hand-held blow dryer turned to a cool setting, to lift the hair from the scalp. While some people find it easy to hold the mirror in one hand and the dryer in the other, many do not. For the scalp examination in particular, then, you might ask your spouse or a friend to assist you.

Step 9

Sit down and prop up one leg on a chair or stool in front of you as shown. Using the hand-held mirror, examine the inside of the propped-up leg, beginning at the groin area and moving the mirror down the leg to your foot. Repeat the procedure for your other leg.

Step 10

Still sitting, cross one leg over the other. Use the hand-held mirror to examine the top of your foot, the toes, toenails, and spaces between the toes. Then look at the sole or bottom of your foot. Repeat the procedure for the other foot.

Figure 18–4.   The American Cancer Society's recommended method of skin self-examination.

cacy of any particular method with any certainty. Berwick and colleagues reported that self-examination may be of some value in identifying early melanomas although they admitted that more research is probably necessary before any particular skin self-examination technique could be promoted.[22]

A study of 1,344 people in New South Wales, Australia, recorded that 12 percent had noticed one or more signs suggestive of abnormality in the previous year, using the ABCDE classification mentioned above.[23] The positive predictive value of the ABCDE classification in that study was 4.2 percent.

Because the true natural history of melanoma is not known, we are not in a position to recommend a screening interval (ie, how frequently a person should examine their skin with a structured self-examination technique). Nevertheless, in Australia (which has never recommended a particular self-examination technique nor a specific screening interval for self-examination), a substantial shift in the detection of early melanoma among the population has been effected by merely increasing the individual's awareness of the signs that might indicate the need to see a doctor. This has been achieved by ongoing public awareness programs, including dramatized case studies in top-rated television programs.

Professional Screening

Surveillance of High-Risk Groups

People with a family history of melanoma and dysplastic nevi who have a large number of nevi, both common acquired and dysplastic, are at very high risk for developing a melanoma over a lifetime. Being recognized as people at high risk allows such individuals to enter regular surveillance programs. In such a program, the use of standardized sets of photographs of the nevi for comparison over time are of value in following the patient. One set of photographs is all that is necessary for the detection of any change over time at regular visits.

As yet, there is not enough information to be sure of the screening interval although most people attend screening programs at 6- to 12-month intervals. These specialized clinics tend to detect tumors earlier than such tumors might otherwise be detected.

Opportunistic Screening

Opportunistic screening takes advantage of the fact that a patient is consulting a doctor for something and takes that opportunity to examine the patient's skin for skin cancer. Most people see a medical practitioner at regular intervals; the frequency of their visits increases with age, as does the risk of skin cancer. Data also suggest that with increasing age, more skin cancers (both melanomas and nonmelanoma skin cancers) occur in the light-exposed areas that are easily examined during a normal medical consultation.[24,25]

In Queensland, Australia, 23 percent of melanomas were recognized by a doctor before the patient noticed anything wrong.[26] Rigel and colleagues reported that a full body examination substantially improved the detection of melanomas that would not have been discovered by a partial skin examination.[27]

How reliable are professionals at examining the skin and detecting skin cancer under these conditions? It has been reported that skin cancer specialists had an overall sensitivity of 81 percent, a specificity of 99 percent, and a positive predictive value of 73 percent for detecting melanoma in a hospital-based skin cancer clinic in 1955 to 1982.[28] On the other hand, inspection by dermatologists in the "skin cancer fairs" run by the American Academy of Dermatology showed a positive predictive value for dermatologists of 35 to 40 percent.[29]

Correct diagnosis (positive predictive value) of nonmelanoma skin cancer is highest for BCC (on the order of 90 percent for dermatologists) but is substantially lower for SCC, for which the positive predictive value was just over 50 percent.[30] For family medical practitioners, the positive predictive value for BCC was 68 percent and was 15 percent for SCC.[30]

Cassileth and colleagues simulated the diagnostic situation in a task involving the classification of photographs and showed that only 38 percent of nondermatologists correctly diagnosed four or more of six melanomas, compared to 92 percent of dermatologists.[31] Only 42 percent of nondermatologists could identify dysplastic nevi, compared to 96 percent of dermatologists. These differences in the ability to diagnose for melanoma and other pigmented lesions between specialists and others less well trained have been noted in a variety of studies over time. Thus, although opportunistic screening (or case finding) does seem attractive, its effectiveness depends very much on the level of training as well as the desire of the individual practitioners to undertake it in practice.

Population-Based Screening

As yet, there are no published data regarding the cost-effectiveness of population-based screening for either nonmelanoma skin cancer or melanoma, even in Australia, which has the highest rate of skin cancer in the world (Figure 18–5). The American Academy of Der-

matology, in association with the American Cancer Society, has had annual skin cancer fairs since 1985. Dermatologists screen members of the population, who attend on a voluntary basis. An evaluation of 4,458 persons who may have had melanoma showed a positive predictive value of 17 percent under these screening conditions.[32] Of those persons with a confirmed melanoma, 39 percent indicated that without the free program they would not have considered having a physician examine their skin.

Unfortunately, these fairs do not constitute true population-based screening. Carefully controlled population-based screening requires the recruitment

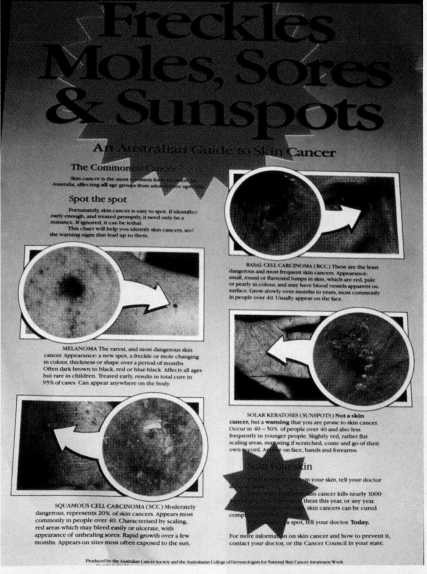

Figure 18–5. Poster placed in pharmacies and other places in Australia, recommending self-examination of the skin and what to look for. (Reproduced with permission from the Anti-Cancer Council of Victoria.)

of all of the population at risk, not just those who might see or hear an advertisement or decide they need their skin checked. As yet, no one has been able to evaluate a system in which the whole population has been involved. Such an evaluation would mean analyzing not only what tumors were detected, but also how many people received unnecessary medical attention, the cost of administering such a screening program, and whether the program were likely to affect current mortality rates in the community in the long-term.

Technology-Assisted Screening

The main role of technology in assisting or improving the diagnosis has been with pigmented tumors. The most widely promoted and used instrument is the dermatoscope (Figure 18–6), used in epiluminescence microscopy.[33] This is a technique that reduces the air-skin interface by applying oil to the skin and allows inspection of the subcorneal epidermis and dermis with an illuminated magnification instrument. Characteristic melanocytic patterns for benign lesions are well described, as are features suggesting risk of malignancy, such as radial streaming, pseudopods, dots and globules, blue/white veil, and asymmetrical pigmentary patterns (Figures 18–7 to 18–10). Whole books are written on this subject and are recommended to those who are likely to use the dermatoscope on a regular basis.[33]

Diagnostic accuracy has been shown to be reduced (even among dermatologists) when clinicians are initially using the instrument and have not been specially trained in its use.[34] Following spe-

cialized training, diagnostic accuracy has been reported to improve to slightly better than visual inspection when used by dermatologists. However,

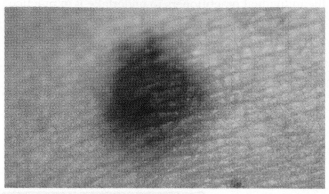

Figure 18–7. A benign melanocytic nevus, seen clinically. (Courtesy of Dr. John Kelly, Melbourne)

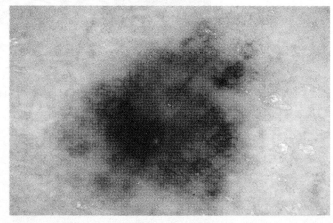

Figure 18–8. A benign melanocytic nevus, seen by epiluminescence microscopy. (Courtesy of Dr. John Kelly, Melbourne)

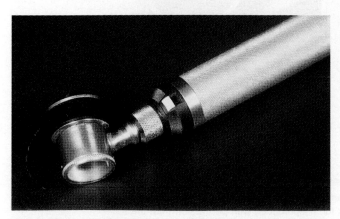

Figure 18–6. The dermatoscope (epiluminescent microscope).

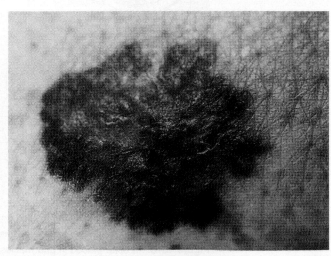

Figure 18–9. A superficially spreading melanoma, seen clinically. (Courtesy of Dr. John Kelly, Melbourne)

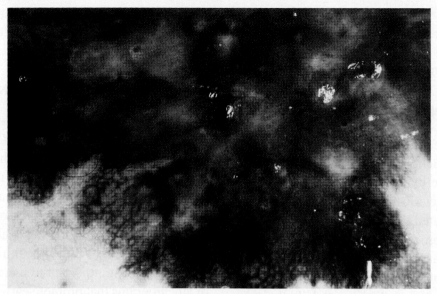

Figure 18–10. A superficially spreading melanoma, seen by epiluminescence microscopy. (Courtesy of Dr. John Kelly, Melbourne)

its main role for the vast majority of physicians who now use it appears to be in excluding malignancy rather than in detecting it.

Epiluminescence microscopy has been used for images that have been digitalized in many computerized imaging systems that are being developed and used in a number of countries (Figure 18–11). Numerous software programs that analyze particular features of the digitalized images are being developed. They are used in two ways. The initial use is in determining, on a single view, the likelihood of a

particular lesion being malignant and therefore requiring excision. A variety of software computing techniques have been used for image analysis, including neural networks, to improve both sensitivity and specificity in the detection of melanoma. The second use is in comparing the same lesion in a person over time—in other words, looking for evidence of change. With the increasing sophistication and understanding of computerized image analysis, the possibility of increased sensitivity to change while maintaining a high level of specificity at the same

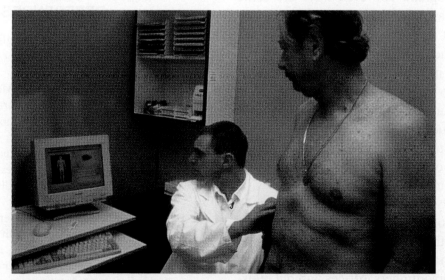

Figure 18–11. Digitalized computer imaging of epiluminescence microscopy used in the diagnosis of melanoma. (Courtesy of Dr. Harald Kittler, Vienna)

time is very attractive. This technology is still in the development phase, and despite a number of particular systems being promoted at a commercial level, their role remains rather tentative.

EVALUATION OF EARLY DETECTION

The long-term outcome of successful early detection programs is a reduction in the morbidity and mortality related to the tumors that are being detected. As pointed out previously, morbidity includes not only morbidity related directly to the tumor but also that related to the procedures required for treatment.

The earliest changes include an increase in public knowledge about skin cancer and the need to seek attention when an abnormality is noted. At the same time, there should be an increase in the knowledge and skill of medical practitioners regarding the correct diagnosis and treatment of skin cancer.

Where data are collected, a successful program will lead initially to an artificial increase in the incidence of tumors as more people attend for treatment.[35] For melanoma, this may be manifest also as an increasing proportion of people having tumors removed in the early thin curable stage and a decreasing proportion (and absolute number) having thick tumors treated. Eventually, a decrease in mortality due to both melanoma and SCC will be recorded if the program is successful.

These are the positive outcomes of a successful early detection program. However, there are some other potential measures of outcome that need to be taken into account as a balance to the positive outcomes. These include measures of the costs of a program, both to the individual and to the community. There also needs to be an assessment of cost in terms of the number of unnecessary procedures that occur as a result of an education program (ie, the number of benign lesions removed). Another cost is personal cost in anxiety or other forms of distress caused by the treatment of malignant and benign lesions.

Where mortality is involved, cost-benefit can be expressed as the cost of a life saved or person-years of life saved. In the treatment of lesions such as BCC (which are not lethal and many of which are treated in private practitioners' offices without registration of the tumor), assessment of outcome can be difficult and may require specifically designed community-based prospective studies evaluating the effect of education programs.

CONCLUSION

There is much that can be done to prevent problems related to melanoma, SCC, and BCC. The superficial nature of these tumors makes them susceptible to early detection, but since they are not symptomatic in their early stages, they do not attract expert attention except through vigilance and/or organization on the part of the public and the medical profession. From the point of view of public health and resource allocation, it is most important to increase the specificity of any programs that promote early diagnosis, lest too much unnecessary concern and cost be precipitated. As always, prevention is better than cure, so programs to reduce solar UVR exposure should also receive support, particularly as these have been estimated to be highly cost-effective.[36] Behavioral studies suggest that while specific interventions with target groups can be effective in the short term at least, comprehensive ongoing public programs that involve relevant professionals (physicians, teachers, recreational staff, etc), structural change (shade structures, policy development [such as rescheduling outdoor activity], etc), community development and resourcing, and campaigns in the mass media will be necessary to succeed in reducing the incidence of skin cancer.

REFERENCES

1. Gies HP, Roy CR, Elliott G, Zongli W. Ultraviolet radiation protection factors (UPF) for clothing. Health Phys 1994;67:131–9.
2. Hill D, White V, Marks R, et al. Melanoma prevention: behavioural and non-behavioural factors in sunburn among an Australian urban population. Prev Med 1992;21:654–69.
3. Hill D, Borland R. Methodological issues in research on primary and secondary prevention of malignant melanoma. In: Mackie RM, editor. Pigment cell 11. Basel: Karger; 1996. p. 1–21.
4. Buller DB, Borland R. Skin cancer prevention for children: a critical review. Health Educ Behav 1999; 26:317–43.
5. Rodrigue JR. Promoting healthier behaviors, attitudes, and beliefs toward sun exposure in parents of young children. J Consult Clin Psychol 1996;64:1431–6.

6. Lowe JB, Balanda KP, Stanton WR, Gillespie A. Evaluation of a three-year school-based intervention to increase adolescent sun protection. Health Educ Behav 1999;26:396–408.

7. Lombard D, Neubauer TE, Canfield D, Winett RA. Behavioral and community intervention to reduce the risk of skin cancer. J Appl Behav Anal 1991; 24:677–86.

8. Segan CJ, Borland R, Hill DJ. Development and evaluation of a brochure on sun protection and sun exposure for tourists. Health Educ J 1999;58:177–91.

9. Dey P, Collins S, Will S, Woodman C. Randomised controlled trial assessing effectiveness of health education leaflets in reducing evidence of sunburn. BMJ 1995;311:1062–3.

10. Borland R, Hocking B, Godkin G, et al. The impact of a skin cancer control educational package for outdoor workers. Med J Aust 1991;154:686–8.

11. Miller DR, Geller AC, Wood MC, et al. The Falmouth Safe Skin project: evaluation of a community program to promote sun protection in youth. Health Educ Behav 1999;26:369–84.

12. Hill D, White V, Marks R, Borland R. Changes in sun-related attitudes and behaviours and reduced sunburn prevalence in a population at high risk of melanoma. Eur J Cancer Prev 1993;2:447–56.

13. Thompson SC, Jolley D, Marks R. Reduction of solar keratoses by regular sunscreen use. N Engl J Med 1993;329:1147–51.

14. Green A, Williams G, Neale R, et al. Daily sunscreen application and betacarotene supplementation in prevention of basal-cell and squamous-cell carcinomas of the skin: a randomised controlled trial. Lancet 1999;354:723–9.

15. Giles G, Armstrong BK, Burton RC, et al. Has mortality from melanoma stopped rising in Australia? Analysis of trends between 1931 and 1994. BMJ 1996;312:1121–5.

16. Staples M, Marks R, Giles G. Skin cancer trends in Australia 1985–1995: evidence of the effectiveness of sun protection campaigns. Int J Cancer 1998; 78:144–8.

17. Weinstock MA. Non-melanoma skin cancer mortality in the United States, 1969 through 1988. Arch Dermatol 1993;129:1286–90.

18. Breslow A. Thickness, cross-sectional areas and depth of invasion in the prognosis of cutaneous melanoma. Ann Surg 1970;172:902–8.

19. Burton RC, Armstrong BK. Recent incidence trends imply a nonmetastasizing form of invasive melanoma. Melanoma Res 1994;4:107–13.

20. Frost CA, Green AC. Epidemiology of solar keratoses. Br J Dermatol 1994;131:455–64.

21. Keefe M, Dick DC, Wakeel RA. A study of the value of the seven-point checklist in distinguishing benign pigmented lesions from melanoma. Clin Exp Dermatol 1990;15:167–71.

22. Berwick M, Begg CB, Fine JA, et al. Screening for cutaneous melanoma by skin self-examination. J Natl Cancer Inst 1996;88:17–23.

23. Hennrikus D, Girgis A, Redman S, Sanson-Fisher RW. A community study of delay in presenting with signs of melanoma to medical practitioners. Arch Dermatol 1991;127:356–61.

24. Rosenblatt L, Marks R. Deaths due to squamous cell carcinoma in Australia: is there a case for a public health intervention? Australas J Dermatol 1996; 37:26–9.

25. Hersey P, Sillar RW, Hawe CG, et al. Factors related to the presentation of patients with thick primary melanomas. Med J Aust 1991;154:583–7.

26. Green A. Incidence and reporting of cutaneous melanoma in Queensland. Australas J Dermatol 1982;23:105–9.

27. Rigel DS, Friedman RJ, Kopf AW, et al. Importance of complete cutaneous examination for the detection of malignant melanoma. J Am Acad Dermatol 1986; 14:857–60.

28. Grin CM, Kopf AW, Welkovich B, et al. Accuracy in clinical diagnosis of malignant melanoma. Arch Dermatol 1990;126:763–6.

29. Koh HK, Caruso A, Gage I, et al. Evaluation of melanoma/skin cancer screening in Massachusetts: preliminary results. Cancer 1990;65:375–9.

30. Nixon RL, Dorevitch AP, Marks R. Squamous cell carcinoma: accuracy of clinical diagnosis and outcome of followup in Australia. Med J Aust 1986;144: 235–9.

31. Cassileth BR, Clark WH Jr, Lusk EJ, et al. How well do physicians recognise melanoma and other problem lesions? J Am Acad Dermatol 1986;14:555–60.

32. Koh HK, Norton LA, Geller AC, et al. Evaluation of the American Academy of Dermatology's national skin cancer early detection and screening program. J Am Acad Dermatol 1996;34:971–8.

33. Menzies SW, Crotty KA, Ingvar C, McCarthy WH. An atlas of surface microscopy of pigmented skin lesions. Sydney: McGraw-Hill Book Co.; 1996.

34. Binder M, Schwarz M, Winkler A, et al. Epiluminescence microscopy: a useful tool for the diagnosis of pigmented skin lesions for formally trained dermatologists. Arch Dermatol 1995;131:286–91.

35. Pehamberger H, Binder M, Knollmayer S, Wolff K. Immediate effects of a public education campaign on prognostic features of melanoma. J Am Acad Dermatol 1993;29:106–9.

36. Carter R, Marks R, Hill D. Could a national skin cancer primary prevention campaign in Australia be worthwhile? An economic perspective. Health Promotion Int 1999;14(1):73–82.

Index

In this index, *italic* page numbers designate figures; page numbers followed by "t" designate tables; *See also* cross-references designate related topics or more detailed subtopic breakdowns.